How well do you know your pharmacology?
Use our online study aid to find out.

Congratulations on purchasing the perfect study tool!

Pharmacology–An Illustrated Review is a two-part package that will be invaluable for your course and exams. In addition to the wealth of illustrations and information in this book, you also get access to 400 review questions online at **WinkingSkull.com**.

These questions (200 from the book plus 200 more) have answer explanations for right and wrong answers. Test yourself and get immediate feedback, quickly identifying areas of mastery or for further study.

Use the scratch-off code below to get started today!

Thieme's new illustrated *Review Series* will help you master the essentials of the basic sciences — *Pharmacology, Physiology, Anatomy, Biochemistry, Microbiology & Immunology,* and *Pathology.*

To find out more about this essential series, visit **www.thieme.com/IllustratedReview**

Get started today!

D1091850

Scratch off the panel below to reveal your access code and then log on to www.WinkingSkull.com to get started.

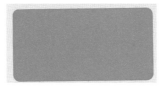

This book cannot be returned if the access code panel is scratched off.

Pharmacology
An Illustrated Review

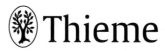

Pharmacology
An Illustrated Review

Mark A. Simmons, PhD

Professor of Pharmacology
Department of Integrative Medical Sciences
College of Medicine, and
Department of Pharmaceutical Sciences
College of Pharmacy
Northeast Ohio Medical University
Rootstown, Ohio

Pharmacology Graduate Program
School of Biomedical Sciences
Kent State University
Kent, Ohio

Thieme
New York • Stuttgart

Thieme Medical Publishers, Inc.
333 Seventh Ave.
New York, NY 10001

Vice President and Editorial Director, Educational Products: Anne T. Vinnicombe
Developmental Editor: Julie O'Meara
Production Editor: Megan Conway
Senior Vice President, International Sales and Marketing: Cornelia Schulze
Director of Sales: Ross Lumpkin
Chief Financial Officer: Sarah Vanderbilt
President: Brian D. Scanlan
Compositor: Manila Typesetting Company
Printer: Transcontinental Interglobe Printing Inc.

**QV
18.2
S592p
2012**

Library of Congress Cataloging-in-Publication Data
Simmons, Mark A.
Pharmacology: an illustrated review / Mark A. Simmons.
    p. ; cm. – (Illustrated review series)
    Includes index.
    Summary: "Pharmacology: An Illustrated Review covers the facts and concepts you must master for class-room and USMLE success—as well as key knowledge for daily clinical practice. Thieme's new illustrated Review Series serves an important dual purpose for medical students–both concise course review and high-yield USMLE test preparation. Covering all the basic science subjects that you will take in medical school and that will be found on the USMLE Step 1, the series features unparalleled color illustrations, a streamlined format, and hundreds of print and online study questions and answers–all designed to increase your mastery of the topic, promote classroom success, and boost your confidence for the exam! Combining targeted reviews of the basic sciences with a multitude of exam questions for easy reinforcement and retention, these efficient-to-study books put success at your fingertips"–Provided by publisher.
    ISBN 978-1-60406-205-2 (pbk. : alk. paper) 1. Pharmacology–Examinations, questions, etc. 2. Pharmacology–Atlases. 3. Pharmacology–Outlines, syllabi, etc. I. Title. II. Series: Thieme illustrated review series.
    [DNLM: 1. Pharmacological Phenomena–Atlases. 2. Pharmacological Phenomena—Examination Questions. 3. Pharmacological Phenomena–Outlines. QV 18.2]
    RM301.13.S56 2012
    615.1076—dc23

                                                                                          2011028084

Important note: Medical knowledge is ever-changing. As new research and clinical experience broaden our knowledge, changes in treatment and drug therapy may be required. The authors and editors of the material herein have consulted sources believed to be reliable in their efforts to provide information that is complete and in accord with the standards accepted at the time of publication. However, in view of the possibility of human error by the authors, editors, or publisher of the work herein or changes in medical knowledge, neither the authors, editors, nor publisher, nor any other party who has been involved in the preparation of this work, warrants that the information contained herein is in every respect accurate or complete, and they are not responsible for any errors or omissions or for the results obtained from use of such information. Readers are encouraged to confirm the information contained herein with other sources. For example, readers are advised to check the product information sheet included in the package of each drug they plan to administer to be certain that the information contained in this publication is accurate and that changes have not been made in the recommended dose or in the contraindications for administration. This recommendation is of particular importance in connection with new or infrequently used drugs.

Some of the product names, patents, and registered designs referred to in this book are in fact registered trademarks or proprietary names even though specific reference to this fact is not always made in the text. Therefore, the appearance of a name without designation as proprietary is not to be construed as a representation by the publisher that it is in the public domain.

Printed in Canada

5 4 3 2 1

ISBN 978-1-60406-205-2

To the teachers who cultivated my interest in pharmacology,
To the colleagues who have collaborated with me in teaching and research,
To the students who have made the teaching of pharmacology so rewarding, and
To Robin, my eternal inspiration.

Contents

Preface ix

I General Principles of Pharmacology

1 Pharmacokinetics...1
2 Mechanisms of Drug Action and Pharmacodynamics...20
3 Pharmacogenetics and Other Special Considerations 27
Questions & Answers.. *31*

II Drugs Acting on the Peripheral Nervous System

4 The Peripheral Nervous System 35
5 Cholinergic Agents 44
6 Adrenergic Agents 54
Questions & Answers.. *64*

III Drugs Acting on the Central Nervous System

7 Neuropharmacological Principles..67
8 Anesthetic Drugs...75
9 Anxiolytic and Sedative-Hypnotic Drugs 82
10 Antidepressant and Antimanic Drugs 86
11 Anticonvulsant Drugs..91
12 Antipsychotic Drugs..98
13 Opiate Receptor Agonists and Antagonists 102
14 Treatment of Neurodegenerative Diseases...110
15 Drugs of Abuse 118
Questions & Answers.. *127*

IV Drugs Acting on the Endocrine and Reproductive Systems

16 Drugs Used in the Treatment of Hypothalamic, Pituitary, Thyroid,
   and Adrenal Disorders..136
17 Drugs Used in Reproductive Endocrinology...157
18 Insulin, Hypoglycemic, and Antihypoglycemic Drugs..170
Questions & Answers.. *178*

Contents

V Drugs Acting on the Renal and Cardiovascular Systems

19 Renal Pharmacology 181
20 Antihypertensive Drugs 191
21 Drugs Used in the Treatment of Heart Failure 203
22 Antianginal Drugs 208
23 Antiarrythmic Drugs 213
24 Drugs Acting on the Blood 223
25 Antihyperlipidemic Drugs 236

Questions & Answers 242

VI Drugs Acting on the Respiratory and Gastrointestinal Systems

26 Drugs Acting on the Respiratory System 249
27 Drugs Acting on the Gastrointestinal System 259

Questions & Answers 279

VII Antimicrobial Drugs

28 Principles of Antimicrobial Therapy 281
29 Antibacterial Drugs 287
30 Antiviral Drugs 313
31 Antifungal and Antiparasitic Drugs 324

Questions & Answers 334

VIII Autocoids and Analgesic, Antipyretic, and Antiinflammatory Drugs

32 Autocoids and Related Drugs 340
33 Analgesic, Antipyretic, and Antiinflammatory Drugs 351

Questions & Answers 362

IX Cancer Chemotherapy and Toxicology

34 Cancer Chemotherapy and Immunosuppressants 365
35 Toxicology and Poisoning 388

Questions & Answers 393

Index 397

Preface

Pharmacology, the study of the effects of drugs on the body, is one of the most important disciplines that must be mastered to be successful in the practice of medicine or the biomedical sciences. The prevention or treatment of almost every disease involves the use of drugs. Furthermore, many patients seek medical help as a result of drug side effects or toxicities.

Pharmacology—An Illustrated Review covers the facts of pharmacology and integrates the concepts that you must master for success in the classroom and for the USMLE. It provides a concise study aid for pharmacology courses. It can also be used as a succinct source of key knowledge for daily clinical practice.

This book is in a streamlined bullet-point format and includes hundreds of full-color illustrations that demonstrate pharmacological processes and modes of action. For each pharmaceutical agent or group of agents, mechanisms of action, pharmacokinetics, uses, contraindications, and side effects are discussed.

Sidebars connect pharmacological concepts in the text with normal function (orange), fundamental biochemical, genetic, and embryologic processes (green), and disease and treatment (blue).

For self-testing, the text includes both factual and USMLE-style questions. All of the questions are accompanied by explanatory answers. The 200 questions and answers in the text are supplemented by an additional 200 questions and answers online at WinkingSkull. com via the scratch-off code in the book. The questions provide intensive practice, offer immediate feedback, and allow you to quickly identify areas for further study. I tell the students in my pharmacology courses that if they can answer the questions in this book and online correctly, they will have no problem with the pharmacology portions of the licensing exams.

As you use this book, please send comments or suggestions you have for improvement to IllustratedReview@thieme.com.

Acknowledgements

I would like to thank the following reviewers for their feedback: A. B. Al-Mehdi (Temple University School of Medicine), Barrie Ashby (University of South Alabama College of Medicine), Edward Pankey (Tulane University School of Medicine), Catherine Howard (Tulane University School of Medicine) , Brian Katz (Northeast Ohio Medical University), Michael Kaufmann (University of Chicago Medical Center), Anthony Sassong (Massachusetts General Hospital and Harvard Medical School), Mia Smucny (University of California—San Francisco), Yasmeen Tandon (Metro Health Hospital, Cleveland, OH), and Kelly Wright (John H. Stroger, Jr., Hospital of Cook County). I would also like to thank the editorial staff at Thieme, who have made significant contributions to this work. In particular, I wish to thank Julie O'Meara, the Developmental Editor, who has organized and improved the text and illustrations, and has been indefatigable in the quest for clarity and quality; Megan Conway, the Production Editor, who has worked tirelessly on the production of this volume; and Anne Vinnicombe, Vice President and Editorial Director of Educational Products at Thieme, for her unwavering support and resolute demand for quality and consistency in this volume and throughout the review series.

Mark A. Simmons

1 Pharmacokinetics

Pharmacokinetics is concerned with the movement of drugs into and out of the body and includes the principles of absorption, distribution, metabolism, and elimination. Knowledge of a drug's pharmacokinetic profile allows the clinician to select the correct agent, mode of administration, and dosing regimen to achieve a timely effect.

1.1 Routes of Drug Administration

Enteral

Enteral administration is the term used to describe drugs given via the gastrointestinal (GI) tract. Oral administration (PO) is by far the most common enteral route. The predominant site of absorption for drugs given orally is the duodenum, due to its large surface area. Drugs may also be absorbed in the stomach. Several factors influence the absorption of drugs given orally:

— Stomach acid can destroy many drugs unless coated with an acid-resistant material.
— Digestive enzymes (e.g., pepsin, gelatinase, gastric amylase, and lipases) may break down drugs.
— The presence of food in the stomach may delay or decrease absorption of the drug.

Parenteral

In parenteral administration a drug is delivered by injection; therefore, the drug bypasses the GI tract. This method is used for medications that are poorly absorbed in the GI tract or when rapid onset of action or tight control of pharmacokinetic parameters (e.g., plasma concentration) is required.

Other Methods of Drug Administration

Other methods of drug administration are *topical, transdermal, and by inhalation.* See **Table 1.1** for a comparison of the different routes of drug administration and **Fig. 1.1** for the time course of plasma concentration with each route.

1.2 Absorption of Drugs

Factors that Affect Absorption

Drugs given intravenously (IV) gain direct access to the bloodstream and so their absorption is complete. Drugs given by other methods have to cross biological membranes to reach the bloodstream, leading to partial absorption. The amount and rate of absorption are critical factors in therapeutics.

Absorption of a drug from the site of administration to the bloodstream depends on both the properties of the drug and physiological variables. The factors that govern whether a drug crosses a biological membrane include size, charge, and hydrophobicity. In general, low molecular weight, nonionized, water-soluble molecules are more readily absorbed.

The mechanisms by which molecules can cross biological membranes include passive diffusion and active transport.

— *Passive diffusion* is the most common method of absorption and occurs when a concentration gradient exists across a membrane such that the drug will move from the side with a high concentration to that with the lower concentration. Water-soluble drugs and those with low molecular weights are able to diffuse directly through pores in cell membranes. Lipid-soluble drugs dissolve readily in the lipid bilayer of cell membranes, thus gaining entry to the cell.

Pepsin

Pepsin is an endopeptidase, formed from the proenzyme pepsinogen. Its precursor, pepsinogen, is released from chief cells in the stomach when food is ingested and is responsible for cleaving proteins into peptides. Gastrin and vagus nerve stimulation cause the release of hydrochloric acid (HCl), which converts pepsinogen to pepsin.

Drug absorption and food in the stomach

Certain drugs can cause irritation to the stomach unless they are taken with food. Food delays absorption until the drug (e.g., aspirin) reaches the duodenum, where it is more easily tolerated. Other drugs (e.g., ampicillin) must be taken on an empty stomach, as food may decrease their absorption.

Table 1.1 ▶ Routes of Drug Administration		
Route	**Advantages**	**Disadvantages**
Enteral		
Oral	Convenient Cost-effective Relatively safe Desired therapeutic concentration is achieved gradually	Often low bioavailability following first-pass metabolism by liver More difficult to adjust plasma concentration Requires a functional GI tract Requires compliance by patients
Rectal	Useful when patient is vomiting Can be used in the unconscious patient Limited first-pass metabolism Relatively painless Tolerated well in children	Not well accepted Irregular absorption can compromise safety Irritation to rectal mucosa
Sublingual (buccal)	Rapid absorption Avoids first-pass metabolism	Only useful for small amount of drug Requires prolonged contact with mucosa Unpleasant taste
Parenteral		
Intravenous	Allows for rapid administration of a precise amount of drug Avoids first-pass metabolism Dosage is easily adjusted Suitable for large volumes Very useful in the unconscious patient No issues with compliance by patients	Drug cannot be recalled once administered More complications from administration (e.g., infection and hematoma) Adverse reactions more likely, so monitoring by clinician is vital IV access often difficult to establish
Intramuscular	Relatively easy to administer Fairly rapid absorption under normal circumstances May be used to deliver depot injections, where the active compound of a drug is released consistently over time	Painful Can cause nerve damage Can cause bleeding, so contraindicated in bleeding disorders Can only be used for relatively small injection volumes
Subcutaneous	Easy to administer Slow and constant absorption Minimal pain involved May be used to deliver depot injections, where the active compound of a drug is released consistently over time	Can only be used for very small volumes of drug Potential tissue irritation
Other Methods		
Topical	Applied to various surfaces, commonly the skin, eyes, nose, and vagina, to produce a local effect	May cause irritation
Transdermal	Controlled release preparations may be used via this mode of application Can achieve systemic effects	Rate of absorption variable May cause irritation
Inhalation	Rapid absorption Ideal for drugs that can be administered as an aerosol Ideal for treating lung disease, as drug is essentially exerting a local effect	Variable systemic distribution (not considered a disadvantage for the current drugs administered by this route) May cause irritation of the respiratory tract

Abbreviations: GI, gastrointestinal; IV, intravenous.

— *Active transport* occurs when a drug is moved against a concentration gradient or when the properties of the drug do not allow it to penetrate the cell by diffusion. Transmembrane carrier proteins with high structural specificity are responsible for active transport, utilizing energy from adenosine triphosphate (ATP) hydrolysis. The rate of carrier-mediated transport may show saturation at high solute concentrations because the number of carrier proteins is finite, and the cycling of carrier proteins is limited.

Effect of Ionization on Drug Absorption

Most drugs exist as weak acids or weak bases; however, un-ionized forms will be absorbed more readily. The fraction of drug in the un-ionized form depends on the pH of the environment. This can be determined using the Henderson-Hasselbalch equation.

For a weak acid, A, the equation is as follows:

$$pH = pK_a + Log\ [A^-]/[HA]$$

Fig. 1.1 ▶ **Mode of administration and time course of plasma drug concentration.**
Drugs given intravenously (*red*) reach their peak plasma drug concentration almost immediately, but this declines rapidly as the drug is distributed and eliminated. Drugs given intramuscularly (*green*) take longer to reach their peak plasma concentration, followed by drugs given subcutaneously (*blue*). Drugs taken orally (*purple*) are the slowest to reach their peak plasma concentration, the value of which is determined by bioavailability following first-pass metabolism.

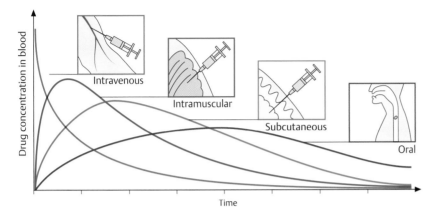

where

pH = $-\log_{10}$ [H⁺] (pH units)

pK_a = $-\log_{10}$ equilibrium constant (pH units)

[A⁻] = concentration of the unprotonated, or ionized, form of the acid

[HA] = concentration of the protonated, or un-ionized, form of the acid

For a weak base, B, the equation is as follows:

$$pH = pK_a + Log\ [B]/[BH^+]$$

where

pH = $-\log_{10}$ [H⁺] (pH units)

pK_a = $-\log_{10}$ equilibrium constant (pH units)

[B] = concentration of the unprotonated, or un-ionized, form of the base

[BH⁺] = concentration of the protonated, or ionized, form of the base

When the pH equals the pK_a, the drug is 50% ionized and 50% un-ionized. When the pH is less than the pK_a the protonated forms HA and BH⁺ predominate; conversely, when the pH is greater than the pK_a, the unprotonated forms A⁻ and B predominate. At gastric pH, acidic drugs will tend to be un-ionized and are absorbed well through the stomach, whereas basic drugs will tend to be ionized in the stomach and be absorbed only when they reach the duodenum, where they will exist in their more un-ionized form.

Bioavailability (*F*)

Bioavailability (*F*) is the fraction of the administered dose of a drug that reaches the systemic circulation in an unchanged form. It is calculated by comparing the plasma concentration over time achieved by giving an IV dose (where all of the drug reaches the plasma) with the plasma concentration over time following administration of the same dose of a drug given by another route (e.g., orally). Absorption and first-pass metabolism are the main influences on bioavailability. *First-pass metabolism* is the metabolism of a drug that occurs during its first pass through the liver immediately following its absorption in the GI tract. It principally affects drugs that are taken orally, but can also affect drugs that are administered rectally to a lesser extent. The parenteral administration of drugs avoids first-pass metabolism.

Portal circulation

A portal system is one in which veins from one capillary bed drain into another capillary bed, instead of emptying into the heart. The hepatic portal system is one such example of this. In this system, the hepatic portal vein, formed from the superior mesenteric and splenic veins, drains blood from the stomach, intestines, pancreas, and spleen. This nutrient-rich blood drains into the hepatic sinusoids, and the substrates it contains are then metabolized by hepatocytes. Blood leaves the liver via the hepatic vein, which empties into the inferior vena cava, then into the right atrium of the heart. This system ensures that ingested substances are metabolized before entering the systemic circulation.

1.3 Drug Distribution

Factors that Affect Distribution

Following its absorption, a drug is distributed in the bloodstream before it leaves this compartment and enters the extracellular fluid and/or the cells of tissues (**Fig. 1.2**). This process is primarily affected by the blood flow to a particular tissue, the permeability of capillaries to the drug, and the degree of drug binding to proteins in plasma and tissues. A drug will tend to move from the bloodstream to tissues along a concentration gradient until equilibrium is established. When blood levels of a drug fall, the process reverses, and the drug is eliminated from the tissues.

Blood Flow

Initial distribution will tend toward those tissues with a higher blood flow (brain or central nervous system [CNS], liver, and kidneys), then gradually be redistributed to those that are less vascular (skin, bone, and adipose tissue).

Permeability of Capillaries

Capillary endothelial cells that line blood vessels are, in general, separated by junctions that allow drugs to pass between them quite readily (**Fig. 1.3**). In the liver, these junctions are larger than usual, allowing drugs to pass even more readily. This is useful as the liver is the major site of drug metabolism. Conversely, the capillary endothelial cells of the brain have very tight junctions between them, which, along with glial cells, form the blood–brain barrier. For drugs to enter the brain, they must diffuse through the endothelial cells (i.e., lipophilic drugs), or they may be transported across the endothelial cell membrane via a carrier molecule.

Plasma Protein Binding

Drugs that are bound to plasma proteins (usually albumin but also α_1 acid glycoprotein) cannot be distributed into tissues or eliminated and so are pharmacologically inactive. However, they act as a reservoir such that when the concentration of free drug in plasma falls (due to redistribution, metabolism, or elimination), the bound drug proportionally dissociates from albumin to maintain a constant free-drug concentration.

Drugs bind with vastly different affinities for albumin. Competition for binding occurs when two drugs with a high affinity for albumin are given at the same time. This will increase plasma free-drug concentration, which could lead to increased side effects or toxicity. This is a common cause of drug interactions.

Table 1.2 lists the drug types that bind to albumin and α_1 acid glycoprotein and gives examples of such drugs.

Table 1.2 ▶ **Plasma Protein Binding**		
Plasma Protein	**Drug Type**	**Examples**
Albumin	Acidic drugs Neutral drugs	Warfarin, naproxen, phenytoin, sulfamethoxazole
α_1 acid glycoprotein	Basic drugs	Alprenolol, amitryptiline, imipramine, lidocaine
Note: Plasma protein binding is reversible.		

Volume of Distribution (V_d)

Volume of distribution is a pharmacological term that is defined as the volume in which a drug would need to be uniformly distributed to produce the same concentration throughout the body as found in plasma. It is an arbitrary value that is useful as a guide when comparing the relative concentration of the drug in plasma with the rest of the body and should not be thought of as an actual physical volume of fluid. A low V_d (e.g. 4 L) indicates that the drug is mainly

---

■ Albumin

Serum albumin is the most abundant plasma protein in the body. It is synthesized by the liver and is an important transport molecule for endogenous substances, such as steroid hormones, bilirubin, bile salts, free fatty acids, and calcium. It also acts as a transporter of many drugs. Albumin plays a critical role in regulating blood volume by maintaining the oncotic pressure of blood, which allows fluid to be retained in the vascular compartment. The concentration of albumin falls in liver disease, kidney disease (e.g., nephrotic syndrome, where kidney damage causes proteins to leak into urine), in inflammatory states, and in malnutrition.

■ α_1 acid glycoprotein

α_1 acid glycoprotein (AAG) is an acute-phase protein whose levels are increased in acute inflammatory states and tissue injury. Like albumin, AAG is synthesized in the liver and acts as a transport protein for endogenous substances, such as steroid hormones, and for many drugs.

■ Reflection coefficient

Reflection coefficient is a number between 0 and 1 that describes the ability of a membrane to prevent diffusion of a solute relative to water. If the reflection coefficient is 1, the solute is completely impermeable. Serum albumin has a reflection coefficient through endothelium that is close to 1. This explains why albumin is retained in the vascular compartment and exerts an oncotic effect. If it is 0, the solute is equally as permeable as water and will not exert any oncotic effect, i.e., it will not cause water to flow.

■ Hypoalbuminemia

Lower than normal levels of albumin in the blood (hypoalbuminemia), and hence decreased plasma protein binding, may occur in the following conditions: liver disease (e.g., hepatitis, cirrhosis, or hepatocellular necrosis), ascites, nephrotic syndrome, malabsorption syndromes (e.g., Crohn disease), extensive burns, and pregnancy.

Fig. 1.2 ► Distribution following different modes of administration.
Drugs given intravenously, transdermally, intramuscularly, sublingually, and buccally enter the venous circulation following administration and reach the general circulation after passing through the heart and lungs. Oral drugs are absorbed from the stomach or duodenum into the portal circulation, where they undergo first-pass metabolism in the liver before reaching the venous and then general circulation. Drugs given rectally are mainly transported directly to the venous circulation, but some of the drug enters the portal circulation to the liver. Drugs given by inhalation have a local effect on the lungs and may also reach the general circulation (e.g. general anesthetics).

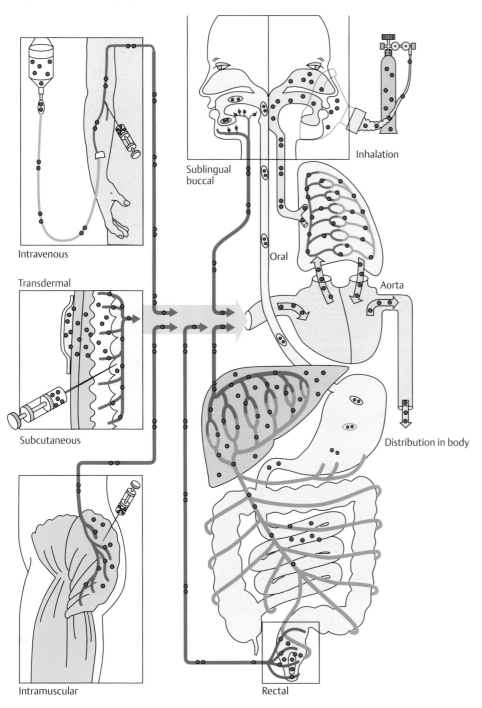

Intravenous

Transdermal

Subcutaneous

Intramuscular

Sublingual buccal

Inhalation

Oral

Aorta

Distribution in body

Rectal

Fig. 1.3 ► **Blood–tissue barriers.**
The penetrability of the capillary wall depends on the tissue. In cardiac muscle (*top right*), there is endocytotic and transcytotic activity (*arrowheads* in micrographs) that transports fluid and macromolecules into and out of the interstitium. Drugs that are in the fluid will also be transported, regardless of their physiochemical properties. In the endocrine glands (e.g., the pancreas, *lower right*) and the gut, the endothelial cells have fenestrations (*arrowheads*) that are closed by diaphragms. These diaphragms, along with the basement membrane, can readily be penetrated by low-molecular-weight substances (i.e., most drugs), but macromolecule penetration will depend on molecular weight and ionization. The liver (*lower left*) has large fenestrations that are not closed by diaphragms or basement membranes, so drugs are able to move freely into the interstitium. Finally, the central nervous system (CNS, *top left*) has no pores, fenestrations, or transcytotic activity, so drugs must either diffuse or be transported through the endothelial cells to gain access. (AM, actomyosin; D, Disse space; E, erythrocyte; G, insulin storage granule; Z, tight junction. Solid black line in schematic drawings are basement membranes.)

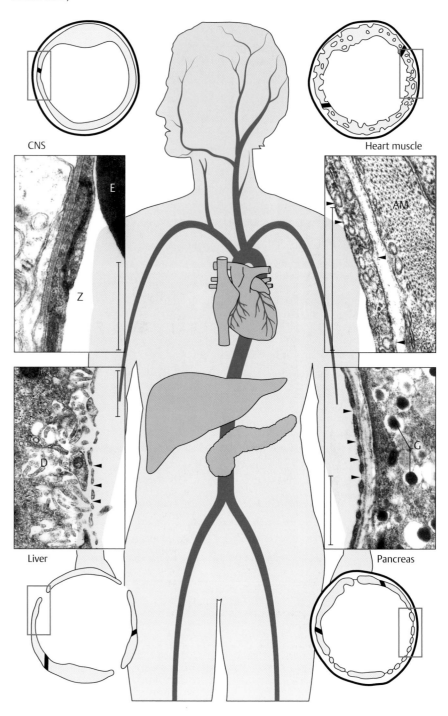

distributed in plasma, whereas a larger V_d (> 10 L) means that the drug has been distributed to additional compartments (e.g. interstitial or intracellular fluid). In reality, a drug will not be exclusively contained within one fluid compartment but distributed unevenly throughout one or more of them. **Figure 1.4** illustrates the compartments for drug distribution. **Table 1.3** lists the physiochemical features of drugs that cause them to predominate in a certain compartment and provides examples.

Fig. 1.4 ► **Fluid compartments for drug distribution.**
Drugs may be distributed to different body compartments depending on their physiochemical properties. See Table 1.3 for examples of drugs in each compartment.

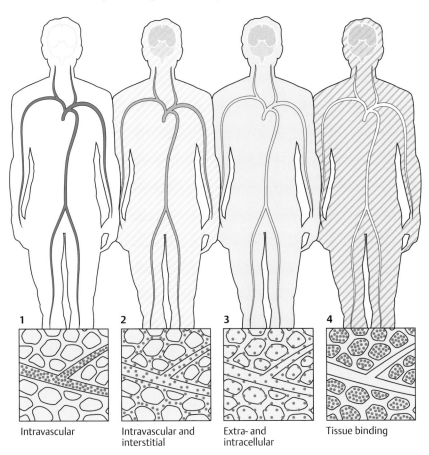

1	2	3	4
Intravascular	Intravascular and interstitial	Extra- and intracellular	Tissue binding

Table 1.3 ► Features of Drugs That Cause Them to Predominate in Each Fluid Compartment		
Fluid Compartment	**Drug Features**	**Examples**
Intravascular (plasma) (4 L) (Fig. 1.4–1)	High molecular weight Bound to plasma albumin	Heparin Warfarin Benzodiazepines Penicillin Sulphonamides Tetracyclines
Interstitial fluid (14 L) (Fig. 1.4–2)	Low molecular weight Hydrophilic	Epinephrine Amikacin
Intracellular fluid (42 L) (Fig. 1.4–3)	Low molecular weight Hydrophobic	Ethanol
Tissue binding (49 L) (Fig. 1.4–4)	Binds to high affinity site in those tissues High lipid solubility	Digoxin (myocardial and skeletal muscle) Thiopental (adipose tissue) Tetracyclines Lead (bone and teeth)

The apparent volume of distribution of a drug relates to the amount of drug administered to the plasma concentration according to the equation

$$V_d = \text{Dose (mg)/plasma concentration (mg/L)}$$

Calculating the Amount of Drug to Administer from V_d

The V_d is used to calculate the amount of drug needed to achieve a desired plasma concentration by rearrangement of the above equation:

$$\text{Dose (mg)} = \text{plasma concentration (mg/L)} \times V_d \text{ (L)}$$

This assumes, for simplicity, that the bioavailability of the drug is complete, distribution is instantaneous, and the drug is not being eliminated.

Effect of V_d on the Half-life of a Drug

For a drug to be eliminated, it must be present in its free form in plasma so that it may pass through the liver or kidney for excretion in bile or urine. The higher the volume of distribution, the less a drug is contained in the plasma compartment, so its half-life is prolonged.

1.4 Metabolism of Drugs

Drug metabolism usually inactivates therapeutic agents, transforming them into derivatives that are more readily excreted. However, metabolism can also produce active agents from inactive prodrugs, or can produce toxic metabolites.

The liver and intestinal wall are the main sites of metabolism, but drug metabolism can also occur in the kidneys, lungs, and gonads.

Phase 1 Metabolism

Metabolism generally consists of a phase 1 reaction that converts a drug to a less active form, followed by a phase 2 conjugation reaction (**Fig. 1.5**). Phase 1 metabolism involves the oxidation, reduction, or hydrolysis of a drug, making it more polar by adding or exposing a functional group ($-OH$, $-NH_2$, $-SH$, $-COO^-$). These functional groups can then act as the site of conjugation in phase 2 metabolism.

Oxidation Reactions

In the liver, the most important site of metabolism is the microsomal enzyme system. This includes the mixed function oxidases located in the smooth endoplasmic reticulum. Pharmacologically, the most important of these is the cytochrome P-450 family of enzymes (**Fig. 1.6**).

Each cytochrome P-450 enzyme is denoted by the abbreviation CYP followed by a number related to the family, then an upper case letter related to its subfamily, followed by a number to specify the particular enzyme. Each enzyme has the capacity to catalyze the metabolism of many drugs with some overlap between them for substrates. More than 50% of drugs are catalyzed by the CYP3A family, with ~30% by CYP2D6 and 15% by CYP2C. This system can be induced or inhibited by drugs, which creates a huge potential for drug interactions (**Fig. 1.7**).

■ Drug–Grapefruit Interactions

Grapefruit juice is a powerful inhibitor of CYP3A4-mediated drug metabolism. This can lead to elevated plasma concentrations of many drugs, including benzodiazepines, codeine, and amiodarone (a potent antiarrhythmic drug), and the possible toxicity of these drugs.

Fig. 1.5 ▶ Process of metabolism.

Drugs and other endogenous and exogenous substances undergo biotransformations that ultimately allow them to be excreted in urine or bile. (UDP-GlcUA = urinidine diphosphate glucuronate; UDP = uridine diphosphate.)

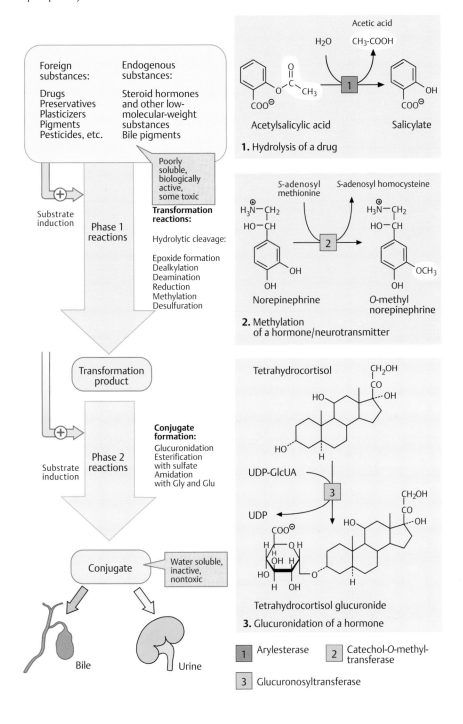

1. Hydrolysis of a drug

2. Methylation of a hormone/neurotransmitter

3. Glucuronidation of a hormone

1	Arylesterase
2	Catechol-O-methyl-transferase
3	Glucuronosyltransferase

Fig. 1.6 ▶ **Cytochrome P-450 synthesis in the liver.**
Inducer substances activate transcription factors in the CYP gene, producing more cytochrome P-450. Cytochrome P-450 enzymes are then able to metabolize substrates unless they are acted upon by an inhibitor. Inhibitors bind to cytochrome P-450 enzymes with high affinity and cause the substrates of cytochrome P-450 enzymes to be metabolized more slowly. (mRNA, messenger RNA).

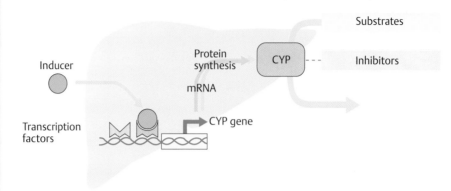

Fig. 1.7 ▶ **Substrates, inducers, and inhibitors of cytochrome P-450 enzymes.**
Inducer substances can be environmental, endogenous substances, or they may be drugs themselves. The cytochrome enzyme that they induce is then able to metabolize specific substrates (drugs) more rapidly, so these drugs may not reach their effective therapeutic concentration. Inhibitors interfere with substrate metabolism and may cause toxic accumulation of a drug in the body. (HIV, human immunodeficiency virus; SSRIs, selective serotonin reuptake inhibitors.)

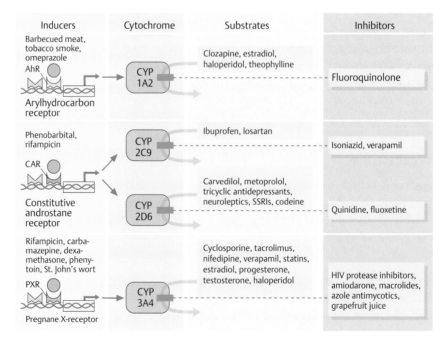

The cytochrome P450-dependent oxidation reactions include:

— aromatic and aliphatic hydroxylation

— alkyl oxidations and desulfuration

— oxidative deamination

— N-dealkylation from nitrogen, oxygen, and sulfur

— sulfoxidation

— epoxidation

When a drug is oxidized, oxygen is reduced to water as a byproduct. This type of reaction requires energy in the form of NADPH to drive the conversion the enzyme cytochrome P-450 reductase.

Some drugs are metabolized by noninducible, nonmicrosomal enzymes. Examples include monoamine oxidase (in mitochondria) in the metabolism of sympathomimetic amines, e.g., epinephrine, norepinephrine, dopamine; alcohol dehydrogenase (in cytosol) in the metabolism of ethanol; and xanthidine oxidase (in cytosol) in the catabolism of purines and xanthines.

Reduction Reactions

Reduction reactions generally require anaerobic conditions and may be catalyzed by bacteria in the gut or urinary tract. Microsomal enzymes can also reduce drugs under appropriate conditions. Examples of reduction reactions include the formation of nitrites from organic nitrates and amine formation from the reduction of nitro ($-NO_2$) containing compounds.

Hydrolysis Reactions

Drug hydrolysis predominantly occurs in plasma and cellular cytosol as a result of chemical or enzymatic reactions. Examples of enzymes that catalyze these reactions include esterases, which metabolize acetylcholine, atropine, and procaine; amidases, which metabolize procainamide and lidocaine; and peptidases, which metabolize insulin and vasopressin. Metabolites produced by these reactions are usually more water soluble than the parent compound and may be excreted in this form or processed further by conjugation.

Phase 2 Metabolism

Drug conjugations are referred to as phase 2 reactions because they often occur after initial drug oxidation, reduction, or hydrolysis; however, drugs can bypass phase 1 metabolism and go straight to phase 2. Conjugated compounds are generally inactive, especially glucuronide, sulfate, and glutathione conjugates, which are highly water soluble and readily excreted in urine.

Table 1.4 lists the types of phase 2 conjugation reactions and gives examples of drugs that undergo each type of conjugation.

Table 1.4 ▶ **Phase 2 Conjugation Reactions**		
Type of Conjugation	**Method of Conjugation**	**Examples**
Glucuronidation*	Glucose is used to form uridine diphosphate glucuronic acid (UDPGA), which transfers a glucuronide to the functional group of the drug in the presence of glucuronyl transferase	Majority of drugs Steroid hormones Bilirubin
Sulfation	Catalyzed by sulfotransferases	Estradiol Acetaminophen
Amino acids	Conjugated by glycine and glutamine	Simple aromatic acids (e.g., salicylates)
Glutathione	Catalyzed by glutathione S-transferase	Acetaminophen
Acetylation	Catalyzed by acetyltransferases	Limited to drugs with primary amino groups (e.g., sulfonamides)
Methylation	Catalyzed by N-methyl-transferases, catechol-O-methyltransferase (methylates, dopamine, methyldopa, and L-dopa), and a thiopurine methyltransferase	Azathioprine 6-mercaptopurine Thioguanine

*This is the only phase 2 reaction that can be induced by other pharmacological agents and has a potential for drug interactions.
Note: All conjugations, except glucuronindation, are catalysed by transferases, located mainly in the cystol.

1.5 Elimination of Drugs

Elimination of drugs and their metabolites mainly occurs in urine and feces, although many other minor routes of elimination exist, such as saliva, sweat, tears, breast milk, and expired air (from the lungs).

Renal Elimination

To undergo renal elimination, a drug must be filtered or actively transported into the urine and must resist reabsorption back into plasma and subsequent reentry into the systemic circulation.

Glomerular Filtration

Drugs are filtered into the urine from plasma depending on their molecular weight, ionization, and degree of protein binding.

— Low-molecular-weight and/or ionized drugs are more readily filtered.
— Drugs that are highly bound to plasma proteins are too large to be filtered.

Drugs that are filtered in the glomerulus and not reabsorbed are eliminated at a rate that equals creatinine clearance (125 mL/min).

Active Transport in the Proximal Tubule

Drugs that are acids or bases in plasma can be actively secreted into the tubular lumen against a concentration gradient by anionic and cationic transport systems. This process requires energy.

Reabsorption in the Distal Tubule

Un-ionized drugs are able to passively diffuse back into plasma, especially if they are lipid soluble and there is a favorable concentration gradient. The ionization of a drug is affected by changes in urinary pH. For example, if urine is made more alkaline by administration of bicarbonate, weak acids will become more ionized, thereby slowing their reabsorption and increasing their elimination (see Henderson-Hasselbalch equation page 3).

Creatinine

Creatinine is formed in a nonenzymatic reaction from creatine phosphate in skeletal muscle. It is excreted with minimal reabsorption in the kidneys, and its clearance rate is an excellent indication of glomerular filtration and therefore renal function.

Hepatic Elimination

Conjugated drugs (mainly glucuronic acid derivatives) are actively secreted into bile. Unconjugated drugs are liberated in the small intestine by bacterial enzyme hydrolysis and reabsorbed into the portal circulation. This is the enterohepatic cycle. Some of the drug escapes reabsorption and appears in feces. Antibiotic-induced decreases in intestinal bacterial flora will decrease the hydrolysis of conjugated drugs thus interfering with enterohepatic cycling and decreasing the drug concentration below its therapeutic range (e.g., steroids used for contraception).

1.6 Drug Interactions

Drug interactions may occur at any stage between absorption and elimination, but competition for plasma albumin binding and induction/inhibition of the CYP-450 enzymes (**Fig. 1.8**) are by far the most common interactions. **Table 1.5** lists some common mechanisms of interactions and gives examples of drugs that can cause them.

Fig. 1.8 ▶ **Drug interactions involving cytochrome P-450 enzymes.**
In patients taking cyclosporine (an immunosuppressant drug used to prevent organ rejection), concomitant use of rifampicin (an antibiotic) or St. John's wort (a herbal drug, used to treat depression) will induce CYP3A4, increasing cyclosporine metabolism and elimination. In this case, plasma levels of cyclosporine are not maintained at the therapeutic level, leading to transplant rejection. Conversely, if itraconazole (an antifungal agent) is taken with cyclosporine, CYP3A4 is inhibited, and cyclosporine metabolism and elimination are slowed, leading to toxic accumulation in the kidneys.

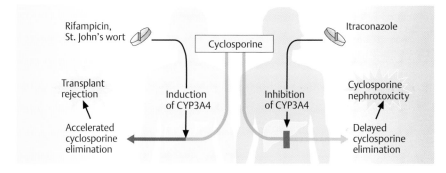

Table 1.5 ▶ Stage and Mechanism of Drug Interactions		
Stage	**Mechanism of Interaction**	**Drug Example(s)**
Absorption	Change in GI pH Changes in GI motility Changes in GI perfusion Chelation Inactivation of drug by adsorption	H_2 blockers, antacids Laxatives, anticholinergics Vasodilators Tetracycline, calcium Activated charcoal
Distribution	Competition for plasma albumin binding Changes in perfusion Changes in V_d	Warfarin, NSAIDs, nifedipine Vasodilators, ACE inhibitors Diuretics
Metabolism	Increased by inducers of CYP-450 Decreased by inhibitors of CYP-450 Increased by inducers of glucuronidation	Carbamazepine, rifampin, phenytoin Erythromycin, ketoconazole, fluoxetine Rifampin
Elimination	Changes in urinary pH Competition for binding to active transporters in the proximal tubule	Bicarbonate Salicylate, furosemide, penicillin G

Abbreviations: ACE, angiotensin-converting enzyme; GI, gastrointestinal; NSAIDs, nonsteroidal antiinflammatory drugs.

1.7 Determinants of Plasma Concentration and Dosing

The rate of drug dosing depends primarily on its rate of elimination. Most drugs are removed from plasma by processes that are concentration-dependent (i.e., metabolism, secretion, and filtration) and result in "first-order" kinetics of elimination.

First-Order Elimination

With first-order kinetics,

- A constant percentage of the drug is eliminated per unit of time. This is known as the elimination rate constant (K_e).
- The elimination half-life ($t_{1/2}$) is the time it takes for the plasma concentration to be reduced by 50%. It is constant and is independent of the dose.
- Half-life is related to K_e by the following:

$$t_{1/2} = 0.693/K_e$$

- Clearance (CL) is the volume of fluid from which the drug is eliminated per unit of time.

$$CL = V_d \times K_e$$

Substituting $0.693/t_{1/2}$ for K_e gives

$$CL = (0.693 \times V_d/t_{1/2})$$

- A plot of log plasma concentration against time is a straight line (**Fig. 1.9**). The y-intercept is an extrapolated value and would be the plasma concentration of drug at time 0 assuming instantaneous distribution.
- Most drugs exhibit first-order kinetics unless they are given in very high doses.

Fig. 1.9 ▶ **First-order elimination.**
With first-order kinetics, a constant percentage of the drug is eliminated per unit of time. Note that plasma concentration is plotted on a logarithmic scale.

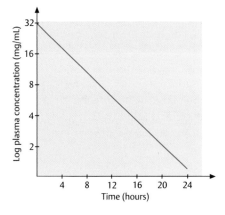

Zero-Order Elimination

With zero-order kinetics,

- A constant amount of drug is eliminated per unit of time regardless of its concentration. This usually occurs because the route of elimination has become saturated.
- The half-life is not constant but depends on the concentration, i.e., the higher the concentration, the longer the half-life.
- Drugs in this category will demonstrate first-order kinetics whenever the drug concentration falls substantially below the saturation level of the elimination process.
- Examples of drug that exhibit zero-order kinetics include ethanol and heparin, plus other drugs at high doses (e.g., salicylates such as aspirin).

1.8 Pharmacokinetics of Drug Administration in Practice

It is important that clinicians understand the factors that affect the total amount of drug in the body, how much drug is in plasma, and how this changes over time so that an appropriate therapeutic regimen can be devised. To illustrate these concepts, we will discuss the two different types of drug administration: continuous IV infusion and repeated dosing.

Kinetics of Continuous IV Infusion

If a drug is given by IV infusion, a constant amount of the drug enters plasma, and a constant percentage is eliminated (cleared from the blood) per unit of time (if elimination is first-order); that is, plasma concentration and elimination are proportional such that any increase in plasma concentration of a drug will lead to an increase in its elimination. At the start of an IV infusion, plasma drug concentration will rise until it reaches the point where elimination exactly matches administration. At this point, the plasma concentration will remain constant and is referred to as the steady-state concentration (C_{ss}) (**Fig. 1.10**). For drugs that are given by continuous IV infusion, the equation for calculating C_{ss} is

$$C_{ss} = R_0/CL,$$

where
R_0 = the infusion rate
CL = clearance (mL/min)

- Note that the time to reach steady-state concentration is solely determined by the half-life. It takes roughly four half-lives for a drug to be eliminated from the body, and because steady-state concentration and elimination are proportional, it takes about four half-lifes to reach steady-state concentration.
- Increasing the rate of infusion does not increase the rate at which the steady-state concentration is reached; rather, it will increase the rate at which any given concentration of drug in the plasma is achieved.

Fig. 1.10 ► **Time for drug to reach plasma steady-state concentration and be eliminated.**
When a drug is given by IV infusion, 50% of plasma steady-state concentration (C_{SS}) is achieved after one half-life and 75% after two half-lifes; C_{SS} is complete after approximately four half-lifes. If the infusion is stopped, the drug is eliminated in these same proportions (i.e., 50% is eliminated after one half-life and so on until it is almost completely eliminated after four half-lifes).

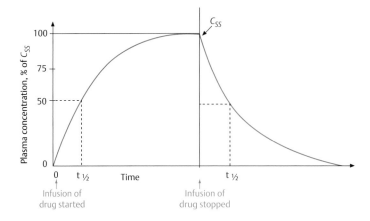

Kinetics of Repeated Dosing

Fixed-Dose/Fixed-Time-Interval Regimens

The most common drug-dosing regimen is to take a drug orally one or more times per day; however, such a repeated dosing regimen introduces issues related to fluctuations in plasma drug concentration. With any fixed-dose/fixed-time-interval regimen, a steady-state concentration is ultimately reached as before, but it is not achieved in a smooth, exponential way as for the IV infusion, but rather by way of fluctuating around a mean (**Fig. 1.11**). This is because most intermittent doses of drugs are given in fewer than four half-lifes (i.e., before the preceding dose has been completely eliminated), so the drug will accumulate until the steady state is achieved. The magnitude of the peaks and troughs around the mean will depend on the dosing interval (see **Table 1.6**). Smaller doses at shorter intervals will minimize these fluctuations but will not alter the steady-state concentration or the rate at which it is attained.

Table 1.6 ► **Effect of Dosing Interval on Time To Reach Steady-State Concentration, the Degree of Fluctuation of Plasma Drug Concentration, and the Most Useful Mode of Administration to Combat These Variables**

Half-life (Hours)/ Dosing Interval	Time to Reach C_{SS}	Plasma Concentration Fluctuation	Mode of Administration
< 4	Short	Large	IV infusion Sustained-release preparation
6–24	Medium	Medium	Usually oral fixed dose at interval equal to $t_{1/2}$
> 24	Long	Small	Sustained-release preparation ± loading dose

Abbreviation: C_{SS}, steady-state concentration; IV, intravenous.

Fig. 1.11 ▶ **Accumulation: dose, dose interval, and fluctuation of plasma level.**
When a large dose of a drug is given once per day, the plasma concentration shows a large fluctuation. Toxic levels are obtained (*pink area*) at peak plasma concentrations and subtherapeutic levels (*green area*) are obtained at the trough. If the drug is given in smaller, more frequent doses, the peaks and troughs are smaller. The mean steady-state concentration will be obtained in four half-lives, independent of the frequency of dosing.

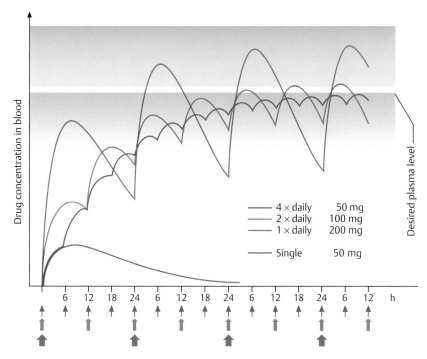

For drugs that are taken orally on a fixed-dose/fixed-time-interval regimen, the equation for calculating the steady-state concentration is

$$C_{ss} = [F \times (D/T)]/CL,$$

where

C_{ss} = Steady-state concentration (mg/mL)
F = Bioavailability
D = Dose (mg)
T = Dosing interval (min)
CL = clearance (mL/min)

Note:

— To change the steady-state concentration, it is generally better to increase the frequency of dosing rather than the amount of drug given to avoid toxic effects related to larger excursions around the mean concentration (i.e., larger peak and trough values).
— For orally administered drugs, bioavailability must be taken into account in the calculation of steady-state concentration.
— No simple prediction of steady-state concentration can be made for drugs eliminated by zero-order kinetics. In this case toxic concentrations can accumulate more quickly and be eliminated more slowly than drugs that follow first-order kinetics.

Use of a Loading Dose

It is often desirable to achieve the steady-state concentration more quickly than four half-lives, especially if the half-life of the drug is long. In these cases, a loading dose (*LD*) can be used. Loading doses can be given as a single bolus injection, but the high initial plasma concentrations achieved can sometimes lead to adverse effects. These adverse effects may be avoided by staggering the loading dose over a short period, which allows time for some redistribution of the drug to occur. Loading dose (mg) is calculated as follows:

$$LD = (V_d) \times (\text{desired } C_{ss})$$

For an orally administered loading dose, bioavailability must be considered.

Irregular Dosing Regimens

Irregular dosing occurs to an extent during fixed-dose/fixed-time-interval regimens because patients do not take a drug dose during the night. It also commonly occurs when patients do not adhere strictly to the prescribed dosing interval. As a consequence of irregular dosing, plasma drug concentrations often fall below the therapeutic level (**Fig. 1.12**).

Table 1.7 summarizes the factors that should be considered when choosing a dosing regimen.

Table 1.7 ▶ Summary of Factors to Consider When Choosing a Dosing Regimen	
Factor	Comments
Steady-state plasma concentration (C_{ss})	This will be the desired therapeutic plasma concentration and will lie within the therapeutic index.
Clearance (*CL*)	This is the same as creatinine clearance in a healthy adult patient (125 mL/min).
Half-life ($t_{1/2}$)	This dictates the time taken to reach the steady-state concentration and therefore the dosing interval.
Therapeutic index (*TI*)	The therapeutic index is a means of comparing the amount of a drug required to attain the therapeutic level in 50% of patients to the amount that is lethal to 50% of patients. A large *TI* allows for a variety of dosing regimens. A small *TI* often necessitates that a drug is given intravenously (IV), by IV infusion, or as a sustained-release preparation.
Bioavailability (*F*)	This must be factored in when considering all methods of administration of drugs except for IV (100% bioavailability). It is especially important in determining oral dosing regimens.
Volume of distribution (V_d)	This will affect the concentration of free drug in plasma, which, in turn, determines how much is available for elimination. V_d is usually constant and can be largely ignored when calculating a dosing regimen, but it gains in significance in disease states.
Route of administration	This is determined by patient factors and the biochemical properties of the drug.
Drug interactions	Clinicians should always consider drug interactions, especially the most serious and clinically relevant ones.

Fig. 1.12 ► **Plasma concentration of drugs with irregular dosing.**
Irregular dosing, such as occurs with the increased nocturnal dosing interval with fixed-dose/fixed-time-interval regimens or due to missed doses (poor patient compliance), results in the plasma drug concentration falling below the desired therapeutic level (*pink areas*). It then takes several doses to reach the desired therapeutic level once again. Note that the arrows signify when each dose of drug is taken and the question mark (?) represents a missed dose.

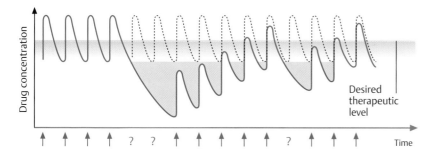

Drug Dosage in Renal Disease

Renal disease must be taken into consideration when drugs are excreted primarily (> 50%) unchanged by the kidney.

— The initial dose is the same as for any patient, but because clearance is decreased, the maintenance dose is decreased or the dosing interval is increased in proportion to the decrease in renal clearance of creatinine. In doing this, the percentage of drug eliminated by the kidney remains unchanged.

Drug Dosage in Hepatic Disease

Hepatic disease has the potential to affect the pharmacokinetics of many drugs; however, because hepatic reserves are large, disease has to be severe for changes in drug metabolism to occur. The mechanisms by which the pharmacokinetics may be altered include the following:

— Reduced hepatic blood flow reduces first-pass metabolism of drugs taken orally.
— Reduced plasma protein binding may affect both distribution and elimination.
— Plasma clearance of a drug is reduced if it is eliminated following metabolism and/or following excretion into bile.

A dose reduction will be necessary in hepatic disease, but it should be calculated for each individual patient.

Nephrotoxic drugs

An example of a nephrotoxic drug is gentamicin, an aminoglycoside antibiotic used to treat severe bacterial infections. It is excreted in unchanged form, mostly by glomerular filtration, in the kidney. In renal impairment, gentamicin will accumulate in the kidney causing destruction of kidney cells (nephrotoxicity). When gentamicin is prescribed, the dosage and treatment period should be minimal, and plasma concentration should be closely monitored.

2 Mechanisms of Drug Action and Pharmacodynamics

Pharmacodynamics are the pharmacological principles that describe drug effects on the body, explaining both mechanism of action and dose–response relationship.

2.1 Drug–Receptor Interactions

Most drug effects are produced by interaction with specific plasma membrane or intracellular receptors, leading to molecular changes that produce a given response (**Fig. 2.1**). These receptors are mainly proteins or nucleic acids. Binding is usually reversible and occurs by low-energy forces (hydrogen bonds, hydrophobic bonds, and van der Waals bonds), although a few examples of drug action associated with ionic or covalent binding are known. The binding of a drug to a receptor requires structural specificity and often stereospecificity (specificity for one stereoisomer of the drug).

Drugs may also exert their effects by physical or chemical interactions that do not involve receptors. Examples include antacids that work by neutralizing gastric pH; chelators that bind to heavy metals, inactivating them; and osmotic diuretics that act by absorbing water into the lumen of the kidney to maintain osmotic balance.

Fig. 2.1 ▶ **Site at which drugs act to modify cell function.**
Drugs cause cellular changes, leading to their physiological effects. They may act at receptors, causing a direct effect (e.g., opening of an ion channel), or receptor binding may activate a signal transduction system, leading to the cellular response. Drugs may also act by altering the activity of a cellular transport system; or by activating or inhibiting enzymes that control intracellular processes. They may also act on DNA to damage it or to alter the transcription of proteins.

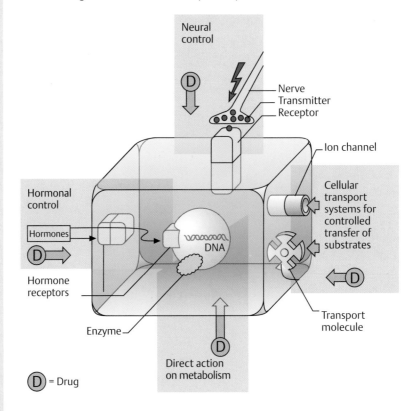

Receptors and Their Signal Transduction

Types of Receptors

— *Ligand-gated ion channels* are specialized membrane pores made up of multisubunit proteins. Binding of ligands, e.g., endogenous compounds or drugs, to these receptors opens or closes the pores thus changing the permeability of Na^+, K^+, Cl^-, or other ions (**Fig. 2.2**).

— *G protein–coupled receptors* (GPCRs). Guanine-nucleotide-binding proteins (G proteins) are transducers of information between ligand–receptor binding to GPCRs and the formation of several intracellular second messengers that culminate in a cellular response. The mechanisms of G protein signal transduction are discussed below.

— *Voltage-dependent ion channels* normally open or close in response to changes in the membrane potential, but they can also function as receptors for drugs. For example, the calcium channel blockers bind to voltage-dependent Ca^{2+} channels and block Ca^{2+} entry into cells when stimulated. This causes decreased contractility in target tissues, such as cardiac and smooth muscle.

— *Enzyme-linked membrane receptors*. When a drug binds to this type of receptor, it causes an enzyme to become "switched on" intracellularly. This enzyme then catalyzes the formation of other signal proteins that ultimately lead to the cellular response (**Fig. 2.3**).

— *Intracellular receptors*. Lipid-soluble drugs diffuse through cell membranes and bind either in the cellular cytosol or in the nucleus. Gene expression is altered, and protein synthesis is either increased or decreased, which causes the cellular response (**Fig. 2.4**). This mechanism is the slowest, and effects can usually be measured in terms of hours rather than minutes or seconds.

Fig. 2.2 ▶ **Ligand-gated ion channel.**
An example of a ligand-gated ion channel is the nicotinic cholinergic receptor on the motor end plate. When two acetylcholine (Ach) molecules bind to this receptor simultaneously (at the α-subunits) and the inner pore opens, Na^+ enters the cell and K^+ leaves the cell. This causes membrane depolarization and action potential propagation, resulting in muscle contraction.

Fig. 2.3 ▶ **Enzyme-linked membrane receptor.**
Insulin binding to the tyrosine kinase receptor causes the enzyme to phosphorylate tyrosine residues in proteins. These proteins can then signal other proteins to be formed, resulting in glucose uptake into cells.

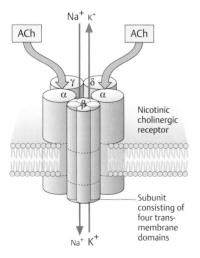

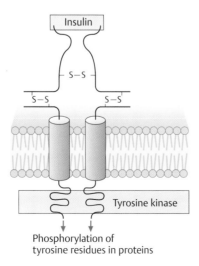

Fig. 2.4 ► **Intracellular receptor.**
Lipophilic substances, such as steroid hormones and thyroid hormones, can diffuse through the cell membrane and interact with receptors in the cytoplasm or nucleus. The hormone-receptor complex then alters gene transcription, causing the synthesis of effector proteins. The hormone-receptor complex interacts with DNA in pairs; these may be identical (homodimeric) or nonidentical (heterodimeric) pairs.

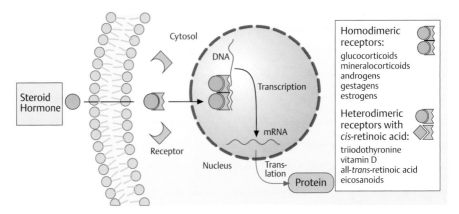

G Protein Signal Transduction

Heterotrimeric G-proteins couple to membrane receptors, e.g., α-adrenergic receptors. When the receptor binds a ligand, this causes the α-subunit of the G protein to split from the β and γ subunits (**Fig. 2.5**). The now free subunits then interact with other proteins in the membrane that may produce second messengers. These second messengers are cyclic AMP (cAMP), diacylglycerol (DAG), and inositol 1, 4, 5-triphosphate (IP$_3$).

Fig. 2.5 ► **G-protein-mediated effect of an agonist.**
(1) This shows the G-protein-coupled receptor in the resting state. (2) When an agonist binds to the G-protein-coupled receptor, it causes the receptor and G-protein to change conformation. The α-subunit exchanges guanosine triphosphate (GTP) for guanosine diphosphate (GDP) and dissociates from the other subunits, where it interacts with an effector protein (adenylate cyclase or phospholipase C) (3). This effector protein can then stimulate or inhibit second messenger molecules to produce a physiological effect. The α-subunit then hydrolyses the bound GTP to GDP and reassociates with the other subunits (4).

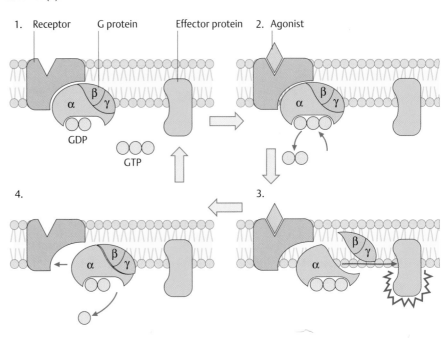

– G_s proteins activate cAMP.
– G_i proteins inhibit cAMP.
– G_q proteins activate phospholipase C, which increases DAG and IP_3.

When G proteins are activated, GTP replaces GDP on the α-subunit. Following activation of G-proteins, GTP is rapidly degraded to inactive GDP by the activity of the α-subunit GTPase.

Adenylate cyclase system. Ligands that bind to a GPCR that activates G_s stimulate adenylate cyclase to convert ATP to cyclic AMP (cAMP) (**Fig. 2.6 A**). Cyclic AMP then activates protein kinase A which prophorylates proteins, resulting in the physiologic response. Cyclic AMP is degraded to 5'AMP by phosphodiesterases. Ligands that bind to a GPCR that activates G_i inhibit adenylate cyclase (↓ cyclic AMP), therefore protein kinase A is not activated, and proteins are not phosphorylated.

DAG and IP_3 system. GPCRs may also couple to G_q. G_q activates the enzyme phospholipase C, which produces the second messengers IP_3 and DAG from phosphatidylinositol 4,5-bisphosphate (PIP_2) (**Fig. 2.6 B**).

Hydrophilic IP_3 diffuses from the membrane to the endoplasmic reticulum and releases Ca^{2+}. The Ca^{2+} released can then cause physiologic effects in the following ways:

– Activation of protein kinase C (with DAG) leading to the phosphorylation of proteins
– Binding to calmodulin with the resultant complex mediating further effects, e.g., production of nitric oxide (NO).

Lipophilic DAG has two functions:

– Activation of protein kinase C. This process is Ca^{2+}-dependent.
– Formation of arachidonic acid (an eicosanoid precursor) following its degradation by DAG lipase.

Fig. 2.6 ▸ **G proteins, second messengers, and effects.**
G-proteins can stimulate or inhibit adenylate cyclase. If activated, adenylate cyclase stimulates the second messenger, cyclic adenosine monophosphate (cAMP) to cause phosphorylation of proteins, which then exert the physiological effect (A). Similarly, G-proteins can activate phospholipase C and its second messenger substances to cause the physiological effect (B). G-proteins can also cause ion channels to open. The movement of ions may then initiate an action potential, or it may normalize intracellular ion content (C). (ATP, adenosine triphosphate; DAG, diacylglycerol; IP_3, inositol triphosphate)

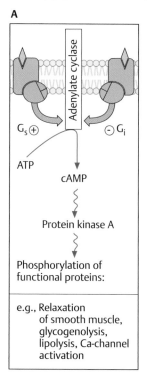

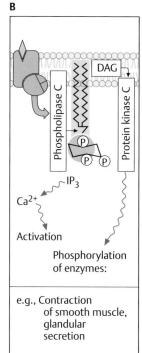

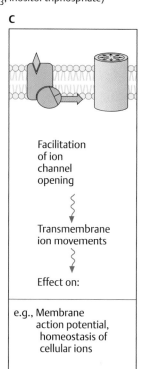

Other effects of G proteins.   G proteins may also interact directly with ion channels to alter ionic conductance and cellular excitability (**Fig. 2.6 C**).

Table 2.1 gives examples of each of the types of receptors above and substances that bind to these receptors.

Table 2.1 ▶ Types of Receptors	
Type of Receptor	**Examples**
Ligand-gated ion channels	Nicotinic receptors (bind ACh) Glutamate receptor $GABA_A$ receptor
G-protein-coupled receptor	Muscarinic receptors (bind ACh)
Voltage-dependent ion channels	Ca^{2+} channels on cardiac or smooth muscle
Enzyme-linked membrane receptor	Tyrosine kinase receptor (binds insulin)
Intracellular receptors	Steroid hormones Thyroid hormone (thyroxine)

Abbreviations: $GABA_A$, gamma-aminobutyric acid, type A; ACh, acetylcholine.

Drug Classification Based on Interaction with Receptors

Agonists

Agonists bind to a receptor, causing a change in its conformation that leads to a cellular response. The magnitude of the response for any given concentration of drug is determined by its *efficacy*, which is the maximum effect a given drug can produce, and by its *affinity*, which is the propensity of a drug to bind to a receptor.

— Full agonists are drugs of high intrinsic efficacy.
— Partial agonists are drugs with efficacy lower than full agonists.
— Tissue factors (receptor number and/or receptor coupling to transduction mechanisms) may cause markedly different relative responses for the same partial agonist when applied to different tissues.
— Partial agonists may antagonize the effects of full agonists at sufficient concentrations and may have greater affinity than full agonists for the same receptor.

Inverse Agonists

Inverse agonists are drugs that cause an effect opposite that of conventional agonists. This action is inhibited by specific antagonists for the receptor. This action implies tonic (ongoing) receptor or signal transduction activity in the tissue. An example is Ro15–4513, which is an inverse agonist of the benzodiazepine receptor. It binds to gamma-aminobutyric acid (GABA) receptors, causing anxiety rather than sedation (produced by benzodiazepines).

Antagonists

Antagonists bind to a receptor, usually with high affinity, but they do not produce an intrinsic cellular response (they lack efficacy). They block the effects of agonists. If given simultaneously with agonists, competitive antagonists compete for binding to the receptor (**Fig. 2.7**). Their respective affinities and concentration will determine which predominates. Noncompetitive antagonists either prevent the agonist from binding to the receptor or prevent the agonist from activating the receptor. This cannot be overcome by increasing the agonist concentration.

Fig. 2.7 ▶ **Competitive antagonism.**
Agonists and competitive antagonists compete for receptor binding. Their affinities for the receptor and their concentration will determine which one predominates; therefore, an increase in agonist concentration can overcome the blockage of the competitive antagonist and allow it to reach its maximal effect.

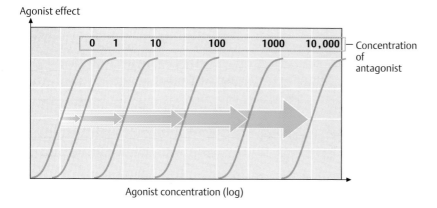

2.2 Dose–Response Relationship

Responses to drugs may be graded (response magnitude is proportional to dose) or quantal (response is all or none). Comparisons between drugs are usually made based on the median effective dose that produces a response in 50% of patients, the ED_{50} (**Fig. 2.8**).

Potency

Potency refers to the amount of drug required to produce an effect of a given intensity. It is convenient to set this intensity value at the EC_{50}, which is the median effective concentration that corresponds to 50% of the maximal response. The higher the potency of a drug, the lower the concentration needed to reach EC_{50}. Often potency and toxicity are linked because the toxic response is an extension of the therapeutic effect; therefore, a more potent drug is not necessarily a better drug.

Fig. 2.8 ▶ **Safety of a drug as determined by quantal dose-response curves.**
This graph illustrates the ED_{50} which is the dose that provides a therapeutic effect (e.g., vasodilation) in 50% of patients, the TD_{50}, which is the dose producing a toxic effect in 50% of patients (e.g., arrhythmia), and the LD_{50}, which is the lethal dose in 50% of patients.

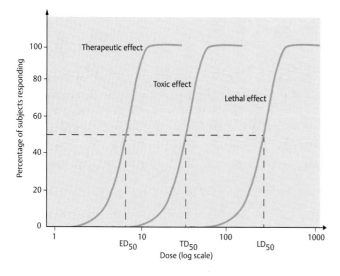

Therapeutic Index

The therapeutic index is a means of comparing the amount of a drug required to attain the therapeutic level in 50% of patients to the amount that is lethal to 50% of patients. It is expressed as the ratio LD_{50}/ED_{50}. A high therapeutic index is preferable, as the margin of safety between the dose that would be sufficient to achieve therapeutic levels and that which would produce toxic effects is high.

Certain Safety Factor

The certain safety factor is defined as the $LD_1:ED_{99}$, that is, the amount that would be lethal to just 1% of patients compared with the amount that would elicit a therapeutic effect in 99% of patients. It is another estimate of risk that indicates the degree of overlap of the lethal and therapeutic effect curves.

3 Pharmacogenetics and Other Special Considerations

The pharmacokinetics and pharmacodynamics of a drug may be altered by genetic conditions, age-related conditions, and pregnancy, altering the drug effects and influencing drug choice and dosing regimens.

3.1 Pharmacogenetics

Pharmacogenetics is concerned with hereditary differences that contribute to variations in responses to drugs. Although pharmacogenetic disorders are inherited, they may not be recognized until the individual is challenged with the drug and exhibits an abnormal response (**Fig. 3.1**). Some common examples of pharmacogenetic disorders are listed in **Table 3.1**.

Table 3.1 ▶ **Pharmacogenetic Disorders**	
Disorder	**Cause**
Abnormally Low Amounts of Enzymes or Defective Proteins	
Succinylcholine apnea	Caused by an atypical plasma cholinesterase, resulting in prolonged muscle relaxation and apnea after administration of succinylcholine
Acetylation polymorphism	Rapid and slow acetylators differ by a single autosomal gene. Slow acetylation is a recessive trait. The phenotype determines the rate of N-acetylation of drugs such as isoniazid and sulfonamides. Drug-induced lupus erythematous is more common in slow acetylators following exposure to hydralazine and procainamide due to their slow metabolism.
Hemolytic anemia	Glucose-6-phosphate dehydrogenase deficiency, an X-linked defect, may result in hemolytic anemia after exposure to primaquine and certain other oxidizing drugs.
Abnormalities in cytochrome P-450	Debrisoquine-4-hydroxylase deficiency was one of the first adverse effects attributed to low levels of a form of cytochrome P-450 (CYP 2D6), which metabolizes many drugs.
Increased Resistance to Drugs	
Heritable insensitivity to warfarin anticoagulants	This condition is probably related to abnormal proteins which synthesize vitamin K-dependent clotting factors. Affinity is decreased for warfarin, but not for vitamin K.
Responses Indirectly Related to Drug Metabolism	
Induction of drug-metabolizing enzymes	This increases heme biosynthesis through increased activity of aminolevulinic acid synthetase. This may result in various types of porphyria in people who are slow to metabolize heme precursors.

3.2 The Pediatric Patient

Children are not just small adults. To appropriately treat the pediatric patient, the clinician must appreciate that children differ physiologically and psychologically from adults.

When prescribing drugs for children,

— A "child" usually refers to someone 12 years of age or under.
— Dosages of drugs for children are usually expressed per kilogram of body weight to account for age and weight differences.
— If possible, avoid painful intramuscular injections.

Glucose-6-phosphate dehydrogenase

Glucose-6-phosphate dehydrogenase catalyzes the conversion of glucose to ribose 5-phosphate in the pentose phosphate pathway. Nicotinamide adenine dinucleotide phosphate (NADPH) and H^+ are also produced. Ribose 5-phosphate is a precursor of nucleotide biosynthesis, and NADPH is involved in the biosynthesis of fatty acids and in protecting cells from oxidative damage.

Porphyria

Porphyrias are a rare group of diseases in which there are errors in the pathway of heme biosynthesis. This causes the precursors of heme, porphyrins, to build up in the body. Porphyrias primarily affect the nervous system (acute porphyria) and skin (cutaneous porphyria). Symptoms of acute porphyria include colicky abdominal pain with vomiting or constipation, peripheral neuritis (especially motor), seizures, and mental disturbances, such as psychosis, depression, and anxiety. Skin manifestations include itching, blistering, erythema (redness of the skin), and skin edema. Treatment for both types of porphyria involves avoiding/treating precipitating factors. Acute porphyria may also require the administration of pain medication, IV fluids to correct electrolyte imbalances and treat dehydration, and the IV injection of hemin or hematin (heme arginate) which are forms of heme. Cutaneous porphyria may require repeated blood draws to reduce the iron content of the body which reduces porphyrins, activated charcoal to absorb excess porphyrins and facilitate faster excretion, and beta carotene (a vitamin A precursor) to promote healthy skin.

Drug-induced lupus erythematous

Drug-induced lupus erythematous (DIL) is an autoimmune disease caused by the chronic use of certain drugs, most commonly hydralazine (an antihypertensive drug), procainamide (an anticonvulsant drug), and isoniazid (an antibiotic). DIL is thought to be caused by slow acetylation of the drug by a portion of the population. Symptoms are similar to those caused by systemic lupus erythematous (SLE), the more common and more serious form of lupus. These include joint pain (arthalgia), swelling, and stiffness; muscle pain (mylagia), fatigue, pericarditis (inflammation of the pericaridium surrounding the heart), and pleuritis (inflammation of the pleura surrounding the lungs). Treatment involves discontinuing the causal drug, NSAIDs (nonsteroidal antiinflammatory drugs) to treat pain and inflammation, and corticosteroids to treat inflammation.

Fig. 3.1 ► **Genetic variants in pharmacokinetics.**
Azathioprine and mercaptopurine (immunosuppressant drugs) are metabolized more slowly in people with a genetic disorder affecting the enzyme thiopurine methyltransferase (TPMT). This causes toxic plasma drug levels to accumulate, resulting in damage to bone marrow.

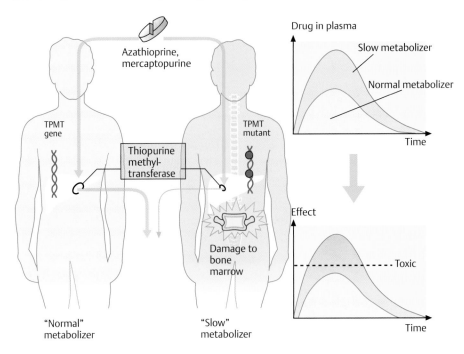

3.3 The Elderly Patient

In addition to the physiological changes that occur as a person ages, chronic diseases are more common. The use of multiple drugs, or *polypharmacy*, is also more common in this population. Polypharmacy can increase the chance of adverse reactions and drug interactions, leading to morbidity and mortality. It has also been shown to decrease compliance.

When prescribing drugs for the elderly,

1. *Minimize polypharmacy.*
— Avoid excessive or inappropriate consumption of drugs, but do prescribe adequately when necessary.
— Review and simplify drug regimens periodically.

2. *Consider the form of the drug.*
— Some elderly patients may have difficulty swallowing tablets, so prescribe liquid preparations when possible.

3. *Consider sensitivity.*
— As we age, our target organs, especially the central nervous system, are more susceptible to drugs, so all drugs should be used with caution.

4. *Reduce the dose.*
— It is prudent to assume at least mild renal impairment when prescribing for any elderly patient. Generally, the doses given should be lower than for healthy adults.
— Dose reduction should be proportional to creatinine clearance in more severe cases.
— Drugs with long half-lifes should be avoided.

Acute illness may lead to a rapid decline in renal function, especially if coupled with dehydration. This is particularly relevant when prescribing drugs with a narrow therapeutic index (e.g., digoxin, a cardiac glycoside used to treat heart failure).

3.4 The Pregnant Patient

During pregnancy, any drug given to the mother that crosses the blood–brain barrier will also cross the placenta and exert an effect on the unborn child. Some of these effects can be predicted from our understanding of the pharmacokinetics of the drug given, but others cannot. The clinician should assess the risks to the unborn child of a drug for use during pregnancy.

When prescribing a drug for a pregnant patient, consider

1. *Stage of development of the unborn child*
— A severe consequence of a drug given in the first trimester would be malformation of the unborn child, as this is when organ development is occurring (**Fig. 3.2**). After the first trimester, drugs may cause functional disturbances, as the child has formed but is growing and maturing. Drugs given at term or during labor may affect the neonate.

2. *Ability of the drug to pass through the placenta*
— The placental syncytiotrophoblast forms a diffusion barrier between the maternal circulation and the capillaries of the fetal umbilical cord (**Fig. 3.2**). However, it is permeable to most drugs (especially low-molecular-weight, non-ionized, non-protein-bound drugs), so any systemically-acting drug given to the mother during pregnancy can reach the fetus.

Fig. 3.2 ► **Pregnancy: fetal damage due to drugs.**
The sequelae of a drug taken during pregnancy depends on the stage of fetal development and the ability of the drug to cross the placenta.

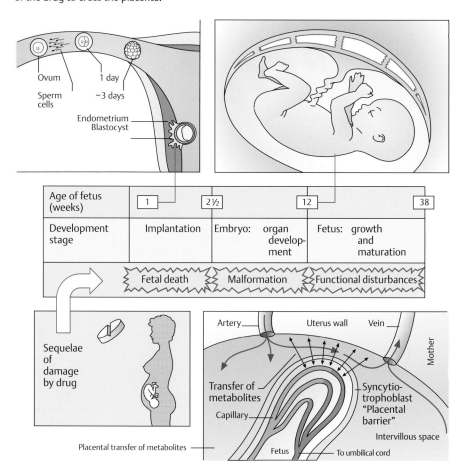

Physiological changes in pregnancy

Maternal physiology changes during pregnancy. In the cardiovascular system, blood volume increases (> 50% of pre-pregnancy levels), heart rate increases (10–15%), stroke volume increases (30%), cardiac output increases (up to 60%), and blood pressure (especially diastolic) drops in the first and second trimesters but rises to nonpregnant levels at term. In the respiratory system, ventilation increases (40%), and oxygen consumption increases (20%). In the kidneys, glomerular filtration increases (60%), renal plasma flow increases (50–70%), and there is glycosuria (as glucose reabsorption mechanisms become saturated). In the GI tract, there is decreased esophageal tone, decreased gastric acid production, increased mucus production, and decreased gut motility. These physiological parameters return to normal after parturition.

Physiology of Neonates

The physiology of neonates differs from that of older children and adults. Notably, neonates have immature active transport systems for organic anions and cations, an immature liver microsomal system for drug metabolism, a lower glomerular filtration rate; a reduced ability to glucuronidate phase 1 metabolism products causing delayed elimination of drugs, and a differing target organ sensitivity to drugs.

3. *Teratogenicity of the drug*
— Drugs that are known teratogenic agents are listed in any pharmacopeia and the clinician should become familiar with these. This will allow for an educated analysis of the risk of teratogenesis to be made. Unfortunately, the teratogenic potential of new drugs often cannot be established.

4. *The effect on the fetus of discontinuing the drug*
— The clinician must also consider the effect on the unborn child of discontinuing a drug (this may happen if the mother continues receiving the drug, but the child is born, thus severing its supply). The child may suffer from withdrawal effects and should be treated accordingly.

3.5 The Breastfed Child

The physiology of a neonate (child younger than 30 days old) is markedly different from older children and adults. Low-molecular-weight, non-ionized, non-protein-bound drugs passively diffuse into breast cells and may be ingested by the neonate via breast milk (**Fig. 3.3**). A drug that is considered relatively safe during pregnancy due to its relative inability to cross the placenta may be more readily secreted into breast milk and is therefore not safe for the breastfed infant (e.g., chloramphenicol can accumulate to toxic levels in breastfed infants causing bone marrow suppression).

Fig. 3.3 ▶ **Lactation: maternal intake of drugs.**
Drugs taken by a nursing mother can be secreted in breast milk and ingested by the baby. The effect that this has on the baby will depend on the extent of drug transfer into the milk (which determines the dose to the baby) and how the baby metabolizes and eliminates the drug.

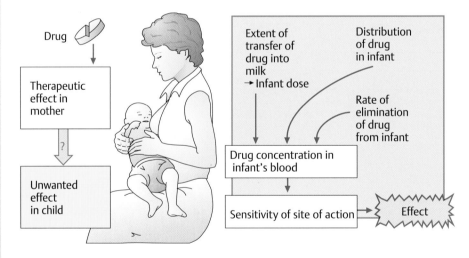

Review Questions

1. What is the term used to describe the fraction of a drug dose that reaches the systemic circulation?
   A. Plasma half-life
   B. Bioavailability
   C. Enterohepatic cycling
   D. Biotransformation
   E. Biliary excretion

2. A new antiarrhythmic agent is given intravenously to a patient with premature ventricular contractions in a dose of 500 mg. The electrocardiogram (ECG) is monitored, and blood samples are taken for analysis of plasma concentrations. The following concentrations were reported from the laboratory (see table, below). The ECG tracing showed changes in myocardial conduction for 30 minutes after administration that were indicative of the toxic effect of the drug. The patient's premature ventricular contractions were not apparent on the ECG until 5 hours after the drug was given intravenously. The information from the drug company contains no data on the metabolism or renal clearance of the drug. The patient has no pre-existing liver or kidney disease. What is the apparent volume of distribution (V_d) of the drug?

Time after Administration (hours)	Concentration of Free Drug (µg/mL)
0.5	4.5
1	4.0
2	3.4
3	2.8
4	2.4
5	2.0
6	1.7
7	1.4
8	1.3

   A. 40 L
   B. 100 L
   C. 200 L
   D. 400 L

3. The patient in question is sent home with an oral preparation of the drug. You have decided to maintain the average plasma concentration halfway between the toxic and minimal therapeutic plasma concentrations and to give the drug every 8 hours. What would be the dose within 50 mg that the patient would take?
   A. 100 mg   D. 800 mg
   B. 200 mg   E. 1 g
   C. 350 mg

4. A patient who has been taking secobarbital (a barbiturate that induces the liver microsomal enzyme system) for several weeks is stabilized on warfarin (an oral anticoagulant that is inactivated by side-chain hydroxylation). The patient then discontinues the secobarbital but continues to take the warfarin. How should the patient's warfarin dose be changed?
   A. The dose should be increased
   B. The dose should be decreased
   C. The dose should not be changed

5. For a drug that is eliminated by a first-order process, which parameter is dependent upon the dose?
   A. Clearance
   B. Elimination rate constant
   C. Steady-state plasma concentration
   D. Elimination half-life
   E. Time required to reach steady-state plasma concentration

6. A patient with seizures is started on phenytoin, 300 mg daily. Frequent plasma-level monitoring is done as part of a clinical study. After 5 days, phenytoin concentration in plasma is stabilized below the desired range, and the patient still has seizures. The dose is increased to 450 mg daily. It now takes 9 days for plasma levels to stabilize, and although seizures are controlled, the drug concentration in plasma is higher than predicted, and the patient shows signs of phenytoin toxicity. Which one of the following is the most likely explanation for the higher than predicted drug concentration?
   A. The enzymes that hydroxylate phenytoin are saturated, so its biotransformation is no longer a first-order process.
   B. There is accumulation of an active metabolite.
   C. Phenytoin is not very water soluble, so its distribution becomes limited at higher plasma concentrations.
   D. Phenytoin has induced the cytochrome P-450 enzymes, increasing its own biotransformation.
   E. The patient has a genetic inability to parahydroxylate phenytoin.

7. The total body clearance of theophylline in an adult weighing 70 kg is 48 mL/min. If theophylline is administered by continuous intravenous (IV) infusion at a rate of 60 mg/hour, the steady-state plasma concentration (C_{ss}) will be about
   A. 1 mg/dL
   B. 2 mg/dL
   C. 5 mg/dL
   D. 10 mg/dL
   E. 20 mg/dL

8. A 53-year-old man has swollen ankles, shortness of breath, and fatigue upon mild exercise. He is observed to have severe pitting edema of the lower extremities, distended neck veins with prominent pulsation, a sinus tachycardia of 105 beats/min at rest, and a normal blood pressure. He is diagnosed as being in congestive heart failure. It is noted, however, that his renal function is relatively normal (creatinine clearance = 115 mL/min). If treatment is begun with oral digoxin ($t_{1/2}$ = 36 hours) with a usual daily maintenance dose of 0.125 mg, how long should you wait before increasing the dose if his initial response appears inadequate?
   A. Approximately 2 hours
   B. Approximately 1 day
   C. Approximately 2 days
   D. Approximately 1 week

9. A patient with impaired renal function (creatinine clearance = 40 mL/min) is being treated for a urinary tract infection with a cephalosporin antibiotic. The drug is normally excreted unchanged by the kidneys with a clearance rate approximately equal to creatinine clearance (120 mL/min). The typical oral dose of the drug is 240 mg every 6 hours. Which of the following dosing regimens would be appropriate for this patient to achieve the same drug level as a patient without normal renal function?
   A. 80 mg every 18 hours
   B. 120 mg every 6 hours
   C. 240 mg every 12 hours
   D. 80 mg every 6 hours
   E. 240 mg once a day

10. Which one of the following statements is true concerning the dose–response curves in the graph?

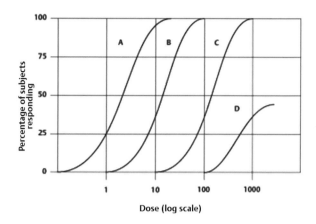

A. Curves A, B, and C represent responses to weak agonists, with C being the most potent.
B. Curve A represents the responses to a full agonist, and curves B and C represent the responses to the agonist in the presence of two concentrations of a competitive antagonist.
C. Curves A, B, and C show that the three drugs are acting at different receptors because their potencies are different.
D. Curve D shows the response to agonist A in the presence of a competitive inhibitor.
E. Curve D represents an agonist with a high intrinsic efficacy, as the dose needed for a given effect is larger than that of agonists A, B, or C.

11. Which of the following provides information about the sensitivity of a population to a drug?
   A. Graded dose–response curve
   B. Quantal dose–response curve
   C. Therapeutic index
   D. Efficacy

12. An experiment was performed to determine the median effective dose required to produce hypnosis in 50% of the population (ED_{50}) and the median lethal dose for 50% of the population (LD_{50}) of a drug. The ED_{50} was found to be 1 mg. The LD_{50} was found to be 300 mg. What is the therapeutic index for this drug?
   A. < 1
   B. 1
   C. 3
   D. 30
   E. 300

13. The following table shows the drug dosages that produce a therapeutic effect (bronchodilation), a toxic effect (cardiac arrhythmia), and death in 1%, 50%, or 99% of patients. What is the median effective dose for 50% of the population (ED_{50})?

% of Patients Showing Effect	Dose Causing Bronchodilation (mg)	Dose Causing Cardiac Arrhythmia (mg)	Dose Causing Death (mg)
1%	1 mg	200 mg	2000 mg
50%	15 mg	750 mg	6000 mg
99%	200 mg	900 mg	9000 mg

A. 1 mg
B. 15 mg
C. 200 mg
D. 750 mg
E. 6000 mg

14. What is the median lethal dose for 50% of the population (LD_{50})?
A. 1 mg
B. 15 mg
C. 200 mg
D. 750 mg
E. 6000 mg

15. At a dose of 200 mg, what percentage of patients experienced an adverse effect?
A. 1%
B. 10%
C. 50%
D. 75%
E. 99%

16. If a patient overdoses on 9 g of the drug, what is the probability that the patient will die?
A. 1%
B. 10%
C. 50%
D. 75%
E. 99%

Answers and Explanations

1. **B** Bioavailability is the fraction of the administered dose of a drug that reaches the systemic circulation in an unchanged form (p. 3).
A. Plasma half-life is the time it takes for the drug level in the blood to decrease from its peak to one half of its peak.
C. Enterohepatic cycling occurs when conjugated drugs (mainly glucuronic acid derivatives) are actively secreted into bile, and unconjugated drugs are liberated in the small intestine by bacterial enzyme hydrolysis and reabsorbed into the portal circulation.
D. Biotransformation is the process by which drugs are metabolized to (usually) less active forms for excretion.
E. Biliary excretion occurs when drugs are delivered to the bile and then excreted.

2. **B** V_d = dose (mg)/plasma concentration (mg/L) = 500 mg/4.5 mg/L ≈ 100 L (p. 8).

3. **C** Toxic effects were observed at 0.5 hour, when the plasma concentration was 4.5 µg/mL, and a therapeutic effect lasted until 4 hours, at which time the level was 2.4 µg/mL. Halfway between these two is ~3.5 µg/mL. The apparent volume of distribution of the drug was calculated from the initial dose given intravenously and its plasma concentration after 30 minutes as follows: V_d = dose (mg)/plasma concentration (mg/L) = 500 mg/4.5 mg/L ≈ 100 L. The amount of drug (taken orally) needed to achieve a desired plasma concentration by rearrangement of this equation is: Dose = plasma concentration (mg/L) × V_d (L) = 3.5 mg/L × 100 L = 350 mg (p. 8).

4. **B** Induction of liver microsomal enzymes by secobarbital increases the metabolism of warfarin. Discontinuation of the secobarbital will lead to decreased microsomal enzyme activity, lower metabolism of warfarin, increased warfarin levels, and increased anticoagulant activity. Thus, the patient's dosage will have to be decreased to maintain the same degree of anticoagulant activity (p. 10).

5. C The only one of these that is dependent upon the dose is the steady-state plasma concentration, which equals $[F \times (D/T)]/CL$, where F is bioavailability, D is dose, T is dosing interval, and CL is clearance (p. 17).

6. A Zero-order kinetics of elimination usually occur because the route of elimination has become saturated. In this case, phenytoin originally exhibited first-order kinetics when the drug concentration was below the maximum rate of the elimination process. As elimination was saturated, the time to steady-state peak level, as well as the achievement of a higher than predicted drug level, was observed. Only answer A addresses these findings; none of the other answers can explain them (p. 14).

7. B For drugs that are given by continuous IV infusion, the equation for calculating C_{ss} is $C_{ss} = R_0/CL$, where R_0 is the infusion rate, and CL is clearance. $C_{ss} = (60 \text{ mg/h})/(48 \text{ mL/min}) = (1 \text{ mg/min})/(48 \text{ mL/min}) = 0.02 \text{ mg/mL} = 2 \text{ mg/dL}$ (p. 15).

8. D The time to reach steady-state concentration (C_{ss}) is solely determined by the half-life ($t_{1/2}$). Because it takes roughly four half-lifes for a drug to reach steady-state concentration (C_{ss}), for a drug with $t_{1/2} = 36$ hours, 4×36 hours = 144 hours, or ~1 week, is required to reach steady-state concentration (C_{ss}). Steady-state concentration coincides with the desired therapeutic concentration of a drug (p. 15).

9. D $C_{ss} = [F \times (D/T)]/CL$, where C_{ss} is the steady-state concentration, F is bioavailability, D is dose, T is dosing interval, and CL is clearance. Because clearance is decreased in this patient to approximately one third of its normal value (= creatinine clearance), the maintenance dose must be decreased by one third or the dose interval increased 3-fold to achieve the same steady-state drug concentration (p. 17).

10. B Because a competitive antagonist competes with the agonist for binding to the receptor, more of the agonist drug is required to elicit a given response in the presence of a competitive antagonist. This results in the dose–response curve being shifted to the right (p. 25).
A. Curves A to C do not represent responses to a weak agonist because they all show 100% responses, which would not occur with a weak agonist. Also C is the least potent, not the most potent.
C. Variations in potency do not indicate that different receptors are affected.
D. A competitive antagonist does not reduce the maximal response, but instead increases the amount of agonist needed to obtain the same response.
E. Curve D, which does not reach a 100% response, represents a lower, not higher, efficacy for the agonist.

11. B A quantal dose–response curve plots the proportion of a population that responds to different concentrations of a drug (p. 25).
A. A graded dose–response curve plots the magnitude of a response as a function of the dose.
C. The therapeutic index is the ratio LD_{50}/ED_{50}, where LD_{50} is the drug dose that is lethal to 50% of the population and ED_{50} is the median effective dose for 50% of the population.
D. Efficacy is the maximum effect a given drug can produce.

12. E The therapeutic index is the ratio LD_{50}/ED_{50}. In this example, the therapeutic index would therefore be 300 (300/1), meaning that 300 times the median effective dose (ED_{50}) would need to be given to produce a lethal effect for 50% of the population (p. 26).

13. B The ED_{50} is the dose that causes bronchodilation, in this case, in 50% of patients. This is achieved with a dose of 15 mg (p. 26).

14. E The LD_{50} is 6000 mg (p. 26).

15. A At a dose of 200 mg, only 1% of the patients experienced cardiac arrhythmia, the adverse effect (p. 26).

16. E At a dose of 9000 mg (or 9 g), 99% of patients will die (p. 26).

4 The Peripheral Nervous System

The peripheral nervous system (PNS) is composed of afferent and efferent neurons that lie outside the brain and spinal cord. It regulates and coordinates body physiology in conjunction with the endocrine system. The actions of the PNS are mediated by neurotransmitters acting on a diverse array of receptors at effector organs. Pharmacological agents act on the efferent nerves of the PNS by either mimicking or blocking the effects of these neurotransmitters.

4.1 Divisions of the Peripheral Nervous System

Autonomic Nervous System

Efferent neurons of the autonomic nervous system (ANS) innervate the viscera and are responsible for involuntary homeostatic control of the organs. The ANS is subdivided into the sympathetic and parasympathetic nervous systems, which are summarized in **Table 4.1**. The relative innervations of target organs by each subdivision are depicted in **Fig. 4.1**.

Table 4.1 ▶ **Summary of the Divisions of the Autonomic Nervous System**		
	Parasympathetic Division	**Sympathetic Division**
Region of spinal cord from which preganglionic neurons emerge	Cranial and sacral – Cell bodies of preganglionic neurons are in the midbrain, pons, and medulla giving rise to the autonomic components of cranial nerves III, VII, IX, and X – Cell bodies of preganglionic neurons are in S2-S4	Thoracolumbar – Cell bodies of preganglionic neurons are in T1-L3
Length of preganglionic neurons	Long	Short
Length of postganglionic neurons	Short	Long
Location of ganglia	Near target organs	Sympathetic chain ganglia (located parallel to the spinal cord on both sides) Abdominal prevertebral ganglia Adrenal medulla
Neurotransmitters and receptors	Preganglionic neurons release acetylcholine, which acts at nicotinic receptors. Postganglionic neurons release acetylcholine, which acts at muscarinic receptors.	Preganglionic neurons release acetylcholine, which acts at nicotinic receptors. Postganglionic neurons release norepinephrine, which acts at adrenergic receptors.
General functions	Principally concerned with maintenance, conservation, and protection of body resources (anabolic).	Principally involved with expenditure of body resources or energy (catabolic).
Comments	A functioning parasympathetic system is necessary to sustain life as it maintains essential bodily functions. Parasympathetic nerves can act in isolation from the system as a whole, producing discrete effects at specific end organs.	The sympathetic system is not strictly necessary to maintain life. It is capable of a mass response, the emergency "flight or fight response." The neuronal basis of this widespread response lies in the wide divergence of preganglionic axons within the sympathetic chain ganglia.

Embryology of the adrenal gland

The adrenal cortex, which comprises 80% of the adrenal gland, is derived from mesothelium; the adrenal medulla, which comprises 20%, is derived from neural crest cells as are the neurons of the sympathetic nervous system. The adrenal medulla is innervated by preganglionic sympathetic nerves and is pharmacologically similar to a sympathetic ganglion. However, because the chromaffin cells of the adrenal medulla lack axons, the adrenal medulla responds to preganglionic secretion of acetylcholine by secreting the hormones epinephrine (and norepinephrine to a lesser extent) into the bloodstream.

Quadriplegia

Quadriplegia is caused by spinal cord injury at the level of the cervical spine. A ventilator may be required if the injury involves C3–C5, as these spinal nerves control the diaphragm (via the phrenic nerve), which is the major muscle that allows us to breathe. However, quadriplegic patients can survive because the cranial nerves (ANS preganglionic parasympathetic nerves) remain intact and can coordinate vital bodily functions despite the patient's having no voluntary control from below the level of injury.

Fig. 4.1 ▶ **The autonomic nervous system (ANS).**
The ANS comprises a parasympathetic division and a sympathetic division. Parasympathetic preganglionic neurons arise in the cranial and sacral region of the spinal cord and are relatively long compared with the parasympathetic postganglionic neurons. Sympathetic preganglionic neurons arise in the thoracolumbar region of the spinal cord and are relatively short compared to sympathetic postganglionic neurons.
Both pre- and postganglionic parasympathetic neurons release acetylcholine as their neurotransmitter substance. Sympathetic preganglionic neurons also release acetylcholine, but postganglionic neurons release norepinephrine. The exception to this is sweat glands, which are innervated by sympathetic fibers but release acetylcholine from postganglionic neurons.

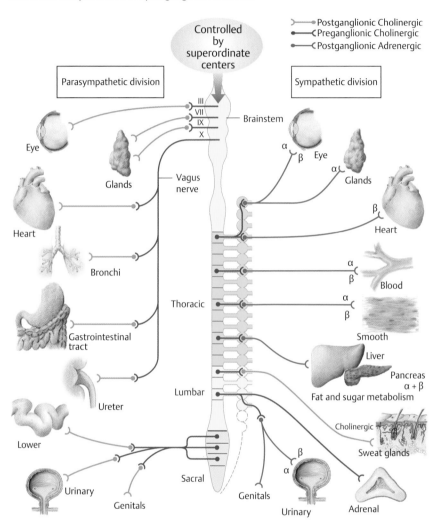

Horner Syndrome

Horner syndrome may occur due to an interruption of the sympathetic nerve supply to the face through a disease of or injury to the brainstem or thoracolumbar region of the spinal cord, for example, by stroke, tumors, carotid artery dissection (tearing of the lining of the artery), or spinal cord injury. It may also be idiopathic (cause not known). Horner syndrome causes miosis (pupillary constriction), enophthalmos (a sunken eye), ptosis (drooping of the upper eyelid), and anhidrosis (loss of sweating) on the affected side of the face. Treatment for Horner syndrome is directed at the underlying cause.

Chapter 5 covers cholinergic agents and Chapter 6 covers adrenergic agents.

Somatic Nervous System

Efferent neurons of the somatic nervous system innervate skeletal muscle and are responsible for voluntary movements. The axons of these efferent neurons originate in the spinal cord and synapse directly on skeletal muscle.

Drugs that block nicotinic cholinergic receptors on skeletal muscle are covered in the section on "Depolarizing and Nondepolarizing Neuromuscular Blockers of Acetylcholine" in Chapter 5 (p. 49).

The efferent neurons of the parasympathetic, sympathetic, and somatic neurons are shown schematically in **Fig. 4.2**.

Fig. 4.2 ▶ **Efferent neurons of the parasympathetic, sympathetic, and somatic nervous systems.**
Postganglionic neurons that innervate sweat glands release ACh. (ACh, acetylcholine; NE, norepinephrine; EPI, epinephrine.)

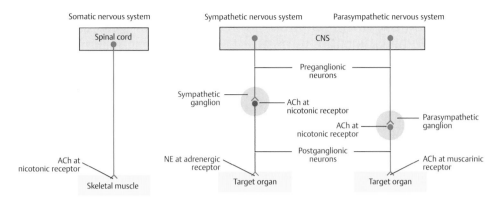

Enteric Nervous System

Enteric neurons include the submucosal and myenteric plexuses in the gastrointestinal (GI) tract. This system possesses all the elements necessary for the short reflex regulation of GI functions, i.e., modification of motility and secretory activity by afferent and efferent nerves entirely within the GI tract. It is able to do this without modulation from the ANS, with the exception of the proximal esophagus and the external anal sphincter.

4.2 Neurotransmitters of the Autonomic and Somatic Nervous Systems

Acetylcholine

Synthesis.   The neurotransmitter acetylcholine (ACh) is synthesized in the nerve terminal from acetate, derived from acetyl coenzyme A, and choline. This reaction is catalyzed by the enzyme choline acetyltransferase. The uptake of choline is the rate-limiting step in acetylcholine synthesis (**Fig. 4.3**).

Storage and release.   Acetylcholine is stored within vesicles in nerve terminals. An action potential causes Ca^{2+} influx through voltage-gated channels and the subsequent release of ACh into the synaptic cleft.

Degradation.   The breakdown of acetylcholine to acetic acid and choline is rapid and occurs via the enzyme acetylcholinesterase. Acetylcholinesterase is located in neuronal membranes and red blood cells. Pseudocholinesterases (nonspecific) or butyrylcholinesterases, which are more widely distributed, can also hydrolyze acetylcholine.

Site of neurotransmission.   ACh is the neurotransmitter released from the following types of neurons:

— Preganglionic neurons that innervate all autonomic (parasympathetic and sympathetic) ganglia
— Postganglionic parasympathetic neurons
— Somatic motor neurons that innervate the neuromuscular junction
— Neurons that innervate the adrenal medulla
— Postganglionic neurons that innervate sweat glands

■ **Neuronal Communication**

Nerve cells communicate with each other through the release of neurotransmitters from the presynaptic nerve terminal. The sequence of events that leads to the response of a postsynaptic neuron or effector organ is as follows:
— Presynaptic action potential
— Influx of Ca^{2+} into the nerve terminal
— Release of the neurotransmitter from the presynaptic terminal
— Neurotransmitter binds to the postsynaptic receptor.
— Transduction of the message to the ion channel
— Integration of signals from various inputs
— Postsynaptic response

Coenzyme A

Pantothenic acid (vitamin B_5) is a precursor of coenzyme A (CoA). CoA participates in fatty acid synthesis and oxidation, as well as the oxidation of pyruvate in the citric acid cycle. A molecule of CoA that has an acetyl group is acetyl coenzyme A (acetyl CoA). Acetate, which is derived from acetyl CoA, combines with choline to form the neurotransmitter acetylcholine (ACh).

Fig. 4.3 ► **Acetylcholine: release, effects, and degradation.**
Acetylcholine is stored in vesicles in the axoplasm of presynaptic nerve terminals. These vesicles are anchored to a cytoskeletal network by the protein synapsin, thus allowing for the accumulation of vesicles near the presynaptic membrane while preventing fusion with the membrane. An action potential causes Ca^{2+} influx into the axoplasm through voltage-gated channels. Ca^{2+} then activates protein kinases that phosphorylate synapsin. This causes the vesicles to become free, fuse with the membrane, and release acetylcholine into the synaptic gap. Acetylcholine attaches to receptors on the postsynaptic membrane and exerts its effects. It is then hydrolyzed by acetylcholinesterase with reuptake of the choline component into the axoplasm.

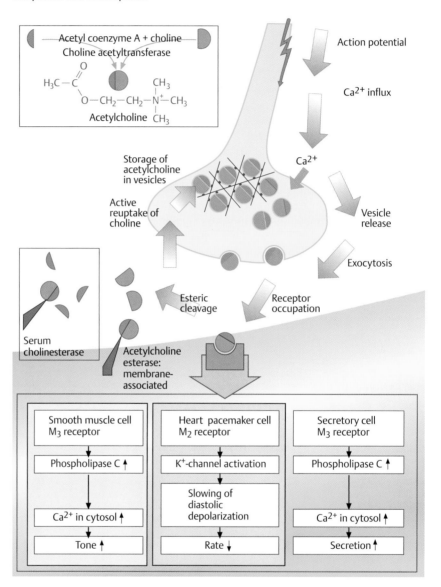

Norepinephrine and Epinephrine

Synthesis

— Norepinephrine (NE) is synthesized in nerve terminals. Tyrosine is converted to dopa by tyrosine hydroxylase (rate-limiting step). Dopa is converted to dopamine by dopa decarboxylase and then dopamine is converted to norepinephrine by dopamine-β-hydroxylase.

- Epinephrine (EPI) (and a lesser amount of norepinephrine) is synthesized in the adrenal medulla. A cytoplasmic enzyme in the adrenal medulla (phenylethanolamine-N-methyltransferase) transfers a methyl group to norepinephrine to form epinephrine (**Fig. 4.4**).

Storage and release
- NE is stored in vesicles within nerve terminals. An action potential at the nerve terminal causes the influx of Ca^{2+} through voltage-gated channels and the subsequent release of NE into the synaptic cleft.
- EPI (80%) and NE (20%) are released from the adrenal medulla following sympathetic stimulation (via ACh).

Degradation
Termination of action is primarily by reuptake (60–90%) into the nerve terminal. Secondary degradation is by monoamine oxidase (MAO) and catechol-O-methyltransferase (COMT).

Site of neurotransmission
- NE is the neurotransmitter released from postganglioinc sympathetic neurons (except sweat glands which release ACh).

Ascorbic acid redox reactions

Ascorbic acid (vitamin C) is involved in many processes in the body, including collagen and bile acid synthesis, activation of neuroendocrine hormones (e.g., gastrin, corticotropin-releasing hormone [CRH], and thyrotropin-releasing hormone [TRH]), iron absorption, and detoxification (via stimulation of cytochrome P-450 enzymes in the liver. Ascorbic acid is oxidized to dehydroascorbic acid via an extremely reactive intermediate, semidehydro-L-ascorbate. The hydrogen ions that are liberated in this oxidation are able to act as donors in hydroxylation reactions throughout the body (which accounts for some of its effects). One such reaction where this occurs is when ascorbic acid acts as a cofactor for dopamine-β-hydroxylase in the synthesis of norepinephrine and epinephrine.

Fig. 4.4 ► Synthesis and termination of norepinephrine and adrenergic transmission.
Postganglionic sympathetic nerve terminals possess varicosities that enable them to lie in close proximity to effector organs. Norepinephrine (NE) synthesis and storage in vesicles occurs in these varicosities. An action potential at the nerve terminal causes the influx of Ca^{2+} and the subsequent release of NE into the synaptic cleft. NE then binds to adrenergic receptors on effector organs, exerting a physiological effect. Note that NE has little effect on the β_2-adrenergic receptors, whereas epinephrine, synthesized in the adrenal medulla, acts at all adrenergic receptors. Approximately 70% of NE is taken back up into the presynaptic nerve terminal and repackaged in vesicles or is inactivated by monoamine oxidase (MAO). In the heart, NE is inactivated by MAO or catechol-O-methyltransferase (COMT).

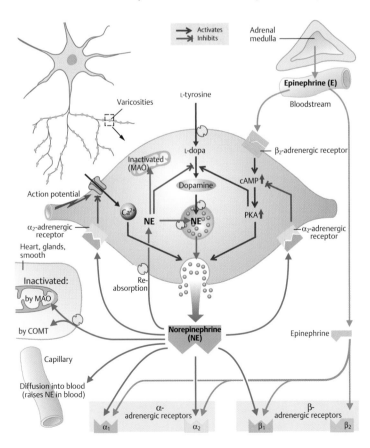

4.3 Neurotransmitter Receptors

There are two broad categories of neurotransmitter receptors in the ANS, cholinergic and adrenergic. The cholinergic receptors can be further broken down into two types, nicotinic and muscarinic receptors.

Cholinergic Receptors

Nicotinic Receptors

Nicotinic receptors are ligand-gated ion channels composed of five protein subunits that combine to form a functional receptor and ion pore. Ligand binding induces Na^+ conductance. The two major subtypes are the muscle type and the neuronal type and they each have different subunit compositions:
- The muscle type is composed of α_1, β_1, δ, and ϵ subunits in a 2:1:1:1 ratio in adults.
- The neuronal subtypes are homomeric or heteromeric combinations of 12 different nicotinic receptor subunits: α_2 through α_{10} and β_2 through β_4.

Location
- Autonomic ganglia
- Neuromuscular junction of somatic nerves and skeletal muscle
- Adrenal medulla

Muscarinic Receptors

Muscarinic receptors are brain G protein-coupled receptors (see pages 21 to 23), which in turn transduce receptor activation by acetylcholine into various intracellular changes. There are five main subtypes of muscarinic receptors. Three primary ones (M_1 to M_3) will be considered here.

Location
- M_1 receptors are found in the CNS.
- M_2 receptors are found in the heart.
- M_3 receptors are found in smooth muscle and glands.

Signal transduction mechanism
- M_1 and M_3 couple to G_q: G_q activates phospholipase which increases DAG and IP_3 (see page 23).
- M_2 couples to G_i: G_i inhibits cAMP (see page 23).

Cholinergic nicotinic and muscarinic receptors are illustrated in **Fig. 4.5**.

Fig. 4.5 ▶ **Acetylcholine receptors.**
(**A**) The nicotinic receptor consists of five protein subunits. Binding of acetylcholine to the two α subunits is thought to change its conformation, allowing for the central pore to open and for the influx of ions into the cell. (**B**) The muscarinic receptor is coupled to intracellular G proteins, which may then transduce excitatory effects via phospholipase C or inhibitory/excitatory effects via adenylate cyclase.

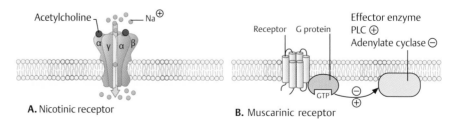

A. Nicotinic receptor   B. Muscarinic receptor

Adrenergic Receptors

Adrenergic receptors are G-protein coupled receptors (GPCRs). There are two main subtypes of adrenergic receptors, α and β.

Location
- α_1 are found on vascular smooth muscle.
- α_2 are autoreceptors at presynaptic terminals of sympathetic neurons.
- β_1 are found in cardiac muscle.
- β_2 are found in the lung.
- β_3 are found in adipose tissue.

Signal transduction mechanism
- α_1 couples to G_q.
- α_2 couples to G_i.
- β-receptors couple to G_s (see page 23).

Table 4.2 provides a summary of ANS receptors.

Table 4.2 ▶ Autonomic Nervous System Receptors				
Major Types of ANS Receptors	**Receptor Subclassification**	**Location of Receptor**	**Neurotransmitter Acting On the Receptor**	**Signal Transduction Mechanism**
Cholinergic receptors	Nicotinic	Autonomic ganglia Neuromuscular junction of somatic nerves and skeletal muscle Adrenal medulla	ACh	Nicotinic receptors open Na^+ and K^+ channels
	Muscarinic	M_1: CNS M_2: Heart M_3: Smooth muscle* and glands	ACh	M_1 and M_3: G_q leading to ↑ IP_3 and DAG M_2: G_i leading to ↓ cAMP
Adrenergic receptors	α	α_1: vascular smooth muscle α_2: Autoreceptors at presynaptic terminals of sympathetic neurons	EPI and NE	α_1: G_q leading to ↑ IP_3 and DAG α_2: G_i leading to ↓ cAMP
	β	β_1: cardiac muscle β_2: lung β_3: adipose tissue	EPI and NE	β-receptors: G_s leading to ↑ cAMP

* Effects on smooth muscle are the most important in terms of autonomic responses.
Abbreviations: cAMP, cyclic adenosine monophosphate; IP_3, inositol triphosphate; EPI, epinephrine.

4.4 Physiologic Responses of the Autonomic Nervous System

Drugs that act on the ANS alter the physiological responses of the endogenous system. Understanding the normal sympathetic or parasympathetic responses of the various organs is important to understanding the actions of drugs that affect the ANS. Most organs receive dual innervation from both the sympathetic and parasympathetic divisions, which generally have opposing effects (**Fig. 4.6**).

Disorders of CNS autonomic control

Disorders involving central autonomic control may manifest as hyperactivity (e.g., hypertension and arrhythmias) or as autonomic failure (e.g., orthostatic hypotension, impotence, or GI tract dysmotility). In general, autonomic hyperactivity tends to occur acutely, whereas autonomic failure is more typical of chronic neurodegenerative disease (e.g., multiple sclerosis).

Fig. 4.6 ▶ Physiological responses of the autonomic nervous system.
The effects of parasympathetic and sympathetic stimulation on organs throughout the body are shown. Many organs are innervated by both systems, with each having a different effect; however, an exception to this is blood vessels, which only receive innervation by sympathetic postganglionic neurons. (cAMP, cyclic adenosine monophosphate; CNS, central nervous system; DAG, diacylglycerol; IP$_3$, inositol triphosphate; VIP, vasoactive intestinal polypeptide.)

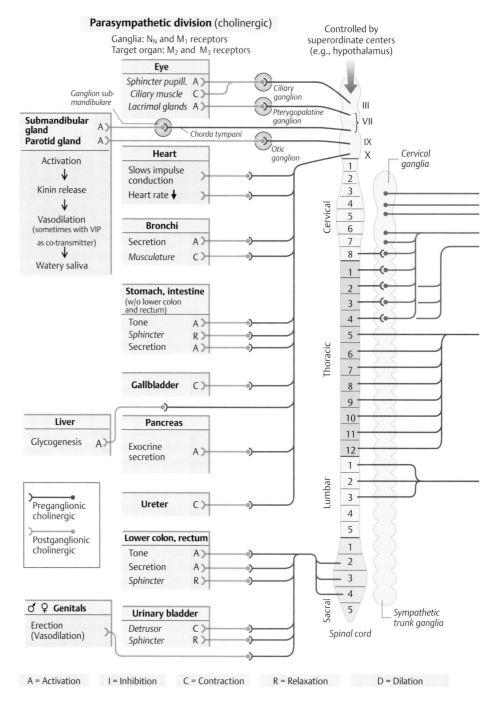

Fig. 4.6 ▶ (Continued)

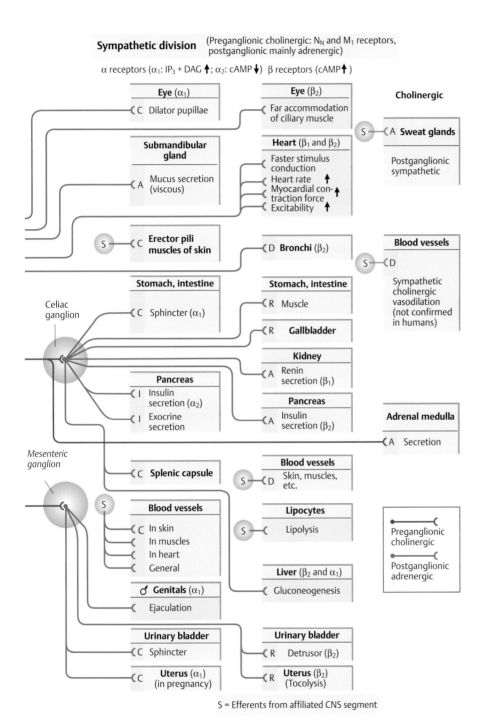

Sympathetic division (Preganglionic cholinergic: N_N and M_1 receptors, postganglionic mainly adrenergic)

α receptors ($α_1$: IP_3 + DAG ↑; $α_2$: cAMP ↓)   β receptors (cAMP ↑)

Eye ($α_1$)
- C Dilator pupillae

Eye ($β_2$)
- Far accommodation of ciliary muscle

Cholinergic

S — A **Sweat glands**

Postganglionic sympathetic

Submandibular gland
- A Mucus secretion (viscous)

Heart ($β_1$ and $β_2$)
- Faster stimulus conduction
- Heart rate ↑
- Myocardial contraction force ↑
- Excitability ↑

S — C **Erector pili muscles of skin**

- D **Bronchi ($β_2$)**

Blood vessels

S — D

Sympathetic cholinergic vasodilation (not confirmed in humans)

Celiac ganglion

Stomach, intestine
- C Sphincter ($α_1$)

Stomach, intestine
- R Muscle

- R **Gallbladder**

Kidney
- A Renin secretion ($β_1$)

Pancreas
- I Insulin secretion ($α_2$)
- I Exocrine secretion

Pancreas
- A Insulin secretion ($β_2$)

Adrenal medulla
- A Secretion

Mesenteric ganglion

- C **Splenic capsule**

Blood vessels

S — D Skin, muscles, etc.

S

Blood vessels
- C In skin
- In muscles
- In heart
- General

Lipocytes

S — Lipolysis

♂ **Genitals ($α_1$)**
- Ejaculation

Liver ($β_2$ and $α_1$)
- Gluconeogenesis

Preganglionic cholinergic

Postganglionic adrenergic

Urinary bladder
- C Sphincter

Urinary bladder
- R Detrusor ($β_2$)

- C **Uterus ($α_1$)** (in pregnancy)

- R **Uterus ($β_2$)** (Tocolysis)

S = Efferents from affiliated CNS segment

5 Cholinergic Agents

5.1 Cholinergic Agonists

Cholinergic agonist drugs are termed *parasympathomimetics* (or *cholinomimetics*), as they mimic the effects of the neurotransmitter acetylcholine (**Fig. 5.1**) in the parasympathetic nervous system. They can be either direct- or indirect-acting.

- Direct-acting parasympathomimetics bind directly to cholinergic receptors.
- Indirect-acting parasympathomimetics inhibit the enzyme acetylcholinesterase, thereby increasing the concentration of acetylcholine in the synaptic cleft. They are further subdivided into reversible and irreversible agents.

Fig. 5.1 ▶ **Direct and indirect parasympathomimetics.**
Direct parasympathomimetics (e.g., carbachol and arecoline) mimic the effects of acetylcholine (ACh) at effector organs but are not hydrolyzed by acetylcholinesterase (AChE), allowing for their therapeutic use. Indirect parasympathomimetics (e.g., neostigmine, and physostigmine) inhibit AChE, thus raising the concentration of ACh at all cholinergic receptors.

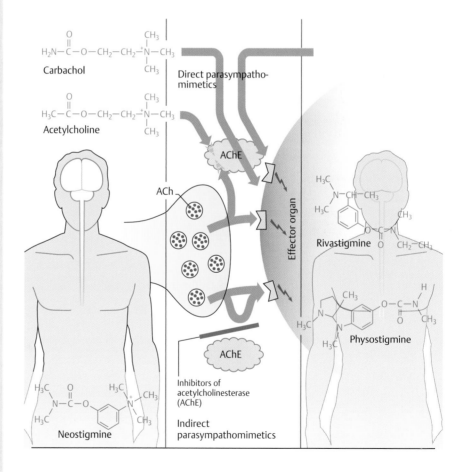

Table 5.1 summarizes the effects of acetylcholine activation in the parasympathetic system and therefore the effects of parasympathomimetic drugs.

Table 5.1 ▸ Effects of Acetylcholine Activation in the Parasympathetic System and the Effects of Parasympathomimetic Drugs	
System/Parameter	Effects
Cardiovascular system	↓ heart rate and velocity of conduction ↓ blood pressure Vasodilation of arterioles
Respiratory system	↑ bronchoconstriction
Gastrointestinal tract	↑ gastrointestinal motility and peristalsis
Urinary tract	↑ contraction of ureter and bladder smooth muscle Relaxation of the sphincter
Eye	↑ contraction of ciliary muscle and iris
Secretions	↑ salivation ↑ lacrimation ↑ gastrointestinal secretions ↑ bronchial secretions ↑ sweating

Direct-acting Parasympathomimetics

Direct-acting parasympathomimetics are chemical analogues of acetylcholine; therefore, they have actions similar to acetylcholine. They differ in their degree of selectivity for nicotinic versus muscarinic receptors. Some direct-acting parasympathomimetic agents are illustrated in **Fig. 5.1**. These agents are less susceptible to degradation by acetylcholinesterases and serum esterases than acetylcholine.

Side effects. General side effects of direct-acting parasympathomimetics include salivation, lacrimation, urination, diarrhea, vomiting, bronchorrhea, bronchospasm, and bradycardia.

Contraindications
— Peptic ulcers (due to increased gastric acid production)
— Asthma (due to bronchoconstriction)
— Cardiac disease (due to decreased heart rate and velocity of conduction)
— Parkinson disease (worsens tremors)

Methacholine
Mechanism of action. Strong muscarinic (little nicotinic) action

Primary open-angle glaucoma

Glaucoma refers to a group of eye diseases that cause damage to the optic nerve. Primary open-angle glaucoma is the most common form of glaucoma. In this case, drainage of the aqueous humor is prevented due to blockage of the drainage channels between the cornea and the iris. The resultant buildup of aqueous humor raises intraocular pressure, causing damage to the optic nerve. The symptoms include the gradual loss of peripheral vision, which progresses to tunnel vision. Drug treatment is aimed at reducing intraocular pressure by decreasing the production of aqueous humor (e.g., β-blockers [timolol], α-agonists [apraclonidine]), and/or increasing the drainage of the aqueous humor (e.g., lantanoprost, pilocarpine).

Sjögren syndrome

Sjögren syndrome is an autoimmune disease causing keratoconjuctivitis sicca (diminished tear production) and xerostomia (dry mouth). It is also associated with rheumatoid arthritis (in 50% of cases) and lupus. Lymphocytes and plasma cells infiltrate secretory glands and cause injury. Diminished tear production causes dry, itchy, gritty eyes, while diminished saliva production makes swallowing difficult and increases the likelihood of development of dental caries. Rheumatoid arthritis causes joint pain, swelling, and stiffness. Treatment for dry eyes involves the use of artificial tears. Dry mouth may be relieved by artificial saliva, taking frequent sips of water, and chewing gum to stimulate saliva flow. If this is insufficient, pilocarpine may be used to stimulate saliva production. Nonsteroidal antiinflammatory drugs (NSAIDs) are used for rheumatoid arthritis. Other drugs that may be useful include hydroxychloroquine (an antimalarial drug) and immunosuppressants (e.g., methotrexate and cyclosporine).

Pharmacokinetics. Partially susceptible to ester hydrolysis

Uses
— Diagnosis of asthma (by inducing bronchial hypersensitivity)

Side effects
— Light-headedness, itching, headache

Carbachol

Mechanism of action. Strong nicotinic (little muscarinic) action

Pharmacokinetics. Not susceptible to ester hydrolysis by serum esterases or acetylcholinesterase

Uses
— Used as a miotic to treat glaucoma if pilocarpine is ineffective

Side effects
— Few side effects at ophthalmologic doses

Bethanechol

Mechanism of action. Strong muscarinic (little nicotinic) action

Pharmacokinetics
— Not susceptible to ester hydrolysis by serum esterases or acetylcholinesterase

Uses
— Treatment for urinary retention (stimulates the smooth muscle of the bladder)
— Used to increase GI motility postoperatively and for gastric atony following bilateral vagotomy (stimulates the smooth muscle of the GI tract)

Note: Bethanechol should not be used for urinary retention or to increase GI motility if there is a mechanical obstruction.

Side effects. General side effects of cholinergic stimulation include decreased blood pressure, bronchospasm, nausea, abdominal pain, diarrhea, sweating, and flushing

Pilocarpine

Mechanism of action. Strong muscarinic action

Pharmacokinetics
— Crosses the blood–brain barrier
— Not susceptible to ester hydrolysis by serum esterases or acetylcholinesterase

Uses
— Glaucoma
— Sjögren syndrome (to increase the secretion of saliva)

Side effects
— Same as for bethanechol

Indirect-acting Parasympathomimetics (Anticholinesterases)

Indirect-acting parasympathomimetics inhibit acetylcholinesterase (AChE), thereby increasing concentrations of acetylcholine and enhancing cholinergic function (**Fig. 5.1**). The effects are the same as those seen following activation of nicotinic and muscarinic receptors.

Side effects. All of the side effects seen with direct-acting parasympathomimetics (salivation, lacrimation, urination, diarrhea, vomiting, bronchorrhea, bronchospasm, and bradycardia) plus muscle weakness, cramps, convulsions, coma, and cardiovascular and respiratory failure, caused by the increased nicotinic component.

Physostigmine

Mechanism of action. Physostigmine is a reversible blocker of AChE.

Pharmacokinetics
— Can enter the central nervous system (CNS)
— Slowly hydrolyzed by AChE
— Effects last 4 to 6 hours

Uses
— Atropine poisoning
— Glaucoma
— Myasthenia gravis (rarely)

Neostigmine

Mechanism of action. Neostigmine is a reversible blocker of AChE.

Pharmacokinetics
— Excluded from the CNS because it is polar
— Slowly hydrolyzed by AChE
— Effects last 4 to 6 hours

Uses
— Myasthenia gravis
— Reverses the effects of nondepolarizing (competitive) muscle relaxants

Pyridostigmine and Ambenonium

Mechanism of action. These agents are reversible blockers of AChE.

Pharmacokinetics
— Slowly hydrolyzed by AChE
— Effects last 4 to 8 hours

Uses
— Treatment of myasthenia gravis, especially in patients who have become tolerant to neostigmine

Edrophonium

Mechanism of action. Edrophonium is a reversible blocker of AChE.

▎ Myasthenia gravis

Myasthenia gravis is an autoimmune disease in which there are too few functioning acetylcholine receptors at the neuromuscular junction. Patients with this condition often present in young adulthood with muscle fatigue that may progress to permanent muscle weakness. Often the eye muscles are the first to be affected causing ptosis (drooping of the eyelids) and diplopia (double vision). It is treated with neostigmine or similar agents to improve muscle contraction and muscle strength. Corticosteroids, e.g., hydrocortisone, or immunosuppressant drugs, e.g., azathioprine or cyclosporine, may also be given to inhibit the immune system.

Pharmacokinetics
— Rapidly reversible binding to AChE
— Short-acting (10 to 20 minutes)

Uses
— Useful in diagnosis of myasthenia gravis and "cholinergic crisis"

Parathion and Isoflurophate

Mechanism of action.   These agents are irreversible blockers of AChE.

Pharmacokinetics
— Covalently binds to ester site on acetylcholinesterase
— Very slowly released from AChE by hydrolysis (hence "irreversible")
— Removed from AChE by oxime reactivators, such as pralidoxime (2-PAM), along with atropine (to prevent muscarinic effects)

Uses
— Primarily used as an insecticide
— Sometimes used topically to treat glaucoma
— Component of nerve gas for biological warfare

5.2 Cholinergic Antagonists

Drugs are available to block neuronal and muscle nicotinic receptors, as well as muscarinic receptors. Drugs that block peripheral neuronal nicotinic receptors are termed *ganglionic blocking agents* and are infrequently used. Agents that block nicotinic receptors on skeletal muscle can be depolarizing or nondepolarizing. Depolarizing blockers persistently activate the receptors, leading to receptor desensitization and thereby blocking the effects of acetylcholine. Nondepolarizing blockers are antagonists at muscle nicotinic receptors and thus block the effects of acetylcholine without depolarization. Muscarinic receptor antagonists differ mainly in their relative activities in the CNS and PNS.

Nicotinic Receptor Antagonists: Ganglionic Blocking Agents

Hexamethonium and Trimethaphan

Mechanism of action.   These agents block the nicotinic receptors of both sympathetic and parasympathetic ganglia, but they are not effective at the nicotinic receptor of skeletal muscle.

Pharmacokinetics.   Trimethaphan is only effective intravenously and has a short half-life.

Uses
— Hexamethonium is an experimental agent.
— Trimethaphan is used clinically in surgery or in emergencies to reduce blood pressure.

Side effects.   These depend on the relative balance of sympathetic and parasympathetic influences and are unpredictable.

Nicotinic Receptor Antagonists: Depolarizing Neuromuscular Blockers of Acetylcholine

Succinylcholine

Mechanism of action.   Succinylcholine persistently activates nicotinic receptors, leading to initial target stimulation followed by persistent desensitization (**Fig. 5.2**).

Pharmacokinetics.   Neuromuscular blockage appears within 1 minute of injection and lasts up to 30 minutes.

Uses.   Succinylcholine is used to produce skeletal muscle relaxation during surgery.

Side effects
— Muscle pain
— Increased intraocular pressure
— Hyperkalemia (high plasma K^+)

Nicotinic Receptor Antagonists: Nondepolarizing Neuromuscular Blockers of Acetylcholine

Curare and Vecuronium (and All Other "Curoniums")

Mechanism of action.   These agents act as competitive antagonists at nicotinic receptors, thus blocking the effects of acetylcholine without depolarization.

Pharmacokinetics
— Given intravenously
— These drugs vary in duration of action by 1 to 3 hours.

Uses.   Curare, vecuronium, and related drugs are used to produce skeletal muscle relaxation during surgery.

Side effects
— Respiratory paralysis at toxic doses

Muscarinic Receptor Antagonists

— Muscarinic receptor antagonists are active at all muscarinic receptors throughout the body and as such have low organ specificity (**Fig. 5.3**).

Atropine

Mechanism of action.   Atropine is a competitive antagonist at muscarinic receptors.

Pharmacokinetics
— Orally absorbed
— Readily enters the CNS and therefore has both PNS and CNS actions

Uses.   Preanesthetic agent (when reductions of bronchial secretions are necessary)

Fig. 5.2 ▶ **Action of the depolarizing neuromuscular blocking agent succinylcholine.**
Succinylcholine is structurally like a double acetylcholine (ACh) molecule, and as such it can act as an
agonist at motor end plate nicotinic receptors. It is unlike ACh, however, in that it is not hydrolyzed by
acetylcholinesterase, but rather is degraded more slowly by plasma cholinesterase. This allows it to
accumulate in the synaptic cleft and cause persistent depolarization of the motor end plate, which is
accompanied by the persistent contraction of skeletal muscle fibers.

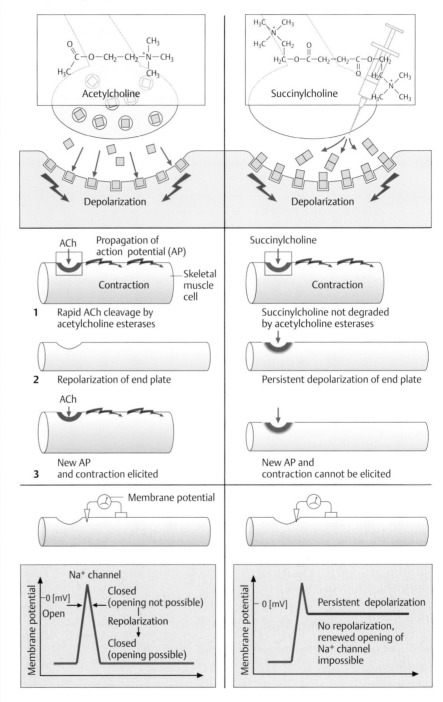

Fig. 5.3 ▶ Muscarinic receptor antagonists.

These agents act on all muscarinic receptors and have low organ selectivity. The mode of administration is therefore important for targeted treatment, as it determines distribution (as indicated by the shading) and organ concentration (indicated in red). (ED, effective dose.).

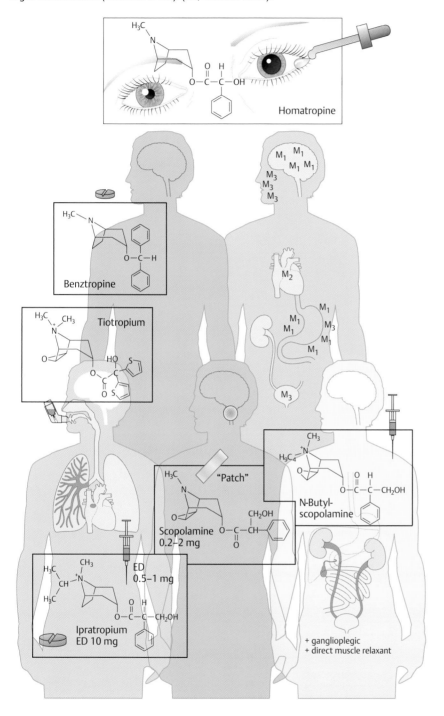

Side effects

— Typical anticholinergic effects are dry mouth, mydriasis (excessive dilation of the pupil), cycloplegia (paralysis of the ciliary muscle of the eye), constipation, difficulty in urination, and decreased sweating. There is little direct effect on blood pressure. Larger doses will increase the heart rate and speed conduction of impulses through the atrioventricular node.
— Very toxic in children

Contraindications

— Glaucoma

Scopolamine

Mechanism of action.   Scopolamine is a competitive antagonist at muscarinic receptors.

Uses

— Motion sickness

Side effects

— Same anticholinergic side effects as atropine but may cause more sedation

Homatropine, Cyclopentolate, and Ipratropium

Mechanism of action.   These agents are synthetic atropine analogues that act as competitive antagonists at muscarinic receptors.

Pharmacokinetics

— Fewer CNS effects than atropine

Uses

— Dry eyes substitutes (homatropine and cyclopentolate)
— Bronchodilation in asthma (ipratropium)

Side effects

— Mydriasis (excessive dilation of the pupil) and cycloplegia (paralysis of the ciliary muscle of the eye)

Benztropine

Mechanism of action.   Benztropine is a competitive antagonist at muscarinic receptors.

Pharmacokinetics

— Stronger CNS effects than atropine but less peripheral action

Uses

— Parkinson disease

Side effects

— Same anticholinergic side effects as atropine

Glycopyrrolate

Mechanism of action.   Glycopyrrolate is a competitive antagonist at muscarinic receptors. It has fewer CNS effects than atropine (as it cannot cross the blood–brain barrier) but similar actions in the PNS, resulting in blockage of vagal inputs to the heart and decreased secretions.

Pharmacokinetics.   Glycopyrrolate is a quaternary ammonium compound that does not cross the blood–brain barrier.

Uses
— Adjunctive agent in anesthesia (to reduce bronchial secretions)

Side effects
— Same anticholinergic side effects as atropine

Table 5.2 summarizes the cholinergic antagonists and their mechanism of action.

Table 5.2 ▶ **Summary of Cholinergic Antagonists**	
Drug(s)	**Mechanism**
Nicotinic antagonists	
Ganglionic blocking agents: Hexamethonium and trimethaphan	These agents block the following receptors: —Nicotinic receptors of pre- and postganglionic parasympathetic ganglia —Nicotinic receptors of preganglionic sympathetic ganglia Note. Not effective at the NMJ
Depolarizing neuromuscular blocker: Succinylcholine	Desensitization of nicotinic receptors at the NMJ
Nondepolarizing neuromuscular blockers: Curare and vecuronium (and all other "curoniums")	Competitive antagonists of ACh at nicotinic receptors of the NMJ
Muscarinic antagonists	
Atropine, scopolamine, homatropine, cyclopentolate, ipratropium, benztropine, and glycopyrrolate	Competitive antagonists of ACh at muscarinic receptors
Abbreviations: ACh, acetylcholine; NMJ, neuromuscular junction.	

■ Botulinus toxin

Botulinus toxin is a neurotoxin produced by *Clostridium botulinum*. It is highly potent and can be lethal in very small amounts. It works by preventing the release of acetylcholine at the neuromuscular junction, thereby causing paralysis of muscles. In its purified form (Botox), this paralysis of muscles is temporary (3 to 4 months) and is used cosmetically to soften the appearance of wrinkles. It is also used therapeutically in the treatment of cervical dystonia (a neuromuscular disorder of the head and neck), severe hyperhydriasis (excessive sweating), achalasia (failure of the lower esophageal sphincter to relax), migraine, and other conditions.

6 Adrenergic Agents

Drugs that mimic or enhance the actions of norepinephrine or epinephrine in adrenergic neurotransmission are termed *sympathomimetics*. These include the endogenous catecholamines, synthetic catecholamines, and directly- and indirectly-acting synthetic sympathomimetic drugs.

Drugs that inhibit adrenergic function are termed *sympatholytics*. These include the adrenergic receptor antagonists and drugs that deplete catecholamines.

6.1 Catecholamine Sympathomimetics

Endogenous Catecholamines

Norepinephrine

Norepinephrine is also discussed on pages 38 and 39.

Mechanism of action.   Norepinephrine stimulates α_1-, α_2-, β_1-, and β_2-adrenergic receptors.

Effects

— Arterioles in the skin and mucosa, as well as splanchnic, renal, and coronary vascular beds, are directly constricted (α_1 and α_2). See **Fig. 6.1**.
— Total peripheral resistance (TPR), diastolic and systolic blood pressure (BP) increase. Increased BP activates baroreceptors to reflexly decrease sympathetic tone and to increase vagal activity.
— The direct effect on β_1-adrenergic receptors of the heart to increase heart rate, force, and velocity of contractions is offset by this reflex vagal slowing of the heart rate (**Fig. 6.2**).
— Glycogenolysis occurs in the liver and skeletal muscle (β_2) and lipolysis occurs in adipose tissue (β_2 and β_2). This is illustrated in **Fig. 6.3**.

> ### Baroreceptor reflex
>
> The baroreceptor reflex allows the body to compensate rapidly for changes in arterial pressure. It is mediated by receptors sensitive to mechanical stretch that are located in the carotid sinuses and in the walls of the aortic arch. The carotid sinus baroreceptors respond to both increases and decreases in arterial pressure; aortic arch baroreceptors only respond to increases in arterial pressure. Decreased arterial pressure causes carotid sinus baroreceptors to experience a reduced amount of stretch. This decreases the rate of action potential firing of the glossopharnygeal nerve (cranial nerve [CN] IX), which innervates the carotid sinus. Impulses from CN IX are then relayed to the vasomotor center in the medulla oblongata, which increases sympathetic outflow. This results in increased heart rate, contractility, and stroke volume. This also results in venoconstriction, which reduces the capacitance of veins thus increasing preload and cardiac output (via the Frank-Starling mechanism) and vasoconstriction of arterioles.

Fig. 6.1 ► **Effects of catecholamines on vascular smooth muscle.**
Differences in signal transduction are responsible for the opposing effects of α- and β-adrenergic receptor activation by epinephrine or norepinephrine. Binding to α_1 causes stimulation of phospholipase C (PLC) and inositol triphosphate (IP_3) and the release of Ca^{2+}. Ca^{2+} and calmodulin then activate the enzyme myosin kinase, which phosphorylates myosin, leading to vasoconstriction. Binding to α_2-adrenergic receptors also activates PLC via different subunits on G proteins. Binding to β_2-adrenergic receptors activates adenylate cyclase, which increases cyclic adenosine monophosphate (cAMP) production intracellularly. Myosin kinase is inhibited by cAMP, leading to vasodilation.

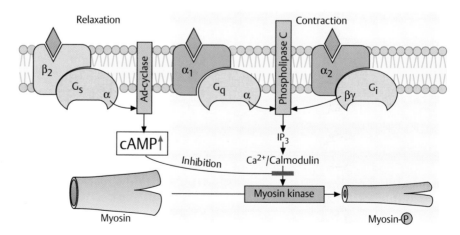

Fig. 6.2 ► **Cardiac effects of catecholamines.**
Stimulation of β receptors in cardiac muscle increases cyclic adenosine monophosphate (cAMP), which then opens "pacemaker" channels. This hastens diastolic depolarization and reduces the threshold for action potential generation, resulting in an increase in conduction velocity, and thus increased heart rate. cAMP also activates protein kinase A, which phosphorylates various Ca^{2+} transport proteins, leading to more Ca^{2+} entering the cell and more Ca^{2+} being released from the sarcoplasmic reticulum. This results in greater contraction of heart muscle. The necessary accompanying increased rate of heart muscle relaxation is caused by the phosphorylation of troponin and phospholamban.

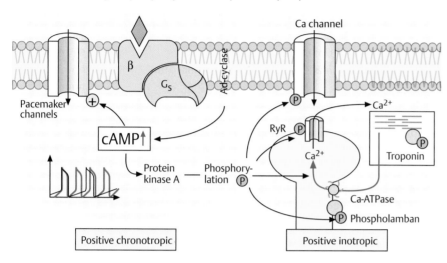

Fig. 6.3 ► **Metabolic effects of catecholamines.**
Stimulation of β receptors increases cyclic adenosine monophosphate (cAMP). This causes glycogenolysis in the liver and skeletal muscle, with glucose being released into the bloodstream. Lipolysis occurs in adipose tissue, causing the hydrolysis of triglycerides to fatty acids (and glycerol). These fatty acids are also released into the bloodstream.

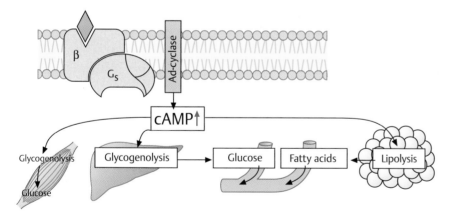

Epinephrine

Epinephrine is also discussed on page 39.

Mechanism of action. Epinephrine stimulates α_1-, α_2-, and β_2-adrenergic receptors (**Fig. 6.4**).

Pharmacokinetics

— Given by intravenous (IV) infusion as it has poor enteral absorbability (**Fig. 6.5**).

Fig. 6.4 ► **Interaction between epinephrine and the β₂-adrenergic receptor.**
Epinephrine and other adrenergic receptor agonists typically share a phenylethylamine structure. The hydroxyl group on the side chain (*pink*) has an affinity to both α and β receptors. Substitution on the amino group (*blue*) decreases the affinity to α but increases the affinity to β receptors. Increasing the bulk of this amino substitute favors the β₂ receptor. Both hydroxyl groups on the aromatic ring (*purple*) also contribute to affinity. If these hydroxyl groups are at positions 3 and 4, the ligand will have a greater affinity to α receptors, but if they are at positions 3 and 5, they will have greater affinity to β receptors.

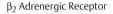

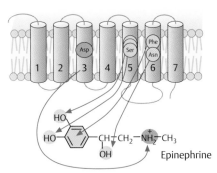

Fig. 6.5 ► **Structure–activity relationship of epinephrine.**
Epinephrine and other catecholamines have poor lipophilicity and so have poor absorbability and penetrability through lipid membranes. This is caused by the hydroxyl group; thus, deletion of one or more of the hydroxyl groups will improve penetrability. Substances without one or more of the aromatic hydroxyl groups will have increased indirect sympathomimetic activity. A change in the position of one or more of the aromatic hydroxyl groups or their substitution prevents inactivation by catechol-*O*-methyltransferase (COMT). Introduction of a small alkyl residue on the carbon atom adjacent to the amino group prevents the breakdown of epinephrine by monoamine oxidase (MAO).

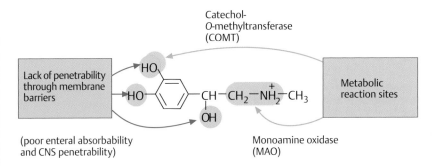

Effects

— With small doses or with slow infusion, vasodilation occurs (skeletal muscle), and diastolic BP decreases (β₂ effect).
— With larger doses, vasoconstriction (skin and splanchnics) occurs, and TPR is increased (α effect). See **Fig. 6.1**.
— The direct effect on β₁ receptors of the heart is the same as for norepinephrine: increased heart rate, force, and velocity of contraction. These effects combine to increase cardiac output. At large doses, it causes reflex vagal slowing of the heart and decreased cardiac output despite direct effects (**Fig. 6.2**).

Uses

— Often added to local anesthetic preparations to produce local vasoconstriction which decreases local bleeding and increases the duration of action of the anesthetic.
— Used clinically to treat anaphylaxis (parenterally) and bronchospasm (subcutaneously) and for minor bleeding (topically).

Dopamine

Dopamine is a precursor in the formation of norepinephrine and epinephrine in the peripheral nervous system.

Mechanism of action. Dopamine acts on dopamine receptors and on α_1- and β_1-adrenergic receptors (**Fig. 6.6**) in the peripheral autonomic nervous system.

Effects
- Increases BP and heart rate (β_1 effect)
- In the CNS, it acts as a neurotransmitter, especially in the extrapyramidal motor system.

Pharmacokinetics
- Given by IV infusion as it is not orally effective

Uses
- Can be given to boost cardiac output in shock or heart failure

Synthetic Catecholamines

Isoproterenol

Mechanism of action. Isoproterenol acts directly on all subtypes of β-adrenergic receptors with no α action.

Effects
- Increases heart rate, force of contraction, and cardiac output with no reflex vagal activation (direct β_1 effects).
- Vasodilation, resulting in decreased diastolic BP and decreased TPR (β_2 effects).

Uses
- Torsades de points (with Mg^{2+}). See call-out box on p. 217.
- Cardiac arrest or complete heart block (rarely)
- Asthma or COPD (rarely)

Fig. 6.6 ▶ **Dopamine as a therapeutic agent.**
Dopamine can be given as an infusion to treat circulatory shock with impaired renal blood flow. In this case, binding to the D_1 receptor causes dilation of the renal and splanchnic arteries, thus increasing renal blood flow and reducing cardiac afterload. At higher doses, dopamine will stimulate β_1 receptors, resulting in cardiac stimulation, and at progressively higher doses, it will also stimulate α_1 receptors. This will produce vasoconstriction, which would be undesirable in this case.

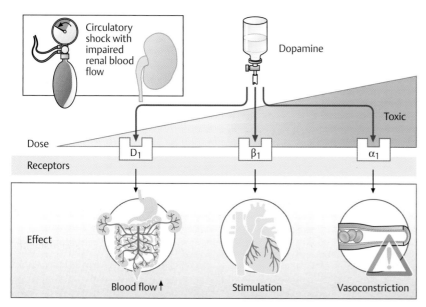

Dobutamine

Mechanism of action. Dobutamine is a direct-acting, selective β$_1$-adrenergic receptor agonist.

Pharmacokinetics

- Given by IV infusion

Effects

- Increases contractility and heart rate (contractility > heart rate)

Uses

- Severe congestive heart failure

6.2 Noncatecholamine Sympathomimetics

Noncatecholamine sympathomimetics may exert effects by direct or indirect actions. Direct sympathomimetics act to stimulate α- or β-adrenergic receptors. Indirect sympathomimetics may release stored norepinephrine from nerve terminals or may block reuptake mechanisms (many do both).

Direct-acting Sympathomimetics

Phenylephrine, Methoxamine, and Metaraminol

Mechanism of action. These agents are direct-acting α-adrenergic receptor agonists.

Effects

- Increases BP

Uses

- These drugs may be used to restore blood pressure during spinal or general anesthesia, in hypotensive emergencies, or after overdose of an antihypertensive medication.
- Nasal decongestant (phenylephrine)

Clonidine

Mechanism of action. Clonidine is a selective α$_2$-agonist (**Fig. 6.7**).

Fig. 6.7 ▶ **Inhibitors of sympathetic tone.**
Clonidine is an α$_2$ agonist that is lipophilic and so is able to penetrate the blood–brain barrier. Stimulation of central α$_2$ receptors suppresses sympathetic impulses in the vasomotor center of the medulla oblongata, resulting in reduced arterial pressure. Methyldopa is an amino acid and as such is able to cross the blood–brain barrier. Methyldopa is decarboxylated in the brain to α-methyldopamine and is then hydroxylated to α-methylnorepinephrine (NE). The decarboxylation step requires dopa decarboxylase; thus reducing the amount of the enzyme available to convert L-dopa to NE.

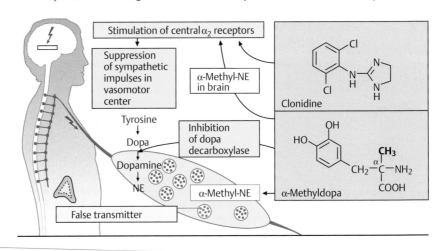

Effects
— Acts in the CNS to decrease sympathetic outflow to periphery

Uses
— Hypertension

Metaproterenol, Terbutaline, and Albuterol

Mechanism of action.   These agents are direct-acting β_2-adrenergic receptor agonists.

Effects
— Bronchodilation
— Minimal cardiac effects

Uses
— Asthma
— Sometimes used to inhibit uterine contractions in premature labor

Mixed-acting Sympathomimetics

Amphetamine, Methamphetamine, and Ephedrine

Mechanism of action.   These agents act as agonists at adrenergic receptors, cause the release of endogenous norepinephrine and inhibit its reuptake.

Pharmacokinetics
— Orally effective

Effects
— Increase BP, heart rate, and contractility
— Bronchodilation
— Mydriasis without cycloplegia
— Nasal decongestion
— Also act as stimulants in the CNS

Uses
— Attention deficit hyperactivity disorder (amphetamine) (see page 123)
— Nasal decongestant (ephedrine, but this was discontinued due to CNS stimulatory actions)
— Drug of abuse (methamphetamine)

Tolerance
— Readily develops to the CNS stimulant effects, appetite suppression, and mood elevation.

Tyramine

Mechanism of action.   Tyramine causes the release of norepinephrine from sympathetic nerve terminals.

Effects
— Increases BP

Uses
— No therapeutic uses

Drug interactions.   Tyramine may precipitate hypertensive crisis when ingested with MAO inhibitors (pp. 87–88).

6.3 Drugs Inhibiting Sympathetic Function (Sympatholytics)

α-Blockers

Phenoxybenzamine and Phentolamine

Mechanism of action.   These agents are antagonists at both α_1 and α_2 receptors.
- Phenoxybenzamine is an irreversible, noncompetitive antagonist.
- Phentolamine is a competitive antagonist.

Effects.   These agents block vasoconstriction caused by sympathetic nerve stimulation or sympathomimetic drugs, producing a fall in BP.

Uses
- Used during treatment of pheochromocytoma to prevent the effects of epinephrine released from tumor

Side effects
- Postural (orthostatic) hypotension, reflex tachycardia, miosis, nasal stuffiness, and inhibited ejaculation

Prazosin, Terazosin, and Doxazosin

Mechanism of action.   These agents are selective blockers of α_1 receptors.

Uses
- Hypertension

Side effects
- Benign prostatic hypertrophy

Note: The first dose may produce a precipitous hypotensive effect.

β-Blockers

Propranolol, Nadolol, and Timolol

Mechanism of action.   These agents are nonselective β-receptor antagonists (block both β_1- and β_2-adrenergic receptors).

Uses
- Hypertension, angina, and cardiac arrhythmias. They are also used to reduce the incidence of myocardial reinfarction (**Fig. 6.8**).
- Glaucoma
- Treatment of the peripheral effects of hyperthyroidism
- Prophylactic agents for migraine headache

Side effects
- Hypotension, bradycardia, increased airway resistance, decreased response to hypoglycemia, and fatigue

Note: Use with caution in patients with heart disease, asthma, or diabetes (may mask the tachycardic sign of hypoglycemia in diabetics taking insulin).

Acebutolol, Atenolol, Esmolol, and Metoprolol

Mechanism of action.   These agents are cardioselective β_1-adrenergic receptor antagonists (50 times more potent for β_1).

Effects.   These agents are designed to have less effect on bronchial smooth muscle than the nonselective agents (**Fig. 6.9**).

Pheochromocytoma

Pheochromocytoma is a rare, benign tumor of the adrenal medulla (90% unilateral) that produces catecholamines. Signs and symptoms include hypertension, cardiomyopathy, weight loss, hyperglycemia, and periods of crisis, lasting ~15 minutes, characterized by fear, headache, palpitations, sweating, nausea, tremor, and pallor. Treatment involves reduction of blood pressure with phenoxybenzamine and propranolol, followed by surgery to remove the tumor.

Fig. 6.8 ► Beta-blockers: effect on cardiac function.
Beta-blockers antagonize epinephrine and norepinephrine at β receptors. They reduce cardiac work to its base ("coasting") level and ensure that it cannot be stimulated above this level. As a consequence of this reduced cardiac work, oxygen consumption in cardiac muscle is reduced. Beta-blockers also reduce heart rate and blood pressure and protect the failing heart against excessive sympathetic stimulation. However, exercise capacity is reduced because the heart cannot respond in the normal way to β_1 stimulation.

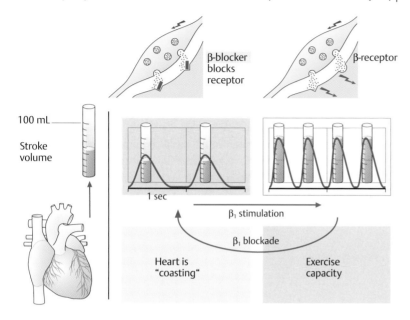

Fig. 6.9 ► Beta-blockers: effect on bronchial and vascular tone.
Beta-blockers cause bronchoconstriction in healthy individuals. In asthmatic patients, β-blockers may cause bronchospasm, leading to acute respiratory distress. Beta-blockers also cause partial vasoconstriction of blood vessels as β_2-mediated vasodilation is blocked, but α-mediated vascular tone is maintained.

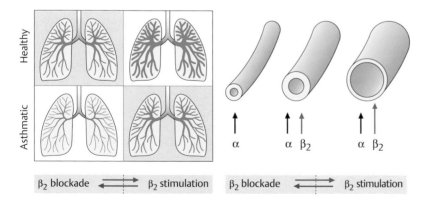

Labetalol

Mechanism of action.   Labetalol is an α_1 antagonist, a nonselective β antagonist, and a weak β_2-adrenergic receptor agonist.

Uses
— Used to treat hypertension and clonidine withdrawal syndrome

Side effects
— Postural (orthostatic) hypotension (α) as well as β side effects listed above

6.4 Drugs that Deplete Catecholamines

Reserpine

Mechanism of action. Reserpine prevents the storage and reuptake of norepinephrine thus causing neuronal depletion of norepinephrine. It also depletes stores of epinephrine, dopamine, and serotonin (**Fig. 6.10**).

Effects. CNS effects include sedation.

Uses
— Hypertension

Guanethidine

Mechanism of action. Guanethidine blocks action potential propagation at fine terminals and acts like reserpine to deplete norepinephrine (**Fig. 6.10**). It must be taken up by nerve endings; thus, the effect is blocked by reuptake inhibitors (tricyclic antidepressants and cocaine).

Uses. Hypertension (rarely used)

Fig. 6.10 ▶ **Inhibitors of sympathetic tone.**
Reserpine prevents norepinephrine (NE) storage and causes the depletion of NE, dopamine, and serotonin by inhibiting a membrane transporter in storage vesicles. Free NE can then be degraded by monoamine oxidase. No epinephrine is released from the adrenal medulla. Guanethidine is taken up by the vesicular amine transporters and stored instead of NE, but it does not function as NE. It also blocks action potentials by stabilizing the axonal membrane. (CNS, central nervous system; DA dopamine; 5HT, 5-hydroxytryptamine.)

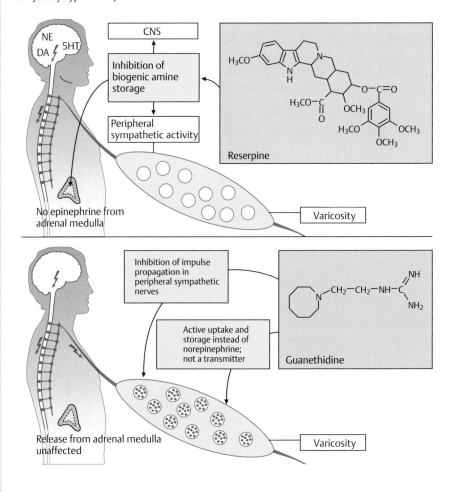

Table 6.1 Summarizes the receptor activation of adrenergic agonists and antagonists.

Table 6.1 ► Interactions of Drugs with Adrenergic Receptors	
Drug	**Receptor Affected**
Agonists	
Norepinephrine	$\alpha_1, \alpha_2, \beta_1, \beta_2$
Epinephrine	$\alpha_1, \alpha_2, \beta_1, \beta_2, \beta_3$
Dopamine	α_1, β_1
Isoproterenol	β_1, β_2
Phenylephrine	α_1
Clonidine	α_2
Albuterol Terbutaline	β_2
Antagonists	
Phentolamine Phenoxybenzamine	α_1, α_2
Propranolol Nadolol Timolol	β_1, β_2
Prazosin	α_1
Yohimbine	α_2
Atenolol Metoprolol	β_1

Review Questions

1. Atropine blocks the action of
   A. dopamine
   B. norepinephrine
   C. serotonin
   D. acetylcholine
   E. histamine

2. Drugs that possess antimuscarinic activity are contraindicated in patients with
   A. glaucoma
   B. diarrhea
   C. hypertension
   D. gout

3. A 52-year-old woman became angry with her spouse and ingested a bottle of pesticide containing parathion, an organophosphate compound. She was brought to the emergency room within 30 minutes. A nasogastric lavage was performed immediately. The patient's symptoms progressed to include miosis, diaphoresis, salivation, lacrimation, defecation, and bronchorrhea. Which of the following drug pairs would comprise part of the treatment for this poisoning episode?
   A. Atropine and pralidoxime
   B. Nitroglycerin and hydrochlorothiazide
   C. Phenylephrine and isoproterenol
   D. Propranolol and theophylline
   E. Tubocurarine and lidocaine

For questions **4** to **8**, refer to the pathway for catecholamine synthesis that follows. **A** to **D** represent the enzymes involved in the steps of that pathway.

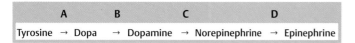

A	B	C	D
Tyrosine → Dopa → Dopamine → Norepinephrine → Epinephrine			

4. Dopa decarboxylase catalyzes which step in the pathway above?

5. Dopamine-β-hydroxylase catalyzes which step in the above pathway?

6. Tyrosine hydroxylase catalyzes which step in the above pathway?

7. Phenylethanolamine-N-methyltransferase (PMNT) catalyzes which step in the above pathway?

8. The rate-limiting step in catecholamine synthesis is:

9. Direct inhibition of norepinephrine release is accomplished via
   A. α_1-adrenergic receptor stimulation
   B. α_2-adrenergic receptor stimulation
   C. β_1-adrenergic receptor stimulation
   D. β_2-adrenergic receptor stimulation

10. Antihypertensive action of clonidine in the central nervous system (CNS) occurs via
    A. activation of α_1-adrenergic receptors
    B. activation of α_2-adrenergic receptors
    C. activation of β_1-adrenergic receptors
    D. activation of β_2-adrenergic receptors
    E. activation of muscarinic receptors

11. Which of the following blocks the blood pressure effects of norepinephrine but does not interfere with the presynaptic actions of norepinephrine to modulate its own release?
    A. Dopamine
    B. Terbutaline
    C. Prazosin
    D. Pindolol

12. A 54-year-old man with benign prostatic hypertrophy is experiencing uncontrollable leakage of small amounts of urine. Drug treatment to reduce prostatic hypertrophy is initiated, but it will take several weeks to alleviate the overflow incontinence. Which of the following agents will act directly in the bladder to decrease outflow obstruction and increase urinary flow rates so that a more rapid therapeutic response may be obtained?
    A. Clonidine
    B. Epinephrine
    C. Doxazosin
    D. Pyridostigmine
    E. Yohimbine

13. An alternative approach to that taken in question 12 may be to activate the postganglionic parasympathetic responses of the bladder. Which of the following drugs would have this effect?
    A. Atropine
    B. Bethanechol
    C. Succinylcholine
    D. Trimethaphan
    E. Tubocurarine

The following information refers to Questions **14** to **17**.

In a dog anesthetized with pentobarbital, recording electrodes are placed on

    I   Carotid sinus baroreceptor nerve fibers

    II Splanchnic (sympathetic) nerve fibers (preganglionic)

    III Inferior cardiac (sympathetic) nerve fibers (postganglionic)

    IV Vagal (parasympathetic) nerve fibers

Answer choices A to E show the changes (if any) in firing rates that would be expected to occur at nerves I to IV following the administration of the <u>last</u> drug in each series of drugs listed in questions 14 to 17. Presume that sufficient time for the actions of the premedicating agents has been allowed and that the last agent is then given intravenously.

	I	II	III	IV
A.	⇔	⇔	⇔	⇔
B.	⇑	⇓	⇓	⇑
C.	⇔	⇓	⇓	⇑
D.	⇓	⇑	⇑	⇓
E.	⇑	⇓	⇔	⇑

Key. ⇑ = increase of nerve activity; ⇓ = decrease nerve activity; ⇔ = no change in neural firing.

14. Propranolol and atropine, then phenylephrine

15. Propranolol, atropine, and reserpine, then phenylephrine

16. Propranolol, atropine, reserpine, and hexamethonium, then phenylephrine

17. Propranolol, atropine, reserpine, hexamethonium, and phenoxybenzamine, then phenylephrine

Answers and Explanations

1.   **D** Atropine is a muscarinic cholinergic receptor antagonist. Of the listed agents, acetylcholine is the only one that is an agonist at cholinergic receptors. Thus, atropine blocks the actions of acetylcholine at the muscarinic subtype of cholinergic receptor (p. 49).
    A. Dopamine is an agonist at dopaminergic receptors.
    B. Norepinephrine is an agonist at adrenergic receptors.
    C. Serotonin is an agonist at serotonin receptors.
    E. Histamine is an agonist at histamine receptors.

2.   **A** Antimuscarinic anticholinergics may worsen glaucoma and are therefore contraindicated in patients with this condition (p. 52).
    B. Antimuscarinic anticholinergics tend to produce constipation, an effect that would be helpful in diarrhea, therefore it is not contraindicated for this condition.
    C and **D**. Antimuscarinic anticholinergics have little or no effect on blood pressure and gout.

3.   **A** Treatment for organophosphate poisoning involves giving atropine to block the muscarinic effects plus pralidoxime to reactivate acetylcholinesterase thereby permitting acetylcholine degradation (p. 48).
    B. Nitroglycerine is a venodilator and hydrochlorothiazide is a thiazide diuretic. Neither are indicated for organophosphate poisoning.
    C. Phenylephrine is a direct-acting α adrenergic receptor agonist. Isoproterenol is a β_1 and β_2 adrenergic receptor agonist. Neither are indicated for organophosphate poisoning.
    D. Propranolol is a nonselective β adrenergic receptor antagonist. Theophylline is a drug used in asthma therapy that acts in many different ways, including being a β receptor agonist. Neither are indicated for organophosphate poisoning.
    E. Tubocurarine is a nondepolarizing neuromuscular nicotinic receptor antagonist. Lidocaine is a local anaesthetic agent.

4.   **B** Dopa decarboxylase catalyzes the conversion of dopa to dopamine (p. 38).

5.   **C** Dopamine-β-hydroxylase catalyzes the conversion of dopamine to norepinephrine (p. 38).

6.   **A** Tyrosine hydroxylase catalyzes the conversion of tyrosine to dopa (p. 38).

7.   **D** Phenylethanolamine-N-methyltransferase (PMNT) catalyzes the conversion of norepinephrine to epinephrine (p. 39).

8.   **A** The rate-limiting step in catecholamine synthesis is conversion of tyrosine to dopa by tyrosine hydroxylase (p. 38).

9.   **B** Activation of α_2 receptors located on presynaptic terminals of sympathetic neurons inhibits the release of norepinephrine (p. 41, table 4.2).
A. Stimulation of α_1-receptors causes vasoconstriction.
C. Stimulation of β_1-receptors increases heart rate, force, and velocity of contraction.
D. Stimulation of β_2- receptors causes brochodilation.

10.   **B** Clonidine is a selective α_2 agonist that acts in the CNS to decrease sympathetic outflow to the periphery. This decreased sympathetic tone leads to decreased blood pressure by lowering total peripheral resistance (p. 58).

11.   **C** Norepinephrine increases blood pressure by activation of α_1 receptors thereby producing vasoconstriction. Its release is regulated by presynaptic α_2 receptors. Prazosin is an α_1-receptor antagonist that blocks the blood pressure effects of norepinephrine but does not interfere with its presynaptic actions (p. 60).
A. Dopamine increases blood pressure by acting on α_1-receptors to produce vasoconstriction.
B. Terbutaline is a β_2 -receptor agonist used as a bronchodilator that produces minimal effects on blood pressure.
D. Pindolol is a nonselective β -adrenergic receptor antagonist.

12.   **C** Urinary outflow is regulated by norepinephrine acting on α_1-adrenergic receptors on the bladder sphincter causing contraction. Doxazosin is an antagonist at α_1-adrenergic receptors and will therefore cause dilation of the bladder sphincter, decreasing outflow obstruction, and increasing urine flow rates (p. 60).
A. Clonidine is a selective α_2 agonist that acts in the CNS to decrease sympathetic outflow to the periphery. This decreased sympathetic tone leads to decreased blood pressure by lowering total peripheral resistance. It does not decrease outflow obstruction and increase urinary flow rates.
B. Epinephrine stimulates α_1, α_2 and β_2 adrenoceptors and so would contribute to the contraction of the bladder sphincter, not lessen it (via α_1 effects).
D. Pyridostigmine is an indirect-acting parasympathomimetic that inhibits acetylcholinesterase, thereby increasing concentrations of acetylcholine, and enhancing cholinergic function. It does not decrease outflow obstruction and increase urinary flow rates.
E. Yohimbine is an α_2-receptor antagonist. It has no important clinical use.

13.   **B** Bethanechol is a direct-acting parasympathomimetic at muscarinic receptors on the bladder sphincter and detrusor muscle. Activation of these receptors will cause relaxation of the sphincter and contraction of the detrusor muscle that expels urine, thus increasing urinary flow (p. 46).
A. Atropine is a muscarinic cholinergic receptor antagonist which would have the opposite effects to bethanechol.
C. Succinylcholine is a nicotinic receptor antagonist at the neuromuscular junction.
D. Trimethaphan blocks nicotinic receptors of both sympathetic and parasympathetic ganglia.

14.   **B** Propranolol is a nonselective β adrenergic receptor antagonist. Atropine is a muscarinic cholinergic receptor antagonist. These agents are given to prevent reflex changes in cardiac output in response to phenylephrine (pages 49 and 60). Phenylephrine will increase blood pressure by direct activation of α_1-adrenerigc receptors. This will increase the baroreceptor firing rate (I) and activate the baroreceptor reflex, leading to decreased sympathetic outflow (II, III) and increased parasympathetic outflow (IV).

15.   **B** The addition of reserpine, which prevents storage and causes depletion of neuronal norepinephrine, will have no effect on the response to phenylephrine, which acts directly on α_1-adrenergic receptors (p. 62).

16.   **E** Hexamethonium is a ganglionic blocking agent that blocks nicotinic receptors of both sympathetic and parasympathetic ganglia, so there will be no change in postganglionic sympathetic nerve activity (p. 48).

17.   **C** Phenoxybenzamine is an irreversible noncompetitive antagonist at both α_1- and α_2-adrenergic receptors. It will thus prevent phenylephrine from having any effect (p. 60).

7 Neuropharmacological Principles

7.1 General Features of Central Neurotransmitters

Most drugs that act on the central nervous system (CNS), except perhaps general anesthetics and ethanol, have specific effects on certain neurotransmitter systems, some of which have been discussed in the previous unit. They can be classified according to their action at a given synapse as excitatory (generally depolarizing), inhibitory (generally hyperpolarizing), or modulatory (conditional). Modulatory actions explain why a given neurotransmitter does not necessarily produce the same effect at all sites; for example, norepinephrine relaxes bronchial smooth muscle but increases contraction of the heart.

7.2 Specific Central Neurotransmitters

This section discusses neurotransmitters that specifically act on the CNS. The effects of these and other CNS neurotransmitters, as well as their receptors, are summarized in **Fig. 7.1**.

Dopamine

Dopamine is also discussed on page 57.

Receptors

There are five types of dopamine receptors located on postsynaptic cells and as autoreceptors on dopamine neurons. Termed D_1 to D_5, these are G-protein coupled receptors (**Fig. 7.2**).

Pathways and Functions

The major relevant functions of dopamine are correlated with the three major dopaminergic tracts in the brain:

— *Nigrostriatal:* Dopamine-containing neurons in the substantia nigra project to the striatum (caudate and putamen). This tract is concerned with initiation and execution of movement. The loss of neurons in the substantia nigra leads to Parkinson disease.
— *Mesolimbic-mesocortical:* Dopamine-containing neurons in the ventral tegmental area project to the amygdala and cortex. These tracts are involved in emotions and the organization of thoughts; they are implicated in schizophrenia and addictive disorders.
— *Tuberoinfundibular:* Dopamine-containing neurons in the arcuate nucleus of the hypothalamus project to the portal vessels of the infundibulum, where dopamine inhibits prolactin secretion. Dopamine receptor antagonists can therefore cause mild hyperprolactinemia.

Norepinephrine

Norepinephrine is also discussed on pages 38, 39, and 54.

Pathways

The largest norepinephrine-containing nucleus in the brain is the locus ceruleus of the caudal pons. Ascending and descending fibers from the locus ceruleus are part of the reticular activating system, which is responsible for behavioral arousal and levels of awareness.

Functions

Norepinephrine may be involved in depression, anxiety, and panic disorders.

■ **Synaptic plasticity**

Neurons are not static, and, in addition to the primary responses to drugs, they undergo several longer-term synaptic changes in response to drugs. These changes may include receptor downregulation, receptor upregulation, and changes in intracellular signal transduction processes. Currently, synaptic plasticity is not exploited as a mechanism of drug action, but it is a definite result of drug use, especially long-term use, and may contribute to the clinical development of tolerance and dependence.

■ **Parkinson disease**

Parkinson disease is a chronic, progressive, age-related neurodegenerative disease resulting from the loss of dopamine-containing neurons in the substantia nigra. Symptoms usually start between 60 and 70 years of age and include a "pill-rolling" tremor, rigidity (limbs resist extension throughout movement), and bradykinesia (slow execution of movement and speech), resulting in a mask-like face and shuffling gait. There are many drug treatment options for Parkinson disease. Levodopa is a dopamine precursor that is converted to dopamine in the brain by dopa decarboxylase. Levodopa is often used in combination with carbidopa, a drug that prevents the peripheral conversion of levodopa to dopamine by inhibiting dopa decarboxylase. Dopamine agonists (e.g., bromocriptine) mimic the effects of dopamine in the brain. Catechol-*O*-methyltransferase (COMT) inhibitors (e.g., entacapone) are used to prevent the peripheral breakdown of levodopa. Monoamine oxidase B (MAO-B) inhibitors (e.g., selegiline) prevent the breakdown of dopamine in the brain. Anticholinergic drugs (e.g., benztropine) may be given as an adjunct for the tremor (see Chapter 14).

Fig. 7.1 ▶ Neurotransmitters in the central nervous system.
Most receptors for neurotransmitters in the CNS are metabotropic (G-protein mediated), and the effects seen are due to differences in ion conductance and signal transduction via second messengers. (ADH, antidiuretic hormone; AMPA, α-amino-3-hydroxy-5-methylisoxazole-4-propionic acid; ATP, adenosine triphosphate; cAMP, cyclic adenosine monophosphate; DAG, diacylglycerol; IP_3, inositol 1,4,5-triphosphate; mGlu, metabotropic glutamic acid; NMDA, N-methyl-D-aspartate; PIP, phosphatidylinositol 4-phosphate; GHIH, growth hormone inhibiting hormone; SRIF, somatotropin release-inhibiting factor.)

Transmitter	Receptor subtypes	Receptor types	Effect — Ion conductance				Effect — Second messenger	
			Na^+	K^+	Ca^{2+}	Cl^-	cAMP	IP_3/DAG
Acetylcholine	Nicotinic	ionotropic	↑	↑	↑			
	Muscarinic: M_1,	metabotropic						↑
	M_2, M_3	metabotropic		↑			↓	
ADH (= vasopressin)	V_1	metabotropic						↑
	V_2	metabotropic					↑	
Dopamine	D_1, D_5	metabotropic					↑	
	D_2	metabotropic		↑	↓		↓	
GABA (= gamma-aminobutyric acid)	$GABA_A$,	ionotropic				↑		
	$GABA_B$	metabotropic		↑	↓		↓	
Glutamate (aspartate)	AMPA	ionotropic	↑	↑				
	Kainic acid	ionotropic	↑	↑				
	NMDA	ionotropic	↑	↑	↑			
	mGlu	metabotropic					↓	↑
Glycine	–	ionotropic				↑		
Histamine	H_1	metabotropic						↑
	H_2	metabotropic					↑	
Norepinephrine, epinephrine	$\alpha_{1(A-D)}$	metabotropic		↑				↑
	$\alpha_{2(A-C)}$	metabotropic		↑	↓		↓	
	β_{1-3}	metabotropic					↑	
Opioid peptides	μ, δ, κ	metabotropic		↑	↓		↓	
Oxytocin	–	metabotropic						↑
Serotonin (5-hydroxytryptamine)	$5\text{-}HT_1$	metabotropic		↓			↓	
	$5\text{-}HT_2$	metabotropic						↑
	$5\text{-}HT_3$	ionotropic	↑	↑				
	$5\text{-}HT_{4-7}$	metabotropic					↑	
Somatostatin (GHIH)	SRIF	metabotropic		↑	↓		↓	
Tachykinin	NK1–3	metabotropic						↑

Amino acids
Catecholamines
Peptides
Others

● = ligand-gated ion channel (ionotropic) receptor
● = G-protein coupled (metabotropic) receptor
↓ = inhibits
↑ = promotes

Fig. 7.2 ▶ **Dopamine release, inactivation, and pharmacological uses.**
Dopamine is released from dopaminergic neurons following an action potential. It then binds to two major types of receptors: D_1-like (subtypes D_1 and D_5), which increase cyclic adenosine monophosphate (cAMP), and D_2-like (subtypes D_2, D_3, and D_4), which decrease cAMP, so the differing effects of dopamine-binding depend on signal transduction. Dopamine's action is terminated by reuptake into neurons, where it is stored in vesicles for reuse, or it is degraded by catechol-O-methyltransferase (COMT) or monoamine oxidase (MAO). D_2 agonists are used to treat Parkinson disease and to inhibit prolactin release, whereas D_2 antagonists are used as antiemetics and in the treatment of schizophrenia.

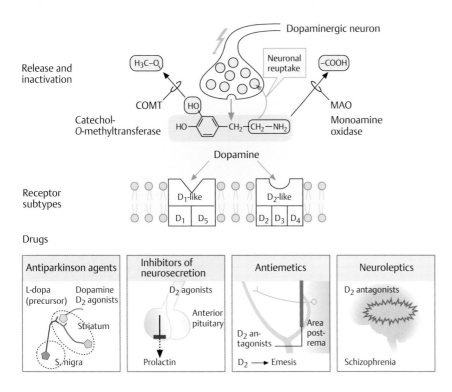

Serotonin

Serotonin (5-hydroxytryptamine [5-HT]) is also discussed on page 340.

Synthesis

Serotonin is synthesized from tryptophan by tryptophan hydroxylase and metabolized by oxidative deamination via monoamine oxidase.

Receptors

Serotonin receptors are located both pre- and postsynaptically. Major groups, 5-HT_1 to 5-HT_7, have been identified, and there are further subtypes. They are all G-protein coupled receptors except 5-HT_3, which is a ligand-gated ion channel.

Pathways

Cell bodies are located in the raphe nuclei of the brainstem. Descending systems innervate all spinal cord levels. Ascending systems innervate the cerebellum, substantia nigra, limbic system, and cortex.

Functions

Ascending systems are involved in the promotion of sleep, in determining mood, and in mental illness (through interactions in limbic areas). Descending 5-HT systems may be involved in modulating pain perception. **Figure 7.3** illustrates some of the actions of serotonin and how various pharmacological agents influence serotonin levels to produce their effects.

Fig. 7.3 ▶ **Serotonin actions as influenced by drugs.**
The effects of serotonin are complex because of the number of receptor subtypes and the differing, and sometimes opposing, effects at each subtype. In blood vessels, for example, serotonin acts on 5-hydroxytryptamine type 2 (5-HT$_2$) receptors to produce vasoconstriction, but it can also act via 5-HT$_{2B}$ receptors to cause the release of vasorelaxant mediators from vascular endothelium, resulting in vasodilation. In the bowel, serotonin acts on 5-HT$_4$ receptors to increase gut motility. Serotonin is involved in many aspects of brain functioning, and as such, many of its central actions are affected by drugs. Serotonin agonists are used to treat migraine and are used recreationally as psychedelic drugs. Fluoxetine, which blocks serotonin reuptake, is used as an antidepressant. Ondansetron, which is an antagonist at the 5-HT$_3$ receptor, is used to treat emesis induced by cytotoxic drugs.

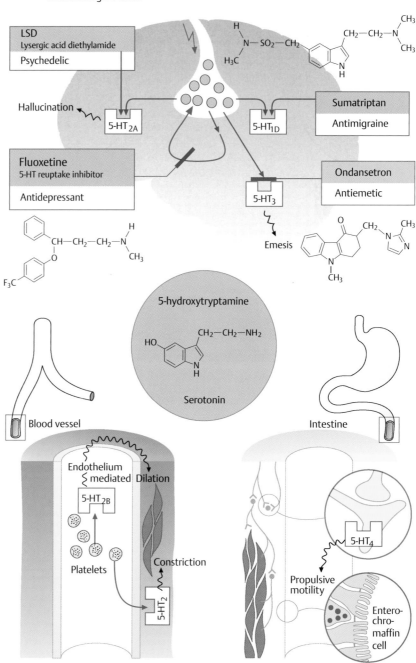

Acetylcholine

This neurotransmitter was discussed in depth on pages 37 and 38 in relation to its action in the peripheral nervous system, but acetylcholine also has an important role as a neurotransmitter in the CNS.

Receptors

Both nicotinic and muscarinic receptors are found in the brain, but 95% of acetylcholine receptors in the brain are muscarinic. Acetylcholine may have excitatory or inhibitory actions in the brain.

Pathways

Acetylcholine neurons are mainly interneurons throughout the cortex.

Functions

The result of loss of cholinergic neurons depends on the site. A global loss throughout the cortex results in senile dementia of the Alzheimer type, degeneration of acetylcholine neurons in the lateral horn of the spinal cord results in amyotrophic lateral sclerosis (ALS), and degeneration of cholinergic and gamma-aminobutyric acid (GABA) neurons in the striatum results in Huntington disease.

Glutamate and Aspartate

Amino acids are the major transmitters in the CNS in terms of percentage of synapses at which they are transmitters.

Synthesis

Glutamate and aspartate are synthesized from glucose and other precursors by several routes (**Fig. 7.4**).

Receptors

Glutamate and aspartate both act on glutamate receptors in the brain. There are two types of glutamate receptors: ionotropic and metabotropic.

Ionotropic Glutamate Receptors.   There are three types of inotropic glutamate receptors; they are classified according to the amino acid that is most potent at that receptor:

— *N*-methyl-ᴅ-aspartate (NMDA)
— α-amino-3-hydroxy-5-methylisoxazole-4-propionic acid (AMPA)
— Kainate

These receptors are said to be excitotoxic, as their prolonged activation increases the entry of cations, including Ca^{2+}, into the cell. High intracellular Ca^{2+} levels trigger a cascade of events leading to neurotoxicity.

Metabotropic Glutamate Receptors.   These are G-protein coupled glutamate receptors.

Pathways

Nearly all of the neuronal pathways delineated thus far for glutamate are corticofugal, that is, from the cortex and hippocampus to other parts of the brain. Antagonists of these receptors are potential antiepileptic agents.

Functions

Glutamate and aspartate are powerful excitatory amino acid transmitters that are eventually neurotoxic.

▬ Huntington disease

Huntington disease is an autosomal dominant neurodegenerative disorder that usually starts in middle age. Its onset is insidious, but the course of the disease progresses with chorea (involuntary, continuous jerky movements), personality change, dementia, and death. There is no cure or any treatment to prevent progression of this disease.

Free GABA can be transaminated by GABA-T to form succinic semialdehyde (only if α-ketoglutarate is the acceptor of the amine group). Succinic semialdehyde is oxidized to succinic acid by succinic semialdehyde dehydrogenase (SSADH) to reenter the Krebs cycle. This transforms α-ketoglutarate into glutamate. GABA can be packaged into synaptic vesicles for release and is picked up by glial cells. GABA-T transaminates to glutamate. Glial cells lack GAD, so glutamate is transformed by glutamine synthetase to glutamine before being transported back to the nerve ending (**Fig. 7.4**). Glutaminase converts glutamine back to glutamate. GABA-T and SSADH are attached to mitochondria. Glutaminase, GAD, and glutamine synthetase are cytoplasmic. GAD occurs only in neurons, glutamine synthesis only in glia, and glutaminase in both.

Fig. 7.4 ▶ Glutamate, glutamine, and gamma-aminobutyric acid (GABA).
Glutamate and GABA are important neurotransmitters synthesized and metabolized in the brain. To regulate their quantity in the extracellular space, glial cells supply glutaminergic and GABAergic neurons with the precursor, glutamine. In glutamate neurons, glutamine is hydrolyzed to glutamate, which is stored in vesicles and released when the nerve is stimulated. In GABA neurons, glutamate is hydrolyzed to glutamate and then converted to GABA. Both types of neurons take up their respective transmitter for reuse. Both transmitters are also taken back up into glial cells, where they are ultimately converted back to glutamine.

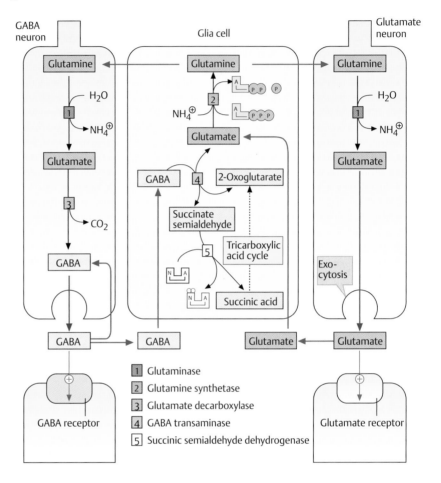

The Krebs cycle (also known as the citric acid cycle/tricarboxylic acid cycle) is one of the metabolic pathways involved in the conversion of carbohydrates, fats, and proteins into carbon dioxide, water, and adenosine triphosphate (ATP) in aerobic organisms. Throughout the cycle, many compounds are produced that are the precursors for other substances needed in the body.

GABA

Synthesis

Glucose is probably the principal in vivo source of GABA. There is a GABA "shunt" of the Krebs cycle whereby α-ketoglutarate is transaminated to glutamic acid by GABA aminotransferase (GABA-T). Glutamic acid is decarboxylated by glutamic acid decarboxylase (GAD) to GABA (**Fig. 7.4**). This process converts glutamate, the principal excitatory neurotransmitter, into the principal inhibitory neurotransmitter, GABA. There is 200 to 1000 times more GABA in the brain than dopamine, norepinephrine, serotonin, or acetylcholine.

Receptors

— $GABA_A$ receptors are postsynaptically located, multisubunit ligand-gated ion channels. Activation leads to opening of the Cl^- channel and synaptic inhibition.
— $GABA_B$ are G-protein coupled receptors located on presynaptic terminals. Activation results in decreased release of GABA and other neurotransmitters from the terminal on which these receptors are located.

Pathways

- GABA is the neurotransmitter of inhibitory interneurons found throughout the cerebral and cerebellar cortices.
- It is also found in neurons projecting from the globus pallidus and substantia nigra to the thalamus and from the striatum to the globus pallidus and substantia nigra.

Functions

GABA accounts for most of the inhibitory action in the CNS. It is also involved in inhibitory motor control in the spinal cord and is thus directly responsible for the regulation of muscle tone. Drugs that enhance GABA-mediated neurotransmission (e.g., benzodiazepines and barbiturates) are used as anxiolytic, sedative, and anticonvulsant drugs.

Glycine

Synthesis

Glycine is formed from serine by the enzyme serine hydroxymethyltransferase.

Pathways

Glycine is released by the inhibitory interneurons that are activated by Ia muscle afferents.

Receptors

Glycine binds to glycine receptors. These receptors can be blocked by strychnine.

Functions

- Inhibitory motor control in the spinal cord

Table 7.1 provides a summary of the CNS neurotransmitters.

Table 7.1 ▶ Summary of Central Neurotransmitters					
CNS Neurotransmitter	Classification	Receptors	Signal Transduction	Functions	Diseases/Disorders
Dopamine	Modulatory	D_1–D_5	G-protein coupled receptors	Initiation and execution of movement Emotions and organization of thought Inhibition of prolactin	Parkinson disease Schizophrenia and affective disorders
Norepinephrine	Modulatory	Adrenergic receptors	G-protein coupled receptors	Behavioral arousal and levels of awareness	Depression, anxiety, and panic disorders
Serotonin	Modulatory	5-HT_1 to 5-HT_7	Most are G-protein coupled receptors 5-HT_3 is a ligand-gated ion channel	Ascending systems: Promotion of sleep, in determining mood and in mental illness Descending 5-HT systems Modulating pain perception	Depression, emesis
Acetylcholine	Modulatory	95% are muscarinic, but there are nicotinic receptors	Muscarinic receptors are G-protein coupled Nicotinic receptors are ligand-gated ion channels	Primarily in interneurons	Alzheimer disease Amyotrophic lateral sclerosis Huntington disease
Glutamate	Excitatory	Ionotropic glutamate receptors Metabotropic glutamate receptors	Ligand-gated ion channels G-protein coupled	Major excitatory neurotransmitter in CNS	Epilepsy, schizophrenia
GABA	Inhibitory	$GABA_A$ $GABA_B$	Ligand-gated ion channels G-protein coupled	Most inhibitory action in the CNS Inhibitory motor control in the spinal cord Regulation of muscle tone	Huntington disease
Glycine	Inhibitory	Glycine receptors	Ligand-gated ion channels	Inhibitory motor control in the spinal cord	

Abbreviations: CNS, central nervous system; GABA, gamma-aminobutyric acid; 5-HT, 5-hydroxytryptamine.

Neuropeptides

Neuropeptide neurotransmitters (comprising 3–100 amino acids) are found in much lower concentrations than amino acid and amine transmitters. They are formed by cleavage of larger molecules and are frequently colocalized with other peptides or with amino acid or amine transmitters. They have no reuptake mechanisms and are generally broken down by peptidases. Neuropeptides are frequently colocalized in, and coreleased from, neurons that also contain one of the smaller molecule neurotransmitters mentioned above.

Table 7.2 lists some common drug-sensitive sites in synaptic transmission. The drugs and the conditions for which they are given are discussed in more detail in the following chapters in this unit.

Table 7.2 ▶ **Drug-sensitive Sites in Synaptic Transmission**		
Site	**Example**	**Therapeutic Use**
Electrically excitable ion channels (includes voltage-dependent Na^+, K^+, and Ca^{2+} channels)	Na^+ channels blocked by local anesthetics	Pain reduction
Chemically regulated ion channels (includes ligand-gated channels that are nicotinic cholinergic, glutamate, and $GABA_A$ receptors)	Benzodiazepines increase Cl^- conductance of the $GABA_A$ receptor	Treatment of anxiety
Presynaptic synthetic pathways	Levodopa to increase dopamine levels	Parkinson disease
Transmitter reuptake mechanisms in neurons and glia	SSRIs	Treatment of depression
Extracellular and glial degradative enzymes	Acetylcholinesterase inhibitors block acetylcholine hydrolysis	Alzheimer disease
G-protein coupled membrane receptors (include norepinephrine, dopamine, serotonin, muscarinic cholinergic, $GABA_B$, and neuropeptide receptors)	Morphine	Pain reduction
Abbreviations: GABA, gamma-aminobutyric acid; SSRI, selective serotonin reuptake inhibitor.		

8 Anesthetic Drugs

Anesthesia is defined as the lack of sensation. The ideal general anesthetic agent would produce unconsciousness, analgesia, amnesia, and muscle relaxation, with no untoward side effects or toxicities (**Fig. 8.1**). Anesthetics developed to date are not ideal and are administered in combination with numerous other preoperative and postoperative medications in order to achieve the desired effects listed above (see **Table 8.1**).

Table 8.1 ▶ Adjuncts to Anesthetics		
Desired Effect	**Drugs Used (Intravenously)**	**Example(s)**
Induction of anesthesia	Ultra short-acting barbiturate	Thiopental, thiamylal, and methohexital
Muscle relaxation	Depolarizing and nondepolarizing neuromuscular blocking agents	Succinylcholine, pancuronium
Analgesia	Short-acting, intravenous opiates	Fentanyl
Amnesia	Short-acting benzodiazepines (doses given are higher than anxiolytic doses)	Diazepam, midazolam, and lorazepam
Autonomic stabilization	Anticholinergic drugs Antiadrenergic drugs	Atropine and glycopyrrolate Esmolol

8.1 Inhalation Agents

The major anesthetic gases include several halogenated hydrocarbons (halothane, isoflurane, enflurane, desflurane, and sevoflurane) and nitrous oxide. These agents act in the brain to produce surgical anesthesia, but the precise mechanism of action for these agents and specific receptors with which these agents interact are not known. The pharmacokinetics of these agents is unique because they are administered as gases and exert their pharmacologic effects when in gaseous form. Thus, the important factor for determining the level of anesthetic effect is the partial pressure or tension of the anesthetic gas. The standard for anesthetic dosing is the minimal alveolar concentration (MAC), which is the alveolar concentration, expressed as a percentage of inspired gas, at which 50% of the patients fail to respond to a noxious stimulus.

Fig. 8.1 ▶ **Goals of surgical anesthesia.**
Commonly used agents as adjuncts to the general anesthetics include drugs that more selectively produce muscle relaxation, analgesia, loss of consciousness, amnesia, and autonomic stabilization.

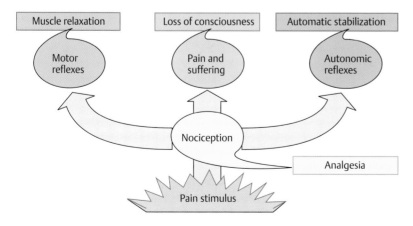

Factors influencing the rate of induction of inhalation anesthesia

Table 8.2 discusses the factors influencing the rate of induction of inhalation anesthesia.

Table 8.2 ► Factors Influencing the Rate of Induction of Inhalation Anesthesia	
Factor	**Explanation**
Concentration of gas in inspired air	The higher the concentration of anesthetic in inspired air, the more rapid the increase in tension of anesthetic in the blood and therefore the brain.
Ventilation rate and depth	Increased ventilation rate and depth lead to an increased rate of induction of anesthesia.
Blood solubility	The solubility of an anesthetic agent in the blood is a very important factor in determining the rate of induction of inhalation anesthesia. The blood:gas partition coefficient is the ratio of the concentration of anesthetic in the blood to the concentration of anesthetic gas at equilibrium. Note that anesthetic molecules that are dissolved in the blood are not exerting a partial pressure and therefore not contributing to anesthesia. Thus, an agent that has high blood solubility will show a slower increase in anesthetic tension and therefore a slower induction rate. Agents that are not soluble in the blood will have a rapid rate of induction.
Blood flow	Uptake of anesthetic into tissues is dependent on blood flow to those tissues, so highly perfused organs will see a more rapid rise in anesthetic tension.
Tissue solubility	In general, anesthetic gases are soluble in fatty tissues; therefore, the rate of rise of anesthetic tension in adipose tissue is slower than in lean tissues, such as the brain.*

* The brain is a lean, well-perfused organ; therefore, the rate of rise of anesthetic tension in the brain is rapid.

Effects

— All of the inhalation agents produce unconsciousness, amnesia, and analgesia. They also decrease blood pressure, depress respiration, and increase intracranial pressure (with the exception of nitrous oxide). The relative analgesic and muscle relaxant effects and side effects are summarized in **Table 8.3.**

— The use of halogenated agents has been associated with rare cases of hyperkalemia and malignant hyperthermia, both of which require aggressive treatment.

▌ Malignant hyperthermia

Malignant hyperthermia is a rare complication of anesthesia with any volatile anesthetic but most commonly with halothane. The anesthetic produces a substantial increase in skeletal muscle oxidative metabolism, which consumes oxygen and causes a buildup of carbon dioxide. The body also loses its capacity to regulate temperature which rises rapidly (e.g., 1°C/5 min). This can lead to circulatory collapse and death. Signs include muscular rigidity with accompanying acidosis, increased oxygen consumption, hypercapnia (increased carbon dioxide), tachycardia, and hyperthermia. Malignant hyperthermia may be treatable if dantrolene, a drug that reduces muscular contraction and the hypermetabolic state, is given promptly. Susceptibility to malignant hyperpyrexia is an autosomal dominant trait.

Table 8.3 ► Summary of Analgesia, Muscle Relaxation, and Side Effects of Inhalation Agents			
Agent	**Analgesia**	**Muscle Relaxation**	**Agent-specific Side Effects**
Halothane	++	+	Sensitizes myocardium to catecholamines increasing possibility of arrhythmias Hepatotoxicity
Enflurane	++	++	May increase seizure activity
Isoflurane	++	++	Decreased blood pressure Respiratory depression
Desflurane	++	++	May cause cough and laryngospasm, as it is an irritant to the upper respiratory tract
Sevoflurane	++	++	None of note
Nitrous oxide	++++	No effect	Contraindicated in cases of occluded middle ear and pneumothorax, as air pockets in the body may expand as larger amounts of nitrous oxide replace nitrogen

Nitrous Oxide

Uses

- Nitrous oxide is a good analgesic (produces superior analgesia than halogenated agents without decreases in blood pressure or depressed respiration).
- It does not produce surgical levels of anesthesia except with very high doses when oxygenation is inadequate. It is therefore not used alone as an anesthetic agent but can be used as the sole agent for analgesia. It is frequently combined with one of the other anesthetic agents.

Side effects

- It is always administered with 30 to 35% oxygen, as it can cause diffusion hypoxia.
- Long-term exposure to trace concentrations may cause pernicious anemia and an increased incidence of spontaneous abortions.

8.2 Intravenous Anesthetic Agents

Propofol

Mechanism of action.   The mechanism of action of propofol is not completely understood, but it enhances gamma-aminobutyric acid (GABA)–mediated neuronal inhibition (via $GABA_A$ receptors), and it also blocks Na^+ channels (**Fig. 8.2**).

Pharmacokinetics

- Given intravenously (IV)
- Metabolized rapidly by the liver
- Rapid induction of anesthesia and recovery

Uses

- General anesthesia

Note: Propofol is a poor analgesic, so it must be supplemented with an opiate.

Side effects

- Hypotension (due to decreased vascular resistance)

Ketamine

This is a "dissociative anesthetic" similar to the street drug phencyclidine (angel dust). Dissociative anesthetics make the patient feel dissociated from the environment.

> **■ Diffusion hypoxia with nitrous oxide**
>
> When nitrous oxide administration is terminated at the end of anesthesia, the concentration of nitrous oxide in the alveoli is lower than the blood. Consequently, it diffuses along this concentration gradient and floods into the lungs, displacing oxygen and nitrogen in the process. This causes a temporary diffusion hypoxia (lack of oxygen). To counteract this, patients are given 100% oxygen until the nitrous oxide is removed from the lungs by expiration.

Uses
— Induction and maintenance of general anesthesia; it is not widely used due to side effects

Effects.   At anesthetic doses, it produces catatonia, analgesia, and amnesia.

Side effects
— Disorientation and hallucinations

Barbiturates

Thiopental, Thiamylal, and Methohexital

Pharmacokinetics
— Unconsciousness occurs within the circulation time from arm to brain and is then maintained with an inhalation agent.
— Termination of CNS action of the barbiturate is by redistribution of drug from the brain to other tissues (**Fig. 8.3**).

Fig. 8.2 ► **Termination of IV anesthetic agent effects by redistribution.**
After an IV anesthetic is given, a high concentration accumulates rapidly in the brain because the brain has a high blood flow compared with other tissues in the body. The drug then redistributes to other tissues, and the concentration in the brain falls. Thus, the effects of the drug (anesthesia) subside before the drug has been eliminated. (CNS, central nervous system.)

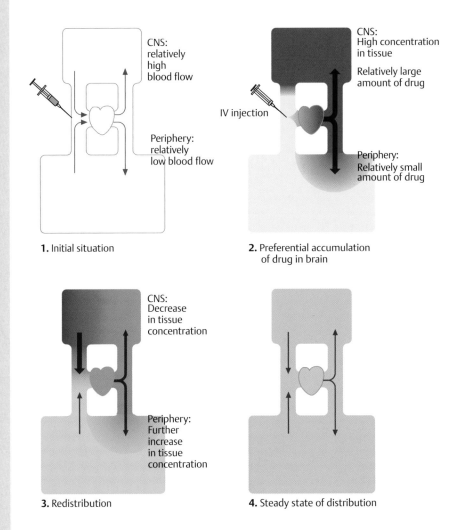

CNS:
relatively
high
blood flow

Periphery:
relatively
low blood flow

1. Initial situation

IV injection

CNS:
High concentration
in tissue

Relatively large
amount of drug

Periphery:
Relatively small
amount of drug

2. Preferential accumulation
of drug in brain

CNS:
Decrease
in tissue
concentration

Periphery:
Further
increase
in tissue
concentration

3. Redistribution

4. Steady state of distribution

Uses
— Induction of anesthesia

Side effects
— Respiratory and cardiovascular depression

Benzodiazepines

These drugs are discussed in detail in Chapter 9.

Diazepam, Midazolam, and Lorazepam

Pharmacokinetics
— Given IV.

Uses. These agents are used as anesthetic premedications to produce sedation and amnesia.

8.3 Local Anesthetics

Local anesthetics act directly on nerve axons to reversibly block nerve conduction. They produce a lack of sensation in the area innervated by those nerve fibers. The methods by which local anesthetics can be administered are outlined in **Table 8.4.**

Table 8.4 ▶ Methods of Local Anesthesia Administration		
Methods of Local Anesthetic Administration	**Technique**	**Clinical Situation**
Topical	Applied to skin or mucous membranes	Typically used prior to injection of anesthetics to make the procedure less painful Also used prior to eye surgery and endoscopy
Infiltration	Inject dilute solution and let diffuse (e.g., subcutaneous or submucosal)	Very common in dentistry to anesthetize most teeth
Nerve block	Inject close to the nerve trunk, proximal to the intended area of anesthesia	Very common in dentistry to anesthetize mandibular teeth Can be useful in cases where pain sensation to a limb needs to be blocked (e.g., following femur fracture)
Spinal	Inject anesthetic in the subarachnoid space	Chronic pain or surgery
Epidural	Inject within the vertebral canal but outside the dura	Very commonly used in labor and delivery

Lidocaine, Articaine, and Bupivacaine (Amides); Benzocaine, Procaine, and Tetracaine (Esters)

Mechanism of action. Local anesthetics exist in two forms in the body: as an uncharged base and as a charged acid. Only the uncharged base can cross nerve membranes. However, once inside the axon, the charged form is active. Local anesthetics interfere with the propagation of action potentials in nerve axons by blocking Na^+ channels from the cytoplasmic side of the channel (**Fig. 8.4**).

■ **Vasoconstrictors in local anesthetics**

Epinephrine is added to local anesthetic solutions to produce vasoconstriction at the site of injection. This decreases systemic absorption and prolongs the duration of action. Epinephrine should be used with caution in patients with cardiac disease, high blood pressure, hyperthyroidism, and other vascular diseases. Epinephrine is absolutely contraindicated in digital or penile blocks and around the nose or ears, as the ischemia produced may lead to gangrene.

■ **Facial palsy with dental injections**

The parotid salivary gland lies laterally to the ramus of the mandible and encloses the five branches of the facial nerve (cranial nerve VII). It is a wedge-shaped structure that wraps around the posterior border of the ramus. If a dentist is inaccurate when giving an inferior alveolar nerve block, some of the local anesthetic may penetrate the capsule of the parotid gland, causing anesthesia of the facial nerve. Symptoms include a drooping mouth and inability to blink on the affected side. The patient's affected eye should be taped closed to prevent drying and contamination with airborne debris until anesthesia subsides and the symptoms resolve.

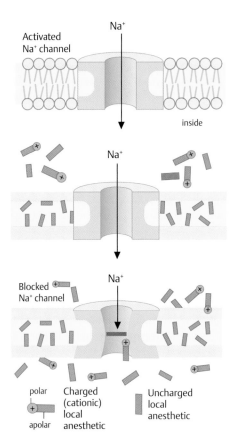

Fig. 8.3 ▶ Effects of local anesthetics.
Local anesthetics block the inner gate of the Na⁺ channels in nerve cells, preventing Na⁺ influx and action potential initiation and propagation. Charged (cationic) local anesthetic is thought to block the sodium channel by becoming incorporated into the phospholipid membrane or channel protein. Uncharged local anesthetic may also become incorporated into the apolar region of the channel protein. (CNS, central nervous system.)

Pharmacokinetics

— Local anesthetics differ mainly in their rate of onset and duration of action (**Table 8.5**).
— Termination of action at the site of injection is by diffusion of the active drug into the systemic circulation followed by metabolism. Ester local anesthetics are inactivated primarily by hydrolysis via esterases in plasma and the liver. Amide local anesthetics are metabolized primarily by the liver.

Table 8.5 ▶ Rate of Onset and Duration of Action of Some Common Local Anesthetic Agents		
Local Anesthetic Agent	**Rate of Onset**	**Duration of Action***
Lidocaine	Rapid	Short
Articaine	Rapid	Intermediate
Bupivacaine	Slow	Long
Procaine	Rapid	Short
Tetracaine	Slow	Long
* The duration of action is prolonged when combined with epinephrine.		

Side effects

The toxic effects of local anesthetics are dependent on the amount of drug that gains entry into the systemic circulation.

— *CNS effects:* These include stimulation, restlessness, and tremor that may lead to clonic convulsions. This is followed by depression and death due to respiratory failure. Direct systemic injection may lead directly to death.

— *Cardiac effects:* Direct effects on the myocardium include decreased electrical excitability, decreased conduction rate, and a negative inotropic effect. Sudden cardiac death may occur.

— *Hypersensitivity:* This is rare, but it can cause dermatitis, asthma attacks, or fatal anaphylactic reactions. Allergy is more frequent with esters.

9 Anxiolytic and Sedative-Hypnotic Drugs

Central nervous system (CNS) depressants are used to relieve anxiety (anxiolytic), to produce sedation (sedative), or to induce sleep (hypnotic). They are also anticonvulsants, centrally acting muscle relaxants, and drugs that produce amnesia. Physical and psychological dependence develops with prolonged use of these agents.

Benzodiazepines

There are many benzodiazepines in use, varying mainly in potency and pharmacokinetics (i.e., onset and duration of action). Depending on these properties, specific agents are used to treat insomnia, anxiety, epilepsy, and for anesthetic induction.

Diazepam, Midazolam, Temazepam, Triazolam, Flurazepam, Clonazepam, Oxazepam, Lorazepam, and Alprazolam

Mechanism of action.   The benzodiazepines potentiate the actions of gamma-aminobutyric acid (GABA) by increasing the flow of Cl^- ions through the $GABA_A$ receptor (**Fig. 9.1**). Many benzodiazepines have active metabolites.

Effects.   Benzodiazepines act almost exclusively in the CNS. The only peripheral effects are coronary vasodilation after certain benzodiazepines are injected intravenously (IV) and neuromuscular block after very high doses.

   Note: Benzodiazepines have a higher therapeutic index than barbiturates. This is because benzodiazepines act by facilitating the effects of endogenous GABA, whereas barbiturates facilitate the effects of endogenous GABA and have direct GABA-like effects, thus producing more CNS depression.

— Diazepam has a direct muscle relaxant effect in addition to CNS actions.
— Alprazolam has an additional antidepressant effect.
— Triazolam may result in rebound anxiety following cessation of administration.

Uses.   **Table 9.1** lists the primary use for each of the benzodiazepine drugs, which is related to their duration of action.

Table 9.1 ▶ Summary of Benzodiazepine Uses		
Benzodiazepine Agent	**Duration of Action**	**Use(s)**
Midazolam	Short	Anesthetic induction
Triazolam		Insomnia
Temazepam	Intermediate	Insomnia
Clonazepam		Anticonvulsant
Oxazepam		Anxiolysis
Lorazepam		Anxiolysis
Alprazolam		Anxiolysis
Diazepam	Long	Anxiolysis
Flurazepam		Insomnia

Side effects
- Incoordination, dizziness, drowsiness, and decreased cognitive function
- Fatal overdose can occur when combined with ethanol.

Flumazenil

Mechanism of action. Flumazenil is a relatively specific competitive antagonist at benzodiazepine receptors.

Uses
- Overdose or poisoning with benzodiazepines

Nonbenzodiazepine Benzodiazepine Receptor Agonists

Eszopiclone, Zaleplon, and Zolpidem

Mechanism of action. These agents are structurally unrelated to the benzodiazepines but bind to a specific subclass of benzodiazepine receptor found in the brain. They have poor muscle-relaxing or anticonvulsant activity.

Uses. They are used exclusively to treat insomnia.

Tolerance, Dependence, and Withdrawal
- Tolerance develops to the effects of these agents.
- Physical dependence can occur.
- Withdrawal symptoms are generally opposite to the effects of the drugs: anxiety, insomnia, and convulsions in severe withdrawal.

Barbiturates

Barbiturates as drugs of abuse are discussed on page 122.

Thiopental, Phenobarbital, Thiomylal, Methohexital, Amobarbital, Pentobarbital, and Secobarbital

Mechanism of action. Barbiturates increase the chloride conductance of the $GABA_A$ receptor by facilitating the action of GABA. They also have direct GABA-like effects (see **Fig. 9.1**).

Pharmacokinetics
- Barbiturates have a low therapeutic index, so overdose (accidental or deliberate) is a problem with these agents (see note in Benzodiazepine section on p. 82). They are also used recreationally.
- These agents induce cytochrome P-450 microsomal enzyme activity, which increases the rate of their own metabolism, as well as other drugs metabolized by this system.
- They also induce δ-aminolevulinic acid (δ-ALA) synthetase, the rate-limiting step in heme biosynthesis. Thus, barbiturates are contraindicated in patients with acute intermittent porphyria, porphyria variegata, or a positive family history of these porphyrias (see callout box on page 27).

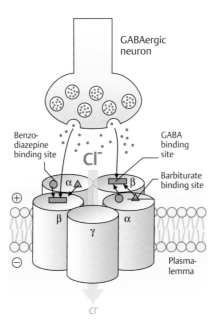

Fig. 9.1 ► **Mechanism of action of benzodiazepines and barbiturates.**
Gamma-aminobutyric acid (GABA) is the main inhibitory neurotransmitter in the central nervous system (CNS). When GABA is released from GABAergic neurons, it binds to the β subunit of the pentameric GABA receptor, leading to opening of the chlorine channel, Cl^- influx, neuronal hyperpolarization, and decreased excitability. Benzodiazepines bind to the α subunits of the $GABA_A$ receptor, enhancing the binding and effects of GABA. Barbiturates also bind to the α subunits of the $GABA_A$ receptor. They increase the length of time that the chlorine channel is open when acted upon by GABA.

Uses

Table 9.2 summarizes the use of each of the barbiturate drugs.

Table 9.2 ► **Summary of Barbiturate Uses**		
Barbiturate Drug	**Duration of Action**	**Use(s)**
Thiopental Methohexital Thiomylal	Ultra-short acting	Anesthetic induction
Amobarbital Pentobarbital Secobarbital	Intermediate*	Insomnia
Phenobarbital	Long	Anticonvulsant
* Intermediate-acting drugs are more prone to abuse.		

Side effects

— Incoordination, dizziness, drowsiness, and decreased cognitive function occur with intensity proportional to potency and dose.
— Fatal overdose may occur by suppression of the neurogenic and hypoxic drive for respiration.

Alcohol

Alcohol is discussed in detail on pages 119–122.

Ethanol

Ethanol is the most widely used sedative-hypnotic.

Mechanism of action.   The mechanism of action is unknown.

Uses.   Used as a solvent, germicide, and for several topical applications.

Other Sedative-Hypnotic and Anxiolytic Drugs

Buspirone

Mechanism of action.   Buspirone is a 5-hydroxytryptamine type 1A (5-HT$_{1A}$) receptor agonist.

Pharmacokinetics.   Buspirone has a selective anxiolytic action with a slow therapeutic onset (action may be delayed up to 2 weeks).

Uses.   Buspirone is used in the treatment of anxiety.
   Note: Buspirone does not potentiate the effects of ethanol or other CNS depressants; thus, it is useful for treating anxiety in alcoholics.

Side effects
— Headache, dizziness, and nervousness

Doxylamine and Diphenhydramine

Mechanism of action.   Doxylamine and diphenhydramine are H$_1$ antihistamines that are able to penetrate into the CNS, causing sedation.

Uses.   Doxylamine and diphenhydramine are used to treat insomnia.

Side effects
— Drowsiness, dry mouth, headache, and increased appetite

Ramelteon

Mechanism of action.   Ramelteon is a melatonin receptor agonist.

Pharmacokinetics.   Metabolized by CYP-1A2 in the liver.

Uses.   Insomnia.

Side effects
— Dizziness, drowsiness, and decreased alertness

Contraindications.   Ramelteon is contraindicated in combination with fluvoxamine, which is a strong CYP-1A2 inhibitor.

10 Antidepressant and Antimanic Drugs

Antidepressant and antimanic drugs are used to treat the affective disorders. These include major depression, mania, and manic depression. These disorders may be bipolar (cycling back and forth between mania and depression) or unipolar (mania or depression only). **Table 10.1** lists symptoms of depression and mania.

Table 10.1 ▶ **Symptoms of Depression and Mania**	
Affective Disorders	**Symptoms**
Depression	Intense sadness and despair; fatigue, musculoskeletal complaints, sleep disorders, feeling of worthlessness, and loss of joy in living
Mania	Abnormally elevated mood, feelings of grandiosity, decreased sleep, increased talkativeness, and increased activity or agitation

Antidepressant drugs block the reuptake of the biogenic monoamines norepinephrine and serotonin. Their selectivity for different uptake mechanisms varies.

10.1 First-generation Antidepressant Drugs

Tricyclic Antidepressants

Amitriptyline, Nortriptyline, Imipramine, and Desipramine

Tricyclic antidepressants are structurally related to phenothiazines (antipsychotic drugs—see page 100) but have different pharmacological effects.

Mechanism of action. These agents block the reuptake of the biogenic monoamines norepinephrine and seratonin. They also interact with many other receptor types, including muscarinic (M_1), histamine (H_1), and adrenergic (α_1) (**Fig. 10.1**).

- Desipramine is the most potent inhibitor of norepinephrine reuptake. It is 1000 times less potent on serotonin reuptake.
- Amitriptyline blocks both norepinephrine and serotonin reuptake equally.
- Tricyclics also block muscarinic, serotonergic, histaminic, and α-adrenergic receptors. These actions are thought to be related to their side effects.

Uses. Depression

Effects

- Acute effects include drowsiness and decreased blood pressure, but with sustained use will cause an elevation of mood
- Suppression of rapid eye movement (REM) sleep
- Sleep promotion

Side effects

- *Anticholinergic:* dry mouth, blurred vision, urinary retention, and constipation
- *Antiadrenergic:* orthostatic hypotension and delayed cardiac conduction
- Weight gain
- Mania, confusion, and delirium

Acute poisoning with tricyclic antidepressants

Accidental and deliberate overdose of tricyclic antidepresssants occurs frequently and constitutes a serious medical emergency that may result in death. Signs may include excitement, seizures, coma with depressed respiration, hypoxia, hypothermia, and hypotension. Anticholinergic effects are also evident. Because no antagonists are available, treatment includes supportive measures in an intensive care unit setting.

Fig. 10.1 ▶ **Antidepressants.**
Activity profiles of selected first-generation antidepressants (tricyclic antidepressants) and third-generation antidepressants (selective serotonin reuptake inhibitors), including the neurotransmitter affected.

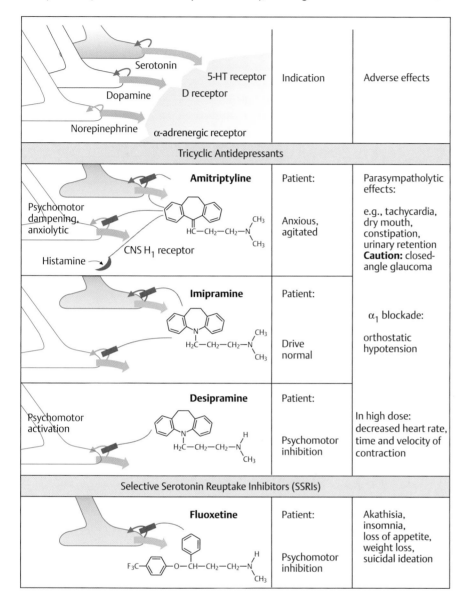

Drug interactions. When tricyclic antidepressants are taken with other drugs, their effects or side effects can be potentiated.

— When they are taken with alcohol, this leads to additive sedation.
— When taken with other anticholinergic drugs, additive anticholinergic effects occur.
— When they are taken with monoamine oxidase inhibitors (MAOIs), severe central nervous system (CNS) toxicity can occur, but this is rare.

Monoamine Oxidase Inhibitors (MAOIs)

Tranylcypromine, Phenelzine, and Isocarboxazid

Mechanism of action. MAOIs inhibit both monoamine oxidase A and B (MAO-A and MAO-B).

Pharmacokinetics

— Phenelzine and isocarboxazid are "suicide" inhibitors of the enzyme. This means that once an MAO molecule binds to one of these drugs, its activity cannot be restored. Restoration of MAO activity depends on synthesis of new enzyme molecules. The exception to this is tranylcypromine, which is reversible.
— MAOIs interfere with hepatic metabolism of many drugs and are not selective for MAO-A or MAO-B.
— The effects of MAOIs take 2 to 3 weeks to become apparent.

Uses. MAOIs are used to treat depression when tricyclic antidepressants are ineffective.

Effects

— Cardiovascular system: postural (orthostatic) hypotension
— Suppression of REM sleep

Side effects

— Hepatotoxicity and CNS stimulation
Note: Acute poisoning causes agitation, hallucinations, hyperreflexia, and convulsions. Treatment is by maintaining vital functions in the hospital setting for approximately 1 week.

Drug interactions

— MAOIs interact with sympathomimetic drugs, leading to hypertensive crisis.
— MAOIs taken with meperidine (an opioid analgesic) can lead to fever, delirium, and hypertension.

10.2 Second-generation Antidepressant Drugs

Second-generation antidepressant drugs were developed in an attempt to eliminate some of the troublesome side effects seen with tricyclic antidepressants, such as cardiac manifestations, orthostatic hypotension, drowsiness, and weight gain.

Bupropion, Mirtazapine, Duloxetine, Amoxapine, Maprotiline, and Trazadone

Mechanism of action. These agents are pharmacologically very similar to tricyclics. They may act as serotonin and norepinephrine reuptake inhibitors.

Uses. Depression

Effects

— *Anticholinergic:* dry mouth, blurred vision, urinary retention, and constipation
— *Antiadrenergic:* postural (orthostatic) hypotension and delayed cardiac conduction
— *Antihistaminergic:* sedation
— Weight gain

Side effects. This generation of antidepressants generally has fewer side effects than tricyclic antidepressants. Exceptions include

— *Bupropion:* seizures and cardiac arrhythmias
— *Amoxapine:* extrapyramidal side effects
— *Maprotiline:* rashes and seizures

Hypertensive crisis with monoamine oxidase inhibitors

Hypertensive crisis may occur within hours of ingestion of tyramine-containing foods, including cheese, certain meats (liver and fermented or cured meats), cured or pickled fish, overripe fruits and vegetables, Chianti wine, and some beers. Hypertensive crisis is characterized by headache, palpitation, neck pain or stiffness, nausea, vomiting, sweating (sometimes with fever or cold, clammy skin), photophobia, tachycardia or bradycardia, constricting chest pain, and dilated pupils. Potentially fatal intracranial bleeding may result from this crisis. Patients should avoid tyramine-containing foods while taking MAOIs and for 2 weeks after treatment with MAOIs is discontinued to avoid precipitating this condition. If hypertensive crisis does occur, then treatment is with intravenous (IV) phentolamine (a non-selective α antagonist agent).

10.3   Third-generation Antidepressant Drugs

Third-generation antidepressants may be safer than tricyclics in overdose situations. Selective serotonin reuptake inhibitors (SSRIs) are not as effective in treating severe depression as first- or second-generation agents.

Fluoxetine, Paroxetine, Sertraline, Fluvoxamine, Citalopram, and Venlafaxine

Mechanisms of action

— Fluoxetine (see also **Fig. 7.3,** page 70), paroxetine, sertraline, and fluvoxamine and citalopram are SSRIs.
— Venlafaxine affects serotonin and norepinephrine reuptake and weakly inhibits dopamine reuptake.

Pharmacokinetics

— Completely absorbed from the gastrointestinal (GI) tract and extensively metabolized in the liver
— Eliminated in the urine and feces
— The therapeutic effect takes 10 to 14 days to develop.
— Long half-life (days)

Uses

— Depression
— Obsessive-compulsive disorder (fuvoxamine and fluoxetine)

Side effects.   Fewer anticholinergic and sedative effects are seen than with tricyclics (they do not interfere with cardiac conduction or cause orthostatic hypotension). Side effects do include the following:

— Headache, tremor, insomnia, diarrhea, and nausea. Diarrhea and nausea diminish or resolve over time.
— They also stimulate the CNS, with agitation the most frequent adverse effect.
— Psychotic reactions may be exacerbated in depressed schizophrenics.
— Liver enzymes are inhibited by fluoxetine and paroxetine but not affected by sertraline.
— Sexual dysfunction and anorgasmia occur in both men and women.
— Generally less weight gain than seen with other classes
— Altered sleep
— Akathisia (a movement disorder charaterized by motor restlessness)

10.4   Antimanic Drug

Lithium Salts

Lithium is an alkali metal ion used to treat mania, manic-depressive illness, and unipolar depression. It has no effects on healthy individuals unless toxic levels are reached. With acute mania, 70 to 80% of patients improve when given lithium.

▮ Serotonin syndrome

Acute intoxication with third-generation antidepressants can cause serotonin syndrome when given with MAOIs. The effects of the syndrome include hyperthermia, rigidity, myoclonus (quick, involuntary muscle jerks), confusion, delirium, and coma.

Mechanism of action.   The mechanism of action for lithium salts is unknown.

Pharmacokinetics

— Completely absorbed from the GI tract
— Eliminated in the urine
— Narrow therapeutic index, so frequent monitoring of serum or urine levels is required to prevent toxicity. This is performed daily during treatment of acute mania.
— There is a lag of 10 to 14 days before treatment becomes effective.

Uses

— Acute mania
— Bipolar manic-depressive illness
— Unipolar depression

Side effects

— Neurologic effects can range from mild side effects such as tremor to muscle twitches or fasciculations, ataxia, and confusion. Severe side effects such as seizures, hallucinations, and delirium may also occur.
— Cardiac effects: flattened or inverted T waves (benign), arrhythmias, and sudden death
— Polydipsia (excessive thirst) and polyuria (excessive urination) are seen, possibly from the inhibition of antidiuretic hormone (ADH) by lithium. This may be disturbing to the patient. Mild polyuria usually occurs early in treatment. Polyuria appearing late may indicate impaired renal function.
— Nephrogenic diabetes insipidus (see p. 189)
— Thyroid enlargement

Note: Acute intoxication is characterized by nausea, vomiting, profuse diarrhea, tremor, coma, and convulsions. Treatment is supportive.

10.5   Obsessive-Compulsive Disorder

Obsessive-compulsive disorder is characterized by obsessive thoughts and compulsive behaviors. Obsessions are unwanted thoughts that run repeatedly through the patient's mind. Compulsions are irresistible urges to perform ritualistic behaviors.

Clomipramine, Fluvoxamine, and Fluoxetine

— Clomipramine is a tricyclic antidepressant agent.
— Fluvoxamine and fluoxetine are SSRIs.

Treatment with these drugs may take up to 10 weeks for a full response. About half of all patients treated with these drugs respond favorably.

11 Anticonvulsant Drugs

11.1 Epilepsy and Seizures

The term *epilepsy* is a collective designation for a group of chronic central nervous system (CNS) disorders characterized by recurrent abnormal discharges of CNS neurons. The abnormal discharge may be limited to a focal area or encompass diffuse areas of the brain. Although the abnormal discharge itself may have no clinical manifestations, such a discharge often leads to a seizure. The epileptic seizure takes many forms, ranging from brief cessations of responsiveness without loss of consciousness to convulsions with accompanying loss of consciousness. **Table 11.1** describes the different seizure types.

Table 11.1 ▶ Types of Seizures

	Seizure Type	Features
Partial seizures (focal, local)	Simple	Motor, somatosensory, autonomic, or psychic symptoms, with loss of consciousness
	Complex	Impaired consciousness at the outset Simple partial seizure followed by impaired consciousness
Generalized seizures (convulsive or nonconvulsive)	Absence Typical	Sudden brief lapses of consciousness with loss of posture
	Atypical	Typical form + brief motor activity or loss of muscle tone
	Myoclonic	Isolated jerking movements
	Clonic	Repetitive jerking movements without muscle rigidity
	Tonic	Muscle rigidity without jerking movements
	Tonic-clonic	Muscle rigidity followed by rhythmic jerking movements
	Atonic	Loss of muscle tone

* Partial seizures can evolve to generalized tonic-clonic.

Misdiagnosis or improper drug selection generally makes epilepsy worse, so it is critical that the correct seizure disorder is identified and that it is treated with the most efficacious drug. If the drug of choice fails to control the seizures, then a follow-up agent is used.

11.2 Antiepileptic Agents

Phenytoin

Mechanism of action. Phenytoin limits the repetitive firing of action potentials in brain neurons by slowing the rate of recovery of voltage-activated Na^+ channels from inactivation (**Fig. 11.1**).

Pharmacokinetics
— Slow, unpredictable absorption
— Ninety percent bound to plasma proteins
— Metabolized in liver to inactive metabolites

Uses
— Effective in all types of epilepsy except absence and atonic seizures
— Trigeminal neuralgia

■ Status epilepticus

Status epilepticus is the term used to describe prolonged seizures (usually lasting 30 minutes or more) or multiple seizures that occur without recovery of consciousness. Status epilepticus constitutes a medical emergency, as the risk of death or brain damage increases the longer the seizures continue. Treatment involves maintaining the patient's airway and giving oxygen, a bolus of glucose (as the brain is a huge consumer of glucose), and intravenous (IV) or rectal diazepam to terminate the seizure. IV diazepam is given in the form of an emulsion to prevent thrombophlebitis (inflammation of a vein due to a blood clot).

Side effects.   Phenytoin is relatively safe, but the following may occur:

— Gingival hyperplasia is the most common side effect in children (20% of patients). Infections are minimized by good oral hygiene.
— CNS: nystagmus, ataxia, vertigo, and diplopia
— Hyperglycemia, osteomalacia, lymphadenopathy, rashes (Stevens-Johnson syndrome [erythema multiforme bullosum]), and hematological reactions (leukopenia, megaloblastic anemia, thrombocytopenia, agranulocytosis, and aplastic anemia). These are allergic reactions that require cessation of therapy.
— Hirsutism
— Fetal abnormalities
— Cardiovascular collapse can occur after IV phenytoin.

Drug interactions

— Metabolism of phenytoin can be increased or decreased by agents that can induce or inhibit cytochrome P-450 enzymes.
— Phenytoin induces hepatic microsomal enzymes; it thus reduces the plasma concentration of drugs that are metabolized by these enzymes, including warfarin, oral contraceptives, carbamazepine, and some antibiotics.
— Drugs that bind to plasma proteins will displace phenytoin, which could result in toxicity.

Carbamazepine

Mechanism of action.   Carbamazepine limits the repetitive firing of action potentials by slowing the rate of recovery of voltage-activated Na^+ channels from inactivation (**Fig. 11.1**).

Fig. 11.1 ▶ **Neuronal sites of action of antiepileptics.**
Antiepileptic drugs act at many neuronal sites to inhibit excitation of the neuron. Gamma-aminobutyric acid (GABA) mimetics enhance the inhibitory effects of GABA at the $GABA_A$ receptor/Cl^- channel. Other antiepileptics block voltage-dependent Na^+ channels, which can inhibit the release of the excitatory neurotransmitter glutamate, or they can act on the neurons themselves to inhibit action potentials. Other drugs block the N-methyl-D-aspartate (NMDA) glutamate receptor or T-type Ca^{2+} channels.

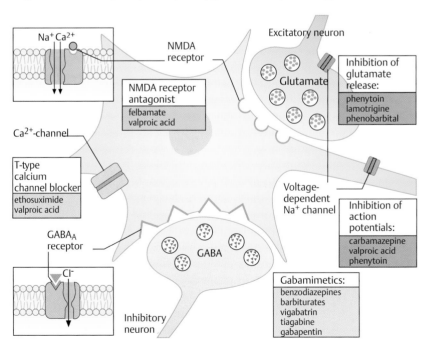

Pharmacokinetics
- Absorption slow and erratic
- Metabolized in liver; may induce hepatic enzymes

Uses
- Generalized tonic-clonic seizures
- Complex partial seizures
- Trigeminal neuralgia

  Note: Carbamazepine is ineffective for absence seizures.

Side effects
- Gastrointestinal (GI) upset
- Vertigo, diplopia, and blurred vision
- Hematological disorders: aplastic anemia, thrombocytopenia (low platelet count), agranulocytosis (failure of bone marrow to produce white blood cells), and leucopenia (low white blood cell count)
- Hypersensitivity

Drug interactions
- Metabolism of carbamazepine can be increased or decreased by agents that can induce or inhibit cytochrome P-450 enzymes.
- Carbamazepine induces hepatic microsomal enzymes; it thus reduces the plasma concentration of drugs that are metabolized by these enzymes, including warfarin, oral contraceptives, and some antibiotics.

Phenobarbital

Mechanism of action.   Phenobarbital is a long-acting barbiturate that potentiates and mimics gamma-aminobutyric acid (GABA; see Chapter 9). It increases the threshold for action potential firing and inhibits the spread of activity from focus (**Fig. 11.1**).

Pharmacokinetics
- Effective orally
- Induces hepatic enzymes

Uses
- Generalized tonic-clonic epilepsy
- Partial seizures
- Prophylaxis or treatment of febrile convulsions

Side effects
- Sedation (tolerance develops)
- Rashes are seen in 1 to 2% of patients. These may be scarlatiniform or morbilliform and are symptomatic of allergic reaction.
- Nystagmus (a rapid, involuntary, oscillatory motion of the eyeball) and ataxia (the inability to coordinate voluntary muscular movement) at excessive doses

  Note: Respiratory depression is not seen with this long-acting barbiturate given orally, but it may be observed after IV injection.

Drug interactions
- Phenobarbital induces hepatic microsomal enzymes; it thus reduces the plasma concentration of drugs that are metabolized by these enzymes including warfarin, oral contraceptives, carbamazepine, and some antibiotics
- Additive effects are seen when phenobarbital is taken with other CNS depressants.
- Valproic acid increases phenobarbital blood levels by inhibiting cytochrome P-450 enzymes.

Febrile convulsions

Febrile seizures (seizures associated with elevated body temperature) are the most common type in children, affecting 2 to 5% between the ages of 6 months and 5 years, with the peak incidence at 18 months. These seizures are not associated with trauma, infection, metabolic disturbances, or a history of seizures, and most last less than 10 minutes. More serious illnesses must be ruled out, but treatment of simple febrile seizures with anticonvulsants is generally not recommended, as the potential drug toxicities associated with these medications outweigh the relatively minor risks associated with the convulsion. There is also no need to specifically cool the child in a cooling bath or to administer an antipyretic drug, e.g., acetaminophen, to reduce the fever. Most febrile convulsions will stop on their own after a few minutes.

Primidone

Mechanism of action.   Mechanism is similar to that of phenobarbital.

Pharmacokinetics.   Primidone is metabolized in the liver to phenobarbital and phenylethylmalonamide (PEMA).

Uses
— Complex partial seizures (primidone is more effective than phenobarbital)
— Generalized tonic-clonic seizures and simple partial seizures
— Frequently combined with phenytoin in refractory cases

Side effects
— Rashes, leukopenia, thrombocytopenia, and systemic lupus erythematosus
— CNS depression

Drug interactions.   Drug interactions are the same as for phenobarbital.

Valproic Acid

Mechanism of action.   Valproic acid increases Na^+ channel inactivation, increases GABA-mediated synaptic inhibition, and inhibits T-type Ca^{2+} channel activation (**Fig. 11.1**). Its anticonvulsant action continues after the drug has been withdrawn.

Pharmacokinetics
— Ninety percent bound to plasma proteins
— Metabolized by the cytochrome P-450 enzymes, but it does not induce these enzymes.

Uses
— Absence seizures, especially of the myoclonic types that are difficult to treat with other drugs. It appears to have an equivalent effect as ethosuximide for absence seizures.
— Combination therapy in the treatment of generalized tonic-clonic seizures and for complex partial seizures

Side effects
— Alopecia (reversible) in 5% of patients
— Transient GI effects in 16% of patients
— CNS: mild behavioral effects, ataxia, and tremor; not a CNS depressant
— Hepatic failure has been reported but is rare.

   Note: Valproic acid should not be used in pregnancy, as it has been shown to be teratogenic in animals.

Drug interactions
— Valproic acid increases blood levels of phenobarbital and primidone by inhibiting their metabolism
— Valproic acid lowers phenytoin levels

Benzodiazepines

Mechanism of action.   Benzodiazepines augment the action of GABA at $GABA_A$ receptors, which are ligand-gated chloride ion channels (**Figs. 9.1** and **11.2**).

Fig. 11.2 ▶ Sites of action of antiepileptics in GABAergic synapse.
Many antiepileptic drugs act on GABA in a number of ways. Some drugs act presynaptically to increase the production of GABA or to reduce its degradation. Others act to inhibit the reuptake of GABA from the synaptic cleft. Progabide mimics the inhibitory effects of GABA at the GABA$_A$ receptor, whereas benzodiazepines act on the GABA$_A$ receptor to enhance the effects of GABA.

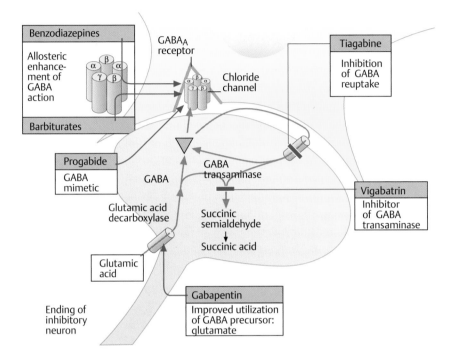

Uses

— Chronic treatment of epilepsy (clonazepam and clorazepate)
— Status epilepticus (lorazepam or diazepam IV)
— Atonic and akinetic seizures, especially as adjuncts
— Absence seizures, but not preferred because of CNS depression

Note: Benzodiazepines do not prevent generalized tonic-clonic seizures

Side effects

— Sedation is the most common side effect.
— Ataxia
— Behavioral problems, such as aggression, anxiety, and restlessness
— Amnesia

Ethosuximide

Mechanism of action.   The mechanism of action for ethosuximide is unknown, but it does enhance CNS inhibition.

Uses.   Ethosuximide is effective only in absence seizures. It is the drug of choice for this condition.

Side effects

— GI irritation: nausea, vomiting, and anorexia (a lack or loss of appetite for food)
— CNS depression: drowsiness, lethargy, euphoria, dizziness, headache, and hiccups
— Rashes: urticaria (hives) and Stevens-Johnson syndrome (rare)
— Blood dyscrasias (an abnormal condition of the blood) (rare)

Gabapentin

Mechanism of action.   The mechanism of action for gabapentin is unknown. Gabapentin is chemically related to GABA but is not an agonist at GABA receptors. It may enhance GABA release (**Fig. 11.2**).

Uses

— Treatment of partial seizures as an adjunctive to other drugs

Side effects

— Sedation, dizziness, ataxia, nystagmus, and tremor

   Note: Gabapentin should be used with caution in children because it may produce adverse psychiatric symptoms, including thought disorders and hostility.

Drug interactions.   This agent does not alter serum concentration of other anticonvulsants.

Felbamate

Uses

— Partial seizures
— Lennox-Gastaut syndrome in children

Side effects

— CNS: insomnia and headache
— GI: anorexia, vomiting, and nausea
— Allergic reactions: hematological and dermatological reactions
— Acute liver failure

Drug interactions.   Felbamate may alter concentrations of other anticonvulsants.

Lamotrigine

Mechanism of action.   Lamotrigine inhibits voltage-dependent Na^+ channels of presynaptic membrane, which decreases the release of excitatory amino acid neurotransmitters.

Uses

— Monotherapy and adjunctive therapy for partial and secondarily generalized tonic-clonic seizures in adults
— Lennox-Gastaut syndrome in both children and adults

Side effects.   Approximately 1 in 1000 people experience severe and potentially life-threatening skin rashes. These are rarely fatal, but children are at higher risk. This can be reduced by slowly increasing the dose.

Topiramate

Mechanisms of action

— Inhibits voltage-dependent Na^+ channels of presynaptic membrane
— Potentiates the action of GABA by a unique mechanism, different from that of the benzodiazepines or barbiturates
— Blocks excitatory amino acid receptors

Uses

— Monotherapy in patients 10 years of age and older with partial onset or primary generalized tonic-clonic seizures
— Adjunctive therapy in partial seizures

■ **Lennox-Gastaut syndrome**

Lennox-Gastaut syndrome is a disorder of childhood characterized by multiple difficult-to-treat seizure types. It is usually accompanied by some form of cognitive impairment. Antiepileptic drugs may control seizures for a time, but tolerance frequently develops.

Side effects

— Mainly involve CNS depression: fatigue, dizziness, ataxia, and decreased cognition
— Hypersensitivity

Tiagabine

Mechanism of action.   Tiagabine is a GABA reuptake inhibitor (**Fig. 11.2**).

Uses

— Adjunctive therapy in partial seizures

Side effects

— Mainly involve CNS depression: fatigue, dizziness, ataxia, and decreased cognition

Levetiracetam

Mechanism of action.   The mechanism of action for levetiracetam is unknown.

Uses

— Adjunctive therapy in partial seizures

Side effects

— Mainly involve CNS depression: fatigue, dizziness, ataxia, and decreased cognition

Zonisamide

Mechanism of action.   Zonisamide prolongs Na^+ channel inactivation and inhibits T-type Ca^{2+} current.

Uses

— Adjunctive therapy in partial seizures

Side effects

— Mainly involve CNS depression: fatigue, dizziness, ataxia, and decreased cognition

Table 11.2 summarizes the drug(s) of choice for each seizure disorder, as well as alternative drugs.

Table 11.2 ► Summary of Antiepileptic Drugs		
Seizure Disorder	**Drug(s) of Choice**	**Alternative Drugs**
Partial, including secondarily generalized	Carbamazepine or phenytoin	Lamotrigine or levetiracetam or topiramate or valproic acid
Typical absence	Ethosuximide	Valproic Acid
Atypical absence	Valproic Acid	Combination of valproic acid and ethosuximide or lamotrigine
Myoclonic	Valproic Acid	Lamotrigine or topiramate
Clonic or tonic	Valproic Acid	Phenytoin
Tonic-clonic	Carbamazepine or phenytoin or valproic acid	Lamotrigine or topiramate
Atonic/akinetic	Valproic Acid	Clonazepam or phenytoin
Recurrent febrile	Diazepam	Phenobarbital
Status epilepticus	Lorazepam or diazepam, followed by phenytoin	Phenytoin or phenobarbital

12 Antipsychotic Drugs

Antipsychotic drugs (neuroleptics) ameliorate the symptoms of psychosis in disorders such as schizophrenia, acute mania, schizoaffective disorders, and borderline personality disorders. In addition, these agents are used as antiemetics and for a variety of other disorders, such as chronic multiple tics, neurogenic pain, Huntington disease (page 71), ballismus, infantile autism, and intractable hiccups. The two major groups of antipsychotic medications are the older typical antipsychotics and the newer atypical agents. They differ in the receptors that they block, the symptoms of schizophrenia that they alleviate, and their side effects.

12.1 Features of Typical and Atypical Antipsychotic Agents

Mechanisms of action

— The primary therapeutic receptor mechanism of action for the typical antipsychotics is thought to be related to their ability to block the D_2 subtype of dopamine receptor on post-synaptic neurons in the dopaminergic pathways in the brain (see page 67). Blockage of D_2 receptors is also implicated in the extrapyrimidal (motor) side effects seen with antipsychotic agents.
— The atypical agents possess $5\text{-}HT_2$ as well as D_2 antagonist properties.
— The atypical antipsychotic aripiprazole is unique in that it is a partial agonist at the D_2 receptor.
— The antipsychotics also block M_1 muscarinic, H_1 histamine, and α_1-adrenergic receptors to varying degrees, which accounts for some of their side effects.

Pharmacokinetics

— Erratic and unpredictable absorption from the gastrointestinal (GI) tract
— Elimination half-life ranges from 20 to 40 hours.
— Very high therapeutic indices
— Flat dose–response cure
— Wide variations in plasma levels occur among individuals.

Effects

— *Neuroleptic*:
  — Spontaneous movement and complex behavior are suppressed, but spinal reflexes remain intact.
  — Reduced initiative, reduced interest in the environment, and reduced displays of emotion or affect.
  — Patients are easily aroused and are capable of answering direct questions; intellectual function remains intact.
  — Psychotic patients become less agitated.
  — Withdrawn patients may become more responsive.
  — Aggression and impulsive behavior are decreased.
  — Hallucinations, delusions, and incoherent thoughts tend to decrease.
— *Extrapyramidal (motor)*:
  — No motor incoordination at usual doses.
  — Spontaneous activity is diminished.
  — Catatonic signs are relieved, or rigidity is induced.
— *Antiemetic*: prevent nausea and vomiting by blocking the effect of emetics that act on D_2 receptors in the chemoreceptor trigger zone (CTZ), an area of the medulla that provides input to the vomiting control center (also in the medulla) to initiate vomiting

Ballismus

Ballismus is a hyperkinetic disorder caused by damage, usually vascular, to the subthalamic nucleus, which is functionally related to the basal ganglia. This ultimately disinhibits neurons in the thalamus leading to excessive activity of the motor cortex. Ballismus is characterized by irregular, flinging movements of the limbs. Treatment, when necessary, involves the use of dopamine-blocking agents (e.g., pimozide, haloperidol, and chlorpromazine), despite the fact that dopamine has not been definitively linked to the disorder.

Extrapyramidal system

The extrapyramidal system (EPS) is the collective name for the neurons, tracts, and pathways that regulate and coordinate movement. Tracts of the EPS mainly originate in the reticular formation of the pons and medulla and receive input from the cortex, basal ganglia, thalamus, and cerebellum. They then act upon cells of the ventral horn of the spinal cord. Because they do not directly innervate motor neurons, the EPS has a modulatory and regulatory function on movement, especially reflexes, postural control, and complex motor functions.

Side effects

- *Extrapyramidal (motor)*:
  - Parkinsonism with bradykinesis, rigidity, and tremor may develop within 1 week to 1 month of initiation of antipsychotic drugs. It is treated with anticholinergics (e.g., benztropine) or amantadine (see pp. 113 and 114).
  - Acute dystonia. This is sustained, often painful muscular spasms in which the patient adopts a twisted posture. It occurs rarely with antipsychotic therapy and is treated with anticholinergic antiparkinsonian agents (e.g., benztropine).
  - Akathisia. This is a strong subjective feeling of distress or discomfort; compelling need to be in constant movement that may start within the first 2 weeks of antipsychotic therapy. It must be distinguished from anxiety or agitation, but if these are ruled out, then the dose of antipsychotic should be lowered or changed
  - Tardive dyskinesia
- *Autonomic nervous system*:
  - Orthostatic (postural) hypotension, impotence, and failure to ejaculate
  - Anticholinergic effects, including dry mouth, blurred vision, nasal stuffiness, urinary retention, palpitations, and toxic-confusional state at high doses
- *Endocrine*:
  - Hyperprolactinemia (increased blood prolactin), which can result in amenorrhea (absence of a menstrual period), galactorrhea (spontaneous flow of milk from the breast, unassociated with lactation following childbirth), infertility, and impotence (inability to develop or maintain an erection)
- *Other*:
  - Sedation
  - Weight gain
  - Agranulocytosis (acute low white blood cell count)
  - Pigmentary degeneration of the retina (rare)
  - Neuroleptic malignant syndrome

Tolerance, dependence, and withdrawal

- Tolerance develops to sedative effects.
- Some signs of dependence may occur.
- Withdrawal may include muscular discomfort and difficulty sleeping.

Drug interactions

- Antipsychotics may potentiate the sedative effects of central depressants and opioid analgesics.
- Antiparkinsonian agents should not be used routinely in combination with antipsychotics, as they potentiate extrapyramidal side effects.

Table 12.1 summarizes of the effects of antipsychotic agents based on the receptors they block.

■ Tardive dyskinesia

Tardive dyskinesia is characterized by involuntary movements and appears only after months or years of treatment with antipsychotic agents. It is less common with atypical agents than typical agents. Stereotypically, the involuntary movements consist of sucking and smacking of the lips, lateral jaw movements, and fly-catching dartings of the tongue. These movements disappear during sleep. Symptoms may persist indefinitely or will sometimes disappear (in weeks to years), especially in younger patients. This condition worsens on withdrawal of antipsychotics and with concomitant use of anticholinergic drugs. There is no adequate drug therapy, so it must be prevented.

■ Neuroleptic malignant syndrome

Neuroleptic malignant syndrome (NMS) is a neurologic disorder that occurs as a result of an idiosyncratic reaction to neuroleptic (antipsychotic) drugs. It usually appears within the first 2 weeks of therapy and presents with fever, muscular rigidity, altered mental status, and autonomic dysfunction (e.g., arrhythmias and fluctuating blood pressure). NMS tends to occur more frequently with typical antipsychotics. The drug management of NMS depends on the symptoms but includes discontinuing the neuroleptic medication, antipyretic drugs (e.g., acetaminophen), dopamine agonists (e.g., bromocriptine), and muscle relaxants (e.g., dantolene sodium). NMS can be fatal, but the prognosis improves with early detection and treatment.

Table 12.1 ▶ Effects of Antipsychotic Agents Based on Receptors Blocked	
Receptor Blocked	**Effects**
5-HT$_2$ receptors in the CNS	Antipsychotic
D$_2$ receptors in the mesolimbic-mesocortical pathway	Antipsychotic
D$_2$ receptors in the nigrostriatal pathway	Extrapyramidal (motor) side effects
D$_2$ receptors in the tuberoinfundibular pathway	Hyperprolactinemia (increased blood prolactin)
D$_2$ receptors in the chemoreceptor trigger zone (CTZ)	Antiemetic
M$_1$ muscarinic	Anticholinergic effects: dry mouth, blurred vision, nasal stuffiness, urinary retention, palpitations
α$_1$-adrenergic	Orthostatic (postural) hypotension, impotence, failure to ejaculate
H$_1$ histamine	Sedation

12.2 Typical Antipsychotics

Phenothiazines

Phenothiazine antipsychotics are divided into 3 chemical classes based on their side chain:

Perphenazine and fluphenazine (piperazine chain)

Uses. These agents are the most potent antipsychotics and antiemetics, but have the highest incidence of extrapyramidal side effects.

Note: typical antipsychotic agents alleviate some of the positive symptoms of schizophrenia (see box "Signs and symptoms of schizophrenia").

Chlorpromazine (aliphatic chain)

Uses

— Chlorpromazine has both antipsychotic and antiemetic efficacy, but adverse effects has made it obsolete in treating schizophrenia.
— Intractable hiccups (drug of choice)

Thioridazine (piperidine chain)

Uses. Thioridazine is the least potent antipsychotic agent and has the lowest incidence of extrapyramidal adverse effects.

Thioxanthenes

Thiothixene

Use. Borderline personality disorders (drug of choice)

Butyrophenones

Haloperidol

Uses. Haloperidol is used extensively, especially for initial stabilization of the psychotic patient.

Side effects. It causes fewer adverse autonomic effects than phenothiazines, however, the induction of tardive dyskinesia and other extrapyramidal adverse effects limits its chronic use.

Pimozide

Uses. This agent prevents the acute exacerbation of chronic schizophrenia and suppresses motor and vocal tics in Tourette syndrome.

Loxapine

Uses. This drug is indicated for the treatment of schizoaffective disorders because its major metabolite, amoxapine, is an antidepressant.

12.3 Atypical Antipsychotics

Clozapine, Olanzapine, Quetiapine, Paliperidone, Risperidone, Ziprasidone, and Aripiprazole

Uses

— Psychotic disorders (olanzapine, quetiapine, paliperidone, risperidone, ziprasidone, aripiprazole). Clozapine is reserved for the treatment of refractory severe psychosis.
— Mania (olanzapine, ziprasidone)

■ Signs and symptoms of schizophrenia

Schizophrenia is characterized by positive, negative, and cognitive signs and symptoms.
Positive: Delusions, hallucinations, agitation, disorganized speech, and disorganized behavior.
Negative: Flattened affect, alogia (lack of unprompted content in normal speech), avolition (lack of drive or motivation), anhedonia (inability to experience pleasure), catatonia, and social isolation.
Cognitive: Disorganized thinking, difficulty concentrating, and memory problems.

— Bipolar disorder (quetiapine, risperidone, aripiprazole)
— Autism (risperidone, aripiprazole)

Note: Atypical antipsychotics improve positive, negative, and cognitive symptoms of schizophrenia.

Side effects

— Atypical agents tend to produce less extrapyramidal reactions and anticholinergic side effects than the typical agents. However, they tend to produce weight gain, leading to type II diabetes and can cause cardiac QT interval prolongation leading to cardiac arrhythmias
— Clozapine may also cause agranulocytosis

Table 12.2 summarizes the differences between typical and atypical antipsychotic drugs.

Table 12.2 ▶ **Prominent Differences Between Typical and Atypical Antipsychotics**						
Antipsychotic Agent	**Receptor Action**	**Symptom Relief in Schizophrenia**	**Extrapyramidal System (EPS) Side Effects (Motor Disorders)**	**Metabolic Disturbances (Weight Gain, Diabetes, Lipid Abnormalities)**	**Agranulocytosis**	**QT Interval Prolongation**
Typical	Primarily D_2 antagonists	Decrease positive symptoms	Greater tendency for EPS side effects	None	None	None
Atypical	5-HT_{2A} and D_2 antagonists	Decrease positive and negative symptoms; improve cognition	Less tendency for EPS side effects	May produce	May produce	May produce
Abbreviation: 5-HT, 5-hydroxytryptamine.						

13 Opiate Receptor Agonists and Antagonists

Opioids or opiates are a class of drugs with opiumlike properties that interact with a set of specific membrane receptors, the opiate receptors. Opioids are used mainly to treat pain.

Pain Modulation

Pain can be modulated at several sites, from its point of origin through the various synaptic junctions in the pain pathways (**Fig. 13.1**). These pathways may correlate with both the perception of pain and the reaction to that sensation. Opioids act in the spinal cord to decrease the sensation of pain (spinal analgesia) and act at higher centers to both decrease the sensation of pain and increase the patient's ability to tolerate the pain (supraspinal analgesia).

Opiate Receptors

There are three major categories of opiate receptors: μ (mu), δ (delta), and κ (kappa). The actions of opioids in current use are interpreted with regard to their actions at μ, δ, and κ receptors, as shown in **Table 13.1.**

Table 13.1 ► Actions Mediated by Opiate Receptors		
Opiate Receptor	**CNS Location***	**Action**
μ	Dorsal horn of the spinal cord, nucleus of the solitary tract, periaqueductal gray region, thalamus, nucleus accumbens, amygdala, cerebral cortex	Supraspinal analgesia Respiratory depression Euphoria Dependence
κ	Dorsal horn of the spinal cord, periaqueductal gray region, hypothalamus	Spinal analgesia Miosis (pupillary constriction) Sedation
δ	Pontine nucleus, nucleus accumbens, amygdala, cerebral cortex	Involved in affective behaviors (related to feelings or mental state)

* Opiate receptors are also found in the enteric nervous system, placenta, vas deferens, and immune system.
Abbreviation: CNS, central nervous system.

13.1 Opiate Agonists

Exogenous Opioid Agonists

Morphine and Related Compounds

Morphine is the standard for comparison among opioids. Many semisynthetic compounds are made by modifying the morphine molecule.

— Diacetylmorphine (heroin) is made by acetylation at the three and six carbon positions.
— Hydromorphone, oxymorphone, oxycodone, and hydrocodone are also made by altering the morphine molecule.

Mechanisms of action

— Morphine and related compounds act at all opiate receptors, but with the highest affinity at μ receptors. Activation of μ receptors decreases the spontaneous activity of neurons in the gut and in the central nervous system (CNS).

Fig. 13.1 ► Pain mechanisms and pathways.
Nociceptors detect painful stimuli and relay nociceptive impulses via Aδ fibers and C fibers to the brain. Impulses that are conveyed to specific areas of the postcentral gyrus produce short, sharp, well-localized pain, whereas impulses conveyed to more than one area of the cortex are perceived as dull, poorly localized pain. Drugs can act at multiple levels of the pain pathway to produce analgesia or alter the perception of pain.

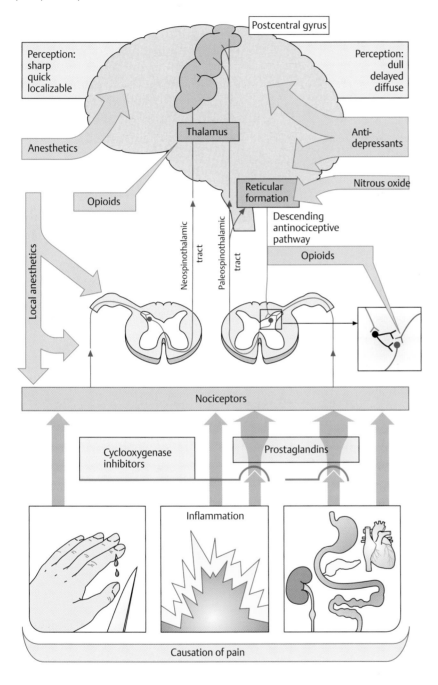

Pain pathways

Pain is transmitted from the periphery by Aδ fibers, activated by noxious heat and mechanical stimuli, and by C fibers, which respond to intense mechanical, chemical, and thermal stimuli. The cell bodies of these nerve fibers are in the dorsal root ganglion. Centrally, they innervate cells in the dorsal horn of the cord. Most of the axons from these cells cross and relay this information to the brain in the spinothalamic tracts. Most of these fibers synapse below the level of the thalamus, but some do go on to the thalamus. The impulses are then relayed to the limbic system and cortex. There are also descending fibers involved in pain, mainly serotonergic fibers from the midbrain raphe nuclei.

— Morphine acts on areas known to be involved in respiration, pain perception, mood, and emotion.
— At the cellular level, all three subtypes of opiate receptors couple to G_i and G_o. Activation of these G proteins by opioid-binding to opiate receptors decrease cyclic adenosine monophosphate levels (cAMP), increase K^+ currents, and decrease Ca^{2+} currents. This results in hyperpolarization and decreased release of neurotransmitters (**Fig. 13.2**).
— Morphine selectively inhibits the excitatory inputs to neurons involved in transmitting information about noxious stimuli without changing the responses to other types of stimuli.

Pharmacokinetics

— Morphine is readily absorbed from the gastrointestinal (GI) tract, nasal mucosa, and lungs.
— Bioavailability of oral preparation ranges from 15 to 50% due to first-pass metabolism in the liver.
— Metabolized by glucuronide conjugation (**Fig. 13.3**)
— Excreted as a glucuronide conjugate in the urine
— Diacetylmorphine (heroin) is rapidly deacetylated in the liver to monoacetylmorphine, which is further deacetylated to morphine.

Endogenous opioids: Endorphins, enkephalins, and dynorphins

Endorphins, enkephalins, and dynorphins are endogenous neuropeptide neurotransmitters that are agonists at opiate receptors. Endorphins are found in the pituitary gland, whereas enkephalins and dynorphins are found throughout the nervous system and gut. Endorphins principally cause pain reduction, but they also produce euphoria, cause the release of sex hormones, and modulate appetite. The release of endorphins during prolonged/strenuous exercise results in the sense of euphoria and well-being accompanying exercise ("runner's high"). Enkephalins and dynorphins are also involved in the regulation and modulation of pain.

Fig. 13.2 ► **Actions of endogenous and exogenous opioids at opiate receptors.**
Endogenous opioids are all cleaved from the precursor peptides proenkephalin, pro-opiomelanocortin, and prodynorphin. Endogenous and exogenous opioids reduce neuronal excitability by increasing K^+ permeability leading to hyperpolarization of the neuronal membrane. Ca^{2+} influx into nerve terminals during excitation is also reduced causing decreased release of transmitter substances and decreased synaptic activity. Stimulant or depressant effects then occur depending on the transmitters and receptors affected.

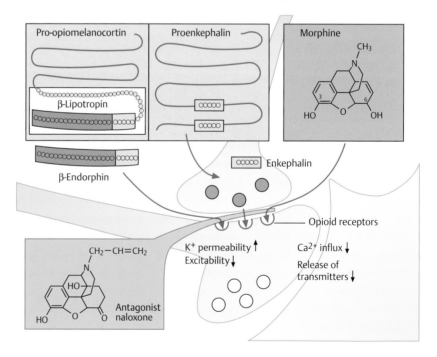

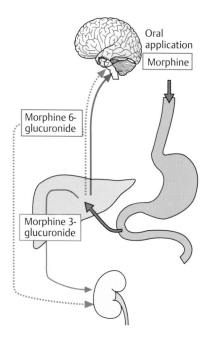

Fig. 13.3 ▶ **Metabolism of morphine.**
Morphine has a free hydroxyl group and is conjugated to glucuronic acid in the liver and excreted renally.

Effects

The effects of opioids are summarized in **Table 13.2.**

Table 13.2 ▶ **Effects of Morphine**		
System	**Effects**	**Explanation/Comment**
CNS	Analgesia without loss of consciousness	Opioids are more selective for pain than other CNS drugs Other sensory modalities remain intact
	Respiratory depression	Direct inhibition of 5-HT$_{4A}$ receptors in the rhythm-generating respiratory neurons in the pre–Boetzinger complex of the brainstem
	Miosis	Excitation at the nucleus of the oculomotor nerve. This is pathognomonic of opiate intoxication (so-called pinpoint pupils)
	Euphoria	
	Antitussive (cough suppressant)	Inhibition of central cough reflex
	Nausea and vomiting	Opiates have a direct action on the chemoreceptor trigger zone in the medulla
	Warmth and drowsiness	
	Itchy nose	
Cardiovascular system	Peripheral vasodilation Inhibition of baroreceptor reflexes Orthostatic hypotension	There is little or no direct effect on the heart
GI system	Constipation	Decreased stomach motility, increased tone and nonpropulsive contractions in the small and large intestine, and increased tone of the anal sphincter
	Increased biliary tract pressure	

Abbreviations: CNS, central nervous system; GI, gastrointestinal.

Abnormal pupillary reactions to drugs

Many drugs cause miosis (constriction of the pupils), including opioids, antipsychotics (e.g., haloperidol), and parasympathomimetic cholinergic drugs (e.g., pilocarpine). Likewise, drugs can cause mydriasis (dilation of the pupils), including anticholinergics (e.g., atropine), hallucinogens (e.g., lysergic acid diethylamide [LSD]), cocaine, and some antidepressant drugs.

Uses

- Acute relief of pain (symptomatic treatment only)
- Chronic treatment of pain
- Antitussives
- Useful in diarrhea to produce constipation. Small amounts of opium tincture or paregoric are ingested. This effect is of particular use following ileostomy or colostomy and in diarrhea and dysentery.

Side effects. Nausea, vomiting, mental cloudiness, dysphoria, constipation, and increased biliary pressure.

Drug interactions. Opioid action is potentiated by phenothiazines, monoamine oxidase inhibitors (MAOIs), and tricyclic antidepressants. Some phenothiazines will enhance the sedative effects of morphine while decreasing the analgesic effects.

Tolerance and dependence. They are characteristics of the opioid drugs.

Contraindications

- It may not be advisable to use opioids in patients with head injury, as mental clouding, vomiting, and miosis may interfere with neurologic assessment of the patient.
- Caution must be used in patients with lung disease due to respiratory depression.

Meperidine

- Meperidine is a synthetic opiate.
- Fentanyl is a meperidine analogue 80 times as potent as morphine.
- Sufentanil is a meperidine analogue 6000 times as potent as morphine.

Mechanism of action. Meperidine acts in the same way as morphine, that is, as an agonist at opiate receptors.

Pharmacokinetics. Meperidine has better bioavailability than morphine: 50% of absorbed meperidine escapes first-pass metabolism.

Effects

- Analgesia
- May cause CNS excitement at toxic doses (unlike morphine)
- Respiratory depression
- Cardiovascular: postural (orthostatic) hypotension but no significant effects
- Smooth muscle: spasmogenic like morphine, but less intense in relation to its analgesia

  Note: Meperidine does not have antitussive or constipating actions.

Uses

- Analgesia

Side effects. The side effects are the same as for morphine, except there is less constipation. The metabolite normeperidine accumulates with repeated dosing. Normeperidine is not an analgesic, but it produces CNS excitation.

Drug interactions. Meperidine may react with MAOIs, causing excitation, delirium, hyperpyrexia, convulsions, and severe respiratory depression.

Methadone and Levo-α-acetylmethadol (LAAM)

Mechanism of action. These agents are synthetic, long-acting opiate agonists with similar pharmacological effects as morphine.

Pharmacokinetics

— Long half-life (1–1.5 days)

Uses

— Analgesia (equally as potent as morphine)
— Treatment of opioid withdrawal symptoms

Side effects

— Constipation and biliary spasm

Propoxyphene (Darvon)

Mechanism of action. Propoxyphene is an agonist at opiate receptors.

Pharmacokinetics. It is not as potent or effective as codeine, but it does have less potential for dependence.

Uses

— Previously used as an analgesic agent but has recently been removed from the market.

13.2 Mixed Opiate Agonist-Antagonists

Pentazocine

Mechanism of action. Pentazocine is a µ-receptor antagonist and a δ- and κ-receptor agonist.

Effects

— Produces analgesia, sedation, and respiratory depression
— May block the analgesia produced by morphine

Uses

— Primarily used as an analgesic, but not effective against severe pain

Side effects

— Respiratory depression
— May cause confusion and hallucinations

Tolerance, dependence, and withdrawal

— Originally thought to have less potential for abuse and released for general use, but then drug abusers combined pentazocine and tripelennamine as a substitute for heroin. Talwin Nx™ (pentazocine and naloxone) includes naloxone to prevent intravenous (IV) use.
— May precipitate withdrawal symptoms in patients who have been receiving opioids

Buprenorphine

Mechanism of action. Buprenorphine is a partial agonist at µ receptors.

Pharmacokinetics

— Given IM or IV

Uses

— Analgesia

Side effects

— Respiratory depression

13.3   Opiate Antagonists

Naloxone, Naltrexone, and Nalmefene

Mechanism of action.   These antagonists bind with high affinity to all opiate receptors but have highest affinity for μ receptors. They act as competitive inhibitors.

Pharmacokinetics
— Naloxone and nalmefene are only effective IV, with nalmefene having a longer duration of action (10 hours versus 1 hour for naloxone).
— Naltrexone is effective orally.

Uses
— Naloxone and nalmefene are used to treat opioid poisoning
— Nalrexone has been tested for treating drug and alcohol addictions

Withdrawal.   In patients dependent on opiates, antagonists will induce withdrawal symptoms.

13.4   Related Compounds

Dextromethorphan

Dextromethorphan is an opioid analogue that is available over the counter but has no analgesic or addictive properties.

Mechanism of action
— Unclear, but may involve μ and κ receptors

Uses
— Antitussive

Tramadol

Tramadol is chemically unrelated to opioids.

Mechanism of action.   Tramadol is a weak opiate receptor agonist. It also inhibits norepinephrine and 5-hydroxytryptamine (5-HT) reuptake. It is only partially inhibited by naloxone. It is equal to or less effective than codeine plus aspirin or to codeine plus acetaminophen.

Uses
— Neuropathic pain

Side effects
— Constipation, nausea, vomiting, dizziness, and drowsiness

Ziconotide

Ziconotide is not an opioid.

Mechanism of action.   Ziconotide is a peptide blocker of neuronal N-type Ca^{2+} channels.

Pharmacokinetics
— Given by intrathecal infusion

Uses
— Management of severe chronic pain

■ **Opioid poisoning**

Opioid poisoning may result from clinical use, abuse, or suicide attempt. Symptoms include coma, pinpoint pupils, and depressed respiration. Overdose is frequently accompanied by other drugs, which may confound the diagnosis and treatment. Treatment involves supporting ventilation and administering naloxone intravenously.

Side effects

— Severe psychiatric symptoms, such as hallucinations, paranoia, and delirium. Drunklike reactions also occur (e.g., dizziness, sleepiness, confusion, incoordination, and mental slowness). These symptoms take days or weeks to resolve after discontinuation.
— Bacterial meningitis

Table 13.3 provides a summary of the primary indications for the opioid analgesics.

Table 13.3 ► Primary Indications for Opioid Analgesics	
Opioid	**Indications**
Morphine and related compounds	Acute pain Chronic pain Cough (codeine)* Diarrhea
Meperidine and analogues	Analgesia Regional analgesia (fentanyl) Preanesthetic (fentanyl)
Methadone and LAAM	Opioid withdrawal
Pentazocine	Analgesia for moderate pain
Buprenorphine	Analgesia
Naloxone and nalmefene	Opioid poisoning
Dextromethorphan	Cough*
Tramadol	Neuropathic pain
Ziconotide	Severe chronic pain

* Opioids and related compounds are used for severe cough when nonopioid cough suppressants have failed.
Abbreviation: LAAM, levo-α-acetylmethadol.

14   Treatment of Neurodegenerative Diseases

14.1   Parkinson Disease

Description

Parkinson disease is a chronic, progressive, age-related neurodegenerative disease resulting from loss of dopamine-containing neurons in the substantia nigra (**Fig. 14.1**). This affects the complex release of excitatory and inhibitory neurotransmitters in the basal ganglia and sub-thalamic nucleus which culminates in excessive inhibition of the thalamus. Inhibition of the thalamus suppresses voluntary movement and accounts for the signs and symptoms of Parkinson disease including

— Pill-rolling tremor that is present at rest and that increases with stress
— Bradykinesia (slow initiation of movements) and decrease of spontaneous movements
— Masked facies
— Increased muscle tone and cogwheel rigidity
— Postural disturbances occurring in later phases. (The patient adopts a stooped position and a festinating gait.)
— Lewy body dementia (LBD) in one third of patients

Lewy body dementia

LBD is the second most common form of dementia after Alzheimer disease. It occurs as a result of abnormal proteins (Lewy body proteins) being deposited throughout the cortex of the brain. If this deposition occurs in the substantia nigra, dopamine stores become depleted, resulting in parkinsonian symptoms. LBD manifests with cognitive impairment and increasing difficulty in performing tasks, as well as memory problems and visual hallucinations. There is no cure for this disease, so treatment aims to reduce symptoms by using cholinesterase inhibitors, levodopa, and antipsychotic (neuroleptic) drugs. Dangerous reactions can occur in 50% of patients taking antipsychotic (neuroleptic) drugs.

Fig. 14.1 ► **Parkinson disease.**
In Parkinson disease, there is death of dopaminergic neurons in the substantia nigra. This causes less dopamine to be available to neurons in the striatum. Ultimately, these changes cause excess inhibition of the thalamus (via gamma-aminobutyric acid [GABA]) and are responsible for the symptoms of Parkinson disease. Treatment aims to increase dopamine in neurons.

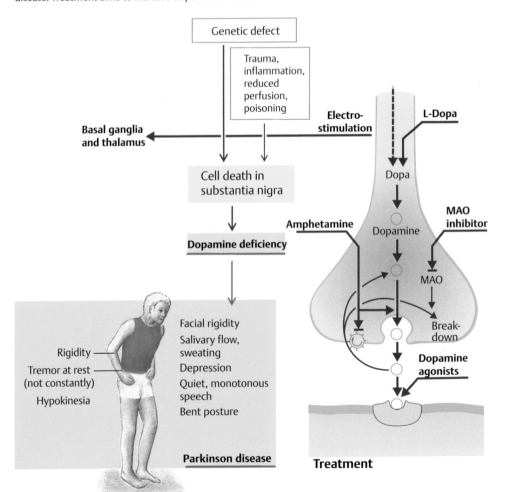

Nigrostriatal Tract and Parkinson Disease

In a normal, healthy person, there is a balance between inhibitory dopamine components and excitatory acetylcholine components in the nigrostriatal tract. In Parkinson disease, however, there is a deficiency of the dopamine component; therefore, the goal of therapy is to restore dopamine levels. Alternatively, you can decrease the acetylcholine component (**Fig. 14.2**).

Antiparkinsonian Drugs

Dopamine cannot be given directly because it is rapidly metabolized in the periphery, has adverse side effects on the cardiovascular system, and very little penetrates the CNS. Strategies to combat the dopamine deficiency include increasing dopamine precursor levels (levodopa), decreasing dopamine breakdown (entacapone, tolcapone, selegiline, and rasagiline), enhancing dopamine release (amantadine), and administering dopamine receptor agonists (bromocriptine, pramepixole, and ropinirole).

Levodopa

Mechanism of action. Levodopa, or L-3,4-dihydroxyphenylalanine (L-dopa), is a precursor in dopamine synthesis. It is formed from L-tyrosine and is transformed to dopamine by aromatic L-amino acid decarboxylase (dopa decarboxylase). Levodopa itself is pharmacologically inert; its effects are a result of decarboxylation to dopamine (**Fig. 14.3**).

Pharmacokinetics

- Levodopa is rapidly absorbed from the intestine by active transport. Administration with meals reduces absorption.
- It has a short plasma half-life of 1 to 3 hours.
- It undergoes peripheral decarboxylation.
- Small amounts enter the central nervous system (CNS).
- It is converted to dihydroxyphenylacetic acid and homovanillic acid and excreted in the urine.

Fig. 14.2 ▶ **Basal ganglia.**
Neurons in the cortex release glutamate, which activates striatal neurons. Neurons within the basal ganglia communicate mainly via the inhibitory neurotransmitter, GABA. Glutamate (an excitatory neurotransmitter) is also released by neurons of the subthalamic nucleus, which acts on neurons in the inner pallidum and substantia nigra to release GABA. GABA is responsible for the inhibitory effect on the thalamus. Dopamine, released from the substantia nigra, may have an excitatory or inhibitory effect on the striatum. Acetylcholine activates striatal neurons.

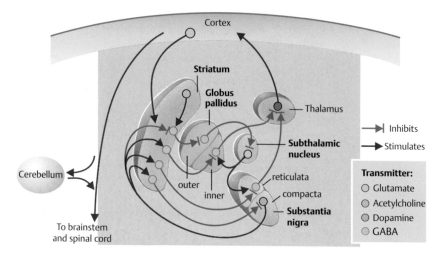

Basal Ganglia

The basal ganglia are made up of the corpus striatum (which is composed of the caudate nucleus and putamen), globus pallidus, subthalamic nucleus, and substantia nigra. It functions to control movement in conjunction with the cerebellum and motor cortex (**Fig. 14.2**).

Control of movements

The pyramidal and extrapyramidal motor systems are involved in the control of movement. The pyramidal system is involved in initiation and termination of movement. Disorders of the pyramidal system are characterized by paralysis and spasticity. The extrapyramidal motor system consists of the basal ganglia (caudate putamen, globus pallidus, subthalamic nuclei, and substantia nigra), with connections to the thalamus, cortex, reticular formation, and spinal cord (**Fig. 14.2**). The extrapyramidal system integrates and coordinates impulses arising in the pyramidal system. Disorders of this system are characterized by dyskinesias.

Effects. **Table 14.1** describes the effects of levodopa.

Table 14.1 ▶ **Effects of Levodopa**	
System	**Effects**
CNS	Relieves bradykinesia and rigidity preferentially over relieving tremor Secondary improvements are seen in posture, gait, ability to modify facial expression, speech, and handwriting. There is no relief of dementia.
Cardiovascular system	Postural (orthostatic) hypotension and cardiac stimulation occur, although tolerance usually develops (mechanism unknown).
Endocrine system	Prolactin secretion is inhibited.* Growth hormone release may also be observed in healthy individuals but not in patients with Parkinson disease.

* Dopamine is a prolactin-inhibiting hormone.
Abbreviation: CNS, central nervous system.

Side effects. **Table 14.2** lists the side effects experienced by most patients who take levodopa.

Table 14.2 ▶ **Side Effects of Levodopa***	
	Side Effects
Short-term	Nausea and vomiting Cardiac arrhythmias
Long-term	Abnormal movements such as tics, grimacing, head bobbing, and oscillatory movements of the limbs are seen in 50% of patients within 2 to 4 months and in 80% of patients by 1 year. No tolerance develops to these effects, and they will worsen if the dose is not reduced. Psychiatric disturbances (serious in 15% of patients): hallucinations, paranoia, mania, insomnia, anxiety, nightmares, and depression False-positive test for ketoacidosis by the dipstick test due to the presence of levodopa metabolites Red-colored urine that changes to black on exposure to air or alkali

* All side effects are seen in the majority of patients. These are reversible and can be controlled by reducing the dose.

Drug interactions

— Pyridoxine, a form of vitamin B_6 found in multivitamins, is a cofactor for dopa decarboxylase and may enhance the metabolism of levodopa.
— Antipsychotics antagonize dopamine receptors and are thus contraindicated with levodopa.
— Reserpine is contraindicated because it depletes dopamine.
— Monoamine oxidase inhibitors (MAOIs) block dopamine breakdown and may exaggerate effects (hypertensive crisis and hyperpyrexia). MAOIs should be withdrawn at least 2 weeks prior to levodopa administration.
— Anticholinergics may slow gastric emptying.

Contraindications.   Care must be exercised in patients with heart disease, cerebrovascular disease, or neurological disease.

Aromatic L-Amino Acid Decarboxylase Inhibitors: Carbidopa and Benserazide

Carbidopa is the only type available in the United States. Benserazide, which is available in Europe and Canada, has similar properties.

Mechanism of action.   These agents inhibit the peripheral production of dopamine from levodopa by inhibiting dopa decarboxylase. This allows more levodopa to be available to the CNS (**Fig. 14.3**).

Uses.   Carbidopa and benserazide are usually administered with levodopa. They confer the following advantages:

— They allow for a dose reduction of levodopa and for a reduced number of doses.
— The effective dose is achieved more rapidly.
— A larger percentage of patients responds favorably.
— Pyridoxine interaction is avoided.

Side effects.   No side effects are seen when these agents are given alone. All side effects are associated with the increased effect of levodopa.

— CNS side effects may appear more frequently or earlier in therapy.
— There are fewer peripheral side effects, such as nausea, vomiting, and cardiac effects.

Entacapone and Tolcapone

Mechanism of action.   Entacapone and tolcapone are selective and reversible inhibitors of catechol-O-methyltransferase (COMT), which is the enzyme responsible for the peripheral breakdown of levodopa. This allows more levodopa to be available in the CNS (**Fig. 14.3**). They act mainly in the periphery.

Uses.   These agents are given as adjunctive therapy to patients experiencing fluctuations in disability related to levodopa and dopa-decarboxylase inhibitor combinations.

Side effects.   These agents do not cause any adverse effects alone, but they enhance the adverse effects of levodopa.

— Acute liver failure may occur with tolcapone.

Drug interactions.   These agents may potentiate the actions of drugs metabolized by COMT (i.e., dopamine, epinephrine, and methyldopa).

Amantadine

Mechanism of action.   Amantadine probably enhances dopamine release in the CNS (**Fig. 14.3**).

Uses

— Used in early stages of parkinsonism or as a supplement to levodopa.

Side effects

— Neurologic: restlessness, irritability, insomnia, and headache at lower doses, progressing to agitation and delirium at higher doses
— Gastrointestinal: nausea and diarrhea

Bromocriptine, Pramipexole, and Ropinirole

Mechanism of action.   These agents are dopamine agonists.

Uses

— Parkinson disease
— Restless leg syndrome (pramipexole and ropinirole)

Side effects

— The same as levodopa

Fig. 14.3 ▶ Antiparkinsonian drugs.
The dopamine precursor levodopa (L-dopa) penetrates the blood–brain barrier (unlike dopamine), where it can directly replenish striatal dopamine levels. Carbidopa inhibits dopa decarboxylase and thus prevents the peripheral production of dopamine that can cause adverse effects (e.g., vomiting). Carbidopa cannot cross the blood–brain barrier; thus, central decarboxylation is unaffected. Bromocriptine is a dopamine agonist in the central nervous system (CNS). Entacapone is a catechol-O-methyltransferase (COMT) inhibitor that prevents the peripheral breakdown of levodopa, allowing more levodopa to be available for the CNS. Benztropine is a muscarinic receptor antagonist that blocks acetylcholine in the striatum and thereby counteracts excessive cholinergic activity that results from dopamine deficiency. Selegiline inhibits the degradation of dopamine by monoamine oxidase type B (MAO$_B$) in the striatum, and amantadine is thought to block central N-methyl-D-aspartate (NMDA) glutamate receptors in the brain, causing a decreased release of acetylcholine in the striatum.

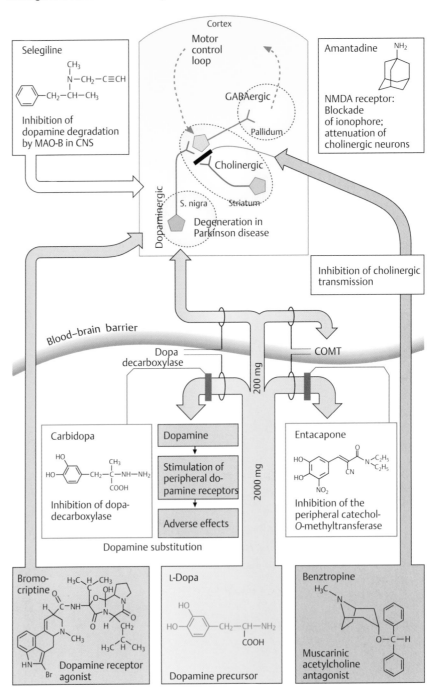

Selegiline and Rasagiline

Mechanism of action.   Selegiline and rasagiline are selective inhibitors of MAO-B, the enzyme involved in dopamine metabolism in the CNS (**Fig. 14.3**).

Side effects.   These agents potentiate the effects of dopamine in the brain but do not potentiate the effects of catecholamines to produce a hypertensive crisis.

Trihexyphenidyl, Benztropine, Procyclidine, and Diphenhydramine

These anticholinergics were the primary agents prior to the introduction of levodopa.

Uses
— Useful in early stages, in patients who are intolerant to levodopa, or as a supplement to levodopa therapy
— More effective in relieving tremor than either rigidity or bradykinesia

Side effects
— Cycloplegia, constipation, and urinary retention
— CNS: confusion, delirium, and hallucinations
— Paralysis of the ciliary muscle of the eye

14.2   Alzheimer disease

Description

Alzheimer disease is a progressive neurodegenerative disorder producing marked atrophy of the cerebral cortex. It is the most common cause of dementia. It produces the following signs and symptoms:

— Impairment of short-term memory
— Impairment of cognition and language
— Increasing difficulty performing the activities of daily living
— Personality changes, e.g., anxiety, depression, aggression, social withdrawal
— Immobility leading to death

Cognitive and memory impairment in Alzheimer disease has been linked to the progressive loss of cholinergic neurons and the subsequent loss of cholinergic transmission within the cerebral cortex. Other neurodegenerative processes may result from damage to neurons due to over-stimulation by glutamate, particularly at N-methyl-D-aspartate (NMDA) receptors.

Alzheimer drugs

Tacrine, Donepezil, Rivastigmine, and Galantamine

Mechanism of action.   These agents are centrally-acting, reversible inhibitors of cholinesterase. They prevent the hydrolysis of ACh thus increasing the concentration of ACh available to neurons.

Uses.   Improves cognition in mild to moderate Alzheimer disease.
Side effects
— Nausea, diarrhea, vomiting.
— Hepatotoxicity (Tacrine only)

Memantine
Mechanism of action.   Memantine is an NMDA receptor antagonist. It protects neurons from damage caused by glutamate.

Uses.   Moderate to severe Alzheimer disease.

Side effects.   Confusion and dizziness

14.3   Spasticity and Muscle Spasms

Spasticity and muscle spasms can result from lesions at various levels of the CNS. Dysfunction in the descending pathways controlling motor neurons results in hyperexcitability of the tonic stretch reflexes. The mechanisms by which drugs can affect skeletal muscle tone are illustrated in **Fig. 14.4.**

Baclofen

Mechanism of action.   Baclofen is a gamma-aminobutyric acid type B ($GABA_B$) receptor antagonist that acts in the spinal cord to hyperpolarize afferent nerve terminals and thus inhibit synaptic transmission.

Uses
— Treatment of spasticity in multiple sclerosis and spinal trauma
— Cerebral palsy (given intrathecally)

   Note: It is not used for stroke.

Side effects
— Sedation, insomnia, dizziness, weakness, and ataxia
— The threshold for seizures is decreased.

Withdrawal
— Causes hallucinations, anxiety, and tachycardia

Fig. 14.4 ▶ **Mechanisms influencing skeletal muscle tone.**
Myotonolytics lower muscle tone by increasing the activity of intraspinal inhibitory neurons. Benzodiazepines augment the action of GABA at $GABA_A$ receptors, which are ligand-gated Cl^- ion channels. Baclofen is an antagonist at $GABA_B$ receptors, which are G-protein coupled. Dantolene acts on muscle cells to reduce Ca^{2+} release from the sarcoplasmic reticulum, causing muscle relaxation. Muscle relaxants themselves also act on muscle cells to cause relaxation. Antiepileptics and antiparkinsonian drugs act centrally to affect muscle tone. These agents are used to treat various spasticity disorders, as well as painful muscle spasms. Convulsants, such as tetanus toxin and strychnine, inhibit glycine, which is an interneuronal synaptic inhibitor. This allows impulses to propagate unchecked along the spinal cord, leading to convulsions.

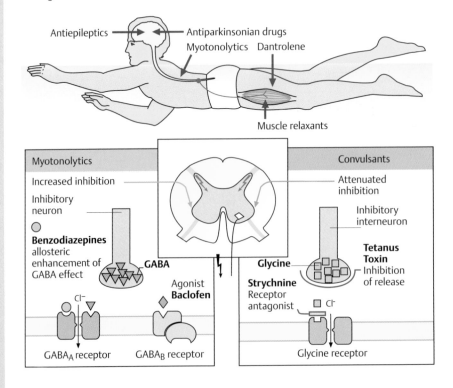

Diazepam

Mechanism of action. Diazepam enhances presynaptic inhibition in the spinal cord.

Uses
- Spinal lesions
- Some cases of cerebral palsy

Dantrolene

Mechanism of action. Dantrolene acts directly on skeletal muscle to apparently decrease Ca^{2+} release from the sarcoplasmic reticulum, thus reducing skeletal muscle contractions (**Fig. 14.5**).

Uses
- Reduces spasticity in paraplegics and hemiplegics
- Cerebral palsy (improvement seen in 50% of cases)

Side effects
- Hepatotoxicity
- Weakness

Fig. 14.5 ▶ Inhibition of neuromuscular transmission and electromechanical coupling.
Acetylcholine (ACh) is released from motor neurons upon stimulation. It then binds to nicotinic receptors in the motor end plate, causing it to depolarize and propagate an action potential to the surrounding sarcolemma. The sarcoplasmic reticulum then releases Ca^{2+}, which causes myofilaments to contract. This electromechanical coupling can be inhibited at different stages. Mg^{2+} and botulinum toxin inhibit acetylcholine release from motor neurons, muscle relaxants inhibit the generation of action potentials, and dantrolene inhibits Ca^{2+} release from the sarcoplasmic reticulum.

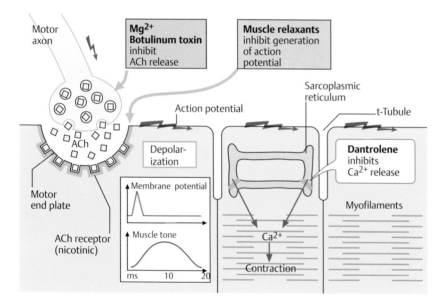

Muscular dystrophy

Muscular dystrophy is a term used to describe a group of inherited muscle diseases. Each individual type of muscular dystrophy has its own genetic defect. The most common type of muscular dystrophy is due to a genetic defect that causes a mutation in dystrophin, part of a protein complex that conveys force from the Z disks to connective tissue on the surface of the fiber. Dystrophin mutations result in degeneration of muscle fibers with increasing muscle weakness. As the disease progresses there will be muscular contractures with loss of mobility of joints. There is no cure for this group of diseases, but drugs are sometimes used to provide symptomatic relief or to slow its progression. Drugs that help with contractures include phenytoin, carbamazepine, and dantrolene. Prednisone, cyclosporin, and azathioprine may also be used to protect muscle cells from damage. Physical therapy is the mainstay of treatment for muscular dystrophy to try to preserve mobility. Surgery may be used for the relief of contractures.

15   Drugs of Abuse

Nonmedical use of drugs includes experimental use, in which a person tries a drug out of curiosity; recreational use, when moderate amounts are used to get "high"; and situational use, when drugs are used in specific circumstances, for example, amphetamines to stay alert. Sometimes these patterns can lead to more frequent use and dependence. Some key terms related to drugs of abuse are defined in **Table 15.1.**

■ Detoxification

Detoxification is the same for all drugs that produce physical dependence. It involves substituting a longer-acting, orally effective, pharmacologically equivalent drug for the abused drug. The patient is stabilized on the substitute, and then it is gradually withdrawn. There is a high recidivism rate among drug abusers. Currently, there are many psychotherapeutic programs after detoxification, but these programs have success rates varying from 10% to perhaps a maximum of 50%.

Table 15.1 ▶ **Definition of Terms**	
Term	**Definition**
Drug abuse	The use, usually by self-administration, of any drug in a manner that deviates from the approved medical or social patterns within a culture.
Drug misuse	Inappropriate use of a drug
Compulsive drug use or compulsive drug abuse	Continued self-administration of a drug despite the fact that the user may be suffering adverse social or medical consequences. In compulsive drug use, the user feels the drug is needed for his or her well-being. There is a continuum of compulsive drug use, from a simple desire to have more drug to a craving and preoccupation with procurement of the drug.
Drug addiction*	According to the World Health Organization, drug addiction is a behavioral pattern of drug use that is characterized by overwhelming involvement with the use of a drug and overwhelming involvement with securing a supply. Along with this, there is a high tendency to relapse after withdrawal. There is some overlap in the definitions of compulsive use and addiction, and it is not always clear when compulsive use becomes addiction.
Tolerance	Decreased responsiveness to a drug with repeated or continued dosing. Cross-tolerance may occur between drugs or between drug classes.
Dependence	Continued use of that drug is required to prevent withdrawal.
Withdrawal	Withdrawal may consist of physical and/or psychological signs and symptoms that occur upon abstinence from a drug.

* There is a difference between addiction and dependence. It is possible for a person to exhibit signs of dependence following withdrawal of a drug, yet not crave the drug.

15.1   Opioids

The pharmacology of these agents is discussed in Chapter 13.

Morphine, Diamorphine (Heroin), Codeine, Meperidine, and Methadone

Effects. The effects of opioids on performance include mental clouding, faulty judgment, and a reduced ability to concentrate. Physical signs of abuse include miosis (pupillary constriction), depression, and apathy.

Tolerance, dependence, and withdrawal. Tolerance, dependence, and withdrawal are characteristic of opioid use.

— Pain relief may be less effective as tolerance develops, even after a single dose. Tolerance develops more slowly to meperidine than morphine.

Opioid withdrawal symptoms are listed in **Table 15.2.**

Table 15.2 ▸ **Opioid Withdrawal Symptoms***	
Early symptoms (10–12 h after withdrawal)	Rhinorrhea (runny nose), perspiration, lacrimation (secretion of tears), and yawning
Intermediate symptoms (18–24 h after withdrawal)	Mydriasism, piloerection, anorexia, and muscular tremors
Peak symptoms (36–72 h after withdrawal)	Restlessness, hot flashes alternating with chills, an increase in both blood pressure and heart rate, an increase in the rate and depth of respiration, fever of 1°C or more, nausea, retching, vomiting, and diarrhea

* Withdrawal from an opioid is generally not life-threatening, although it is almost unbearable. The intensity of the withdrawal symptoms will be in proportion to the amount of drug being used and the duration of the abuse. Withdrawal will be more intense and of a shorter duration after use or abuse of more potent, shorter-acting agents. Likewise, it will be less intense but more prolonged with less potent, longer-acting agents.

15.2 Alcohol

Ethanol Toxicology

Alcohol is rapidly absorbed from the gastrointestinal (GI) tract after oral administration. Its acute effects appear within minutes of ingestion. Ethanol is metabolized in the liver, primarily by alcohol dehydrogenase to acetaldehyde, then by acetaldehyde dehydrogenase to acetate. This metabolism follows zero-order kinetics, which means that a constant amount of ethanol is metabolized per unit of time. The implication of this is that as more ethanol is ingested, the degree of intoxication increases rapidly, as well as the time for the blood level to drop to a nonintoxicating level.

Effects. Effects are listed in **Table 15.3.** See also **Figs. 15.1** and **15.2.**

Table 15.3 ▸ **Effects of Acute and Chronic Intoxication with Ethanol**	
System/Tissue	**Effects**
Acute Intoxication	
CNS	Progressive CNS depression is correlated in time with blood concentrations of ethanol and may include vision and judgment impairments, decreased inhibitions, and muscular incoordination, progressing to staggering gait, slurred speech, and possible coma and death at higher doses.
GI system	Increased salivary and gastric secretions, direct irritation to gastric and buccal mucosa, emesis due to a central effect on the chemoreceptor trigger zone, and irritation of the gastric mucosa. Prolonged use also leads to decreased absorption of folates.
Other	Suppression of antidiuretic hormone (ADH, vasopressin) secretion Increased adrenocorticotropin hormone (ACTH), cortisol, and catecholamine secretion Diuresis due to decreased antidiuretic hormone release Increased consumption of fluids Hypothermia
Chronic Intoxication	
CNS	Wernicke syndrome, Korsakoff psychosis, cerebral atrophy, cerebellar atrophy, and alcoholic polyneuropathy
GI system	Peptic ulcers, esophagitis, gastritis, pancreatitis, and malnutrition
Liver	Steatosis, hepatitis, and cirrhosis (**Figs. 15.1 and 15.2**)
Muscle	Cardiomyopathy and skeletal muscle myopathy
Fetus	Fetal alcohol syndrome
Other	Face puffy, cheeks and nose flushed, eyes bloodshot, palmar erythema, rhinophyma, acne rosacea, and spider nevi

Abbreviations: CNS, central nervous system; GI, gastrointestinal.

▉ Fetal alcohol syndrome

Fetal alcohol syndrome is the term used to describe a spectrum of disorders that can occur in a fetus if a woman drinks alcohol when pregnant. It includes the following: abnormal facial features, growth deficiencies, vision or hearing deficits, and mental disabilities, such as difficulty in learning, memory problems, poor attention span, and poor communication skills.

Fig. 15.1 ▸ **Alcohol catabolism and effects of excess alcohol on the liver.**
In hepatocytes, ethanol is broken down into acetic acid via acetaldehyde. This process utilizes the oxidized form of nicotinamide adenine dinucleotide (NAD⁺), so the requirement for this increases. If alcohol intake is chronic, hepatocytes initially undergo fatty degeneration that is reversible; however, if it continues, cirrhosis occurs as hepatocytes die and are replaced by connective tissue. NADH, the reduced form of nicotinamide adenine dinucleotide.

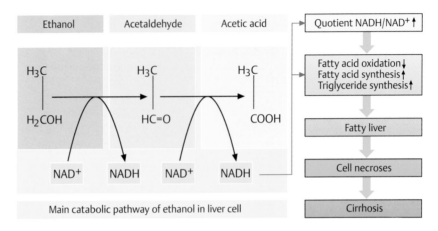

Tolerance, dependence, and withdrawal. Withdrawal symptoms in chronic users of alcohol include tremor, sweating, anxiety, irritability, nausea, vomiting, and insomnia. These symptoms will be mild to moderate in 80 to 85% of patients and more severe in 15 to 20%. Severe withdrawal, known as delirium tremens, is seen in ~1%.

— Benzodiazepines are cross tolerant with alcohol and will alleviate withdrawal symptoms, but they do not have the same stimulating effects on the central nervous system (CNS) as alcohol.
— For serious complications or delirium tremens, replace fluids and electrolytes and treat symptoms. Treat arrhythmias with lidocaine or procainamide, severe tremor with propranolol, and hallucinations and paranoia with a phenothiazine or haloperidol.

Delirium tremens

Delirium tremens is a disorder that occurs as a result of alcohol withdrawal (onset ~72 h after the last drink). Signs include increased pulse, reduced blood pressure, tremors, fits and visual or tactile hallucinations. Treatment is with diazepam.

Fig. 15.2 ▸ **Liver cirrhosis.**
Liver cirrhosis occurs when hepatocytes die and are replaced by connective tissue. Hepatic blood flow is impaired, causing portal hypertension, which in turn causes ascites and the formation of varices. The normal functioning of the liver is reduced, including the elimination of toxins, which can then build up and affect the functioning of the brain.

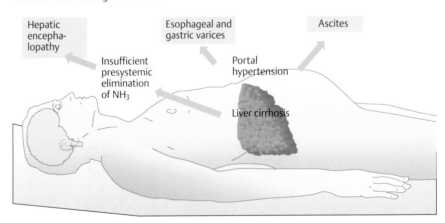

Drugs to Manage Alcoholism

Acute intoxication rarely requires treatment. Management includes supporting ventilation, maintaining temperature, and correcting dehydration, acidosis, or electrolyte imbalance. Gastic lavage (stomach pumping) is rarely necessary.

Chronic intoxication may be treated with the agents listed below.

Naltrexone

Mechanism of action. Naltrexone is an opioid antagonist similar to naloxone but with greater bioavailability and longer duration of action. It apparently blocks the ability of alcohol to activate dopaminergic reward pathways.

Pharmacokinetics
— Orally active, but also available in once-monthly injectable, extended-release form

Side effects
— Nausea and liver damage (in high dosages)

Contraindications
— Liver failure or acute hepatitis

Acamprosate

Mechanism of action
— Unclear

Uses. Acamprosate is also approved for prevention of relapse to alcoholism. Concomitant use of disulfiram appears to increase the effectiveness of acamprosate.

Side effects
— Diarrhea

Disulfiram (Antabuse)

Mechanism of action. Disulfiram is an inhibitor of aldehyde dehydrogenase. If alcohol is taken in the presence of disulfiram, blood acetaldehyde levels increase, producing flushing, dyspnea (shortness of breath), nausea, thirst, chest pain, and palpitations. The effects are intended to be unpleasant so as to discourage alcohol ingestion; however, they can be serious and even life-threatening.

Note: Patients must be informed to avoid alcohol, or their life may be in danger. This includes avoiding sauces, cough syrups, and liquid cold medicines that contain alcohol.

Toxicology of Other Alcohols

Methanol

Metabolism. Methanol is metabolized to formaldehyde by alcohol dehydrogenase. This occurs at about one fifth of the rate of ethanol. It is then further metabolized to formic acid.

Effects
— Metabolic acidosis and organ damage
— Methanol can cause blindness by damaging the optic nerve.

■ Alcoholism and vitamin deficiencies

Alcoholics frequently develop vitamin deficiencies, especially thiamine and niacin. Thiamine (vitamin B_1) is essential for carbohydrate metabolism and is a modulator of neurotransmitter activity. Niacin (vitamin B_3) is a component of nicotinamide adenine dinucleotide (NAD), nicotinamide adenine dinucleotide phosphate (NADP), and the reduced form of NADP (NADPH). It is also the cofactor for numerous dehydrogenases. The reason that alcoholics develop such vitamin deficiencies is multifactorial and includes poor nutrition and the role that alcohol plays in the ability of the body to absorb, metabolize, and store vitamins. Vitamin replacement therefore plays a role in the management of alcoholism.

Treatment. This involves suppressing methanol metabolism by administering ethanol and giving bicarbonate to correct the acidosis. Fomepizole, which is a synthetic parenteral alcohol dehydrogenase inhibitor, may also be used. It prevents the initial metabolism of methanol (and ethylene glycol) to toxic metabolites.

Ethylene Glycol

Metabolism. Ethylene glycol is metabolized to oxalic acid, causing systemic acidosis.

Toxic effects
— Metabolic acidosis and organ damage

Treatment. Same as for methanol poisoning.

15.3 Benzodiazepines

Benzodiazepines are also discussed in Chapter 9.

Diazepam, Midazolam, Temazepam, Triazolam, Flurazepam, Clonazepam, Oxazepam, Lorazepam, and Alprazolam

Intoxication. Intoxication with benzodiazepines produces progressive CNS depression with increasing dose. They may be fatal at high doses due to respiratory depression and cerebral hypoxia.

Tolerance, dependence, and withdrawal
— Tolerance develops to the effects of benzodiazepines.
— Physical dependence can occur.
— Withdrawal symptoms are generally opposite the effects of the drugs: anxiety, insomnia, and convulsions (in severe withdrawal). They can be minimized by slowly decreasing the dose to wean the patient from the drug.

15.4 Barbiturates

Barbiturates are also discussed in Chapter 9.

Thiopental, Phenobarbital, Thiomylal, Methohexital, Amobarbital, Pentobarbital, and Secobarbital

Intoxication
— Same as for benzodiazepines

Tolerance, dependence, and withdrawal
— Tolerance develops to their sedative and hypnotic effects. No tolerance develops to the anticonvulsant actions of barbiturates.
— True physical dependence occurs.
— Moderate withdrawal consists of rebound increases in rapid eye movement (REM) sleep, insomnia, and anxiety. Seizures and delirium can occur in patients taking high doses for long periods. These patients should be withdrawn slowly to avoid these serious complications.

15.5   Quaaludes

Methaqualone

Methaqualone is a former prescription medication that is now synthesized and sold illicitly. It is a CNS depressant with pharmacology similar to barbiturates.

Intoxication

— Same as for benzodiazepines

Tolerance, dependence, and withdrawal

The symptoms and treatments are the same as for barbiturates.

15.6   Stimulants

Mechanisms of action.   Stimulants inhibit the cyclic nucleotide phosphodiesterases, increase cellular Ca^{2+}, and are antagonists at central adenosine receptors.

Caffeine

Effects.   Caffeine decreases fatigue, increases arousal, and improves performance, but it produces insomnia and may have a disruptive effect and worsen performance at very high doses.

Tolerance, dependence, and withdrawal

— No tolerance develops to caffeine.
— A throbbing, diffuse headache is the most common symptom of caffeine dependence.
— Symptoms of withdrawal may include nausea, lethargy, and headache.

Amphetamines and Cocaine

Effects

— CNS actions include euphoria, decreased fatigue, alleviation of sleepiness, and decreased appetite. Amphetamines and cocaine may also increase libido and talkativeness. Restlessness may occur, and the heart rate may increase.
— After prolonged self-administration (a "run") with amphetamines, prolonged sleep, apathy, and depression are common.
— Sympathetic effects may be absent in chronic users.
— Chronic toxicity produces anxiety and confusion, leading to paranoia and psychosis, which is indistinguishable from schizophrenia.

Uses

— Cocaine is sometimes used as a local anesthetic agent.
— Amphetamines are used for attention deficit/hyperactivity disorder (ADHD) and narcolepsy.

Intoxication

— Acute intoxication causes hyperpyrexia, convulsions, and shock. It may result in death. Treatment involves chlorpromazine which will block many of the acute effects of amphetamines, and diazepam to control convulsions. Acidification of the urine will enhance excretion. Death can occur following acute cocaine use by convulsions or cardiac arrhythmias. Chlorpromazine can be used.
— Chronic intoxication may cause toxic syndrome. Signs and symptoms of toxic syndrome include visual, auditory hallucinations, and tactile hallucinations; paranoia and changes in affect. Treatment for paranoid delusions and excitement involves dopamine antagonists (haloperidol). Acidification of the urine will facilitate excretion of amphetamines.

■ **Attention deficit/hyperactivity disorder**

ADHD is characterized by inattention and hyperactive-impulsive behavior. It is a chronic disorder that affects children but may persist in adulthood. Symptoms are usually evident before the child is 7 years old, with the relative amount of inattention or hyperactivity symptoms differing in each case. Attention deficit symptoms include difficulty in sustaining attention during activities, trouble organizing activities, making careless mistakes in schoolwork, lack of listening when spoken to directly, forgetfulness, and often losing things. Hyperactivity symptoms include fidgeting, squirming, inability to remain seated, inappropriate running or climbing, trouble playing quietly, excessive talking, and always being "on the go." ADHD is often accompanied by anxiety and depression, making the diagnosis more complicated. The cause of ADHD is unknown, although it is known to have a strong hereditary element. Maternal smoking, drug use, and exposure to toxins have been shown to increase the likelihood of having a child with ADHD. Treatment involves the use of stimulant medications, such as methylphenidate (Ritalin) and dextromethamphetamine. Nonstimulant medications, such as atomexetine, are also used. Therapy plays an important role in the management of this condition.

■ **Narcolepsy**

Narcolepsy is a chronic sleep disorder that is characterized by sudden attacks of sleep and overwhelming daytime drowsiness. There may also be cataplexy (sudden loss of muscle tone), sleep paralysis (temporary paralysis that occurs when falling asleep or upon waking), hallucinations, and autonomic behavior while sleeping (e.g., talking or performing tasks). People with narcolepsy often have restless nighttime sleep patterns. This condition tends to occur mainly in adolescents and young adults. Damage to hypocretin cells, which regulate wakefulness and the timing of REM sleep, has been implicated as a cause for narcolepsy. Treatment involves the use of stimulant drugs such as modafenil and methylphenidate to help people stay awake; antidepressants to alleviate cataplexy, hallucinations, and sleep paralysis; or sodium oxybate to combat cataplexy.

Tolerance, dependence, and withdrawal
- Marked tolerance develops to amphetamines but not to cocaine.
- Dependence is common and produces an extremely intense drug craving. Physical dependence is minor.
- Withdrawal may include prolonged sleep, laziness, fatigue, overeating, and, occasionally, depression. Craving may persist for years.

15.7   Hallucinogens

Psychedelic Hallucinogens

d-Lysergic Acid Diethylamide (LSD), Psilocybin, and Mescaline

These agents differ primarily in potency. LSD is extremely potent.

Mechanism of action. Their mechanism is unclear, but they are serotonin agonists (see **Fig. 7.3,** page 70).

Intoxication. Psychedelic hallucinogens may produce vivid visual hallucinations and profound changes in thought processes, with confusion alternating with seemingly vivid perceptions and foresight, but these depend greatly on the situation and the individual.

Side effects
- Paranoia, panic reaction, and overt psychosis.
- Synesthesias and "flashbacks" are unique features (seen in up to 15% of users).
  Note: No deaths due to direct drug effects have been reported.

Treatment
- Involves emotional support and antianxiety agents, phenothiazines, or barbiturates in doses to produce sleep

Tolerance, dependence, and withdrawal
- Tolerance and cross-tolerance will occur.
- No dependence or withdrawal

Deliriant Hallucinogens

Phencyclidine and Ketamine

Phencyclidine (PCP) and ketamine are frequently touted as pure tetrahydrocannabinol (THC, the active ingredient in marijuana), LSD, or mescaline.

Intoxication. At low doses, intoxication resembles an acute confused state. At higher doses, serious neurologic, cardiovascular, and psychotic reactions occur.

Side effects. They are mainly psychological and include changes in body image, apparent loss of contact from reality, disorganized thought, and apathy or catatonia. Individuals on PCP may exhibit bizarre and hostile behavior. Use has declined because of unpleasant experiences.

Treatment. Treatment for overdosing involves maintenance of vital functions until the drug effects subside.

Tolerance, dependence, and withdrawal
- Tolerance may develop.
- There is no clear withdrawal syndrome.

15.8   Cannabis

Marijuana and Hashish

The main psychoactive ingredient is tetrahydrocannabinol (THC). Endogenous cannabinoid receptors have been discovered along with an endogenous ligand, anandamide.

Effects
- CNS effects: relaxation, sense of well-being, euphoria, and spontaneous laughter. Short-term memory and capacity to carry out goal-directed behavior are impaired, and there is also motor impairment. THC has variable effects on mood, emotion, and social feelings.
- Heart: tachycardia (paroxysmal atrial tachycardia) may occur.
- Respiratory system: the lungs are adversely affected by smoke.
- Reproductive system: changes in the menstrual cycle, decreased sperm count and motility, and increased number of abnormal sperm
- Amotivational syndrome: no scientific evidence that such a syndrome occurs.

Uses
- Antiemetic in cancer chemotherapy patients

Tolerance, dependence, and withdrawal
- Tolerance develops to the effects of THC.
- Physical dependence does not occur.
- A withdrawal syndrome has not been defined. Many individuals stop using marijuana at will with no craving.

15.9   Tobacco

Nicotine

Mechanism of action.   Nicotine mimics acetylcholine at nicotinic receptors. It also decreases the activity of the enzyme monoamine oxidase (MAO) in the brain, which increases dopamine levels.

Intoxication.   Nicotine causes an alert pattern in the electroencephalogram. It decreases skeletal muscle tone, appetite, and irritability and has a mild euphorigenic effect.

Tolerance, dependence, and withdrawal
- Withdrawal is variable, but increased appetite and inability to concentrate may persist for months. Intense psychological craving to smoke persists for months to years after quitting smoking.

Treatment
- Nicotine replacement therapy: a variety of strategies are available for administering nicotine in place of smoking, including oral (gum or lozenge), transdermal (patches), and intranasal (spray).
- Varenicline, a partial agonist at the $\alpha_2\beta_4$ subtype of nicotinic acetylcholine receptors, stimulates the receptor to relieve cravings and withdrawal while simultaneously blocking nicotine binding, thus reducing the rewarding effect of smoking.
- Bupropion, an antidepressant drug that inhibits dopamine and norepinephrine reuptake, has some efficacy in nicotine addiction. A sustained-release formulation of bupropion is available for treatment of tobacco dependence.

15.10   Inhalants

Nitrous Oxide, Gasoline, Volatile Solvents, and Aerosols

See page 77 for a further discussion of nitrous oxide.

Intoxication

— Acute toxicity may lead to respiratory arrest and cardiac arrhythmias.
— Direct administration of aerosol propellants has resulted in laryngospasm, airway freezing, and suffocation due to an occluded airway.
— Chronic toxicity varies depending on the solvent but is characterized by irreversible tissue damage. This irreversible tissue damage means that solvent abusers are the most difficult group to rehabilitate.

Review Questions

1. The major 5-hydroxytryptamine (5-HT)–containing nuclei in the brain are located in the
   A. interomediolateral column of the spinal cord.
   B. thalamus.
   C. red nucleus.
   D. locus caeruleus.
   E. raphe nuclei.

2. Which of the following changes will increase the rate of induction of surgical anesthesia with an inhalation agent if all other factors remain unchanged?
   A. Increased patient respiration
   B. Increased tissue solubility of anesthetic
   C. Increased weight of patient
   D. Increased blood: gas solubility

3. A patient has just undergone a procedure that required general anesthesia. In the recovery room, the patient's respiration rate and heart rate are noted to be gradually increasing. His blood pressure is 155/90 mm Hg, and his temperature, which was normal before the surgery, is 38°C (100.4°F). These symptoms could be indicative of a reaction to which drug combination?
   A. Morphine/diazepam
   B. Halothane/succinylcholine
   C. Halothane/nitrous oxide
   D. Nitrous oxide/succinylcholine
   E. Morphine/atropine

4. Oxygen is administered to the patient in question 3, and measures are taken to reduce the patient's core temperature. In addition, intravenous administration of a drug is ordered. What is the purpose of this drug?
   A. To dilate peripheral vessels by a direct action on smooth muscle
   B. To decrease respiration via an action in the brainstem
   C. To block muscarinic cholinergic receptors
   D. To provide sedation via depression of the central nervous system
   E. To decrease Ca^{2+} release from the sarcoplastic reticulum of skeletal muscle

5. Local anesthetic agents block nerve conduction by
   A. altering metabolism.
   B. interfering with Na^+-K^+-ATPase.
   C. increasing the resting membrane potential.
   D. blocking Na^+ channels in the nerve membrane.
   E. blocking γ-aminobutyric acid type B ($GABA_B$) receptors.

6. Which is usually lost first after the injection of a local anesthetic?
   A. sense of touch.
   B. sense of pressure.
   C. sense of proprioception.
   D. motor control.
   E. sense of pain.

7. A 7-year-old boy who fell off his bike has a laceration on his right knee that requires sutures. Lidocaine hydrochloride as a 2% solution with epinephrine 1:100,000 is used for local infiltration anesthesia. What is the purpose of the inclusion of epinephrine?
   A. To produce vasoconstriction and increase the duration of action of the local anesthetic
   B. To produce vasodilation and increase absorption of the local anesthetic into the circulation
   C. To decrease the sensitivity of C fibers to the local anesthetic
   D. To decrease the sensitivity of sympathetic nerve endings to the local anesthetic
   E. To produce a higher degree of anesthesia in tissues supplied by end-organs

For questions **8** to **13**, the following are the answer choices:
   A. Voltage-dependent ion channels
   B. Ligand-gated ion channels
   C. Presynaptic synthetic pathways
   D. Transmitter reuptake mechanisms
   E. Extracellular and glial degradative enzymes
   F. G-protein coupled membrane receptors

8. Which is the site of action for lidocaine?

9. Which is the site of action for gamma-aminobutyric acid (GABA) at $GABA_A$ receptors?

10. Which is the site of action for fluoxetine?

11. Which is the site of action for morphine?

12. Which is the site of action for levodopa?

13. Which is the site of action for galantamine?

14. Phenelzine and isocarboxazid are termed "suicide" inhibitors because they
   A. are effective in preventing suicidal behavior.
   B. are apparently irreversible inhibitors of monoamine oxidase.
   C. prevent hallucinations.
   D. decrease monamine levels in the brain.

15. A patient who is unconscious is admitted to the emergency room. She has ingested a combination of ethanol and diazepam. Which of the following might be appropriate therapy?
A. Naloxone
B. Naltrexone
C. Fluphenazine
D. Flumazenil
E. Amphetamine

16. An 18-year-old female patient has been experiencing severe abdominal pain for several days. This has been accompanied by occasional vomiting. The patient is anxious and appears confused. Blood pressure and heart rate are increased. Her urine is red in color. Porphobilinogen, δ-aminolevulinic acid, and porphyrins in urine are increased. How could administering a barbiturate to this patient exacerbate these symptoms?
A. By producing incoordination
B. By producing insomnia
C. By inducing liver enzymes
D. By inducing vomiting
E. By interacting with ethanol

17. A 45-year-old man with a history of alcoholism reports feeling constantly anxious. He says he is always on edge, is irritable, and has difficulty concentrating. Although he finds this tiring, he has not been sleeping well. Because of this patient's history, what would be the most desirable agent to use to treat anxiety?
A. Buspirone
B. Phenobarbital
C. Fluphenazine
D. Diazepam
E. Amphetamine

18. The selective serotonin reuptake inhibitors (SSRIs, e.g., fluoxetine) differ from the tricyclic antidepressants (e.g., amitriptyline) in that they
A. have an immediate onset of antidepressant action.
B. inhibit monoamine oxidase (MAO).
C. have no effect on 5-hydroxytryptamine (5-HT), or serotonin, pathways in the central nervous system.
D. are less likely to produce weight gain.

19. A 32-year-old man developed a decreased need for sleep, increased energy, elevated mood, and hyperactivity. He was diagnosed with a manic disorder, and treatment with an antimanic drug was initiated. After 2 weeks of treatment, the patient developed a mild hand tremor. What does the tremor indicate?
A. Lithium toxicity
B. Lack of sleep
C. Fluoxetine toxicity
D. Chlorpromazine toxicity
E. Fatigue as a result of hyperactivity

20. The therapeutic effects of lithium
A. are observed following the first dose.
B. are antagonized by the administration of chlorpromazine.
C. are observed in normal, nonmanic patients.
D. occur in 70 to 80% of manic patients.

21. You see an adolescent female patient in your office who is being treated for epilepsy. She has hirsutism, her lips are thickened, the mass of skin around her cheekbones is increased, and she has gingival hyperplasia. Which drug would be most likely to cause these effects?
A. Phenytoin
B. Carbamazepine
C. Phenobarbital
D. Ethosuximide
E. Valproic acid

22. Which of the following is very effective for the control of absence (petit mal) seizures?
A. Phenobarbital
B. Phenytoin
C. Valproic acid
D. Carbamazepine

23. Useful therapy for generalized tonic-clonic (grand mal) epilepsy includes
A. phenytoin.
B. ethosuximide.
C. pentazocine.
D. chlorpromazine.

24. A patient who has recently begun treatment for generalized tonic-clonic seizures complains of red, itchy skin. He also says he has been feeling as if he has the flu. His body temperature is 38°C (100.4°F). Upon examination, a multiforme erythematous maculopapular rash is observed on his arms and chest. Which of the following would be the most appropriate therapy?
A. Discontinue the drug treatment immediately.
B. Discontinue the drug treatment immediately, and initiate treatment with valproic acid.
C. Discontinue the drug treatment immediately, and initiate treatment with ethosuximide.
D. Prescribe hydrocortisone cream for the skin lesions.
E. No action is needed, as the rash is common with anticonvulsant therapy.

25. A patient taking thioridazine has xerostomia (dry mouth), tachycardia, dry skin, and urinary hesitancy. In what capacity is thioridazine acting that brings about these effects?
A. As an agonist at muscarinic receptors
B. As an antagonist at muscarinic receptors
C. As an agonist at dopamine receptors
D. As an antagonist at dopamine receptors
E. As a mixed agonist-antagonist at opioid receptors

26. The therapeutic actions of an antipsychotic drug such as chlorpromazine are most likely due to its action as an
    A. antagonist at dopamine receptors on cells receiving mesolimbic innervation.
    B. antagonist at dopamine receptors on cells receiving nigrostriatal innervation.
    C. antagonist of muscarinic receptors.
    D. agonist at opioid receptors.
    E. antagonist at adenosine receptors.

27. A 20-year-old male college student is brought to the clinic by his parents. He has recently stopped attending classes and has refused to answer his cell phone. When questioned, he says that he is afraid that he is being watched and that his classmates are out to get him. He doesn't want them to track him through his phone, but they can call him without using the phone. He has not been showering or eating regularly. Organic and substance abuse disorders are ruled out, and a diagnosis of schizophrenia is made. You must decide whether to treat him with haloperidol or thioridazine. Which statement correctly compares the effectiveness of the drugs and their propensity for producing acute extrapyramidal neurotoxicities?
    A. Haloperidol is more likely to be effective, but it is also more likely to produce extrapyramidal neurotoxicities.
    B. Thioridazine is more likely to be effective, but it is also more likely to produce extrapyramidal neurotoxicities.
    C. The likelihood of effective treatment is equal, but haloperidol is more likely to cause extrapyramidal neurotoxicities.
    D. The likelihood of effective treatment is equal, but thioridazine is more likely to cause extrapyramidal neurotoxicities.
    E. The likelihood of effective treatment is equal, and so is the likelihood of extrapyramidal neurotoxicities.

28. A patient undergoing chronic treatment for schizophrenia, first with a typical antipsychotic and then with an atypical agent, continues to experience episodes of paranoia and hallucinations. It is decided to use clozapine as therapy. Patients being treated with clozapine must have a baseline white blood cell count (WBC) and absolute neutrophil count (ANC) before initiation of treatment, as well as regular WBCs and ANCs during treatment and for at least 4 weeks after discontinuation of treatment. Which of the following may be caused by clozapine, thus necessitating these blood tests?
    A. Agranulocytosis
    B. Weight gain
    C. Orthostatic hypotension
    D. Anticholinergic side effects
    E. Neuroleptic malignant syndrome

29. At 2 weeks of treatment with clozapine, the patient in question 28 has blood tests that reveal an elevated creatine kinase (CK) and white blood cell count (WCC). This could be associated with the development of which of the following?
    A. Akathisia
    B. Acute dystonia
    C. Tardive dyskinesia
    D. Extrapyramidal symptoms
    E. Neuroleptic malignant syndrome

30. Drug-induced parkinsonism may occur during treatment with typical antipsychotic agents. The parkinsonian symptoms can be treated with
    A. anticholinergic drugs.
    B. levodopa.
    C. chlorpromazine.
    D. haloperidol.

31. κ (kappa) opiate receptors mediate
    A. supraspinal analgesia.
    B. respiratory depression.
    C. euphoria.
    D. dependence.
    E. spinal analgesia.

32. Which of the following is converted to a metabolite that is capable of inducing stimulation of the central nervous system (CNS), especially in patients with renal failure?
    A. Acetaminophen
    B. Meperidine
    C. Pentazocine
    D. Naloxone
    E. Naltrexone

33. A 23-year-old man fell from a roof and suffered a ruptured spleen. He has been in a methadone maintenance program for several months and is taking a regular large dose of methadone. Physical examination suggests abdominal bleeding. He is rushed to the operating room for an emergency splenectomy. The anesthesiologist uses sodium thiopental to induce anesthesia and halothane during the surgery. After 1 week, the patient is recovering and is now receiving the same daily dose of methadone he was taking before his accident. That night, pain from the incision keeps him awake, and the resident on duty administers a drug. Within a few minutes, the patient is nauseated, sweating, tremoring, and having intestinal cramps. He also has waves of gooseflesh and involuntary kicking movements of the legs. This is an expected result of administering which of the following drugs to this patient?
    A. Methadone
    B. Codeine
    C. Chloral hydrate
    D. Pentazocine
    E. Diazepam

34. Methadone differs from morphine in that methadone
  A. is not an effective analgesic.
  B. produces a shorter and more tolerable abstinence syndrome than morphine.
  C. is metabolized to morphine.
  D. has a longer half-life.
  E. is selective for κ opioid receptors.

35. A 27-year-old pregnant woman who has had no prenatal care was brought to the hospital in the final stages of labor. A healthy, full-term infant was delivered with no apparent complications. However, within 24 hours, the infant became irritable, cried constantly, and would not nurse. The mother admitted to recent heavy use of illegally obtained oxycodone. Given the history, what are the infant's symptoms most likely indicative of?
  A. Tolerance to oxycodone
  B. Normal response at birth
  C. Opiate withdrawal
  D. Hunger
  E. Bilirubinemia

36. A 65-year-old male retired autoworker complains of tightness in his arms and legs, as well as difficulty walking and going down stairs. He is well nourished and shows no change in facial expressions during the examination. A mild resting tremor of his right hand is noted. Parkinson disease is diagnosed, and treatment is begun with a dopamine receptor agonist. What is the rationale of this therapy?
  A. To increase glucose production in skeletal muscle
  B. To prevent the peripheral decarboxylation of dopamine
  C. To activate dopamine receptors on interneurons in the motor cortex
  D. To mimic the central actions of dopamine in the substantia nigra
  E. To directly stimulate postsynaptic receptors within the striatum

37. An alternative strategy to treat Parkinson disease is to inhibit the metabolism of endogenous dopamine. Which of the following drug combinations inhibit the breakdown of dopamine?
  A. Entacapone and selegiline
  B. Levodopa and carbidopa
  C. Dopa decarboxylase and monoamine oxidase (MAO)
  D. Fluoxetine and sertraline
  E. Bromocriptine and trihexyphenidyl

38. Which of the following is a dopamine receptor agonist?
  A. Levodopa
  B. Bromocriptine
  C. Amantadine
  D. Carbidopa
  E. Benztropine

39. In the treatment of Parkinson disease, which of the following is an alternative approach to increasing dopamine?
  A. Decrease the cholinergic component
  B. Increase the cholinergic component
  C. Decrease the noradrenergic component
  D. Increase the noradrenergic component
  E. Antagonize the serotonergic component

40. For which of the following drugs are miosis, respiratory depression, and lack of bowel sounds the signs of acute intoxication?
  A. Lysergic acid diethylamide (LSD)
  B. Amphetamine
  C. Morphine
  D. Methaqualone

41. Liver damage may result from chronic abuse of
  A. lysergic acid diethylamide (LSD)
  B. ethanol
  C. amphetamine
  D. cocaine

42. Ethanol may have interactions with several other drugs. The interaction of ethanol with other central nervous system (CNS) depressant drugs is characterized by
  A. an enhanced CNS depressant action.
  B. a decreased CNS depressant activity of the other drug.
  C. an increased gastric irritation.
  D. a decreased gastric irritation.
  E. There is no interaction.

43. A patient comes to you complaining of insomnia and nausea. Examination shows a coarse tremor of the extremities, oral temperature of 38.5°C (101.3°F), hyperactive deep tendon reflexes, and orthostatic hypotension. He admits a daily alcohol intake of at least a pint of whiskey and several cans of beer. During the examination, there is a short period of myoclonic jerking of the arms and legs. The patient then volunteers that he had been in jail all night, having been arrested for being drunk and disorderly, though he barely remembers the episode. He has had no drug or alcohol for ~18 hours. Before the patient can be treated, he slumps over, clutching his abdomen. Examination later in the hospital suggests a perforated duodenal ulcer with internal bleeding. The surgeon recommends immediate surgery. During recovery, the patient shows tremor, anxiety, agitation, and muscle twitches. A drug is given that suppresses these signs of alcohol withdrawal. What is the drug?
  A. A vitamin
  B. An opiate receptor blocker
  C. An acetaldehyde dehydrogenase inhibitor
  D. A benzodiazepine receptor agonist
  E. An antimicrobial

44. Upon discharge, the patient in question 43 agrees to seek therapy for his alcohol addiction, including group therapy and a medication. The patient is given a wallet card listing the medication and is warned that, when taking this drug, exposure to alcohol in his diet, in over-the-counter medications, and in toiletries may produce sweating, flushing, headache, nausea, and vomiting. Which drug is prescribed?
   A. A vitamin
   B. An opiate receptor blocker
   C. An aldehyde dehydrogenase inhibitor
   D. A benzodiazepine receptor agonist
   E. An antimicrobial

45. A heavy user of alcohol is in the hospital and scheduled to have his gallbladder removed. He was given pentobarbital to promote sleep the night before the operation. The nurse is surprised to find him still awake after she has doubled the usual dose. What is this an example of?
   A. Addiction
   B. Physical dependence
   C. Psychological dependence
   D. Cross-tolerance
   E. Synergism

46. For which of the following drugs are ataxia and sedation the signs of acute intoxication?
   A. Lysergic acid diethylamide (LSD)
   B. Amphetamine
   C. Morphine
   D. Methaqualone

47. For which of the following drugs are decreased fatigue and increased talkativeness the signs of acute intoxication?
   A. Lysergic acid diethylamide (LSD)
   B. Amphetamine
   C. Morphine
   D. Methaqualone

48. Of the following drugs of abuse, which is most likely to produce the greatest degree of psychological dependence in the largest percentage of users?
   A. Cocaine
   B. Codeine
   C. Heroin
   D. Methadone
   E. Methaqualone

49. For which of the following drugs are anxiety, paranoia, and hallucinations the signs of acute intoxication?
   A. Lysergic acid diethylamide (LSD)
   B. Amphetamine
   C. Morphine
   D. Methaqualone

50. Intoxication with which one of the following agents causes changes in body image, feelings of estrangement, negativism, and hostility?
   A. Barbiturates
   B. Caffeine
   C. Cocaine
   D. Marijuana
   E. Phencyclidine hydrochloride (PCP)

51. A 32-year-old woman has enrolled in a smoking cessation program at work. She has been smoking since she was a teenager. She currently smokes a pack a day but has been unable to quit, despite several tries. Pharmacotherapies she is considering include the nicotine patch, varenicline, and bupropion. How does varenicline differ from the nicotine patch?
   A. Varenicline is a nicotinic receptor antagonist that prevents nicotine from acting at its receptor and blocks the rewarding effects of nicotine.
   B. Varenicline is a partial agonist that stimulates the receptor to relieve cravings and withdrawal while simultaneously blocking nicotine binding.
   C. Varenicline is a nicotine analogue agonist that stimulates the receptor and acts as a replacement for the nicotine found in tobacco.
   D. Varenicline is a selective serotonin reuptake inhibitor that acts as an antidepressant to prevent the negative mood experienced during withdrawal from nicotine.
   E. Varenicline is a dopamine/norepinephrine reuptake inhibitor that acts to increase dopamine in the brain, leading to a decreased craving to smoke.

Answers and Explanations

1. **E** The cell bodies of the main groups of 5-HT-containing neurons are located in the raphe nuclei of the brainstem (p. 69).

2. **A** Because anesthetic induction with inhalation agents is via the lungs, increasing respiration will increase the rate of absorption and thus induction of anesthesia (p. 76).
   B   Increased tissue solubility will decrease the rate of induction.
   C   The rate of anesthetic induction is generally independent of the patient's weight.
   D   Increased blood gas solubility will decrease the rate of induction.

3. **B** Malignant hyperthermia is a rare complication of anesthesia with any volatile anesthetic but, most commonly, with halothane, particularly when it is combined with a depolarizing neuromuscular blocking agent such as succinylcholine. During malignant hyperthermia, there is a substantial increase in skeletal muscle oxidative metabolism, which increases body temperature, consumes oxygen, and leads to a buildup of carbon dioxide (p. 76).

4. **E** Dantrolene is used as a treatment for malignant hyperthermia. This drug acts directly on skeletal muscle to decrease Ca^{2+} release from the sarcoplasmic reticulum. This in turn decreases muscle contraction, metabolism, and the generation of heat, thereby decreasing hyperthermia (pages 76 and 117).

5. **D** Local anesthetics prevent action potential propagation by blocking Na^+ channels in the nerve membrane from the cytoplasmic side of the channel (p. 79).
   A–C, E Local anesthetics do not alter metabolism, interfere with ATPase, increase the resting membrane potential, or block $GABA_B$ receptors.

6. **E** Smaller diameter unmyelinated nerve fibers are most sensitive to block by local anesthetics. Pain fibers are the smallest and so are blocked first (p. 80).
   A–D The loss of the sense of pain is followed by the loss of sensations of cold, warmth, touch, and deep pressure. Proprioceptive and motor fibers are least sensitive.

7. **A** Epinephrine is added to local anesthetic solutions to produce vasoconstriction at the site of injection. Termination of the action of a local anesthetic depends on its diffusion from the site of injection. Vasoconstriction decreases systemic absorption and prolongs the duration of action (p. 79).

8. **A** Lidocaine blocks voltage-dependent Na^+ channels from the cytoplasmic side of the channel (p. 79).

9. **B** Gamma-aminobutyric acid (GABA) acts at $GABA_A$ receptors, which are ligand-gated ion channels. Activation leads to opening of the Cl^- channel and synaptic inhibition (pages 68 and 72).

10. **D** Fluoxetine is a serotonin-specific reuptake inhibitor (SSRI) (p. 89).

11. **F** Morphine acts at opioid receptors (highest affinity for μ receptors), which are G-protein coupled receptors (p. 102).

12. **C** Levodopa is a precursor of dopamine synthesis. It is transformed to dopamine by aromatic amino acid decarboxylase (p. 111).

13. **E** Galantamine is a competitive cholinesterase inhibitor. By inhibiting cholinesterase it increases the concentration of acetylcholine (ACh) in the brain. It is used to treat the symptoms of Alzheimer disease (p. 115).

14. **B** "Suicide" inhibitors are so named because they bind irreversibly to the enzyme, in this case monoamine oxidase, inactivating it. Restoration of enzymatic activity requires synthesis of new enzyme (p. 88).
   A, C The term does not refer to prevention of suicidal behavior or hallucinations.
   D   Phenelzine and isocarboxazid increase monoamine levels in the brain by inhibiting their breakdown by monoamine oxidase.

15. **D** Flumazenil is a relatively specific competitive benzodiazepine receptor antagonist useful in overdose or poisoning. Even in the presence of ethanol, blocking the effect of the benzodiazepine, diazepam may be sufficient to restore consciousness (p. 83).

16. **C** The symptoms are consistent with acute intermittent porphyria, a disorder of porphyrin metabolism. Barbiturates are potent inducers of liver enzymes and will further increase porphyrin synthesis and worsen the disease. Barbiturates are contraindicated in patients with acute intermittent porphyria, porphyria variegata, or a positive family history of these porphyrias (p. 83).

17. **A** Benzodiazepines and ethanol produce similar depressant effects on the central nervous system (CNS). Benzodiazepines are more likely to be abused by patients with a history of CNS depressant abuse. For this patient, an anxiolytic like buspirone that produces less sedation and has a lower propensity for mimicking or enhancing the effects of ethanol is preferable (p. 85).
    B   Phenobarbital is a barbiturate used for anesthetic induction, insomnia, and as an anticonvulsant. It is not used for anxiety and is prone to abuse.
    C   Fluphenazine is an antipsychotic and an antiemetic drug. It is not used to treat anxiety.
    E   Amphetamine is a stimulant drug that would keep the patient awake. Chronic use will lead to anxiety.

18. **D** The SSRIs are less likely than the tricyclic antidepressants to produce weight gain (p. 89).
    A   None of the antidepressant drugs have an immediate onset of antidepressant action.
    B, C The SSRIs do not inhibit MAO, but they do inhibit 5-HT reuptake.

19. **A** Lithium is an antimanic drug with a narrow therapeutic index. Tremor is an indicator of mild toxicity (pages 89 and 90).
    B–E Under these circumstances, tremor does not indicate a lack of sleep, fluoxetine or chlorpromazine toxicity, or fatigue as a result of hyperactivity.

20. **D** Lithium is effective in treating mania in 70 to 80% of patients (p. 89).
    A   The effects of lithium take 1 to 2 weeks to fully develop; they are not seen immediately following the first dose.
    B   The effects of lithium are not antagonized by the antipsychotic drug chlorpromazine. On the contrary, antipsychotic drugs may be used to treat severe acute mania.
    C   Lithium has no effects on nonmanic patients, unless toxic doses are ingested.

21. **A** These are side effects of phenytoin (p. 92).
    B   Carbamazepine side effects include GI upset, hematological disorders, hypersensitivity, vertigo, diplopia, and blurred vision.
    C   Phenobarbital side effects include sedation and rashes. Ataxia and nystagmus may also occur at excessive doses.
    D   Ethosuximide side effects include GI upset, CNS depression, rashes (rarely Stevens-Johnson syndrome) and blood dyscrasias (rarely).
    E   Valproic acid side effects include alopecia, GI upset, ataxia, tremor, and mild behavioral effects.

22. **C** Of the drugs listed, valproic acid is the only one that is effective in absence seizures (p. 94).
    A   Phenobarbital is a barbiturate used to treat generalized tonic-clonic seizures, partial seizure and febrile convulsions.
    B   Phenytoin is effective for all types of seizures except absence and atonic seizures. It is also used for trigeminal neuralgia.
    D   Carbamazepine is used to treat generalized tonic-clonic seizures, complex partial seizures and trigeminal neuralgia.

23. **A** Of the agents listed, phenytoin is the only one used for generalized tonic-clonic seizures (p. 91).
    B   Ethosuximide is the drug of choice for absence seizures.
    C   Pentazocine is an opioid drug used to treat pain.
    D   Chlorpromazine is an antipsychotic agent.

24. **B** The patient is experiencing an allergic reaction to the drug, which may progress to Stevens-Johnson syndrome if the drug is not withdrawn. Of the drugs indicated for use in generalized tonic-clonic seizures, valproic acid is the least likely to lead to Stevens-Johnson syndrome (p. 94).

25. **B** The side effects are characteristic anticholinergic effects (p. 99).

26. **A** The therapeutic efficacy of typical antipsychotics is correlated with their ability to block the D_2 subtype of dopamine receptors. The mesolimbic pathway is the dopaminergic pathway involved in the modulation of behaviors related to schizophrenia (p. 98).
    B   The nigrostriatal dopaminergic pathway is involved in the control of movements and in therapy for Parkinson disease.

27. **C** In general, the antipsychotic agents are similarly effective in treating schizophrenia. The likelihood of extrapyramidal side effects is greater with haloperidol than thioridazine (p. 100).

28. **A** WBC and ANC are measured prior to and during clozapine therapy to detect for bone marrow suppression by the drug and to prevent agranulocytosis (p. 101).

29. **E** Neuroleptic malignant syndrome is an idiosyncratic reaction to antipsychotic drugs that tends to occur more frequently with typical antipsychotics, but it can occur with atypical agents, such as clozapine. It presents with fever, muscular rigidity, altered mental status, and autonomic dysfunction (e.g., arrhythmias and fluctuating blood pressure), leading to elevated CK and WBCs (p. 99).

30. **A** Anticholinergic drugs such as benztropine can be used to treat drug-induced parkinsonism. Benztropine is a muscarinic receptor antagonist that blocks acetylcholine in the striatum and so counteracts excessive cholinergic activity that results from dopamine deficiency (p. 115).

B It would not make sense to treat drug-induced parkinsonism with levodopa to increase dopamine levels because the typical antipsychotics are dopamine antagonists and because this could worsen the symptoms of schizophrenia.

C, D Chlorpromazine and haloperidol are typical antipsychotics that may induce Parkinson-like symptoms.

31. **E** κ (kappa) opiate receptors are found mainly in the spinal cord where they modulate pain sensations (p. 102).

A-D The other choices are mediated by μ receptors.

32. **B** Meperidine is a synthetic opiate agonist, especially at μ receptors. Of the drugs listed, it can induce CNS simulation (p. 106).

A Acetaminophen is an analgesic and antipyretic drug.

C Pentazocine is a mixed opiate agonist-antagonist that is used as an analgesic.

D, E Naloxone and naltrexone are opiate antagonists.

33. **D** The patient's responses are typical signs of opiate withdrawal. Pentazocine is a mixed agonist-antagonist at opiate receptors that may precipitate opiate withdrawal in dependent individuals (p. 107).

34. **D** The half-life of methadone is ~24 hours compared with 4 hours for morphine. This allows once-daily dosing of methadone to prevent opiate withdrawal (p. 107).

A Methadone is an effective analgesic agent (equally as potent as morphine).

B The methadone abstinence syndrome is longer and may not be more tolerable than withdrawal from morphine.

C Methadone is not metabolized to morphine.

E Methadone is not selective for the κ receptor but acts at all three subtypes of opiate receptor.

35. **C** Morphine-like opiate agonist ligands readily cross the placenta and will affect the fetus. In this case, the infant is most likely experiencing opiate withdrawal (p. 119).

36. **E** Parkinson disease results from a degeneration of the dopaminergic neurons in the substantia nigra that project to the striatum. One of the primary therapeutic approaches to Parkinson disease is to restore dopaminergic function, in this case with a dopamine agonist. While the cell bodies of dopamine neurons are in the substanita nigra, these neurons project to the striatum where dopamine is released (p. 111).

37. **A** Entacapone is a catechol-0-methyltransferase inhibitor, and selegiline is an MAO type B inhibitor (p. 113).

38. **B** Of the agents listed, the only one that is a dopamine receptor agonist is bromocriptine (p. 113).

A Levodopa is a precursor of dopamine synthesis. Levodopa is pharmacologically inert, its effects are a result of decarboxylation to dopamine.

C Amantadine probably enhances dopamine release in the CNS.

D Carbidopa inhibits the peripheral production of dopamine from L-dopa by inhibiting dopa decarboxylase.

E Benztropine is a muscarinic receptor antagonist that blocks acetylcholine in the striatum and so counteracts excessive cholinergic activity that results from dopamine deficiency.

39. **A** An alternative approach to restoring dopaminergic function in Parkinson disease is to decrease the cholinergic activity (p. 111).

40. **C** Miosis, respiratory depression, and lack of bowel sounds are the signs of acute intoxication with morphine (p. 105).

41. **B** Chronic use of ethanol, but not the other drugs listed, leads to progressive liver damage that increases with increased ethanol doses and duration of ethanol use (p. 120, Fig. 15.1).

A Chronic abuse of LSD include flashbacks and other psychological problems.

C, D Chronic abuse of amphetamine causes anxiety and confusion, leading to paranoia and psychosis which is indistinguishable from schizophrenia.

42. **A** Ethanol potentiates the sedative and motor incoordinating effects of other drugs that cause CNS depression.

43. **D** Benzodiazepines are cross-tolerant with alcohol and will alleviate withdrawal symptoms, but they do not have the same stimulating effects on the central nervous system as alcohol (p. 120).

A, B, C, E The other drugs do not suppress alcohol withdrawal.

44. **C** Disulfiram, the drug prescribed in this case, is an inhibitor of aldehyde dehydrogenase. Ethanol is metabolized to acetaldehyde by alcohol dehydrogenase. Acetaldehyde is then metabolized to acetate by aldehyde dehydrogenase. Disulfiram inhibits aldehyde dehydrogenase, blocking the conversion of ethanol-derived acetaldehyde to acetate. In the presence of disulfiram, acetaldehyde will accumulate and produce flushing, dyspnea, nausea, thirst, chest pain, and palpitation. The effects are intended to be unpleasant so as to discourage alcohol ingestion; however, they can be serious and even life-threatening (p. 121).

45. **D** Users of ethanol develop tolerance to ethanol and cross-tolerance to other sedative hypnotic agents, such as benzodiazepines and barbiturates, such as pentobarbital (p. 120).

46. **D** Ataxia and sedation are the signs of acute intoxication with methaqualone (p. 123).

47. **B** Decreased fatigue and increased talkativeness are the signs of acute intoxication with amphetamines (p. 123).

48. **A** Psychological dependence consisting of craving and a desire to acquire more of the drug may occur with any of the agents listed, but cocaine has the greatest potential for producing such an effect (p. 123).

49. **A** Anxiety, paranoia, and hallucinations are the signs of acute intoxication with lysergic diethyl amide (LSD) (p. 124).

50. **E** The first two symptoms are characteristic following ingestion of PCP, with the latter two occurring in some individuals and more likely following ingestion of larger doses of the drug (p. 124).
    A–D These symptoms are not typically associated with barbiturate, caffeine, cocaine, or marijuana use.

51. **B** Varenicline is a partial agonist at the α2β4 subtype of nicotinic acetylcholine receptors. It stimulates the receptor to relieve the cravings and withdrawal from nicotine while simultaneously blocking nicotine binding, thus reducing the rewarding effect if the patient does relapse to smoking (p. 125).

16   Drugs Used in the Treatment of Hypothalamic, Pituitary, Thyroid, and Adrenal Disorders

The hypothalamic hormones and their related drugs are discussed in relation to the anterior pituitary hormones that they modulate.

Table 16.1 lists the second messengers used by the hormones discussed in this unit.

Table 16.1 ▶ Second Messengers Used by Hormones	
Hormones	**Second Messenger**
CRH, ACTH, LH, FSH, TSH, PTH, calcitonin, glucagon, ADH (V$_2$ receptors), hCG	↑ Cyclic AMP
Prolactin	↓ Cyclic AMP
GHRH, GnRH, TRH, ADH (V$_1$ receptors), oxytocin	DAG and IP$_3$
Cortisol, aldosterone, testosterone, estrogen, progesterone, calcitriol (vitamin D), thyroid hormones (T$_3$ and T$_4$)	Steroid mechanism
NO	Cyclic GMP
Insulin and IGF-1	Tyrosine kinase

Abbreviations: ACTH, adrenocorticotropic hormone; ADH, antidiuretic hormone; AMP, adenosine monophosphate; CRH, corticotropin-releasing hormone; DAG, diacylglycerol; FSH, follicle-stimulating hormone; GHRH, growth hormone-releasing hormone; GMP, guanosine monophosphate; GnRH, gonadotropin-releasing hormone; hCG, human chorionic gonadotropin; IGF-1, insulinlike growth factor; IP, inositol triphosphate; LH, luteinizing hormone; NO, nitric oxide; PTH, parathyroid hormone; TRH, thyrotropin-releasing hormone; TSH, thyroid-stimulating hormone.

16.1   Pituitary Hormones

Anterior pituitary hormones are secreted or inhibited in response to the action of releasing hormones or inhibiting hormones from the hypothalamus. Posterior pituitary hormones are synthesized in the hypothalamus, stored in the posterior pituitary, and secreted in response to direct neural stimulation (**Fig. 16.1**). **Table 16.2** summarizes the hormonal cascade from the hypothalamus to target organs or the posterior pituitary.

Table 16.2 ▶ Hypothalamic and Pituitary Hormones and their Target Organs		
Hypothalamic Hormone	**Anterior Pituitary Hormone**	**Target Organ(s)**
GHRH	↑ GH	Liver, skeletal muscle, and bone
Somatostatin	↓ GH	Liver, GI tract, and pancreas
CRH	ACTH	Adrenal cortex
GnRH	LH and FSH	Gonads
TRH	TSH	Thyroid gland
PIH (dopamine)	Prolactin	Mammary glands and gonads
Posterior Pituitary Hormones		
Oxytocin		Uterine and other smooth muscle
ADH (vasopressin)		Kidney tubules (mainly); also vascular smooth muscle, liver, and anterior pituitary gland

Abbreviations: ACTH, adrenocorticotropic hormone; ADH, antidiuretic hormone; CRH, corticotropin-releasing hormone; FSH, follicle-stimulating hormone; GH, growth hormone; GHRH, growth hormone–releasing hormone; GI, gastrointestinal; GnRH, gonadotropin-releasing hormone; LH, luteinizing hormone; PIH, prolactin-inhibiting hormone; TRH, thyrotropin-releasing hormone; TSH, thyroid-stimulating hormone.

▮ Hormone receptors

Hormones that are hydrophilic cannot penetrate the plasma membrane; they therefore interact with membrane receptors and exert their effects via second messenger molecules (e.g., cyclic adenosine monophosphate [cAMP], phospholipase C, and Ca^{2+}. Examples of hydrophilic hormones are insulin and adrenocorticotropic hormone (ACTH). Conversely, hormones that are lipophilic (e.g., cortisol and estrogen) are able to pass through the cell membrane and interact with receptors in the cytoplasm or nucleus. In this case, receptor binding alters the gene transcription of proteins to exert the hormones' physiological effects.

Fig. 16.1 ▶ Hypothalamic and pituitary hormones.
Hormones released from the hypothalamus stimulate or inhibit the release of hormones from the anterior pituitary. The pituitary hormones then travel to target tissues, where they exert their physiological effects. Posterior pituitary hormones are synthesized in the hypothalamus and stored in the posterior pituitary until release is stimulated by an action potential. These hormones then travel in the blood to their target tissues. (ACTH, adrenocorticotropic hormone; ADH, antidiuretic hormone; CRH, corticotropin-releasing hormone; FSH, follicle-stimulating hormone; GH, growth hormone; GnRH, gonadotropin-releasing hormone; GHRH, growth hormone–releasing hormone; GRIH, growth hormone-inhibiting hormone (somatostatin); LH, luteinizing hormone; PIH, prolactin inhibiting hormone; TRH, thyrotropin-releasing hormone; TSH, thyroid-stimulating hormone.)

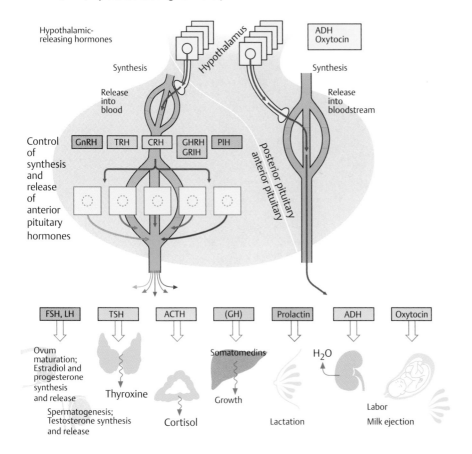

Negative feedback

Negative feedback is when the output of a pathway inhibits inputs to a pathway. This physiological phenomenon is particularly evident in the endocrine system and is an important mechanism in homeostasis.

Growth Hormone

Hypothalamic regulation. Growth hormone release from the anterior pituitary is controlled by two hormones released from the hypothalamus:
- Growth hormone–releasing hormone (GHRH) increases the synthesis and secretion of growth hormone (GH).
- Somatostatin (growth hormone–inhibiting hormone [GHIH]) decreases the sensitivity of the anterior pituitary to GHRH, thus decreasing levels of GH.

Growth hormone receptors

The receptors for GH are found in peripheral tissues and belong to the class 1 cytokine receptor superfamily. These are receptor-associated tyrosine kinase receptors that, upon binding of GH, dimerize and activate the JAK–STAT (Janus kinase–signal transducer and activator of transcription) pathway. The JAK–STAT pathway is a signaling alternative to the second messenger systems. Its activation ultimately causes DNA transcription within the cell.

Factors affecting growth hormone secretion

The major stimuli for GH secretion are deep sleep, hypoglycemia, stress, GHRH, and metabolites (e.g., amino acids and free fatty acids). Secondary stimuli include exercise, glucagon, antidiuretic hormone (ADH), opioids, and pyrogens (fever-inducing substances). GH secretion is inhibited by hyperglycemia and cortisol secretion.

Growth hormone and nitrogen balance

GH creates a positive nitrogen balance in the body. This is mainly due to an increased rate of lipolysis, which provides the energy the body needs while sparing proteins and glucose. Diseases in which there is a negative nitrogen balance, such as acquired immunodeficiency syndrome (AIDS), cachexia (loss of lean body mass that cannot be corrected with increased calorific intake), trauma, and severe burns, can be treated with GH to improve lean body mass and wound healing.

Growth at epiphyseal plates

The epiphyseal plates consist of hyaline cartilage at the end of long bones. Chondrocytes in the epiphyseal plates are constantly undergoing mitosis throughout childhood and adolescence, but ceasing in adulthood. The older cells (at the diaphysis end) are then ossified by osteoblasts. This progressive laying down of bone leads to longitudinal growth. GH acts to increase the mitosis of chondrocytes in the epiphyseal plates..

Carpal tunnel syndrome

Carpal tunnel syndrome is a condition caused by compression of the median nerve within the carpal tunnel of the wrist. It may be caused by anything that produces soft tissue swelling, e.g., pregnancy and rheumatoid arthritis. Symptoms include burning pain, tingling, and numbness in the hand, especially in the thumb, index, middle, and radial half of the ring finger but not the little finger. This pain may be relieved by placing the hand in cold water or by patients "shaking out" their hands. There may also be muscle weakness and wasting. Treatment includes wrist splints, nonsteroidal antiinflammatory drugs (NSAIDs), and corticosteroids (hydrocortisone). Surgical decompression may be necessary if other treatments are ineffective.

Vasoactive intestinal peptide

Vasoactive intestinal peptide (VIP) is a neurocrine peptide secreted by neurons in the mucosa and smooth muscle of the GI tract in response to distention of the stomach and small intestines and vagal activity. It acts to reduce lower esophageal sphincter tone, relax the proximal muscles of the stomach, allowing for entrance of food ("receptive relaxation"), and to increase water and electrolyte secretion in intestine.

Effects. See **Table 16.3.**

Table 16.3 ▶ Effects of Growth Hormone (GH) and Somatomedins*	
Effects Mediated by GH	**Effects Mediated by Somatomedins**

↑ somatomedin synthesis*
 ↑ gluconeogenesis
 ↑ lipolysis
 ↑ protein synthesis
 ↑ amino acid uptake in the gut
 ↓ insulin (causing ↓ glucose uptake into cells)
	↑ protein synthesis resulting in the following effects:
	   ↑ muscle mass
	   ↑ cartilage growth (this causes linear growth)
	   ↑ growth of the internal organs

* Somatomedins are insulinlike growth factors that are intermediaries for some GH actions. Many of the actions of GH occur in association with cortisol.

Disorders
— Deficiency of GH causes short stature with normal body proportions.
— Excess GH leads to gigantism in children and acromegaly in adults.

Somatotropin

Mechanism of action.   Somatotropin is a recombinant form of GH.

Uses
— GH deficiencies in children prior to epiphyseal plate closure (complete ossification)

Side Effects
— Peripheral edema
— Localized muscle pain and weakness
— Carpal tunnel syndrome

Contraindications
— Closed epiphyses
— Active neoplasia

Octreotide and Lanreotide

Mechanism of action.   Octreotide and lanreotide are cyclic peptide analogues of the biologically active portion of somatostatin.

Effects
— These agents mimic the actions of somatostatin to inhibit GH secretion from the anterior pituitary.
— They also inhibit GH secretion from tumors.

Uses
— Acromegaly
— Carcinoid syndrome and vasoactive intestinal polypeptide (VIP)–secreting tumors (octreotide).

Side effects.   Gastrointestinal (GI) side effects, including nausea, diarrhea, and steatorrhea (excess fat in stools), are seen in a majority of patients with acromegaly treated with octreotide. Cholelithiasis (gallstones) is observed in one third of patients with use of octreotide for 6 months or more.

Pegvisomant

Mechanism of action.   Pegvisomant is a GH receptor antagonist that blocks the effects of endogenous GH.

Uses
— Acromegaly in patients unresponsive to surgery, radiation, or octreotide

Adrenocorticotropic Hormone

Hypothalamic regulation.   Corticotropin-releasing hormone (CRH) from the hypothalamus stimulates the release of adrenocorticotropic hormone (ACTH) from the anterior pituitary.

Effects.   The primary target of ACTH is the MC_2 subtype of melanocortin receptor, a G protein–coupled receptor expressed primarily by cells of the adrenal cortex. The MC_2 receptor activates G_s to increase intracellular levels of cyclic AMP, which stimulates the synthesis of corticosteroids, including glucocorticoids, mineralocorticoids, and androgens.

Disorders
— ACTH deficiency causes secondary adrenal insufficiency. This is characterized by fatigue, weakness, anorexia, nausea, and vomiting.
— ACTH excess leads to Cushing syndrome.

Corticorelin

Mechanism of action.   Corticorelin is bovine CRH that acts like the natural hormone.

Uses.   Corticorelin is used to differentiate pituitary ACTH-dependent Cushing disease from ectopic ACTH-secreting tumors (Cushing syndrome). Patients with Cushing disease show normal to increased plasma ACTH and cortisol response, whereas ectopic tumors do not.

Adrenocorticotropic Hormone and Cosyntropin

Mechanism of action.   Cosyntropin is a synthetic peptide consisting of the first 24 amino acids of ACTH. It acts like the natural hormone and is used similarly.

Uses.   These agents are used for the differential diagnosis of primary versus secondary adrenal insufficiency. If there is primary adrenal insufficiency, there will be no response to ACTH; however, if there is secondary adrenal insufficiency due to inadequate ACTH release from the pituitary, administered ACTH will increase plasma glucocorticoids.

Gonadotropins (Follicle-stimulating Hormone and Luteinizing Hormone)

Hypothalamic regulation.   Gonadotropin-releasing hormone (GnRH) released from the hypothalamus stimulates the release of luteinizing hormone (LH) and follicle-stimulating hormone (FSH) from the anterior pituitary.

Effects
— In men, LH stimulates testosterone production by the Leydig cells of the testes. FSH stimulates the Sertoli cells and is critical for maturation of spermatozoa.
— In women, LH stimulates estrogen and progesterone production by the ovaries. FSH stimulates the development of the ovarian follicle (**Fig. 16.2**).

■ Cushing syndrome

Cushing syndrome is a group of signs and symptoms that occur due to high levels of cortisol in the blood. It can be caused by corticosteroid (and ACTH) administration, pituitary adenomas, adrenal gland adenomas/carcinomas, and by excessive intake of alcohol. Signs and symptoms typically include weight gain, particularly to the trunk, with sparing of the limbs; moon face (or moon facies); "buffalo hump" (due to fat deposition on the back); purple striae, especially on the abdomen; sweating; thin skin; and hirsuitism. Treatment depends on the cause.

■ Primary and secondary adrenal insufficiency

Primary adrenal insufficiency occurs when there is impairment or destruction of the adrenal glands. The cause of this may be idiopathic (unknown) or it may be due to autoimmune disease (e.g., Addison's disease), adrenal hyperplasia, or adenoma. Secondary adrenal insufficiency occurs when there is inadequate ACTH secretion from the pituitary to stimulate adrenal hormone production.

Menstrual cycle

The menstrual cycle varies in length from 21 to 35 days. The first half of the cycle is the follicular phase, which begins with menstruation. Following menstruation, in the early follicular phase, FSH induces the production of ~20 follicles. Small amounts of LH are also secreted. Both FSH and LH stimulate enzymes that catalyze the production of androgens that are needed for estrogen synthesis. Estrogens released from follicles cause upregulation of FSH receptors, so the follicle with the highest estrogen content is most sensitive to FSH. This follicle becomes the dominant (graafian) follicle in which an ovum develops. The remaining follicles containing oocytes undergo atresia. In the midfollicular phase, the follicular cells also start to produce progesterone, which causes progressive thickening of the endometrium. In the late follicular phase, increased quantities of FSH and LH are secreted once again. This causes more androgen and estrogen production, which positively feeds back to the hypothalamus, causing an increase in LH. This rapid rise in LH concentration (LH surge) induces ovulation. Just after ovulation, the basal body temperature rises and stays elevated until the end of the cycle. The second half of the cycle is the luteal phase. LH, FSH, and estrogen transform the follicle into a corpus luteum, which secretes large quantities of progesterone, causing further endometrial thickening. If fertilization of the ovum has not occurred, estrogen and progesterone now inhibit FSH and LH both directly and via negative feedback on the hypothalamus and anterior pituitary. This causes a marked drop in plasma estrogen and progesterone concentration, causing constriction of endometrial blood vessels and discharge of the endometrium (menses).

Fig. 16.2 ▶ Hormonal control of the menstrual cycle.
Follicle-stimulating hormone (FSH) and luteinizing hormone (LH) act in the follicular phase to cause follicular growth, estrogen production (causing the selection of a dominant follicle in which the ovum develops), progesterone production (which is primarily responsible for endometrial thickening), and ovulation. Estrogens and progesterone produced in the luteal phase induce endometrial thickening necessary for implantation of the ovum. If this does not occur, feedback inhibition of FSH and LH triggers menstruation.

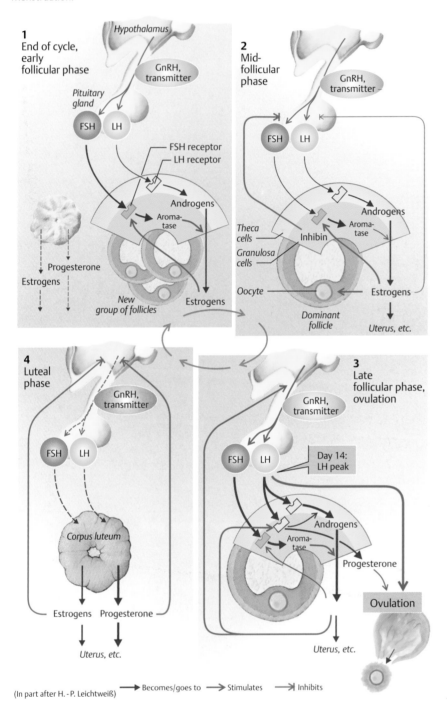

(In part after H. - P. Leichtweiß)　　→ Becomes/goes to　→ Stimulates　⊣ Inhibits

Leuprolide, Goserelin, and Buserelin

Mechanism of action. Leuprolide, goserelin, and buserelin are GnRH agonist analogues. Chronic treatment with one of these agents produces desensitization of the normal response to GnRH. After an initial surge of LH and FSH, the secretion of these hormones decreases.

Pharmacokinetics. These agents are administered intramuscularly in depot form or inhaled intranasally.

Uses

– Endometriosis in women
– Prostatic carcinoma in men

Side effects. These agents may cause bone loss through a prolonged hypoestrogenic state.

Ganirelix and Cetrorelix

Mechanism of action. Ganirelix and cetrorelix are competitive antagonists of GnRH.

Uses. These agents are used to suppress the LH surge and prevent premature follicular luteinization in ovarian-stimulation protocols.

Human Chorionic Gonadotropin and Human Menopausal Gonadotropin (hMG)

Human chorionic gonadotropin (hCG) and human menopausal gonadotropin (hMG) are discussed further in the ovulatory agents section on pages 165 and 166.

Mechanism of action. Both hCG and hMG mimic the effects of gonadotropins.

Pharmacokinetics

– Administered parenterally

Uses

– Used to promote fertility

Thyroid-stimulating Hormone (Thyrotropin)

Hypothalamic control. Thyrotropin-releasing hormone (TRH) is a tripeptide released from the hypothalamus that stimulates thyroid-stimulating hormone (TSH) synthesis and release in the anterior pituitary.

Effects. TSH stimulates the release of thyroid hormones via several mechanisms (see **Table 16.4**).

Table 16.4 ► How Thyroid-Stimulating Hormone (TSH) Increases the Release of Thyroid Hormones
↑ sensitivity of TSH receptors to TSH
↑ thyroglobulin synthesis
↑ thyroid peroxidase and glucose oxidase levels, which increase the iodination of thyroglobulin
↑ activity of the iodide pump
↑ Na^+-K^+ ATPase activity, which increases the capacity for iodide intake
↑ T_3 formation relative to T_4 under acute increases in metabolic demand

■ Endometriosis

Endometriosis is a condition in which endometrial tissue that normally lines the uterus grows outside the uterus. The displaced endometrial tissue (or "implants") responds to FSH and LH during the menstrual cycle as normal endometrial tissue does, causing thickening and then breakdown and bleeding. Surrounding tissue eventually becomes inflamed leading to fibrosis. Symptoms include dysmenorrhea (painful periods); pain during intercourse, bowel movements, or urination; and infertility (usually due to obstruction of the fallopian tubes by scar tissue). Treatment involves the use of NSAIDs for pain, contraceptive hormones to control endometrial buildup, gonadotropin-releasing hormone agonists and antagonists to block the production of FSH and LH, and aromatase inhibitors that block estrogen production. Surgery may be required to remove endometrial implants or hysterectomy in cases of severe endometriosis.

■ Ovarian hyperstimulation syndrome

Ovarian hyperstimulation syndrome occurs when gonadotropins, such as hCG, are given to stimulate ovulation. In ~10 to 25% of patients who are given these drugs parenterally, the ovaries are overstimulated, and fluid leaks from them into the belly and chest following ovulation. Most of the time this produces mild symptoms, such as nausea, vomiting, diarrhea, mild abdominal pain, bloating, and weight gain. However, in a small percentage of cases, these symptoms can be more severe, and there may be additional symptoms, such as shortness of breath (dyspnea), blood clots, electrolyte disturbance, and kidney failure. No treatment may be required if mild, but hospitalization for fluid replacement and management of any serious complications may be necessary for severe cases.

■ Origins of the thyroid gland

The thyroid gland is formed from the pharyngeal arches. During embryonic development, it descends from the foramen cecum of the forming tongue, through the thyroglossal duct, until it reaches its final location in the neck, surrounding the trachea.

Disorders
- TSH deficiency causes secondary hypothyroidism. Symptoms generally mimic those of primary hypothyroidism but are less severe.
- Excess TSH secretion is characterized by goiter and hyperthyroidism.

Protirelin and Thyrotropin

Mechanism of action.   Protirelin is a synthetic peptide identical to TSH. Protirelin and thyrotropin act like the natural hormone.

Uses
- Diagnosis of hypothyroid states (protirelin)
- Given intramuscularly to stimulate iodine 131 (I^{131}) uptake in the treatment of metastatic thyroid carcinoma, but its diagnostic use has largely been replaced by TRH.

Prolactin

Hypothalmic regulation.   Dopamine (prolactin-inhibiting hormone [PIH]) released from the hypothalamus binds to the D_2 subtype of dopamine receptor in the anterior pituitary, which is coupled to G_i and leads to inhibition of adenylate cyclase. This, in turn, causes tonic inhibition of the release of prolactin from the anterior pituitary.

Effects.   Prolactin stimulates the mammary glands to produce milk in the postpartum period.

Disorders.   Loss of PIH after hypothalamic destruction is associated with hypersecretion of prolactin. This causes amenorrhea or galactorrhea.

Cabergoline and Bromocriptine

Mechanism of action.   Cabergoline and bromocriptine are dopamine (PIH) analogue agonists at the D_2 dopamine receptor.

Pharmacokinetics.   Cabergoline has a much longer duration of action (7–14 days) compared with bromocriptine (1–2 days).

Uses
- Prolactin-secreting adenomas
- Amenorrhea or galactorrhea
- Suppression of physiological lactation

Antidiuretic Hormone and Oxytocin

Antidiuretic hormone ([ADH], or vasopressin) and oxytocin are synthesized in the hypothalamus and are transported to the posterior pituitary, where they are stored. Both are peptide hormones consisting of nine amino acids. They differ only in the amino acids at positions 3 and 8, and both have a short half-life (15–30 min) once released into the systemic circulation. Because of their chemical similarities, ADH has slight oxytocic activity, and oxytocin has slight antidiuretic activity. However, oxytocin has no vasoconstricting activity.

See Chapter 17 for a further discussion of oxytocin and Chapter 19 for a discussion of ADH.

Stimuli for ADH synthesis and secretion

ADH is synthesized and released in response to increased plasma osmolality (detected by hypothalamic osmoreceptors), e.g., dehydration; decreased plasma volume (detected by peripheral mechanoreceptors), e.g., hemorrhage (hypovolemia); and decreased blood pressure (detected by baroreceptors). Its release is most sensitive to plasma osmolality, yet larger quantities of ADH are released in response to changes in blood pressure and blood volume.

Table 16.5 summarizes the drugs affecting hypothalamic and pituitary hormone levels.

Table 16.5 ▶ Drugs Affecting Hypothalamic and Pituitary Hormones	
Drug	**Mechanism**
Agonists	
Octreotide, lantreotide	Somatostatin analogues
Somatotropin	GH analogue
Corticorelin	CRH analogue
ACTH, Cosyntropin	ACTH analogue
hCG, hMG	Mimics gonadotropins
Protirelin, thyrotropin	TSH analogues
Cabergoline, bromocriptine	Dopamine (PIH) analogues
Antagonists	
Pegvisomant	GH receptor antagonist
Ganirelix, cetrorelix	Competitive inhibitors of GnRH
Abbreviations: ACTH, adrenocorticotropic hormone; hCG, human chorionic gonadotropin; hMG, human menopausal gonadotropin.	

16.2 Thyroid Hormones

The natural thyroid hormones produced by the thyroid gland are thyroxine (T_4) and triiodothyronine (T_3). The mechanism of their release and degradation is shown in **Fig. 16.3**.

Fig. 16.3 ▶ **Thyroid hormones: release, effects, and degradation.**
TRH from the hypothalamus causes TSH release from the anterior pituitary. The thyroid secretes the hormones thyroxine (T_4) and triiodothyronine (T_3). T_4 is produced in higher quantities than T_3, but T_3 is the more active form. T_4 is converted to T_3 in tissues. T_3 attaches to effector cell receptors, producing its physiological effects. It also causes feedback inhibition of TSH production.

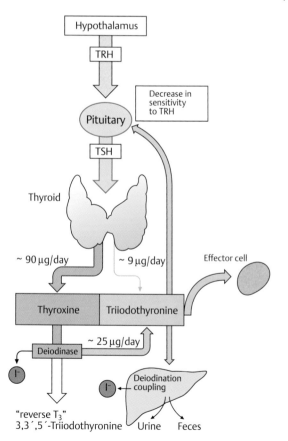

■ Thyroid hormone synthesis

The follicles of the thyroid gland synthesize and store thyroglobulin (TG), a glycoprotein with tyrosine residues. These tyrosine residues are conjugated with iodine (from dietary sources), under the influence of the enzyme thyroid peroxidase, to form monoiodotyrosine (MIT) or diiodotyrosine (DIT). These then undergo a coupling reaction, while still attached to TG, to produce T_3 (MIT + DIT) or T_4 (DIT + DIT). Proteolysis of TG releases free T_3 and T_4 into the circulation.

Mechanism of action. Most cells in the body are responsive to thyroid hormones. Within cells, T_4 is converted to T_3, the active form. T_3 binds to its receptor in the cell nucleus to affect gene transcription.

Effects. See **Table 16.6.**

Table 16.6 ▶ Effects of Thyroid Hormones	
Category	**Effects**
Development	Essential for CNS development
Growth	↑ protein synthesis ↑ bone formation (with GH and somatomedins) ↑ ossification and fusion of growth plates
Metabolic	↑ intestinal absorption of glucose ↑ gluconeogenesis, glycogenolysis, and glucose oxidation ↑ lipolysis ↑ cholesterol turnover and plasma clearance of cholesterol T_3 potentiates the "hypoglycemic" actions of insulin by increasing glucose uptake into muscle and adipose tissue.
Basal metabolic rate (BMR)	↑ BMR ↑ ATP hydrolysis (↑ O_2 consumption and heat as a consequence of the above)
Systemic	Stimulation of adrenergic β-receptors leading to increased heart rate, cardiac output, and ventilation and decreased peripheral vascular resistance. These actions support increased oxygen demand in tissues. T_3 facilitates the actions of cortisol, glucagon, and GH.

Abbreviations: ATP, adenosine triphosphate; CNS, central nervous system; GH, growth hormone.

Pharmacokinetics

— T_4 has a slower onset, is more extensively bound to plasma proteins, and has a longer duration of action than T_3.
— T_3 is four times more potent than T_4.

Treatment of Hypothyroidism

Levothyroxine

Levothyroxine, a synthetic form of the thyroxine (T_4), is the drug of choice for replacement therapy.

Uses

— Hypothyroidism, regardless of etiology, including congenital (cretinism)
— Autoimmune thyroiditis (e.g., Hashimoto thyroiditis)
— Pregnancy and postpartum hypothyroidism
— Thyroid carcinoma (to suppress TSH)

Toxicity. It causes tachycardia, palpitations, restlessness, tremor, and cardiac arrhythmias.

Treatment of Hyperthyroidism and Related Disorders

Propylthiouracil and Methimazole

Mechanism of action. Propylthiouracil and methimazole inhibit thyroid hormone synthesis by inhibiting the peroxidase enzyme that catalyzes the iodination of tyrosine residues in thyroglobulin and couples iodotyrosines to form T_3 and T_4. Effects are not apparent until the thyroid reserve is depleted.

■ **Hypothyroidism (myxedema)**

Hypothyroidism occurs due to decreased levels of plasma T_3 and T_4. Metabolism is slowed producing symptoms such as weight gain, constipation, cold intolerance, lethargy, depression, and dementia. Signs of hypothyroidism include bradycardia, dry skin and face, goiter, congestive heart failure, and edema. This condition may be spontaneously acquired, or it may occur after a thyroidectomy, radioiodine treatment, or following drug therapy (e.g., amiodarone and lithium). It is treated by replacement therapy with levothyroxine. More severe, life-threatening hypothyroidism is called myxedema crisis. This can lead to impaired cognition, somnolence (sleepiness), and coma (myxedema coma). Myxedema can be treated with IV levothyroxine or with liothyronine to achieve a more rapid response.

Pharmacokinetics

- Methimazole is more potent and has a longer duration than propylthiouracil.
- These drugs cross the placenta and are excreted into milk.
- Babies who are exposed to these agents should have thyroid function monitored.

Uses

- Hyperthyroidism

Side effects

- Rash is common.
- Agranulocytosis (acute low white blood cell count) is rare but serious.

Radioiodine (Sodium Iodide, I^{131})

Mechanism of action.   Radioiodine accumulates in the thyroid gland and destroys parenchymal cells. Clinical improvement may take 2 to 3 months.

Uses.   It is the preferred treatment for most patients with hyperthyroidism. Subsequent hypothyroidism occurs in 20 to 80% of patients.

Iodine (Lugol Solution, Potassium Iodide)

Mechanism of action.   Iodine (supraphysiological dose) inhibits thyroid hormone release, but the effect is not sustained (Wolff-Chaikoff effect); therefore, it only produces a temporary remission of symptoms.

Uses

- Thyrotoxicosis
- Prior to thyroid surgery (to decrease vascularity of the gland)
- Following radioiodine therapy

Propranolol, Atenolol, Esmolol, and Metoprolol

The pharmacology of these adrenergic blocking agents was discussed in Chapter 6.

Uses.   These agents are used as adjuncts to treat or prevent thyrotoxicosis.

16.3   Parathyroid Hormone and Other Factors Affecting Bone Metabolism

The major hormones involved in bone mineral homeostasis are parathyroid hormone (PTH) and vitamin D (**Fig. 16.4**). Other endogenous regulators of bone metabolism are calcitonin, glucocorticoids, and estrogens. Numerous exogenous agents are available that affect bone and mineral homeostasis.

Hyperthyroidism (thyrotoxicosis)

Hyperthyroidism occurs when there are elevated levels of T_3 and T_4 in the blood. Patients may develop hyperthyroidism due to adenomas/carcinomas of the thyroid gland or thyroiditis (inflammation of the thyroid), or it may be autoimmune in origin. Signs and symptoms are reflective of a hypermetabolic state and include weight loss, increased appetite, frequent stools, tremor, heat intolerance, increased sweating, tachycardia, tremor, ptosis (lid lag) and thyroid enlargement. Severe hyperthyroidism (thyrotoxic storm) is a medical emergency. Treatment depends on the cause.

Na$^+$- I$^-$ Pump

Iodine (from ingested food) is necessary for thyroid hormone synthesis. Because dietary intake inevitably varies, the thyroid gland must sequester iodine so that adequate amounts are always available for thyroid hormone synthesis. It does this via the Na+-I- pump on the cell membrane. The pump symports two Na+ ions into the cytoplasm for every one I- ion. It is driven by the low intracellular [Na+], via facilitated diffusion, that is maintained by the Na+-K+-ATPase pump. TSH is the major physiological stimulator of the iodide pump. High intracellular levels of iodide inhibit the activity of the pump.

Wolff–Chaikoff effect

The Wolff–Chaikoff effect is a reduction in the synthesis and release of thyroid hormones caused by a large amount of iodine. This effect lasts ~10 days, after which iodine incorporation into TG and thyroid peroxidase function returns to normal. It is widely believed that the resumption of normal functioning is due to downregulation of the iodide pump on the follicular cell membrane. The Wolff–Chaikoff effect is the principle behind the use of iodine for the treatment of hyperthyroidism. Amiodarone may also elicit this side effect, given that it contains iodine.

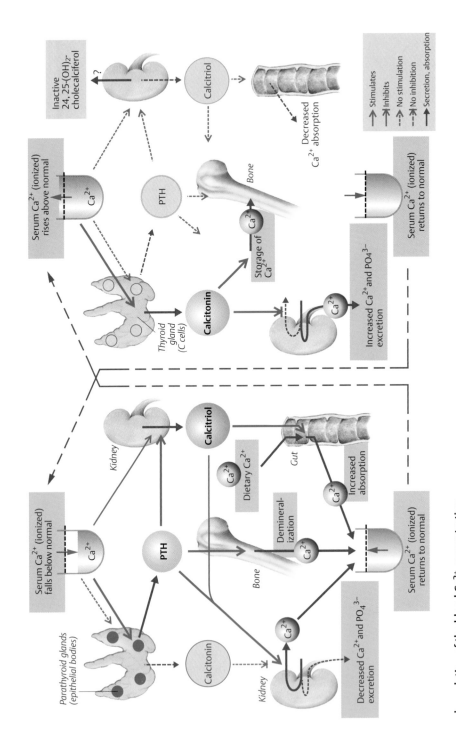

Fig. 16.4 ▶ **Hormonal regulation of the blood Ca²⁺ concentration.**
Ca²⁺ homeostasis is achieved by three main hormones: parathyroid hormone (PTH, from parathyroid gland), calcitonin (from parafollicular cells of the thyroid gland), and calcitriol (mainly produced in the kidney). In low serum Ca²⁺ states, the actions of parathyroid hormone and calcitriol predominate, causing increased Ca²⁺ uptake from the gut and bone and decreased renal excretion. In high serum Ca²⁺ states, the action of calcitonin predominates, causing decreased Ca²⁺ uptake from the gut, increased renal excretion, and storage of excess Ca²⁺ in bone.

Parathyroid Hormone

Regulation of secretion.   PTH is released from the parathyroid glands in response to low plasma Ca^{2+} concentrations.

Effects.   See **Table 16.7.**

Table 16.7 ► Effects of Parathyroid Hormone (PTH)	
Organ/System	**Effects**
Bone	Mobilization of Ca^{2+} and PO_4^{3-} from bone In the longer term, PTH increases the number of both osteoblasts and osteoclasts and increases the remodeling of bone (**Fig. 16.10**).*
Kidney	↑ Ca^{2+} reabsorption ↑ formation of calcitriol which is the active form of vitamin D
GI tract	↑ absorption of Ca^{2+} (effect mediated via calcitriol)

* Daily, intermittent administration of PTH for 1 to 2 hours per day leads to a net stimulation of bone formation. Continuous exposure to elevated PTH leads to bone resorption.
Abbreviation: GI, gastrointestinal.

Teriparatide

Mechanism of action.   Teriparatide is a synthetic polypeptide PTH analogue; it therefore affects calcium homeostasis in the same way as PTH.

Pharmacokinetics
— Given by daily subcutaneous injection

Uses
— Osteoporosis in postmenopausal women at high risk of fracture
— Hypogonadal osteoporosis in men at high risk of fracture

Cinacalcet

Mechanism of action
Cinacalcet activates the Ca^{2+}-sensing receptor of the parathyroid gland, which leads to decreased PTH secretion.

Uses
— Hypercalcemia
— Primary hyperparathyroidism

Vitamin D

The term *vitamin D* refers to cholecalciferol (vitamin D_3) and ergocalciferol (vitamin D_2), which are interchangeable with respect to clinical use. Ergocalciferol is the prescription form of vitamin D and is also used as a food additive. Cholecalciferol is usually used for vitamin D–fortified milk and foods; it is also available in drug combination products. The metabolism of vitamin D is shown in **Fig. 16.5.**

■ Components of bone

The three major components of bone are osteogenic cells (osteoblasts, osteocytes, and osteoclasts), organic matrix, and mineral. The matrix consists of collagen and proteoglycans and accounts for approximately one third of bone mass. The mineral component of bone is calcium phosphate crystals deposited as hydroxyapatite (two thirds of bone mass).

■ Physiological roles of calcium

Calcium is vital to normal body functioning, and its levels must be maintained within tight limits. Calcium is the major structural element of bones and teeth, where it is stored in the form of hydroxyapatite crystals [$Ca_{10}(PO_4)_6(OH)_2$]. It is also involved in neural transmission, muscle contraction, vasodilation and vasoconstriction of blood vessels, activation of vitamin K–dependent clotting factors (II, VII, IX, and X), and secretion of hormones (e.g., insulin).

■ Magnesium and bone metabolism

Magnesium is the fourth most abundant mineral in the body. About half of the body's magnesium is stored in the hydroxyapatite crystals of bone, and the other half is intracellular. The levels of magnesium in the blood are well regulated and tend to follow those of calcium and phosphate. Like calcium and phosphate, magnesium has a role in bone turnover (but to a much lesser extent). Magnesium deficiency may result from severe diarrhea, alcohol abuse, drugs (e.g., diuretics), and diabetic ketoacidosis. It causes parethesias, seizures, arrhythmias, and tetany (due to accompanying hypocalcemia and hypokalemia). Treatment is by replacement of magnesium.

■ Chronic renal failure and renal osteodystrophy

In chronic renal failure, the failing kidneys are unable to perform the necessary 1-α-hydroxylation reactions to produce calcitriol, and they have a reduced capacity to excrete phosphate. This leads to hyperparathyroidism due to hypocalcemia and hyperphosphatemia. Derangement of bone remodeling occurs, which is referred to as renal osteodystrophy. The symptoms of renal osteodystrophy include bone and joint pain, bone deformation, and increased likelihood of bone fractures. Chronic renal failure requires hemodialysis several times per week until renal transplantation can occur. Renal osteodystrophy is treated by calcium and calcitriol, restricting dietary intake of phosphate, and by the administration of medications that bind phosphate, such as calcium carbonate and calcium acetate.

Multiple endocrine neoplasia type I

Multiple endocrine neoplasia type 1 (MEN1) is a rare, inherited disorder that causes multiple tumors (usually benign) in the endocrine glands and duodenum. It affects both genders equally and is usually not detected until adulthood, when tumors start growing. The parathyroid glands are most commonly affected. Tumors in the parathyroid gland cause hyperparathyroidism, which leads to hypercalcemia and its associated symptoms. It also commonly affects the pancreas, causing gastrinomas (from excess gastrin secretion), which, in turn, causes ulcers. These ulcers are more sinister than normal gastric ulcers and are highly prone to perforate. Multiple gastrinomas causing ulcers is referred to as Zollinger–Ellison syndrome. Pancreatic tumors may also cause insulinomas, leading to hypoglycemia; glucagon excess, leading to diabetes; or vasoactive intestinal peptide (VIP), leading to watery diarrhea. Pituitary tumors may also occur, leading to derangement of its hormones. Patients with MEN1 are more likely to develop cancerous tumors in later life. MEN1 can be detected early by gene testing, and individuals affected have a 50% chance of passing the disease to their children. There is no cure for MEN1, but there are various drugs and surgical options to treat the effects.

Fig. 16.5 ▶ **Vitamin D metabolism.**
Ultraviolet light B (UVB) converts 7-dehydrocholesterol to cholecalciferol (vitamin D_3). Ingested vitamin D is fat soluble and is transported to the liver in chylomicrons. All free vitamin D is transported in the blood and liver by a specific vitamin D–binding protein (DBP). The liver converts vitamin D to 25-hydroxycholecalciferol 25-(OH)-D, which is then transported to the kidneys, where it is converted to its active form $1,25\text{-}(OH)_2\text{-}D$, under the influence of parathyroid hormone. The effects of this are increased mineralization of bone, increased calcium and phosphate reabsorption in the kidneys, and increased calcium absorption in the gut. Excess vitamin D is excreted into bile.

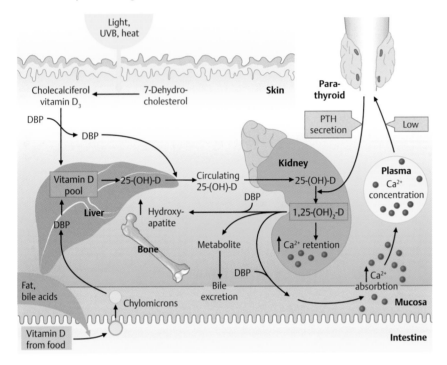

Effects
- *Bone:* The effects of vitamin D on bone are a result of its actions that provide the proper balance of Ca^{2+} and PO_4^{3-} to support bone mineralization.
- *Kidney:* Increased reabsorption of Ca^{2+} and PO_4^{3-}
- *Gastrointestinal tract:* Increased absorption of Ca^{2+}

Ergocalciferol

Uses
- Hypoparathyroidism
- Prophylaxis of vitamin D deficiency

Calcitonin

Calcitonin is produced by the parafollicular cells (C cells) of the thyroid gland. It is released when there is an elevated level of Ca^{2+} in the blood.

Effects
- *Bone:* Decreases bone resorption by inhibiting osteoclast activity (**Fig. 16.6**)
- *Kidney:* Decreases reabsorption of Ca^{2+} and PO_4^{3-}, thus increasing their excretion

Calcitonin (exogenous)

Pharmacokinetics
- Available as a nasal spray

Uses
- Paget disease
- Hypercalcemia
- Osteoporosis

Glucocorticoids

Cortisol

Mechanism of action. Glucocorticoids, e.g., cortisol, enhance bone loss by decreasing Ca^{2+} absorption, increasing Ca^{2+} excretion, and blocking bone formation.

Uses
- Hypercalcemia of malignancy
- Vitamin D poisoning

Side effects. Prolonged administration leads to osteoporosis.

Estrogens and Selective Estrogen Receptor Modulators (SERMs)

Estrogens: Estradiol, Premarin™, Ethinyl Estradiol, Mestranol, and Diethylstilbesterol
- Estradiol esters are administered intramuscularly and by a transdermal patch.
- Premarin™ is a conjugated estrogen that contains estrone and equilin. It is administered orally.
- Ethinyl estradiol and mestranol are synthetic steroid estrogens that are administered orally.
- Diethylstilbestrol is a nonsteroidal synthetic estrogen that is administered orally or parenterally.

Mechanism of action. Estrogens decrease osteoclast activity. The mechanism by which this occurs is unclear, but it may be that the estrogens cause an increase in cytokines (small cell-signaling protein molecules) that support osteoclast formation, or they increase the rate of apoptosis of osteoclasts (**Fig. 16.6**). Estrogens may also decrease other cytokines that decrease osteoblasts.

SERM: Raloxifene

See page 163 and Fig. 17.3 for a further discussion of SERMs.

Uses. Estrogens and SERM agents are used (in the context of bone regulation) to treat post-menopausal osteoporosis. However, estrogens are now only used with caution in patients for whom nonestrogen therapies are not appropriate.

Bisphosphonates

Alendronate, Etidronate, Ibendronate, Pamidronate, Risedronate, Tiludronate, and Zoledronate

Mechanism of action. Bisphosphonates are exogenous regulators of bone metabolism. They are analogues of pyrophosphate that accumulate in bone and prevent bone resorption by inhibiting osteoclast activity (**Fig. 16.4**).

Uses
- Prevention and treatment of osteoporosis

■ Paget disease

Paget disease is a metabolic bone disease which affects 2 to 3% of the population over age 60. It consists of increased bone resorption and new bone formation; however, the newly formed bone is disordered, leading to bowing, stress fractures and arthritis. Additional symptoms may include enlargement of the skull, femur, and clavicle. Nerve compression may occur due to bony overgrowth causing pain, paresthesias, or numbness. Complications include congestive heart failure (due to increased work of the heart) and sarcomas (rarely). Blood biochemistry results show that Ca^{2+} and PO_4^{3-} are usually normal but alkaline phosphatase (ALP) is markedly increased. Because ALP is a by-product of osteoblastic activity, levels of ALP are raised during periods of rapid bone growth (puberty), in bone diseases that cause bone turnover (e.g., Paget disease and osteomalacia), and during calcium derangement (e.g., hyperparathyroidism). Treatment is with a bisphosphonate and/or calcitonin.

■ Bisphosphonates and osteonecrosis of the jaw

Osteonecrosis is death of bone tissue due to a lack of blood supply. Bisphosphonate usage puts patients at risk of developing osteonecrosis of the jaw, which can present following dental extractions. It produces symptoms such as bone pain, swelling, infections, exposed bone, numbness, and loosening of the teeth. This condition usually occurs with IV bisphosphonates, but it can occur when they are taken orally. Patients who are at risk of developing osteonecrosis should have any sources of infection treated before bisphosphonate therapy is initiated to prevent the condition from developing. However, if osteonecrosis does occur, surgical débridement of necrotic bone and areas of infection is necessary.

Fig. 16.6 ▶ **Regulation of bone remodeling.**
Bone remodeling is complex and is initiated by osteoblasts upon stimulation by parathyroid hormone. Osteoblasts interact directly with osteoclast precursors (that form from progenitor cells) via RANKL. Estrogens (and OPG secreted by osteoblasts) block RANKL, thus inhibiting the fusion of osteoclast precursors and their activation to osteoclasts. They also promote osteoclast apoptosis. Bisphosphonates inhibit bone resorption by inhibiting osteoclast activity and promoting apoptosis. Calcitonin inhibits bone resorption by transferring active osteoclasts into a resting state.

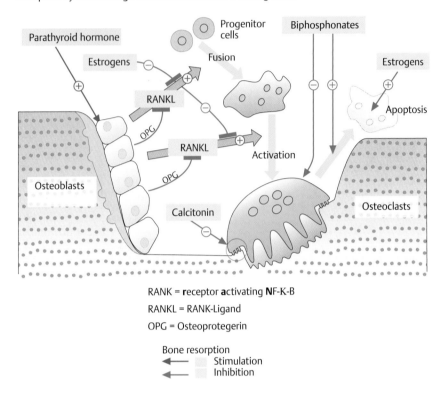

RANK = **r**eceptor **a**ctivating **N**F-K-B
RANKL = RANK-Ligand
OPG = Osteoprotegerin

Bone resorption
◄——☐ Stimulation
◄——☐ Inhibition

Fluoride

Mechanism of action.   Fluoride accumulates in bone and teeth where it slows resorption and promotes calcification.

Uses

— It is added to drinking water to prevent dental caries
— May have a positive effect in osteoporosis

16.4   Adrenocortical Hormones

The adrenocortical steroids, or corticosteroids, are steroid hormones produced by the adrenal cortex (**Fig. 16.7**). They include glucocorticoids, mineralocorticoids, and androgens. The glucocorticoids regulate metabolism and stress responses, and the mineralocorticoids regulate sodium reabsorption. Androgens will be covered on pages 166–168, Chapter 17.

Fig. 16.7 ▶ Hormonal secretions of the adrenal gland.
Stress causes the release of corticotropin-releasing hormone (CRH) from the hypothalamus, which then stimulates adrenocorticotropic hormone (ACTH) release from the anterior pituitary. ACTH acts on all zones of the adrenal cortex, but it predominantly causes the release of cortisol from the fascicular zone. One of the local actions of cortisol is to stimulate the release of norepinephrine and epinephrine from the adrenal medulla, although the main stimulus for this is sympathetic system activation. Cortisol causes negative feedback inhibition of ACTH (predominantly) and CRH.

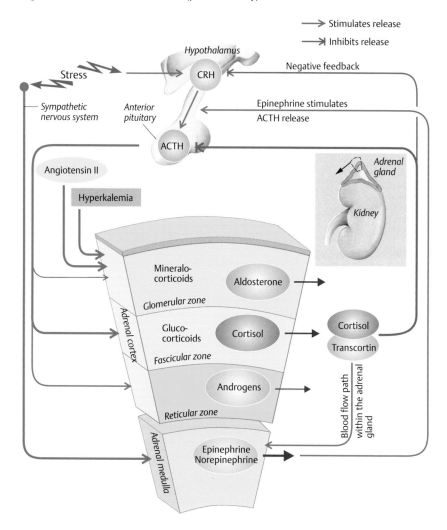

Glucocorticoids

Regulation of secretion. The natural glucocorticoids, cortisol and corticosterone, are synthesized and released in response to ACTH from the anterior pituitary, which is released in response to CRH from the hypothalamus.

Mechanism of action. Glucocorticoids bind to receptors in the cytosol. These receptors then dissociate from heat shock protein complexes, translocate to the nucleus, and bind to specific sites on DNA within the nucleus, altering gene transcription.

Fig. 16.8 ▶ **Glucocorticoids: receptors and second messengers.**
Glucocorticoids act to alter gene transcription, the effects of which are to reduce inflammation. At higher concentrations, they may also act on the cell membrane to reduce the activation capacity of the cell. (ACE, angiotensin-converting enzyme; COX-2, cyclooxygenase-2; hsp, heat shock protein; mRNA, messenger RNA.

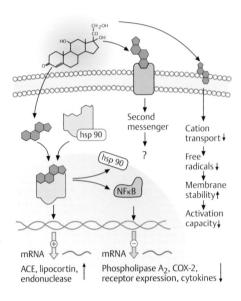

At higher concentrations, glucocorticoids are thought to be integrated into the cell membrane, which alters the physiochemical properties of the cell. The ultimate effect of these changes is that the activation capacity of the cell is reduced (**Fig. 16.8**).

Effects.   **Table 16.8** lists the effects of glucocorticoids. These are further illustrated in **Figs. 16.9** and **16.10**.

Hydrocortisone (Cortisol), Prednisone, Methylprednisolone, Triamcinolone, Dexamethasone, Betamethasone, Beclomethasone, and Fluocinonide

Mechanism of action.   These agents are synthetic glucocorticoids that act like the endogenous hormones.

Table 16.8 ▶ Effects of Glucocorticoids	
Category	**Effects**
Metabolic	↑ hepatic gluconeogenesis ↑ glycogen synthesis ↑ proteolysis ↑ release of amino acids (key enzymes) for gluconeogenesis ↑ lipolysis, which increases fatty acid and ketone body formation ↓ peripheral glucose utilization
Antiinflammatory (see also **Fig. 16.10**)	↓ transcription of most cytokines and chemokines leads to reduced synthesis of these mediators and decreased activation of leukocytes. ↓ transcription of phospholipase A$_2$ and cyclooxygenase-2 (COX-2) results in decreased formation of prostaglandins and thromboxanes (see page 347). ↓ expression of adhesion molecules necessary for leukocyte chemotaxis ↑ expression of antiinflammatory molecules, such as neutral endopeptidase and lipocortins

The effect of corticosteroids on the respiratory burst

The respiratory burst is the rapid release of reactive oxygen species (superoxide radical and hydrogen peroxide) from phagocytes (neutrophils and monocytes) when a microbe is encountered and phagocytosed. It is one of the mechanisms by which phagocytes exert their microbicidal effects and is an important immune defense. The reactive oxygen species are generated by the partial reduction of oxygen in the respiratory chain (electron transport chain). They combine with Cl⁻ to form hypochlorous acid, which dissociates to form hypochlorite ions, which kill the microbes. Cortisol (and exogenous corticosteroids) inhibits the respiratory burst and may predispose an individual to infection.

Fig. 16.9 ▶ Glucocorticoids: principal and adverse effects.
Therapeutic levels of cortisol suppress the inflammatory response. This is useful in treating conditions such as allergy and autoimmune disease and to prevent transplant rejection, where the inflammatory response is unwanted. However, cortisol also produces a number of adverse effects related to its antiinflammatory, mineralocorticoid, and glucocorticoid actions. The relative mineralocorticoid potencies (blue) and glucocorticoid potencies (brown) of some corticosteroids are included.

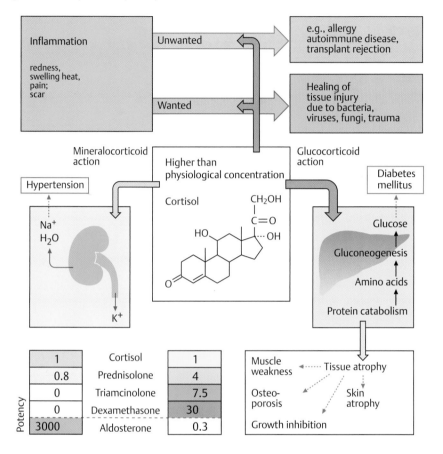

Potency			
1	Cortisol	1	
0.8	Prednisolone	4	
0	Triamcinolone	7.5	
0	Dexamethasone	30	
3000	Aldosterone	0.3	

Fig. 16.10 ▶ Effects of glucocorticoids on the immune system.
Glucocorticoids act on a wide range of cells, including blood cells, endothelial cells, and fibroblasts, as well as receptor proteins and proinflammatory mediators, to reduce inflammation and its spread. (Fc, fragment, crystallizable; IL, interleukin; MHC, major histocompatibility complex; TNF, tumor necrosis factor.)

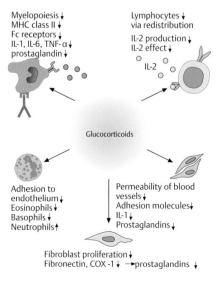

Pharmacokinetics. These agents are effective orally, parenterally, and topically.

Note: Beclomethasone and fluocinonide are for local use only.

Table 16.9 lists the duration of action of these agents.

Table 16.9 ▶ **Duration of Action of Glucocorticoids**	
Duration of Action	**Agent (s)**
Short	Hydrocortisone (cortisol)
Intermediate	Prednisone, methylprednisolone, triamcinolone
Long	Dexamethasone, betamethasone

Uses

— Endocrine
  — Adrenocortical insufficiency (Addison disease)
  — Congenital adrenal hyperplasia (to suppress ACTH release)
— Non-endocrine
  — Rheumatoid arthritis
  — Leukemia
  — Lymphoma
  — Allergic reactions
  — Asthma
  — Inflammatory and autoimmune disorders
  — Immunosuppression for transplantation
  — Collagen disorders
  — Cerebral edema
  — Bacterial meningitis

Side effects. Large doses of glucocorticoids for 1 week or less do not pose problems, but patients with non-endocrine disorders who receive systemic corticosteroids for longer times develop adverse effects, including inhibition of CRH release from the hypothalamus and ACTH release from the anterior pituitary (**Fig. 16.11**). Some of the side effects experienced include

— Hyperglycemia
— Increased susceptibility to infection
— Weight gain (cushingoid features)
— Osteoporosis
— Behavioral and personality changes
— Myopathy
— Ocular effects
— Growth retardation in children

When possible, glucocorticoids should be administered locally, e.g., as an aerosol spray in asthma, to minimize adverse effects, or alternate-day therapy should be used.

■ **Acute adrenal crisis (addisonian crisis)**

Acute adrenal crisis (addisonian crisis) is due to acute insufficiency of adrenal corticosteroids, mainly cortisol. It usually occurs in people with known Addison disease who undergo some form of stress, such as surgery, trauma, or infection, but it may also occur on abrupt cessation of long-term steroids. The main sign of acute adrenal crisis is shock (hypotension, tachycardia, or oliguria), but there may also be acute abdominal pain, diarrhea, vomiting, hypoglycemia, fever, weakness, and confusion. It may progress to seizures, coma, and death if untreated. If there is a high index of suspicion for acute adrenal crisis, treatment should begin before the results of any laboratory tests are known. Treatment involves giving intravenous (IV) fluids, hydrocortisone, antibiotics, and glucose if necessary. In the longer term, the patient can be switched to oral steroids, and the precipitating factor should be treated.

■ **Perioperative steroid coverage**

Patients who have been on long-term steroids or have stopped steroids recently will have some adrenal suppression. Consequently, the perioperative administration of steroids prior to undergoing the stress of surgery is necessary to prevent adrenal crisis, the major effect of which is shock.

Fig. 16.11 ▶ Cortisol release and its modification by glucocorticoids.
Exogenous glucocorticoids cause feedback inhibition of endogenous cortisol production. Depending on the dose, this can cause endogenous cortisol production to decrease or cease completely. If cortisol production is not required by the adrenal cortex, it undergoes atrophy and cannot resume normal cortisol output if exogenous glucocorticoids are abruptly stopped. The dosing regimen of glucocorticoids can minimize adrenocortical atrophy. If they are given when normal cortical secretion is high and feedback inhibition is low (late morning), then the glucocorticoid is eliminated during daytime, and normal cortisol production starts early the following morning.

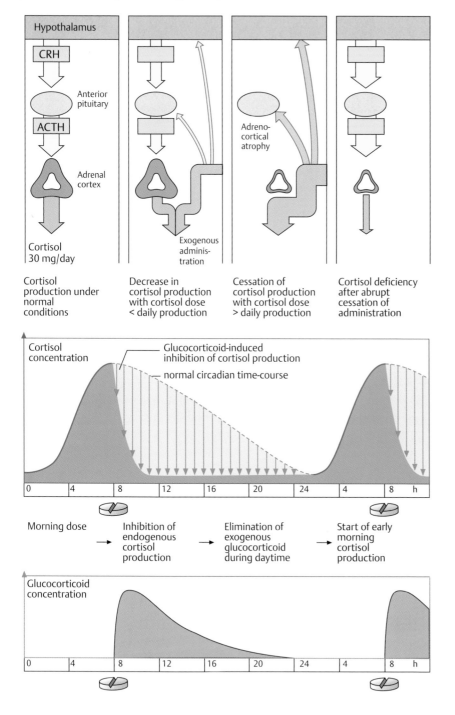

The renin-angiotensin-aldosterone system regulates Na$^+$ balance, fluid volume, and blood pressure. Renin is released by the kidneys in response to reduced perfusion. Renin then stimulates the production of angiotensin II from angiotensin I in the lungs. Angiotensin II causes vasoconstriction and aldosterone secretion from the adrenal glands. Aldosterone causes Na$^+$ (and water) reabsorption, thus increasing fluid volume, blood pressure, and renal perfusion.

■ Cholesterol and steroid
synthesis

Steroid hormones are produced from cholesterol ($C_{27}H_{46}O$). All steroid-producing tissues cleave the side chain of cholesterol between carbons 20 and 22 to form pregnenolone (via cholesterol desmolase). This is the rate-limiting step. In most cases, pregnenolone is then converted to progesterone. In the gonads, progesterone is converted to testosterone via cleavage of the remaining side chain. In many tissues, a 5α-reductase converts testosterone to 5α-dihydrotestosterone (DHT), which is the more active form of the hormone. The ovary also makes testosterone but does not release it. Instead, it aromatizes ring A (resulting in the loss of carbon 19) to form 18 carbon steroids (estradiol, estrone). In the adrenal cortex, hydroxylations produce cortisol and aldosterone. Some conversion of pregnenolone to androgens (especially dehydroepiandrosterone [DHEA]) and estrogens may occur.

Mineralocorticoids

The major mineralocorticoid produced by the adrenal gland is aldosterone. Aldosterone has a very short half-life and is not used therapeutically.

Regulation of secretion.   Aldosterone secretion is regulated by the renin-angiotensin-aldosterone system (see pages 181–183).

Effects.   Mineralocorticoids help maintain normal blood volume by promoting Na$^+$ reabsorption by the distal tubules. K$^+$ and H$^+$ ions are excreted in exchange.

Fludrocortisone

Mechanism of action.   Fludrocortisone is a synthetic corticosteroid that has much greater mineralocorticoid than glucocorticoid activity.

Pharmacokinetics
— Orally effective

Uses
— Used in salt-losing forms of adrenal insufficiency

Spironolactone

See page 188 for further discussion of this agent.

Mechanism of action.   Spironolactone is an aldosterone receptor antagonist.

Uses
— Primary hyperaldosteronism
— Cushing syndrome
— Adrenal adenoma or carcinoma
— Ectopic ACTH-producing tumors

Aminoglutethimide

Mechanism of action.   Aminoglutethimide blocks the conversion of cholesterol to pregnenolone, thereby decreasing secretion of all adrenal cortical steroids.

Uses
— Cushing syndrome
— Adrenal adenoma or carcinoma
— Ectopic ACTH-producing tumors

17 Drugs Used in Reproductive Endocrinology

17.1 Estrogens

The naturally occurring estrogens are the C18 steroids: 17 estradiol, estrone, and estriol, which are secreted by granulosa (follicular) cells within the ovary. 17-estradiol is the major estrogen in premenopausal women, and it maintains reproductive tissues and processes, along with progesterone. Estrogens also have important effects on metabolism, e.g., on transport proteins, clotting factors, electrolyte balance, and serum lipids.

Like other steroids, estrogen binds to receptors in the cytosol and alters DNA transcription.

Effects. See **Table 17.1.**

Table 17.1 ▶ Effects of Estrogen	
Category	**Effects**
Ovulation and reproduction	Supports the growth and maturation of ovarian follicles and endometrium (along with progesterone) and stimulates ovulation ↑ the growth and the motility of the smooth muscle of the uterus and increases uterine blood flow ↓ the viscosity of cervical mucus and makes it more alkaline to support the survival of sperm
Puberty	Initiates ductal development in the breasts Controls the female body configuration (e.g., narrow shoulders and broad hips) and the distribution of fat in the breasts and buttocks
Bone	↑ osteoblast activity ↓ apoptosis of osteoblasts ↓ the number and activity of osteoclasts The net result is an increased formation of bone in the presence of estrogen.
Brain	Estrogen may have a neuroprotective effect to increase neuronal survival and levels of neuronal growth factors and improve cognition.
Cholesterol levels	↓ LDL levels ↑ HDL levels

Abbreviations: HDL, high-density lipoprotein; LDL, low-density lipoprotein.

Estrogens: Estradiol, Premarin, Ethinyl Estradiol, Mestranol, and Diethylstilbestrol

Several types of estrogen preparations are available, and their effectiveness orally when taken depends on the extent of metabolism by the liver.

— Estradiol esters are administered intramuscularly and by a transdermal patch (**Fig. 17.1**).
— Premarin™ is a conjugated estrogen that contains estrone and equilin. It is administered orally.
— Ethinyl estradiol and mestranol are synthetic steroid estrogens that are administered orally.
— Diethylstilbestrol (DES) is a nonsteroidal synthetic estrogen that is administered orally or parenterally.

Note: Estrogens are usually administered in cyclic fashion with a progestin (a natural or synthetic steroid hormone that has progesterone-like activity unless the uterus has been removed).

Uses

— Contraception
— To supplement inadequate production in conditions such as constitutional delay of puberty, ovariectomy, menopause, and osteoporosis
— To correct hormonal imbalance (e.g., dysfunctional uterine bleeding)
— To reverse an abnormal process (e.g., hirsutism or endometriosis) (see page 141)

Fig. 17.1 ▶ **Estradiol, progesterone, and derivatives.**
Exogenous estrogen and progesterone mimic the natural hormones at their receptors. Depot preparations are absorbed slowly and thus have a longer duration of action than the natural hormones. Oral preparations undergo a higher degree of first-pass metabolism in the liver. All three estrogen metabolites are water soluble and are excreted by the kidneys. The main metabolite of progesterone is pregnanediol, which is also excreted by the kidneys. (FSH, follicle-stimulating hormone; GnRH, gonadotropin-releasing hormone; LH, luteinizing hormone.)

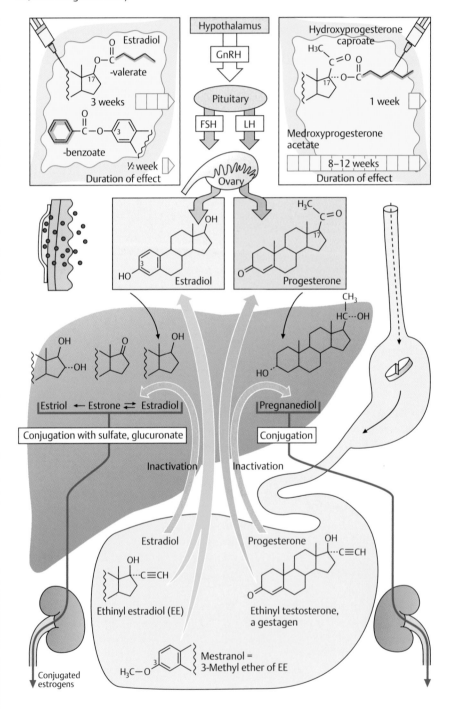

Note: Estrogens are not indicated for treatment or prevention of cardiovascular or neurodegenerative diseases because of possible untoward side effects including breast cancer, stroke, and adverse coronary events.

Side effects
- Nausea and vomiting, breast tenderness, and weight gain due to Na^+ and water retention (usually disappear with continued administration)
- Increased risk of endometrial cancer. This is prevented by the addition of a progestin.
- Reproductive tissue abnormalities and cancers are seen in daughters and sons of women prescribed DES
- Gallstones (due to increased cholesterol caused by estrogen)

17.2   Progestins

Progesterone is a C21 steroid secreted by the corpus luteum, placenta, and ovarian follicle that supports female reproductive tissues and processes (in conjunction with estrogen). It is also an important intermediate in steroid biosynthesis in tissues that secrete steroid hormones. Like other steroids, progesterone binds to intracellular receptors that act in the nucleus to regulate gene transcription.

Effects.   See **Table 17.2.**

Table 17.2 ► **Effects of Progesterone**	
Tissue	**Effects**
Uterus	During the menstrual cycle, progesterone decreases endometrial proliferation and leads to changes that promote implantation of a fertilized ovum. If implantation does not occur, the decline in progesterone at the end of the cycle is the main signal for the onset of menstruation. Maintenance of pregnancy
Breasts	Stimulates lobular-alveolar development Induces differentiation of ductal tissue that has been stimulated by estrogen
Brain	↑ body temperature and is probably responsible for the rise in basal body temperature at the time of ovulation

Progestins: Progesterone, Norethindrone, Ethynodiol, Norgestrel, and Medroxyprogesterone

- Progesterone, the natural hormone, is available in an oily solution for injection (**Fig. 17.1**).
- Norethindrone, ethynodiol, norgestrel (oral), and medroxyprogesterone (oral, parenteral) are synthetic steroids. Some have slight androgenic activity. Synthetic steroids are the most common progesterone preparations.

Uses
- Contraception
- Dysfunctional uterine bleeding
- Dysmenorrhea
- Endometriosis (see page 141)

Side effects
- Decreased high-density lipoprotein (androgenic preparations)

■ Gallstones

The majority of gallstones (75%) are formed when the amount of cholesterol in bile exceeds the ability of bile salts and phospholipids to emulsify it, causing cholesterol to precipitate out of solution. Gallstones may also be caused by an increased amount of unconjugated bilirubin (often in the form of calcium bilirubinate) in the bile ("pigment stones"). Gallstones may be ayraptomatic or they can cause obstruction of a duct causing severe pain, vomiting, and fever. Drugs, e.g., ursodiol, may be used to dissolve small cholesterol gallstones. Ursodiol decreases secretion of cholesterol into bile by reducing cholesterol absorption and suppressing liver cholesterol synthesis. This alters bile composition and allows reabsorption of cholesterol-containing gallstones. As reabsorption is slow, therapy must continue for at least 9 months. Other treatment includes lithotripsy (shock wave obliteration of gallstones that allow the stone fragments to be excreted) or surgical removal of the gallbladder (cholecystectomy).

■ Hormone replacement therapy

The Women's Health Initiative (WHI) is a long-term study by the National Heart, Lung, and Blood Institute that has focused on the health of postmenopausal women. Prior to this study, perimenopausal women were routinely prescribed hormone replacement therapy to alleviate the symptoms of menopause. The WHI found that, compared with the placebo group, women taking estrogen plus progestin had slight increases in breast cancer, heart attacks, strokes, and thromboembolism in the lungs and legs. The benefits were fewer hip fractures and lower occurrences of colon cancer. Women taking estrogen alone had more strokes, more blood clots in the legs, and fewer hip fractures. Estrogen alone had no effect on breast cancer, heart attacks, or colorectal cancer.

17.3 Hormonal Contraception

Estrogen and progesterone are primarily used for hormonal contraception. There are several preparations and modes of administration, which vary in effectiveness. Contraceptive choice largely depends on medical and lifestyle factors.

Combination Oral Contraceptives

A combination of a synthetic estrogen and a progestin is used (e.g., ethinyl estradiol or mestranol combined with norethindrone, ethynodiol, or norgestrel). Monophasic, biphasic, and triphasic preparations are available. In monophasic preparations, each active pill contains the same amount of estrogen and progestin. In biphasic preparations, the estrogen content is the same in each active pill but the level of progestin is increased about halfway through the cycle. In triphasic preparations, the hormone combination changes three times throughout the cycle (approximately every 7 days) (**Fig. 17.2**).

Mechanism of action. Combined oral contraceptive agents act by inhibiting ovulation through feedback inhibition of follicle-stimulating hormone (FSH) and luteinizing hormone (LH) from the anterior pituitary, by thickening cervical mucus, and by inhibition of endometrial proliferation necessary for implantation (**Fig. 17.2**).

Side effects. Most side effects are related to the estrogen component, but cardiovascular changes may be caused by either component. Adverse reactions other than those associated with estrogen therapy include

- Breakthrough bleeding with low-estrogen preparations
- Abnormal glucose tolerance
- Alterations in serum lipids
- Thromboembolic disease (minimal in low-estrogen preparations)
- Increased risk of myocardial infarction (MI) or stroke, particularly in women 35 years of age or older who smoke

Progestin-only Oral Contraceptives

Progestin-only "minipills" contain lower doses of progestin than combination oral contraceptives and are taken daily on a continuous regimen.

Mechanism of action. The contraceptive actions of these agents are due to the formation of impenetrable cervical mucus and to prevention of endometrial implantation. Because these preparations do not inhibit ovulation consistently (**Fig. 17.2**), they are not as effective as combination contraceptives.

Side effects. Unpredictable bleeding is common.

Note: Oral contraception has a 0.3% failure rate with perfect use and 8% with typical use during the first year.

Fig. 17.2 ▶ **Oral contraceptives.**
Oral contraceptives prevent ovulation by feedback inhibition of FSH and LH. The progestin-only minipill primarily acts to increase thick cervical mucus, which is impenetrable to sperm cells. It also inhibits the formation of the endometrial lining, and inconsistently prevents ovulation. Monophasic preparations contain equal amounts of estrogen and progestin. Biphasic preparations have the same estrogen content in each active pill but the level of progestin is increased about halfway through the cycle. Triphasic preparations have three changes to the estrogen and progestin combination throughout the cycle.

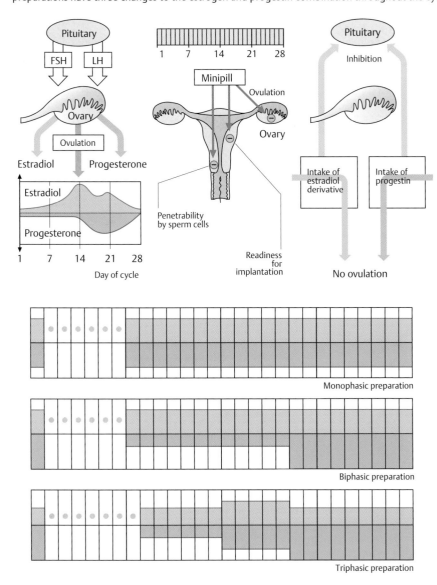

Emergency Contraception

Regimen for emergency contraception
— One progestin-only pill (i.e., levonorgestrel) immediately plus one more after 12 hours (e.g., Plan B™ which is approved by the U.S. Food and Drug Administration.)
— Two combination oral contraceptives immediately plus two more after 12 hours is also effective.

Effectiveness.   Emergency contraceptive regimens provide a 75% reduction in pregnancy.

Side effects.   Nausea, vomiting, and irregular bleeding are common; however, there is less nausea than seen with a progestin-only regimen.

Transdermal Patch Contraceptives

Progestin, Norelgestromin, and Ethinyl Estradiol

Transdermal patches deliver the progestin, norelgestromin, and ethinyl estradiol daily. The patch is applied to the buttocks, upper outer arm, lower abdomen, or upper torso and left on for 3 weeks, followed by a patch-free week to allow for withdrawal bleeding.

Mechanism of action.   The mechanism of action is the same as that for combination oral contraceptives.

Effectiveness.   Generally, transdermal patches are comparable in effectiveness to oral contraceptives; however, women weighing > 90 kg (~198 lb) may experience increased contraceptive failure.

Side effects.   Dysmenorrhea and breast tenderness were more frequent with the patch. Otherwise, the side effects are the same as low-dose oral contraceptives.

Subdermal Implant Contraceptives

Etonogestrel

Etonogestrel (a progestin) is available in a 4-cm–long rod for implantation under the skin of the upper arm. This time-release rod is effective for up to 3 years.

Mechanism of action.   As a progestin, this agent thickens the cervical mucus and produces an atrophic endometrium. Ovulation is suppressed in 97% of cycles.

Effectiveness.   Effectiveness approaches 100%, but it has not been studied in women weighing more than 130% of their ideal body weight.

Side effects.   The major side effect is irregular menstrual bleeding. Others include headache, vaginitis, weight gain, acne, and breast and abdominal pain.

Intravaginal Ring Contraceptives

Etonogestrel and Ethinyl Estradiol

These agents are contained within a flexible polymer ring with an outer diameter of 54 mm and an inner diameter of 50 mm. It is inserted into the vagina for 3 weeks and then removed to allow bleeding.

Mechanism of action.   The mechanism of action is the same as that for combination oral contraceptives.

Effectiveness. Effectiveness approaches 100%.

Side effects. Serum levels of hormones are lower, which minimizes side effects. Both women and men have reported feeling the ring during intercourse.

Intrauterine Contraceptive Devices

Levonorgestrel

Levonorgestrel is a progestin.

Mechanism of action. The mechanism of action is the same as that for progestin-only contraceptives.

Effectiveness. Intrauterine devices (IUDs) are very efficacious and provide 5 to 10 years of continuous contraception.

Side effects. Fewer systemic effects are seen because serum concentrations of hormone are low, but there may still be the following side effects:

— Increased risk of pelvic inflammatory disease related to introduction of bacteria into the genital tract during insertion
— Increased menstrual blood flow and dysmenorrhea

Depot Contraceptive Injections

Medroxyprogesterone Acetate

Medroxyprogesterone acetate is a progestin administered by deep intramuscular injection in the gluteal or deltoid muscle or subcutaneously into the abdomen or thigh. It inhibits ovulation for > 3 months.

Mechanism of action. The mechanism of action is the same as that for progestin-only contraceptives.

Effectiveness. With typical use, 3% of women experience unintended pregnancy.

Side effects. The side effects are the same as those for oral progestin-only contraceptives.

17.4 Estrogen Antagonists

Selective Estrogen Receptor Modulators (SERMs)

Tamoxifen, Toremifene, and Raloxifene

Mechanism of action. Tamoxifen and the related compounds toremifene and raloxifene are partial agonists that inhibit the actions of full agonists such as estradiol at the estrogen receptor (**Fig. 17.3**).

Uses. SERMs are used to treat all stages of breast cancer in both pre- and postmenopausal women, as a palliative treatment for those with advanced disease, and as adjuvant treatment following surgery.

Side effects. Hot flashes, nausea, and vomiting are common.

■ Pelvic inflammatory disease

Pelvic inflammatory disease (PID) is an infection of the fallopian tubes (salpingitis) or ovaries, usually due to sexually transmitted bacteria, e.g., chlamydia. Symptoms include pelvic pain, pain during intercourse or urination, irregular menstrual bleeding, heavy vaginal discharge with an unpleasant odor, fever, fatigue, diarrhea, and vomiting. Untreated PID may cause fibrosis and abscesses in the fallopian tubes. This may lead to ectopic pregnancy, infertility, and chronic pelvic pain. Treatment involves the administration of antibiotics and the avoidance of intercourse until both partners are infection free.

Antiestrogen

Clomiphene

Mechanism of action.   Clomiphene is an antiestrogen with weak estrogenic activity. It acts by binding estrogen receptors and preventing the normal feedback inhibition by estrogen of gonadotropin-releasing hormone and gonadotropin secretion (**Fig. 17.3**). Ovarian stimulation and ovulation result.

Side effects.   They include mild menopausal symptoms, ovarian cyst formation, and multiple births.

Fig. 17.3 ► **Selective estrogen receptor modulators.**
Clomifene is an antagonist at estrogen receptors in the anterior pituitary; because of this, feedback inhibition of gonadotropins by estradiol is suppressed. Raloxifene uses the bone protective effects of estrogen in the prophylaxis and treatment of osteoporosis. Tamoxifen blocks the estrogen stimulus for tumor growth in breast cancer. The relative effects of these agents on cancer and thromboembolism risk, as well as climacteric symptoms (e.g., hot flashes and sweating) and bone mass, are shown.

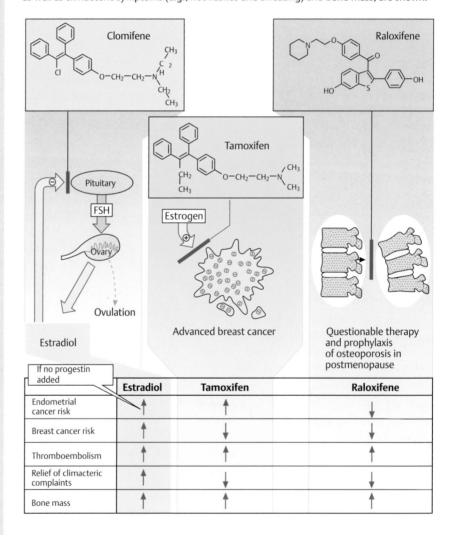

If no progestin added	Estradiol	Tamoxifen	Raloxifene
Endometrial cancer risk	↑	↑	↓
Breast cancer risk	↑	↓	↓
Thromboembolism	↑	↑	↑
Relief of climacteric complaints	↑	↓	↓
Bone mass	↑	↑	↑

17.5 Progesterone Antagonists

Mifepristone

Mechanism of action. Mifepristone (RU 486) is a potent competitive antagonist of progesterone. When administered in the follicular phase of the menstrual cycle, the drug prevents ovulation by inhibiting the effects of progesterone on the pituitary or hypothalamus. When given later, the drug terminates pregnancy by blocking the actions of progesterone on the uterus (**Fig. 17.4**). Mifepristone is also a glucocorticoid antagonist.

Uses

— Contraception
— Medical termination of pregnancy

Fig. 17.4 ▶ **Progesterone receptor antagonist.**
Implantation of the embryo causes the secretion of human chorionic gonadotropin (hCG), which acts on the corpus luteum to secrete progesterone. Progesterone is responsible for maintaining the endometrial lining. Mifepristone is an antagonist of progesterone at its receptors. This agent causes abortion of the embryo due to shedding of the endometrial lining.

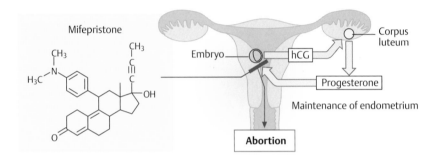

17.6 Ovulatory Agents

Antiestrogen

Clomiphene

See page 164 for a discussion of this agent.

Gonadotropins

Human Chorionic Gonadotropin, Human Menopausal Gonadotropin, Urofollitropin, and Follitropin

Mechanisms of action

— Human chorionic gonadotropin (hCG), which is isolated from the urine of pregnant women, mimics the actions of LH.
— Human menopausal gonadotropin (hMG), or menotropin, which is isolated from the urine of postmenopausal women, contains equal amounts of FSH and LH, as well as other urinary proteins.
— Urofollitropin is highly purified FSH.
— Follitropin is recombinant FSH (rFSH).

Uses
- To induce ovulation
- Cryptorchidism (undescended testicle) to cause the testicle to move to the scrotum, and hypogonadotropic hypogonadism in men (absent or decreased function of the testes) to encourage maturation of leydig cells

Side effects
- Multiple births
- Ovarian enlargement with possible pain and ascites (excess fluid in the peritoneal cavity). This is known as ovarian hyperstimulation syndrome (see page 141).

Prolactin-inhibiting Hormone Agonists

See page 142 for a further discussion of these agents.

Cabergoline and Bromocriptine

Uses
- Infertility (male and female) secondary to hyperprolactinemic states

17.7   Androgens, Anabolic Steroids, and Antiandrogens

The hormone testosterone is produced by the testis, adrenal glands, and ovaries (in small amounts). It has androgenic effects that are important in the development and maintenance of male sex characteristics and anabolic effects to increase muscle size and strength. In cells that contain the 5α-reductase enzyme (skin, prostate, seminal vesicles, and epididymis), testosterone is converted to 5-dihydrotestosterone (DHT), which is the more active form. Like other steroids, testosterone and 5-DHT bind to intracellular receptors that alter gene transcription.

Effects.   See **Table 17.3.**

Table 17.3 ▶ **Effects of Testosterone**	
Androgenic effects	Stimulates the growth of the penis, testes, and scrotum Induces pubic, axillary, and facial hair Thickens the vocal cords and growth of the larynx, producing a lower-pitched voice ↑ libido ↑ activity of sebaceous glands
Anabolic effects	↑ muscle growth and bone mass ↑ production of red blood cells

Synthetic Testosterone Esters

Synthetic agents vary in the ratio of anabolic to androgenic effects. Unaltered testosterone is not suitable for oral or parenteral administration because of its rapid absorption and hepatic metabolism.

Testosterone Cypionate and Testosterone Enanthate

Pharmacokinetics.   These agents are given intramuscularly in oily solutions.

Uses
– Replacement therapy in hypogonadism (primary, secondary, or tertiary)

Synthetic Androgens

Fluoxymesterone, Methyltestosterone, and Danazol
These agents contain 17α-alkyl substitutions to retard hepatic degradation.

Pharmacokinetics
– Orally effective

Uses
– Replacement therapy in hypogonadism (primary, secondary, or tertiary)
– Endometriosis (page 141), fibrocystic breast disease, and hereditary angioneurotic edema (danazol)

Side effects. The substituted androgens produce liver dysfunction.

Anabolic Steroids

Oxymetholone and Oxandrolone
These agents also have 17α-alkyl substitutions. They are weak androgens designed to provide anabolic activity. It is impossible to completely separate androgenic and anabolic effects.

Uses. Anabolic steroids are used in the treatment of constitutional delay of growth.

Side effects
– *Androgenic effects:* acne, facial hair, and deepening of the voice are the earliest effects, followed by priapism (a persistent, usually painful, erection of the penis) and prostatic hyperplasia.
– Gynecomastia
– Cholestatic hepatitis (with 17α-alkylated compounds)
– Atherogenic changes in blood lipids (when taken in large doses, e.g., by athletes)
– Na^+ retention and edema
– Benign and malignant tumors of the liver (rare)

Antiandrogens

Flutamide and Finasteride
Mechanisms of action
– Flutamide is a competitive antagonist of testosterone.
– Finasteride blocks the conversion of testosterone to DHT by inhibiting the enzyme 5α-reductase (**Fig. 17.5**).

Uses
– Finasteride is used in benign prostatic hyperplasia and male pattern baldness.
– Flutamide, in combination with a luteinizing hormone–releasing hormone agonist, is used to treat prostate cancer.

Fig. 17.5 ▶ Testosterone.
Natural testosterone (or its synthetic derivatives) is reduced in target cells to dihydrotestosterone (DHT) by 5α-reductase. DHT has a higher affinity than testosterone for androgen receptors. The liver rapidly metabolizes testosterone to androsterone, which undergoes renal elimination. 5α-reductase inhibitors inhibit the production of DHT and the androgenic activity in tissues where this is active (e.g., the prostate). They have little or no effect on testosterone-dependent tissues (e.g., skeletal muscle). Androgen receptor antagonists inhibit all androgen effects.

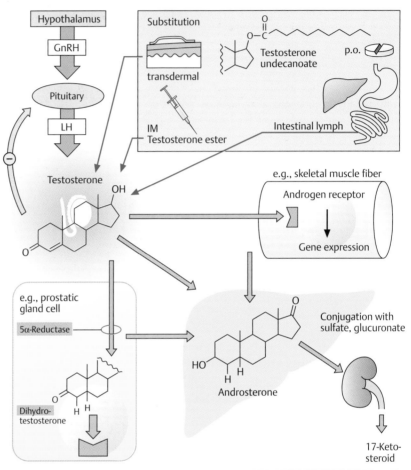

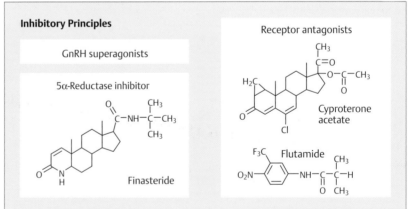

17.8 Drugs Acting on the Uterus

Oxytocin

Oxytocin is a posterior pituitary hormone that can now be synthetically produced for pharmacological use. The uterus is more sensitive to vasopressin than oxytocin except in the third trimester of pregnancy. During the third trimester, uterine oxytocin receptors increase in number, with sensitivity to oxytocin being maximal at term (vasopressin sensitivity decreases in parallel).

Effects
- Stimulates uterine smooth muscle contraction to facilitate parturition (birth)
- Causes myoepithelial cells of the mammary gland to contract and stimulates milk "let-down"
- Oxytocin-containing parvocellular neurons of the hypothalamus send axonal projections throughout the brain to regulate memory and maternal behaviors.

Pharmacokinetics
- Oxytocin is ineffective orally (destroyed by stomach enzymes) and is usually given intravenously or intramuscularly.
- Uterine contractions occur within seconds after intravenous injection and last ~20 minutes.

Uses
- Induction of labor
- Control of postpartum hemorrhage

Side effects
- Transient fall in blood pressure when injected intravenously
- Na$^+$ and water retention

    Note: Do not use oxytocin in patients with uterine abnormalities.

Ergot Alkaloids

Ergot (*Claviceps purpurea*) is a fungus that grows on rye. Extracts of ergot contain a variety of pharmacologically active substances (histamine, tyramine, etc.). Ergot alkaloids per se are derivatives of lysergic acid. Ergot alkaloids have varied actions as agonists or antagonists on tryptaminergic, dopaminergic, and adrenergic receptors.

See Chapter 32 for a discussion of ergot alkaloids in relation to migraine.

Ergonovine

Mechanism of action. Ergonovine is the most potent ergot compound for oxytocic effect with a relatively selective action on the uterus. It is also a partial α-adrenergic receptor agonist.

Pharmacokinetics. Rapid absorption after oral administration provides prompt onset of action.

Effects. Ergonovine can cause forceful, prolonged, or sustained contractions.

Uses
- Prevention and treatment of postpartum hemorrhage (after delivery of the placenta)
- Hastens involution of the uterus (the process where the uterus returns to its normal prepregnant size and state after childbirth)

Methylergonovine

Methylergonovine is a semisynthetic derivative with similar properties as ergonovine.

Anatomy and innervation of the uterus

The uterus is composed of a thick layer of smooth muscle with a central cavity that is lined by glandular epithelium. This cavity is continuous laterally with the fallopian tubes and inferiorly with the lumen of the vagina. The uterus is completely under autonomic control. It is innervated by the inferior hypogastric plexus (sympathetic) and the pelvic splanchnic nerves (parasympathetic from S2 to S4). Afferent signals from the uterus travel with the sympathetic efferents to T10–T12 and L1 spinal cord segments.

18   Insulin, Hypoglycemic, and Antihypoglycemic Drugs

Diabetes Mellitus

Diabetes mellitus is a chronic metabolic disease characterized by hyperglycemia. Insulin-dependent diabetes mellitus (IDDM; type 1) is caused by destruction of the insulin-producing beta cells of the pancreas by antibodies (autoimmune). Non-insulin-dependent diabetes mellitus (NIDDM; type 2) is due to insufficient production of insulin or insulin resistance. The effects of insulin deficiency are shown in **Fig. 18.1,** and **Table 18.1** lists the signs, symptoms, and complications of diabetes mellitus.

<table>
<tr><td colspan="3">Table 18.1 ▶ Signs, Symptoms, and Complications of Diabetes Mellitus</td></tr>
<tr><td>Signs</td><td>Symptoms</td><td>Complications</td></tr>
<tr>
<td>Hyperglycemia

Glycosuria

Poor wound healing

Predilection to infection</td>
<td>Thirst (polydipsia)

Increased frequency of urination (polyuria)

Dehydration

Fatigue

Nausea and vomiting</td>
<td>Microvascular disease:
—retinopathy (can cause blindness)
—nephropathy
—neuropathy

Accelerated atherosclerosis causing strokes, coronary heart disease, and hypertension

Gangrene</td>
</tr>
</table>

18.1   Insulin

Synthesis.   Insulin is produced by the beta cells of the pancreatic islets. Preproinsulin is processed to proinsulin, which is cleaved to form three peptide chains. The A (21 amino acids) and B (30 amino acids) chains of insulin are connected by disulfide bonds and, along with the C peptide, are secreted from the beta cells. The beta cells also secrete amylin, a 37-amino acid peptide.

Mechanism of action.   The insulin receptor is a tyrosine kinase receptor that, upon binding insulin, dimerizes, leading to receptor autophosphorylation and the activation of intracellular signaling molecules. The activated receptor initiates a complex cascade that mediates the effects of insulin (**Fig. 18.2**). Examples include stimulation of the translocation of glucose transporters and increased glycogen synthesis which lowers elevated blood glucose levels. It also stimulates protein synthesis, and lipogenesis.

Uses.   To lower elevated blood glucose levels in type 1 diabetes mellitus, as well as some cases of type 2 diabetes mellitus.

Regular Insulin

Insulin is produced by recombinant DNA techniques.

Pharmacokinetics.   Short half-life (5–10 min).

Fig. 18.1 ► **Effects of insulin deficiency.**
Insulin deficiency causes hyperglycemia. In muscle, glucose uptake is impaired and protein catabolism is increased. Additionally, the uptake of glucose into fat is reduced, glucose conversion to fat is inhibited, and lipolysis is stimulated. The amino acids produced are transported in the blood to the liver, where they are converted to ketone bodies and lipoproteins. Gluconeogenesis is stimulated in the liver, leading to more glucose being transported to the blood than is taken up by the liver. Glucose conversion to glycogen is also inhibited. In the kidneys, glucose is secreted when their capacity to reabsorb glucose is exceeded, along with ketones, water, and electrolytes. (CoA, coenzyme A.)

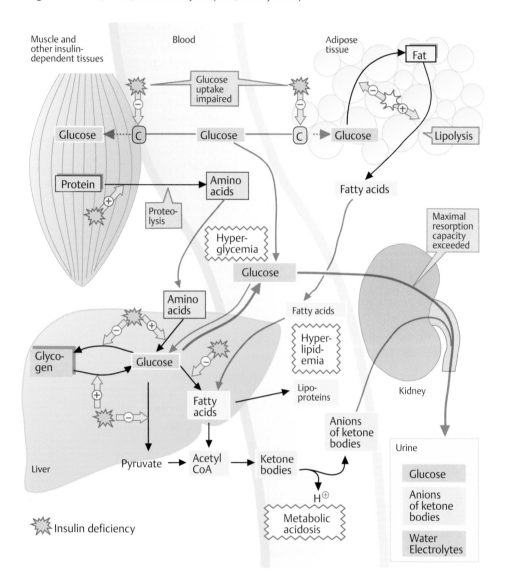

Ketone formation

Ketones provide an alternative source of energy during periods of low glucose after glycogen stores have been consumed. They are formed by the beta oxidation of acetyl coenzyme A (CoA), which is derived from fatty acids, in liver mitochondrial cells. Beta oxidation also yields the reduced form of nicotinamide adenine dinucleotide (NADH) and the hydroquinone form of flavin adenine dinucleotide ($FADH_2$), which then undergoes oxidative phosphorylation, producing adenosine triphosphate (ATP). Acetyl CoA from fatty acid catabolism would normally enter the citric acid cycle, producing energy (via the oxidative phosphorylation of NADH and $FADH_2$). However, in periods of low glucose, oxaloacetate (a citric acid cycle intermediate) is used for gluconeogenesis; thus acetyl CoA is diverted for ketone formation. There are three ketones: acetoacetic acid, β-hydroxybutyric acid, and acetone. Acetone is a result of the spontaneous decarboxylation of acetoacetic acid and is produced in the least quantity of all the ketones. Furthermore, acetone cannot be converted back to acetyl CoA, so it is excreted in urine and exhaled (giving the breath a characteristic "fruity" smell in ketotic states).

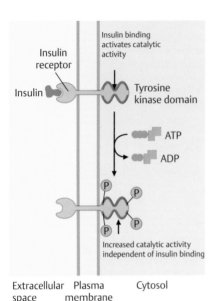

Fig. 18.2 ▸ Signal transduction: insulin.
The insulin receptor is a glycoprotein consisting of two alpha chains, located on the outside of the cell, and two beta chains that are membrane bound and reach into the cytosol. Insulin binds to the exterior alpha chains, which phosphorylates part of the internal beta chains. This activates tyrosine kinase, which then phosphorylates tyrosine groups of a peptide (insulin receptor substrate), which in turn triggers further phosphorylation and dephosphorylation reactions, leading to the physiological effects of insulin. (ADP, adenosine diphosphate; ATP, adenosine triphosphate.)

Gestational diabetes

Gestational diabetes occurs during pregnancy and resembles type 2 diabetes. It is thought to occur in ~2 to 5% of all pregnancies and may improve or disappear after delivery of the baby. Gestational diabetes can be dangerous for both mother and baby. The baby may have macrosomia (high birth weight), congenital cardiac and central nervous system anomalies, and skeletal muscle malformations. They may also have respiratory distress syndrome after birth due to decreased production of surfactant, a substance that causes maturation of the lungs.

Insulin and K^+ balance

K^+ is an important ion in the body, with 98% being intracellular. The ratio of intracellular to extracellular K^+ determines cell membrane potential. Immediate K^+ balance is controlled by intracellular and extracellular potassium exchange driven by the Na^+-K^+-ATPase pump. This is controlled by insulin and β_2 receptors. Long-term K^+ balance is controlled by renal excretion. In hyperkalemic (high-K^+) states, glucose and insulin are used to drive K^+ into cells by increasing the activity of the Na^+-K^+-ATPase pump.

Effects.

— Increased transport of glucose into fat and muscle, increased muscle, and hepatic glycogen synthesis
— Increased K^+ uptake into cells
— Decreased lipolysis and increased triglyceride synthesis
— Decreased protein catabolism, increased amino acid transport, and ribosomal protein synthesis
— Decreased hepatic glucose production (gluconeogenesis)
— Decreased glucagon secretion

Note: The overall effect of insulin is to control hyperglycemia and keto acid formation.

Side effects. Hypoglycemia is the most common adverse effect in patients with well-controlled diabetes. This may be caused by any of the following factors:

— Wrong dose
— Exercise inappropriate for the dose of insulin (exercise increases glucose uptake by insulin-independent mechanisms)
— Not eating at a regular time or eating insufficient amounts
— Drugs enhancing insulin-induced hypoglycemia include anabolic steroids, captopril, ethyl alcohol, and salicylates.
— Beta-adrenergic-blocking drugs that may mask symptoms of hypoglycemia and delay the onset of treatment. These drugs also impair counter-regulatory responses.
— Allergic reactions and localized atrophy are less common with newer, single-component insulin preparations.

Hypoglycemia should be treated with oral glucose (tablets or gel) to relieve the symptoms. Patients and their families may be instructed in the use of a glucagon emergency kit for treating severe hypoglycemic reactions.

Modified Insulin Preparations

Insulin preparations have been developed to delay absorption of insulin and prolong its action, but they act in the same way as regular insulin and have the same side effects. **Table 18.2** provides a summary of the pharmacokinetic properties of different insulin preparations, and **Fig. 18.3** describes two different approaches to insulin replacement.

Table 18.2 ▶ **Pharmacokinetic Properties of Insulin Preparations**				
Type	**Preparations**	**Onset**	**Peak**	**Duration**
Fast-acting insulin	Insulin lispro Insulin aspart Insulin glulisine	5–15 min	1–2 h	4–6 h
Short-acting insulin	Regular insulin	30–60 min	2–4 h	6–10 h
Intermediate-acting insulin	Insulin NPH	1–2 h	4–8 h	10–20 h
Long-acting insulin	Insulin detemir Insulin glargine	1–2 h	None	14–24 h
Abbreviation: NPH, Neutral Protamine Hagedorn.				

Fig. 18.3 ▶ **Methods of insulin replacement.**
In intensified insulin therapy, long-acting insulin is administered late in the evening to generate a basal level. A fast-acting insulin is then injected before meals, the dose being dependent on blood glucose concentration measurement and the meal-dependent demand. This approach allows the patient flexibility in meal times and insulin injection. In conventional insulin therapy, a fixed-dosage schedule is maintained. Insulin (a combination of regular insulin and insulin suspension) is injected in the morning and evening, and carbohydrate ingestion is synchronized with this.

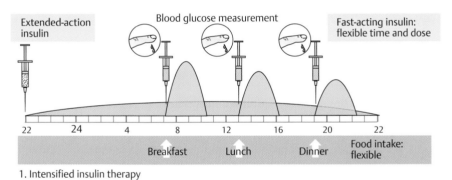

1. Intensified insulin therapy

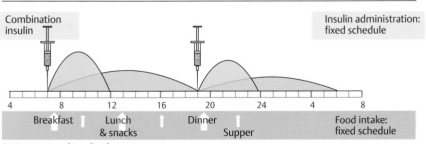

2. Conventional insulin therapy

Fast-acting Insulins: Insulin Lispro, Insulin Aspart, and Insulin Glulisine

— Insulin lispro differs from human insulin by inversion of the B-chain amino acids proline and lysine at positions 28 and 29, respectively.
— Insulin aspart differs from human insulin by replacement of the proline at position 28 (B chain) by aspartic acid.
— Insulin glulisine is formulated by substituting an asparagine for lysine at position 3 and glutamic acid for lysine at position 29 of the B chain.

Intermediate-acting Insulin: Neutral Protamine Hagedorn (NPH) Insulin

NPH insulin is produced by combining insulin with the positively charged polypeptide protamine.

Long-acting Insulin: Insulin Detemir and Insulin Glargine

— Insulin detemir is produced by covalently binding myristic acid to lysine 29 and omitting lysine 30 on the B chain.
— Insulin glargine is produced by replacing the asparagine residue at position 21 of the A chain with glycine and adding two arginine residues to the C terminus of the B chain.

18.2 Oral Hypoglycemic Drugs

Uses. Oral hypoglycemic agents are used in the treatment of type 2 diabetes mellitus, although diet and exercise are the primary treatments for this condition. These agents are ineffective in type 1 diabetes mellitus.

Sulfonylurea Derivatives

Cholporamide, Tolazamide, Tolbutamide, Glimepiride, Glipizide, Glyburide, and Glibenclamide

— *First-generation agents:* Chlorpropamide, Tolazamide, and Tolbutamide
— *Second-generation agents:* Glimepiride, Glipizide, Glyburide, and Glibenclamide

Mechanism of action. These agents block ATP-sensitive K^+ channels on the surface of pancreatic beta cells. This causes membrane depolarization and increased insulin secretion (**Fig. 18.4**).

Side effects

— Hypoglycemia
— Chlorpropamide may cause water retention because of augmentation of antidiuretic hormone action.

Biguanides

Metformin

Mechanism of action

— Decreases hepatic gluconeogenesis and absorption of glucose from the gastrointestinal (GI) tract
— Increases insulin sensitivity of skeletal muscle and adipose tissue

   Note: Metformin does not increase the release of pancreatic insulin; therefore, the risk of hypoglycemia is less than that found for the sulfonylurea agents.

Side effects

— GI disturbances, including diarrhea

Fig. 18.4 ▶ Oral antidiabetics.

Blood glucose concentration depends on the inflow of glucose (mainly from the liver and intestines), and the outflow from the blood into tissues. Metformin and acarbose both inhibit glucose inflow into the blood, and sulfonylureas and thiazolidinedione derivatives positively affect the outflow of glucose into tissues by stimulating insulin secretion and increasing insulin sensitivity, respectively. (PPAR, peroxisome proliferator–activated receptor.)

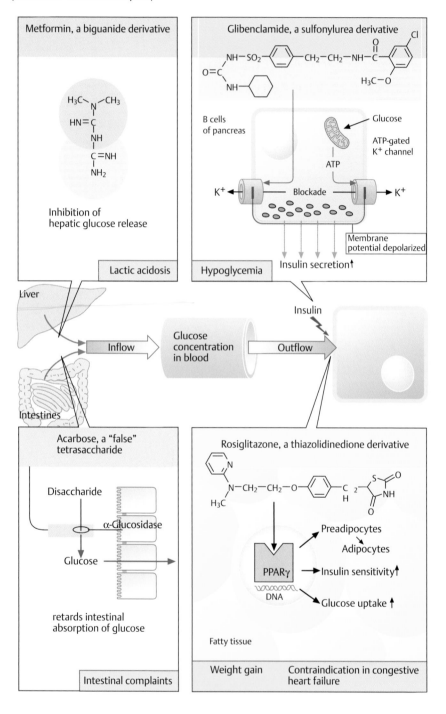

Alpha-Glucosidase Inhibitors

Acarbose and Miglitol

Mechanism of action. These agents are competitive reversible inhibitors of intestinal α-glucosidase, which normally hydrolyzes oligosaccharides, trisaccharides, and disaccharides to glucose and other monosaccharides. They cause delayed absorption of carbohydrates, thereby blunting postprandial hyperglycemia (**Fig. 18.2**).

Pharmacokinetics. These agents are not absorbed systemically.

Side effects
— High incidence of GI pain, discomfort, flatulence, and diarrhea

Thiazolidinediones

Pioglitazone and Rosiglitazone

Mechanism of action. These agents increase insulin sensitivity in tissues, for example, muscle, adipose tissue, and the liver (**Fig. 18.2**).

Side effects
— Edema
— Weight gain

Meglitinides

Nateglinide, and Repaglinide

Mechanism of action. Meglitinides block ATP-sensitive K^+ channels in pancreatic beta cells, leading to membrane depolarization and increased insulin release.

Amylin Analogue

Pramlintide

Mechanism of action. Pramlintide is a synthetic analogue of amylin, a neuroendocrine hormone synthesized by pancreatic beta cells. It mimics amylin effects to delay gastric emptying and to prevent the postprandial rise in plasma glucagon. This improves postprandial glucose control. It may also increase satiety, leading to decreased caloric intake and weight loss.

Pharmacokinetics. It is given by subcutaneous injection with every meal to reduce postprandial hyperglycemia.

Uses
— Type 1 or type 2 diabetes mellitus

Side effects
— Hypoglycemia
— Mild nausea that decreases over time

Glucagon-like peptide 1 (GLP-1) Agonists

Exenatide

Mechanism of action. GLP-1 is a hormone secreted from intestinal L cells in response to nutrient ingestion. It acts on the GLP-1 receptor to stimulate glucose-dependent insulin release and inhibit glucagon secretion. Exenatide is a 39-amino acid peptide that acts as an agonist at the GLP-1 receptor. It lowers blood glucose by mimicking the actions of GLP-1.

Pharmacokinetics.   It is given by subcutaneous injection within 60 minutes before a meal.

Uses.   Exenatide is used as an adjunctive agent to improve glycemic control in patients with type 2 diabetes who are taking metformin, a sulfonylurea, or both.

Side effects
— Hypoglycemia
— Nausea
— Pancreatitis

Dipeptidyl peptidase 4 (DPP-4) Inhibitors

Sitagliptin

Mechanism of action.   DPP-4 is the enzyme that rapidly metabolizes endogenously released GLP-1 in the intestine, terminating its effects. Sitagliptin inhibits the degradation of GLP-1 by DPP-4. It thus enhances the action of GLP-1 to increase insulin release and decrease glucagon levels.

Uses
— Management of type 2 diabetes in combination with metformin and thiazolidinediones

18.3   Antihypoglycemic Drugs

In patients with diabetes who are taking insulin, hypoglycemia may occur from insufficient caloric intake or sudden, excessive physical exertion or an excess of injected insulin. Primary therapy is to raise the glucose level in the blood. In emergency situations, glucagon raises blood glucose levels by increasing the release of glucose from the liver into blood.

Glucagon

Glucagon is a polypeptide produced by the alpha cells of the pancreas.

Mechanism of action.   Glucagon binds to G-protein coupled receptors, mainly in the liver. Signal transduction occurs by means of increased cyclic adenosine monophosphate (cAMP), leading to stimulation of gluconeogenesis and glycogenolysis in the liver and an increase in blood glucose.

Pharmacokinetics.   Glucagon is available as an emergency kit that contains freeze-dried glucagon as a powder and a 1 mL syringe of glycerin. The glycerin is mixed with the glucagon powder prior to injection and may be given intravenously, intramuscularly, or subcutaneously.

Uses
— Hypoglycemic emergency

Side effects
— Nausea and vomiting

Review Questions

1. Which of the following is used to reduce the size of the thyroid prior to surgery?
   A. Propylthiouracil
   B. Levothyroxine
   C. Iodine
   D. Liotrix
   E. Radioactive iodine (^{131}I)

2. A patient is brought to the emergency room with tachycardia, muscle weakness, nervousness, fever, vomiting, extreme sweating, and delirium. Laboratory tests show an elevated serum free tetraiodothyronine, or thyroxine (T_4), and a decreased thyroid-stimulating hormone (TSH) level. To rapidly prevent the synthesis of thyroid hormones, methimazole is given. What is the prescribed action of this drug?
   A. To inhibit tyrosine hydroxylase, thereby decreasing norepinephrine formation
   B. To inhibit thyroid peroxidase, thereby decreasing the formation of thyroxine (T_4) and triiodothyronine (T_3)
   C. To inhibit Ca^{2+} uptake by the endoplasmic reticulum
   D. To increase the secretion of thyroxine
   E. To inhibit growth of parenchymal cells

3. One hour later, the patient in question 2 is given stable iodine as a saturated solution of potassium iodide. What is the purpose of giving high iodide concentrations?
   A. To inhibit thyroid hormone release
   B. To replenish depleted iodine stores
   C. To overcome the thyroid effects of methimazole
   D. To prevent cardiac side effects of methimazole
   E. To replace salts lost by sweating

4. Iodides cannot be used long term to control thyrotoxicosis (hyperthyroidism) because the inhibitory actions of iodide decrease within several weeks. Which of the following treatments can be used to produce a long-term decrease in thyroid hormone levels?
   A. Levothyroxine
   B. Flurouracil
   C. Parathyroid hormone
   D. Calcitriol
   E. Radioactive iodine (^{131}I)

5. Which of the following stimulates conversion of vitamin D precursor to calcitriol at the kidneys?
   A. Levothyroxine
   B. Methimazole
   C. Perchlorate
   D. Parathyroid hormone
   E. Calcitonin

6. A 62-year-old postmenopausal Caucasian woman experienced menopause in her early 50s and has been under hormone replacement therapy with a conjugated estrogen preparation since that time. She is not on any other medications. If the goal of therapy is primarily for prevention of osteoporosis, which of the following therapies might be appropriate?
   A. Estrogen only
   B. Progestin only
   C. A second-generation sulfonylurea
   D. Ergonovine
   E. A Bisphosphonate

7. A 25-year-old man reports becoming exhausted easily and having intestinal pains. The patient also reports being irritable, vomiting for many days, and having a sore throat. Examination shows purple spots on his rib cage and legs. His skin appears tanned even in unexposed areas. The patient has also lost weight. The morning cortisol level after intravenous cosyntropin is unchanged. What would be the primary drug therapy for this patient?
   A. Corticorelin
   B. Aminoglutethimide
   C. Levothyroxine
   D. Hydrocortisone
   E. Mifepristone

8. Although the patient in question 7 reports feeling much better after primary drug therapy, he still feels dizzy when standing. Serum Na^+ is low, and urinary Na^+ is increased. This patient may benefit from the addition of which of the following drugs?
   A. Cortisol (p.o.)
   B. Spironolactone
   C. Dexamethasone
   D. Fludrocortisone
   E. Mifepristone

9. A long-acting synthetic antiinflammatory steroid is
   A. fludrocortisone.
   B. dexamethasone.
   C. prednisone.
   D. cortisol.
   E. aldosterone.

10. Which one of the following is an adverse effect of high-dose estrogen therapy?
    A. Acne
    B. Lymphopenia
    C. Weight loss
    D. Thromboembolism

11. Which of the following is most effective in stimulating protein synthesis in skeletal muscle?
    A. Cortisol
    B. Flutamide
    C. Estradiol
    D. Testosterone
    E. Progesterone

12. An antiandrogen that blocks the prostatic 5α-reductase that catalyzes the conversion of testosterone to dihydrotestosterone and thereby may lead to a reduction in the size of the prostate in men with benign prostatic hypertrophy is
    A. prednisone.
    B. finasteride.
    C. mifepristone.
    D. hydrocortisone.
    E. spironolactone.

13. A known diabetic patient is brought to the emergency room in a deep coma. There is an obvious need for immediate treatment, but the instrument used to determine plasma glucose concentration is not working, and the laboratory cannot supply the result in less than 1 hour. The best emergency procedure is the prompt administration of which of the following?
    A. Crystalline (regular) insulin
    B. Neutral Protamine Hagedorn (NPH) insulin
    C. A second-generation sulfonylurea
    D. Oral glucose
    E. Intravenous glucose

14. A 58-year-old man was found on a routine physical to have a fasting blood glucose level of 200 mg/dL and a positive urine test for glucose. There are no other remarkable signs. He is 70 inches (177 cm) tall and weighs 210 lb (95 kg). What would be the first step in the management of this patient's diabetes?
    A. Prescribe a morning dose of 10 units of Neutral Protamine Hagedorn (NPH) insulin with additional 5 unit doses of regular insulin before each meal.
    B. Place him on a 1200 kcal diet, with a modest exercise program.
    C. Prescribe 500 mg of tolbutamide twice daily.
    D. Prescribe 50 mg of a second-generation sulfonylurea once a day.
    E. Advise him to avoid excess sweets and stress.

15. Which treatment would be administered to the patient in question 14 second if the first treatment is ineffective?
    A. Crystalline (regular) insulin
    B. Neutral Protamine Hagedorn (NPH) insulin
    C. Metformin
    D. Methylphenidate
    E. Intravenous (IV) glucose

Answers and Explanations

1. **C** Iodine is used before thyroidectomy. It is not used for long-term treatment of hyperthyroidism because its effects are temporary (p. 145).
   A, E Propylthiouracil and radioactive iodine (^{131}I) are used to treat hyperthyroidism.
   B, D Levothyroxine and liotrix are used to treat hypothyroidism.

2. **B** The symptoms indicate hyperthyroidism, which is confirmed by the laboratory results. Thus, a drug is needed that will decrease thyroid hormone levels. Methimazole inhibits thyroid peroxidase, decreasing the formation of thyroxine (T_4) and triiodothyronine (T_3), and thus is an effective treatment for hyperthyroidism (p. 144).
   A, C—E None of the other choices describe the mechanism of action of methimazole.

3. **A** Iodine (supraphysiological dose) inhibits thyroid hormone release (p. 145).
   B—E None of the other choices describe the rationale for giving iodine.

4. **E** Radioactive iodine accumulates in the thyroid gland and destroys parenchymal cells thereby producing a long-term decrease in thyroid hormone levels (p. 145).
   A Levothyroxine is the synthetic sodium salt of T_4, or thyroxine and is the drug of choice for replacement therapy of thyroid hormone in hypothyroidism.
   B Flurouracil is a pyrimidine analogue used in treating cancer.
   C Parathyroid hormone is a hormone released from the parathyroid gland and is involved in calcium homeostasis.
   E Calcitriol (1,25 [OH]$_2$D$_3$) is the active form of vitamin D.

5. **D** Parathyroid hormone stimulates the formation of active vitamin D_3, calcitriol (1,25-[OH]$_2$D$_3$), by the kidneys (p. 147).

A Levothyroxine is a synthetic sodium salt of thyroxine and is used to treat hypothyroidism, autoimmune thyroiditis, and thyroid cancer.

B Methimazole inhibits the iodination of tyrosyl residues in thyroglobulin and is used in the treatment of hyperthyroidism.

E Calcitonin acts on bone and kidneys to decrease calcium levels in the blood.

6. **E** Biphosphonates are analogues of pyrophosphate that accumulate in bone and prevent bone resorption in osteoporosis by inhibiting osteoclast activity (p. 149).

A Because the goal is to stop taking estrogens, choice A is not valid.

B Progestin does not have beneficial effects on bone.

C Second-generation sulfonylureas are used to treat type 2 (non-insulin-dependent) diabetes mellitus.

D Ergonovine is an ergot alkaloid used to prevent and treat postpartum hemorrhage and to hasten involution of the uterus.

7. **D** These are signs and symptoms of primary adrenal insufficiency (Addison disease). The lack of cortisol response to intravenous administration of cosyntropin, an adrenocorticotropic hormone (ACTH) agonist, is confirmatory. Treatment is to replace the lack of cortisol with hydrocortisone, a synthetic glucocorticoid, given orally once or twice per day (p. 154).

A Corticorelin, or ovine corticotropin-releasing hormone, is used to differentiate pituitary ACTH-dependent Cushing disease from ectopic ACTH-secreting tumors (Cushing syndrome).

B Aminoglutethimide suppresses the adrenal cortex by inhibiting enzymatic conversion of cholesterol to pregnenolone and inhibiting synthesis of adrenal steroids.

C Levothyroxine is used for replacement therapy in hypothyroidism.

E Mifepristone is a competitive antagonist of progesterone.

8. **D** The symptoms indicate the patient also has a deficiency of the mineralocorticoid aldosterone. Fludrocortisone is a synthetic mineralocorticoid used to treat aldosterone deficiency (p. 156).

A Cortisol is the natural glucocorticoid hormone and is not effective orally.

B Spironolactone is an aldosterone antagonist that would worsen the patients symptoms.

C Dexamethasone is a synthetic glucocorticoid that would be unhelpful in treating the mineralocorticoid aspect of the disease.

E Mifepristone is a competitive antagonist of progesterone.

9. **B** Dexamethasone is a synthetic steroid with a long duration of action (p. 154).

A Fludrocortisone is a synthetic aldosterone analogue used in salt-losing forms of adrenal insufficiency.

C, D Prednisone is an intermediate-acting synthetic steroid, and cortisol is the natural short-acting hydrocortisone.

E Aldosterone is the major mineralocorticoid produced by the adrenal glands. It has a very short half-life and is not used therapeutically.

10. **D** Of the side effects listed, thromboembolism is the one most likely to be seen with estrogen therapy (p. 160).

A and B Acne is often seen in anabolic steroid usage (androgen effects) or progesterone therapy.

B Lymphopenia is not seen with estrogen therapy.

C Estrogen therapy may cause weight gain, not loss.

11. **D** Testosterone is the natural anabolic androgen hormone that stimulates an increase in skeletal muscle (p. 166).

A Cortisol is a natural glucocorticoid whose actions on protein metabolism are mainly catabolic (i.e., increased protein breakdown and decreased protein synthesis).

B Flutamide is a competitive antagonist of testosterone and would therefore block its effects on skeletal muscle.

C, E Estradiol and progesterone are female hormones that do not have anabolic effects on skeletal muscle.

12. **B** Finasteride blocks the conversion of testosterone to dihydrotestosterone by inhibiting the enzyme 5α-reductase and thus has antiandrogenic activity (p. 167).

A, C–E Prednisone and hydrocortisone are glucocorticoids, spironolactone is an aldosterone receptor antagonist, and mifepristone is a progesterone antagonist.

13. **E** This is a hypoglycemic emergency, and the patient is unable to take oral glucose (D). A bolus of dextrose (glucose) should be given, followed by continuous infusion of a dextrose-containing solution.

A–C Insulin and the sulfonylureas are antihyperglycemics and would worsen the patient's condition.

14. **B** The symptoms and complications of type 2 diabetes are worsened by being overweight and leading a sedentary lifestyle. Thus, the initial therapy is to institute lifestyle changes that may be sufficient to decrease blood glucose.

A, C, D are not the initial choices for type II diabetes.

E is an insufficient approach.

15. **C** Metformin is a biguanide that decreases hepatic gluconeogenesis and absorption of glucose from the gastrointestinal tract while increasing insulin sensitivity of skeletal muscle and adipose tissue. Because metformin does not increase the release of pancreatic insulin, the risk of hypoglycemia is less than that found for the sulfonylurea agents (e.g., tolbutamide), which would be a likely third choice for the patient if metformin is ineffective (p. 174).

A, B Insulin is generally not the usual choice for type 2 diabetes mellitus.

D Methylphenidate is a CNS stimulant used to treat ADHD and is not effective in Type II diabetes.

E IV glucose would worsen the condition.

19   Renal Pharmacology

19.1   Overview of Renal Physiology

The major activities of the kidney are eliminating metabolic waste and foreign substances from the body; controlling the excretion of water and electrolytes (salts) to maintain fluid volume, osmolality, and acid–base balance; producing hormones and renin; and aiding in the metabolism of glucose (**Fig. 19.1**).

Renal Transport Systems

The functional unit of the kidney is the nephron. Each section of the nephron and its effects on water and electrolyte excretion are explained in **Table 19.1** and illustrated in **Fig. 19.2**.

Table 19.1 ▶ Effects on Water and Electrolyte Excretion at Different Sections of the Nephron	
Section of the Nephron	**Effects**
Proximal convoluted tubule	Approximately 60 to 70% of the filtered Na^+ and K^+ ions are removed isotonically from the proximal tubule. After passing the length of the proximal tubule, the volume of the filtrate is reduced by 30 to 40% without altering Na^+ or K^+ ion concentrations. Actively transported species include Na^+, K^+, and HCO_3^-. If Na^+ and K^+ ion reabsorption are inhibited at this site, the transport mechanisms remaining in the nephron (loop of Henle and distal convoluted tubule) can fully compensate, and the final urine composition is not altered. HCO_3^- reabsorption and urine pH are primarily controlled in the proximal tubule.
Ascending loop of Henle	Approximately 15 to 20% of the total filtered Na^+ and Cl^- load are reabsorbed at this site by Na^+–K^+–$2Cl^-$ cotransporter.
Distal convoluted tubule	Approximately 8 to 10% of the Na^+ and K^+ load is reabsorbed in the distal convoluted tubule. Active transport mechanisms are present in the distal convoluted tubule for Na^+, K^+, and Cl^-. Cotransport or exchange transport mechanisms exist in the distal convoluted tubule for both Na^+–H^+ exchange and Na^+–K^+ exchange.
Collecting tubule and duct	Na^+–K^+ exchange and, to some extent, Na^+–H^+ ion exchange are controlled by aldosterone and urine Na^+ concentrations. When the Na^+ concentrations increase in the distal tubule, Na^+ ions are absorbed in exchange for K^+ ion and H^+ ion excretion. Increased aldosterone thus increases Na^+ ion retention in the plasma and urinary K^+ excretion. There is a resultant decrease in urine pH (H^+ ion excretion in the urine).

Renin–Angiotensin–Aldosterone Relationship

Renin

Renin is an enzyme released by specialized cells in the proximal convoluted tubule. The enzyme cleaves the inactive peptide, angiotensinogen, into angiotensin I (**Fig. 19.3**). Angiotensin I is then further acted upon by angiotensin-converting enzyme (ACE) in the lung to produce angiotensin II. Angiotensin II is a vasoconstrictor and stimulates aldosterone release from the adrenal cortex. The renin–angiotensin mechanism for aldosterone release is dependent upon the actions of both renin and ACE for the activation of angiotensinogen. Increased quantities of renin are released by the kidneys into the systemic circulation under conditions of

— Low plasma [Na^+]
— Increased sympathetic nervous system stimulation

Ultrafiltration and Starling forces

Ultrafiltration of plasma occurs as plasma moves from glomerular capillaries into Bowman's capsule under the influence of Starling forces. Glomerular filtration is the same mechanism as systemic capillary filtration, i.e., the balance between hydrostatic and oncotic forces across the glomerular membrane determines the direction of fluid movement. Glomerular capillary hydrostatic pressure is the main driving force for ultrafiltration across the glomerular membrane. This is opposed by the hydrostatic pressure in Bowman's capsule and glomerular capillary colloid oncotic pressure.

Glomerular versus systemic capillaries

The glomerular capillaries are much more permeable than average systemic capillaries. Approximately 180 L/day of fluid are filtered across glomerular capillaries, while only 4 L/day of fluid would have been filtered if these were systemic capillaries. The ultrafiltration coefficient (Kf: membrane permeability x surface area) for glomerular capillaries is about 40 to 50 times greater than for systemic capillaries.

Vasa recta

The vasa recta of the kidneys are vessels that branch off efferent arterioles of juxtamedullary nephrons and surround the loop of Henle. The vessels are composed of thin, fenestrated epithelial cells. Each of the vasa recta makes a U-shaped turn in the medulla, and the blood flow through them is very slow. This is fundamental to maintaining the ion gradients in the medulla that are ultimately responsible for the production of concentrated urine. The vasa recta eventually drain into the renal vein. Due to the slow blood flow, the vasa recta are potential sites for thrombosis in hypercoagulable states.

Fig. 19.1 ▶ **Functions of the kidney.**
The kidneys play an important role in excretion, homeostasis, hormone synthesis, and metabolism.
(H, hormone; V, prohormone.)

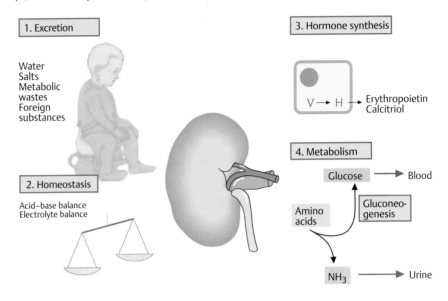

Fig. 19.2 ▶ **Urine formation.**
Urine is formed by the ultrafiltration, secretion, and resorption of substances at different parts of the nephron. The relative quantities are regulated by the kidneys to maintain homeostasis.

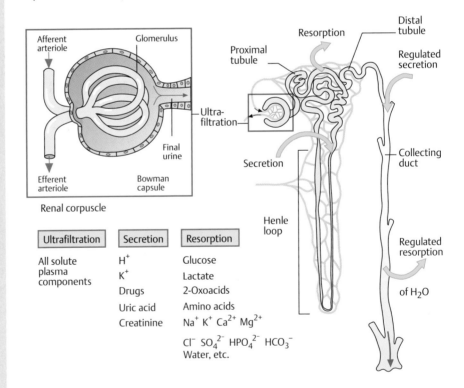

Fig. 19.3 ► **Renin–angiotensin system.**
The kidneys produce renin in response to low blood pressure or low plasma Na⁺ concentration. Renin acts on angiotensinogen in plasma to form angiotensin I. Angiotensin I is converted to angiotensin II in the lungs by the action of angiotensin-converting enzyme (ACE). Angiotensin II acts as a hormone and a neurotransmitter on different organs to produce changes that help restore blood pressure and Na⁺ homeostasis.

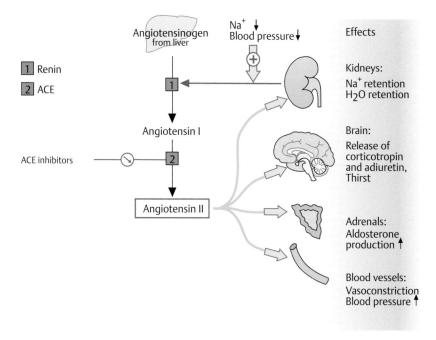

Aldosterone

Aldosterone is secreted from the adrenal cortex and plays an important role in the control of renal Na⁺ excretion and extracellular electrolyte balance. The hormone acts to stimulate Na⁺ reabsorption, Na⁺–K⁺ exchange in the distal tubule, and H⁺ ion secretion in the proximal tubule. The net results of the actions of aldosterone are as follows:

— Na⁺ ion retention
— An increased K⁺ ion excretion
— Mild systemic alkalosis

19.2 Diuretics

Diuretics are the main class of drug used in renal pharmacology. They increase the production of urine by acting in the kidney to alter salt and water excretion. The major indications for use of diuretics are to decrease edema, to treat heart failure, and as antihypertensives.

Most diuretics increase urine flow by altering the reabsorption of Na⁺ ions, and, along with them, Cl⁻ and water, at different sites in the nephron (**Fig. 19.4**). Osmotic diuretics, however, increase urine flow directly. This capacity to increase urine flow is used to treat conditions such as hypertension and congestive heart failure (CHF).

Mannitol in head injury management

Mannitol is widely used to manage head injuries in which there is a need for the acute reduction of intracranial pressure, for example, if the patient shows signs of brain herniation. When given as a bolus, an osmotic gradient is set up such that fluid is drawn out of cells, thus decreasing edema (and intracranial pressure). As an extension of this, circulating blood volume increases, and blood viscosity decreases. This has the beneficial effects of increasing cerebral blood flow and oxygen delivery.

Osmotic diuresis with diabetes

Glucose is normally completely reabsorbed in the proximal tubule of the kidneys. In diabetes, however, high plasma glucose levels exceed the maximum tubular transport capacity (T_m), causing glucose to pass on to the loop of Henle and distal nephron where it causes an osmotic diuresis. Net reabsorption of Na^+ is also reduced (causing hyponatremia), because the large amount of tubular water accompanying the glucose also contains large amounts of Na^+. These factors explain polyuria (excessive urination), polydipsia (excessive thirst), and dehydration that are common presenting symptoms in diabetes.

Diabetic nephropathy

Diabetes mellitus is a leading cause of chronic renal failure. The main pathogenic feature is glomerular disease with thickening of the glomerular basement membrane and glomerulosclerosis. This causes proteinuria to develop and eventually the glomerular filtration rate is irreversibly reduced. Clinically, signs and symptoms include those seen with diabetes and its associated disorders, e.g., retinopathy, neuropathy, hypertension, peripheral vascular disease, coronary artery disease, non-healing ulcers, as well as frothy urine, proteinuria, and edema (if nephrotic syndrome develops [see call-out box page 187]). Diagnosis is made with albuminuria (<300 mg/dL) on two occasions, 3 to 6 months apart, decline in glomerular filtration rate and elevated arterial blood pressure. Treatment involves meticulous glycemic control and ACE inhibitors to slow progression to chronic renal failure. Ultimately dialysis or renal transplantation may be needed.

Fig. 19.4 ► **Renal actions of diuretics.**
Na^+ ions are normally transported into cells from the lumen of the tubules by carrier molecules. They are then secreted into the interstitium by the Na^+-K^+ ATPase pump. Diuretics act at different parts of the nephron to inhibit Na^+ reabsorption. The higher Na^+ load in urine increases its osmolarity, which causes water to be drawn into it and excreted.

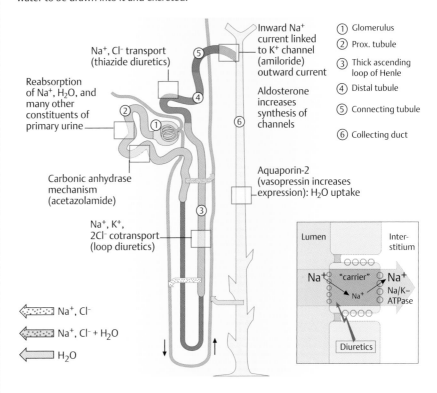

Osmotic Diuretics

Mannitol

Mechanism of action. To be effective, an osmotic diuretic must be freely filtered by the glomerulus and not be reabsorbed from the glomerular filtrate. This increases urine osmolarity and draws water with it without directly affecting Na^+ excretion, so excretion of edema fluid is not increased (**Fig. 19.5**).

Pharmacokinetics. Mannitol is available only as an intravenous (IV) administration dosage.

Uses
— Acute reduction of cerebrospinal or intraocular pressure
— Increased urine flow in cases of acute renal failure
— Dilute toxins in urine

Side effects. These agents can produce fluid overload in patients with inadequate glomerular filtration or dehydration in patients without adequate water replacement.

Fig. 19.5 ▶ **Sodium chloride (NaCl) reabsorption in the proximal tubule and the effect of mannitol.** Mannitol increases the osmolality of the glomerular filtrate. In the proximal tubule this causes reduced reabsorption of water relative to Na⁺. Overall this causes increased urine flow with little increase in Na⁺ excretion.

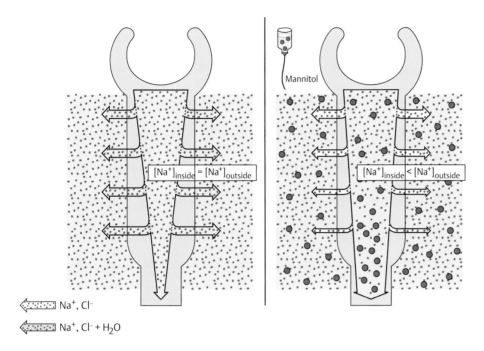

$\Leftarrow\cdots$ Na⁺, Cl⁻

$\Leftarrow\cdots$ Na⁺, Cl⁻ + H_2O

Carbonic Anhydrase Inhibitors

Acetazolamide

Mechanism of action. Carbonic anhydrase inhibitors act in the proximal convoluted tubule to reduce the absorption of HCO_3^- ions from the glomerular filtrate (**Fig. 19.6**). A 90% or greater inhibition of carbonic anhydrase activity must be observed before significant diuresis is observed. Both diuresis and natriuresis (excretion of Na⁺ in urine) are limited because the increased excretion of HCO_3^- in the urine quickly depletes plasma HCO_3^-. This limits their use as diuretics.

Uses
— Treatment of glaucoma (inhibits aqueous humor formation and so reduces ocular pressure)
— Prophylaxis and treatment of acute mountain sickness (mechanism unknown)
— Metabolic alkalosis

Side effects. These include drowsiness and paresthesias (sensations of numbness or tingling of the skin). Serious side effects include metabolic acidosis and formation of kidney stones.

Contraindications
— Liver cirrhosis

Loop (High-Ceiling) Diuretics

Furosemide, Bumetanide, and Ethacrynic Acid

Mechanism of action. The loop diuretics are actively secreted into the proximal convoluted tubule from plasma and act upon the ascending loop of Henle to inhibit the reabsorption of Cl⁻ from the tubular lumen (**Fig. 19.5**) by inhibiting a Na⁺–K⁺–2Cl⁻ cotransporter. These drugs also increase Na⁺, K⁺, and Ca²⁺ excretion, thereby increasing urine volume. Diuresis is independent of acid–base balance. The loop diuretics are the most effective natriuretic and diuretic agents available.

■ **Metabolic acidosis**

Metabolic acidosis occurs when there is excess production of H⁺ in the body, causing blood pH to fall. One of the situations in which this occurs is diabetic ketoacidosis (DKA), when acidic ketone bodies (acetoacetic acid, β hydroxybutyric acid, and acetone) are produced from the breakdown of fat. Bicarbonate ions (HCO_3^-) buffer some of the excess H⁺ ions by binding to them, producing carbonic acid, which then dissociates to form carbon dioxide (CO_2) and water. Centrally, the fall in blood pH stimulates the respiratory center in the medulla to initiate hyperventilation. This hyperventilation (known as Kussmaul respiration) "blows off" CO_2, thus lowering partial pressure of CO_2 (pCO_2), causing blood pH to rise. Renal compensation involves virtually complete reabsorption of HCO_3^-, which replenishes that used to buffer the excess acid and an increase in the excretion of titratable acid and NH_4^+. The availability of titratable acid is very limited, but the kidneys can greatly increase production of NH_4^+.

■ **Kidney stones**

Kidney stones in the renal pelvis and ureters will increase hydrostatic pressure in the Bowman capsule and therefore greatly reduce the glomerular filtration rate. Uric acid kidney stones may sometimes be dissolved by alkalinizing the urine with potassium citrate. Kidney stones that are less than ½-inch in diameter can be fragmented by applying focused ultrasound waves (lithotripsy).

Fig. 19.6 ▸ Action of thiazides, loop diuretics, and carbonic anhydrase inhibitors.
Thiazide diuretics inhibit the Na$^+$–Cl$^-$ cotransporter on the luminal membrane of tubular cells. This leads to reduced reabsorption of NaCl and water. Loop diuretics produce a strong diuresis by inhibiting the Na$^+$–K$^+$–2Cl$^-$ cotransporter in the thick ascending loop of Henle. Carbonic anhydrase (CAH) inhibitors inhibit the production and absorption of bicarbonate in tubular cells. This causes less Na$^+$ reabsorption because fewer H$^+$ ions are available for the Na$^+$–H$^+$ antiporter.

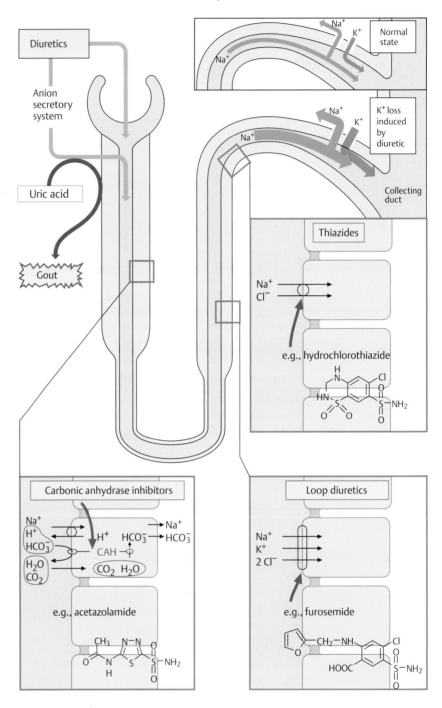

Pharmacokinetics. These agents have a rapid onset of action (within 10–20 min following IV administration).

Uses

- Pulmonary edema due to left ventricular failure
- Chronic congestive heart failure
- Acute oliguria (by maintaining urine formation)
- Hypertension
- Acute hypercalcemia

Side effects. Loop diuretics are more potent than thiazides and thus have more potential for side effects, which may include

- Increased renin production
- Hyperglycemia (mechanism unknown)
- Allergic reactions (these drugs are related to the antibacterial sulfonamides)
- Hypokalemia and dehydration (this can lead to digitalis toxicity and may precipitate skeletal muscle weakness
- Hyperuricemia (excretion of drugs in the proximal convoluted tubules interferes with uric acid excretion and may precipitate gouty arthritis [see page 359 for discussion of gout])

Thiazide Diuretics

Hydrochlorothiazide, Chlorothiazide, and Chlorthalidone

Note: Chlorthalidone is not chemically a thiazide, but has the same mechanism of action.

Mechanism of action. The thiazide diuretics are actively secreted into the proximal convoluted tubule and inhibit Na^+ ion reabsorption in the distal convoluted tubule by inhibiting the Na^+–Cl^- cotransporter. Ca^{2+} ion excretion in the urine is decreased (**Fig. 19.5**). The thiazide diuretics are weak inhibitors of carbonic anhydrase, but diuresis is not dependent upon an inhibition of carbonic anhydrase. Incomplete inhibition of carbonic anhydrase does produce a small increase in urine pH. All thiazide diuretics share a common mechanism of action and common side effects. They differ from each other in potency and duration of action.

Pharmacokinetics. Orally effective.

Uses

- Thiazide diuretics are the standard of therapy in mild to moderate hypertension. They are frequently given along with other antihypertensive medications and can potentiate the action of other antihypertensive drugs. Thiazides are more effective in lowering blood pressure than loop diuretics in patients without edema.
- They may also be used to increase urine flow to dissolve kidney stones.
- Diabetes insipidus (paradoxical antidiuretic effect [see call-out box page 189])

Side effects

- Renal failure due to a decreased glomerular filtration rate
- Hyperuricemia, which may precipitate gouty arthritis
- Hypokalemic alkalosis (due to K^+ loss). This is rarely a problem in normal patients, but it may be problematic in patients with cardiac arrhythmias, especially if they are on digitalis or have severe liver disease.
- Hyperglycemia (decreased glucose tolerance)
- Hypercholesterolemia and hypertriglyceridemia (mild effect)

Pulmonary edema

Pulmonary edema is fluid accumulation in the lungs. Its acute formation constitutes a medical emergency. It is usually caused by left ventricular failure, which renders the heart unable to adequately drain fluid from the lung. Left ventricular failure may be caused by such conditions as myocardial infarction and hypertension. Other causes of pulmonary edema are direct injury to the lung parenchyma, pneumonia, toxins, and high altitude. Signs and symptoms include difficulty breathing, coughing up blood (hemoptysis), anxiety, sweating, pale skin, and pink, frothy sputum. Treatment involves sitting the patient up, oxygen therapy, administering a loop diuretic, nitrate administration, and treating the underlying cause.

Acute renal failure

Acute renal failure produces a sharp rise in urea, creatinine, K^+ (hyperkalemia) and Na^+ (hypernatremia) usually with oliguria (low urine output) or anuria (no urine output). There may also be vomiting, confusion, bruising, or GI bleeding. A metabolic acidosis (usually with a normal anion gap) will occur due to the failure to excrete H^+ as titratable acid and NH_4^+. Acute renal failure may occur due to disease of the kidneys themselves, which may be vascular, septic, neoplastic, due to drugs, or due to pregnancy. Extra renal causes include burns, sepsis, trauma, heart failure, and obstruction. Treatment should be aimed at the underlying cause but hyperkalemia may require urgent correction to avoid cardiac complications (see call out box on page 188). Loop diuretics are given for oliguria/anuria.

Nephrotic syndrome

Nephrotic syndrome results in severe proteinuria (loss of proteins into the urine), hypoalbuminemia, and edema due to the decrease in capillary oncotic pressure. Causes of nephrotic syndrome include glomerulonephritis (inflammation of the glomerulus), diabetes, neoplasia, and drugs. Signs include peripheral edema, ascites, and swelling of the eyelids. Venous thrombosis and emboli may occur due to excretion of certain clotting factors and antithrombin III in the urine. Treatment involves addressing the underlying cause plus the administration of a loop diuretic with a K^+-sparing agent, plasma protein replacement (without salt), and anticoagulation (if necessary).

Potassium-sparing Diuretics

Spironolactone

Mechanism of action. Spironolactone is a competitive antagonist to aldosterone and thus inhibits the synthesis of Na^+ channel proteins and Na^+-K^+-ATPases, which promotes the reabsorption of Na^+, Cl^-, and water.

Uses
— Hypertension: spironolactone is just as effective as thiazides in reducing blood pressure, but it has more side effects.
— Primary aldosteronism (overproduction of aldosterone)
— It may be useful in patients with hyperuricemia, hypokalemia, or glucose intolerance.

Side effects
— Hyperkalemia (high blood K^+)
— Diarrhea, nausea, and vomiting
— Headaches, confusion, and somnolence
— Gynecosmastia

Triamterene and Amiloride

Mechanism of action. These drugs directly interfere with Na^+ transport in the distal convoluted tubule (**Fig. 19.7**). Although the drugs do not act on the renin–angiotensin axis, the net effect on urinary composition is similar.

Uses. Triamterene and amiloride are used to treat hypertension. They are weak diuretics and have little hypotensive action when given alone. However, they are useful when given along with the thiazides to prevent K^+ depletion.

Fig. 19.7 ► **Potassium-sparing diuretics.**
These drugs inhibit Na^+ reabsorption and K^+ secretion in the tubules and proximal part of the collecting duct. This produces a mild diuresis without depleting potassium. Aldosterone increases the synthesis of Na^+ channel proteins and Na^+-K^+-ATPases, which promotes the reabsorption of Na^+, Cl^-, and water. Spironolactone is an antagonist at the aldosterone receptor and inhibits the normal action of aldosterone.

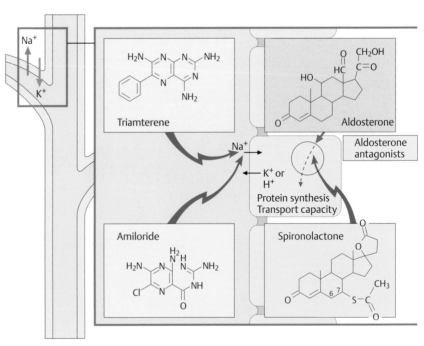

Hyperkalemia

Hyperkalemia (elevated potassium levels) usually occurs due to metabolic acidosis when K^+ is taken up by tubular cells in exchange for H^+ secretion via the H^+-K^+ ATPase antiporter. Hyperkalemia may also be caused by renal failure, severe tissue damage (e.g., rhabdomyolysis [see call-out box page 237]), massive blood transfusions, Addison disease, and potassium-sparing diuretics. Symptoms include palpitations, malaise, and muscle weakness. Severe hyperkalemia (>6.5mmol/L) is a medical emergency as it can cause ventricular fibrillation and sudden death. ECG findings in hyperkalemia include small P waves, widened QRS complexes, and peaked T waves. Treatment is aimed at the underlying cause. In an emergency, calcium gluconate is given intravenously to reduce myocardial excitability; insulin and 50% glucose are given intravenously to shift K^+ into cells (via activity of Na^+-K^+-ATPase); and bicarbonate is given to correct acidosis. Hemodialysis may also be necessary to increase K^+ elimination.

Side effects

— Hyperkalemia

Note: Do not use potassium-sparing diuretics and potassium supplements together.

Over-the-Counter Drugs as Diuretics

Most over-the-counter drugs promoted as diuretic agents contain caffeine (100 mg) and/or ammonium chloride (~500 mg). The drugs have, at best, only a mild diuretic action. Caffeine mildly inhibits Na^+ reabsorption in renal tubules, and ammonium chloride metabolism results in urea formation and excretion of a Cl^- ion. Na^+ passively follows the increased Cl^- load, resulting in mild diuresis.

19.3   Antidiuretic Drugs

Vasopressin

Vasopressin (8-arginine vasopressin), also known as antidiuretic hormone (ADH), is a peptide hormone composed of nine amino acids. It is synthesized in the hypothalamus and transported to its site of release in the posterior pituitary (see also page 142). The main stimuli for vasopressin release are hyperosmolality of the blood and volume depletion.

Two types of vasopressin receptors are known:

— V_1 receptors stimulate contraction of vascular smooth muscles (**Fig. 19.8**).
— V_2 receptors stimulate water reabsorption in the renal tubule through a cyclic adenosine monophosphate (cAMP)–dependent mechanism.

Vasopressin is found in other areas of the brain and may promote learning and improve long-term memory.

Treatment of nephrogenic diabetes insipidus

In nephrogenic diabetes insipidus, the kidneys are unresponsive to vasopressin, and thiazide diuretics cause a paradoxical reduction in polyuria. The mechanism for this effect is uncertain, but it is usually attributed to changes in Na^+ excretion. Thiazides inhibit NaCl reabsorption in the early segments of the distal tubule but have little effect in the thick ascending limb, which is involved in concentrating the urine. In the ascending limb, water is reabsorbed along with Na^+. Although all thiazides share this effect, chlorothiazide is most commonly used to treat this condition.

Fig. 19.8 ► **Vasopressin (antidiuretic hormone [ADH] and derivatives).**
Vasopressin acts on V_2 receptors to promote the reabsorption of water. This occurs due to an increased expression of aquaporins, which increases the permeability of collecting duct epithelium to water. Vasopressin also acts on V_1 receptors on vascular smooth muscle, producing vasoconstriction. Desmopressin is an analogue of vasopressin that produces a varying amount of antidiuretic and vasoconstrictive effects. Nicotine increases and ethanol decreases vasopressin secretion.

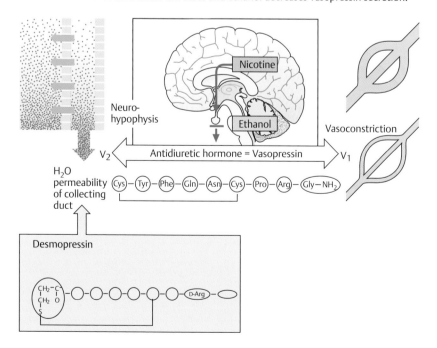

Desmopressin

Desmopressin (1-deamino-8-D-arginine vasopressin) is a synthetic arginine analogue of vasopressin with the highest ratio of antidiuretic:vasopressor activities and the longest duration of action.

Uses

— Diabetes insipidus of pituitary origin (neurogenic diabetes insipidous)
— Primary nocturnal enuresis (bedwetting) in children and adults
— Adjunct in hemophilia therapy (vasopressin increases circulating levels of blood clotting factor VIII)

Side effects

— Vasoconstriction (may be dangerous in patients with angina)
— Contraction and cramps of smooth muscles
— Water intoxication

19.4   Vasopressin Antagonists

Demeclocycline and Lithium Carbonate

Mechanism of action.   Both demeclocycline and lithium antagonize the renal action of vasopressin.

Uses

— Treatment of syndrome of inappropriate secretion of antidiuretic hormone (SIADH)

Syndrome of inappropriate secretion of antidiuretic hormone

SIADH occurs when excessive amounts of ADH are secreted from the posterior pituitary gland. This leads to hyponatremia (low plasma Na^+) and fluid overload. Causes include head injury, meningitis, infections (e.g., brain abscess), pneumonia, and cancer. Treatment involves addressing the cause and using demeclocycline or lithium carbonate for symptomatic control.

20 Antihypertensive Drugs

20.1 Hypertension

Hypertension is a major risk factor for cerebrovascular disease, heart failure, renal insufficiency, and myocardial infarction (see **Fig. 20.1** for the causes and mechanism of hypertension). It is often asymptomatic until organ damage reaches a critical point, so frequent monitoring is vital. Antihypertensive therapy initially consists of lifestyle changes, such as weight reduction, smoking cessation, reduction of salt, saturated fat, and excessive alcohol intake, and increased exercise before drug therapy is initiated.

Indications for Drug Therapy

— Sustained blood pressure elevations > 140/90 mmHg
— When minimally elevated blood pressure is associated with other cardiovascular risk factors (e.g., smoking, diabetes, obesity, hyperlipidemia, genetic predisposition)
— When end-organs are affected by hypertension (e.g., heart, kidneys, and brain)

Drug Management of Hypertension

The following drugs are used in the treatment of hypertension, either as the sole agent or in combination with other agents. Note that the drugs are numbered to reflect the order in which they would most likely be used clinically.

1. Diuretics (mainly thiazides)
2. Angiotensin antagonists: angiotensin-converting enzyme (ACE) inhibitors, angiotensin II receptor antagonists, and renin inhibitors
3. Sympatholytic drugs: β-blockers and mixed antagonists
4. Calcium channel blockers
5. α-adrenergic receptor blocking agents
6. α_2-adrenergic receptor agonists
7. Direct vasodilators

20.2 Diuretics

These drugs are discussed in detail in Chapter 19. The precise mechanism by which diuretics reduce blood pressure is poorly understood; however, antihypertensive effects during the early stage of treatment have been related to a decrease in circulating blood volume and decreased cardiac output, but these parameters return to nearly normal values after a few weeks. Their action may, in part, be related to a depletion or redistribution of Na^+ or a direct arteriolar dilation.

20.3 Angiotensin Antagonists

Angiotensin-converting Enzyme Inhibitors

Captopril, Enalapril, and Lisinopril

Mechanism of action. These agents inhibit ACE (by acting as a false substate), which decreases the conversion of angiotensin I to angiotensin II. In doing so, they prevent the direct effects of angiotensin II on blood vessels (vasoconstriction), as well as preventing aldosterone release from the adrenal cortex (**Fig. 20.2**). ACE inhibitors also prevent the degradation of bradykinin (ACE acts as a kininase). Bradykinin is a vasodilator, and increasing its level may contribute to the effect of ACE inhibitors.

Causes of hypertension

Essential hypertension is when the cause is unknown and accounts for 90% of all cases. The other 10% of hypertension cases are secondary to diseases such as renal artery stenosis, polycystic kidneys, pyelonephritis, glomerulonephritis, diabetes mellitus, Cushing syndrome, Conn syndrome, pheochromocytoma, hyperparathyroidism, coarctation of the aorta, and preeclampsia. Pain can also be a cause of hypertension.

End-organ damage in hypertension

Examples of end organ damage that may result from chronic hypertension include left ventricular hypertrophy, renal failure, peripheral vascular disease, stroke, transient ischemic attacks (TIAs), myocardial infarction, congestive heart failure (CHF), and cerebral encephalopathy.

Baroreceptor reflex

The baroreceptor reflex allows the body to compensate rapidly for changes in arterial pressure. It is mediated by receptors sensitive to mechanical stretch, which are located in the carotid sinuses and in the walls of the aortic arch. Decreased arterial pressure causes carotid sinus baroreceptors to undergo a reduced amount of stretch. This decreases the rate of action potential firing in the carotid sinus nerve, a branch of the glossopharyngeal nerve. The aortic arch is innervated by branches of the vagus nerve and acts in a similar manner. Impulses from baroreceptors are then relayed to the vasomotor center in the medulla oblongata, which increases sympathetic outflow, resulting in increased heart rate, contractility, and stroke volume. It also increases venoconstriction, which reduces the compliance of veins resulting in an increase in venous return to the heart. According to the Frank-Starling mechanism, increased venous return increases filling pressures (preload) such that cardiac output is increased. Increased vasoconstriction of arterioles also occurs.

Fig. 20.1 ▶ Causes and mechanism of hypertension.
This illustration shows the mechanisms by which cardiac output (CO) and/or total peripheral resistance (TPR) are increased in primary and secondary hypertension (renal hypertension, hormonal hypertension, and other forms of hypertension). (ACTH, adrenocorticotropic hormone; ECV, extracellular volume.)

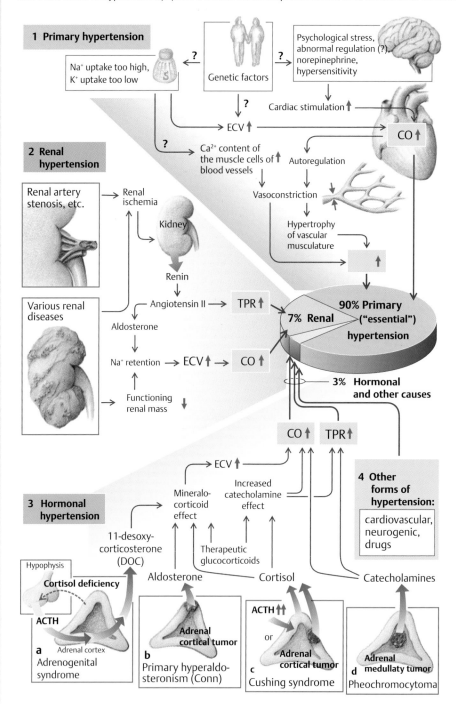

Fig. 20.2 ▶ Renin–angiotensin–aldosterone system and inhibitors.
Angiotensin-converting enzyme (ACE) inhibitors inhibit the ACE in the luminal side of vascular epithelium that is primarily responsible for the conversion of angiotensin I to angiotensin II. They also inhibit kininase II, which contributes to the inactivation of kinins (e.g., bradykinin). The net result is a reduction in blood pressure and in the work of the heart. Angiotensin receptor antagonists produce effects similar to ACE inhibitors, but they do not affect kinin degradation. (BP, blood pressure; CO, cardiac output.)

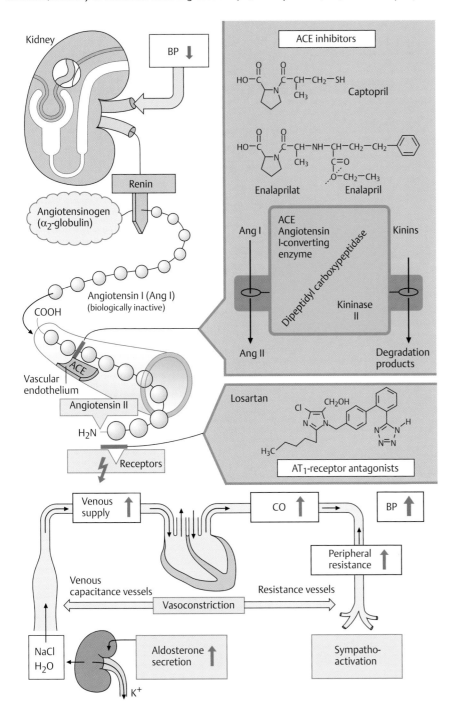

Note: ACE inhibitors are less effective in African American patients unless combined with a thiazide diuretic.

Pharmacokinetics
— Orally effective
— Enalapril is more potent and longer acting than captopril. It is a prodrug that is hydrolyzed in the body to enalaprilat, an active metabolite.

Uses
— Heart failure
— Hypertension (lowers blood pressure in "low-renin" patients). These agents are approved for monotherapy.

Side effects
— Persistent cough
— Hyperkalemia (high plasma K^+ concentration)
— First-dose hypotension
— Taste disturbances

Angiotensin II Receptor Antagonists

Losartan, Valsartan, and Candesartan

Mechanism of action. These agents block the binding of angiotensin II to the AT_1-type angiotensin receptor (**Fig. 20.2**).

Uses and side effects. They are similar to ACE inhibitors, but they do not produce a cough.

Direct Renin Inhibitors

Aliskiren

Mechanism of action. Aliskiren is a relatively new drug that produces a dose-dependent reduction in plasma renin activity, angiotensin I, angiotensin II, and aldosterone, with a concomitant reduction in blood pressure.

Uses and side effects
Direct renin inhibitors are similar to ACE inhibitors.

Note: Drugs that act directly on the renin–angiotensin system, including ACE inhibitors, angiotensin II receptor antagonists, and direct renin inhibitors, can cause injury and death to the developing fetus, and their use in pregnancy should be avoided.

20.4   Sympatholytic Drugs

Sympatholytic drugs are also discussed in Chapter 6.

Beta-Adrenergic Receptor Blocking Agents

Propranolol, Atenolol, Nadolol, Metoprolol, Pindolol, and Timolol

Mechanisms of action
— Propranolol (**Fig. 20.3**), nadolol, pindolol, and timolol are all nonselective β_1- and β_2-blockers.
— Atenolol and metoprolol are more "cardiac" selective β_1-blockers.

Fig. 20.3 ▸ Effects of some β-sympatholytics and their presystemic elimination.
Isoproterenol, a synthetic catecholamine, is an agonist at both $β_1$- and $β_2$-receptors. Pindolol, a partial agonist at β-receptors, is classed as a β-sympatholytic, as it prevents full agonists from achieving their maximal effect. Propranolol blocks Na^+ channel function and so has a "membrane-stabilizing" effect. Atenolol possesses a higher affinity for $β_1$-receptors than $β_2$-receptors and is said to be cardioselective.

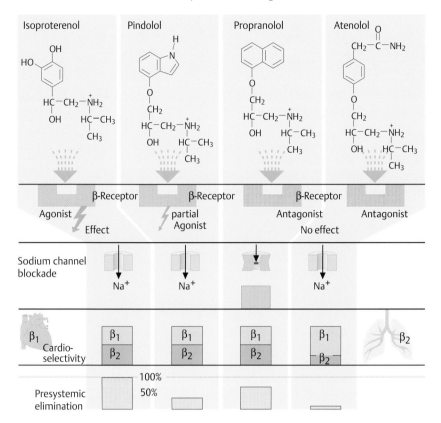

Effects
— Reduces myocardial oxygen consumption by decreasing resting heart rate and myocardial contractility
— Decreases sympathetic tone via central action
— Delays atrioventricular (AV) conduction
— Decreases renin release

Uses
— Effort-induced angina
— Hypertension
— Antiarrhythmias
— Open-angle glaucoma (timolol) (see page 46)

Side effects
They are generally mild, except in patients with accompanying disease, but may include the following:

— Bradycardia
— Dizziness
— Headache

Contraindications
— Asthma/obstructive airways disease due to bronchoconstriction (β_2 effect). Metoprolol or atenolol could be used in asthmatics for treatment of hypertension, but both require caution.
— Congestive heart failure (CHF)/heart block. In these cases, the β_1 effects are unhelpful.

Mixed Antagonists

Labetalol

Mechanism of action.   Labetalol blocks α_1- and β-adrenergic receptors, therefore, it has the combined actions and side effects of both.

Uses
— Hypertension
     Note: There is no evidence that labetalol has an advantage over other β-blockers in the treatment of hypertension with its additional α-blocking capacity.

Calcium Channel Blockers

Calcium channel blockers (also termed *calcium antagonists* and *calcium entry blockers*) are pharmacological agents capable of reducing Ca^{2+} entry through the cell membrane via voltage-dependent, ion-specific channels (slow inward current).

Amlodipine, Nifedipine, Nicardipine, Verapamil, and Diltiazem

— *Dihydropyridine calcium channel blockers:* amlodipine, nifedipine, and nicardipine
— *Nondihydropyridine calcium channel blockers:* verapamil and diltiazem

Mechanism of action.   Two major channel types exist in cardiac and vascular smooth muscle, the T type and the L type. The L-type channel is blocked by calcium channel blockers. Calcium channel blockers differ in their tissue specificity (**Fig. 20.4**).

— The dihydropyridines (amlopidine, nifedipine and nicardipine) inhibit Ca^{2+} entry and smooth muscle contractility with a relative absence of direct effects on the myocardium. The drugs can also prevent or reverse biliary-esophageal spasm.
— Diltiazem and verapamil significantly reduce heart rate, force, and velocity of contraction of the heart in conjunction with smooth muscle relaxation. All calcium channel blockers prevent coronary artery spasm and reduce myocardial oxygen demand.

Uses
— Hypertension (all agents)
— Angina pectoris, both classical and variant types (all agents)
— Supraventricular tachycardia (diltiazem and verapamil only)

Side effects
— Verapamil is markedly negatively inotropic (reduces force of contraction), so it can produce complete AV block if administered in the presence of β-adrenergic receptor blockade.
— Diltiazem is modestly negatively inotropic, so it can be safely administered in conjunction with β-adrenergic receptor blockers.
— With the dihydropyridines, headache and pedal edema are common, resulting from profound vasodilation and fluid retention. Nifedipine may cause reflex tachycardia due to profound vasodilation and is therefore a poor choice of drug in patients with aortic stenosis or severe heart failure. The other agents act more directly on the heart (with less vasodilator activity) so reflex tachycardia is limited.

Excitation-contraction coupling in cardiac muscle

Depolarization of the cardiac muscle cell membrane triggers an action potential which passes through the T-tubules. During phase 2 (plateau) of the action potential, there is increased Ca^{2+} conductance causing inward Ca^{2+} flow. This inward Ca^{2+} flow initiates the release of Ca^{2+} from the sarcoplasmic reticulum (Ca^{2+}-induced Ca^{2+} release). The result of this is an increase in intracellular $[Ca^{2+}]$. Ca^{2+} binds to troponin-C and tropomysin moves out of its blocking position allowing actin and myosin to form cross-bridges. The thick and thin filaments of actin and myosin slide past each other resulting in cardiac muscle cell contraction. The contraction ends when Ca^{2+}-ATPase facilitates the reuptake of Ca^{2+} into the sarcoplasmic reticulum reducing the intracellular $[Ca^{2+}]$. *Note:* The force of contraction of cardiac muscle cells is proportional to the amount of Ca^{2+} release, which varies depending on conditions.

Fig. 20.4 ▶ **Vasodilators: calcium antagonists.**
Calcium channel blockers inhibit Ca^{2+} entry into cells. In smooth muscle cells, this produces arterial vasodilation, which leads to reduced coronary artery spasm, decreased blood pressure, and reduced cardiac work. In heart muscle cells, these agents inhibit cardiac functions, causing decreased heart rate, atrioventricular (AV) conduction, and contractility. Nifedipine acts predominantly on smooth muscle cells to produce vasodilation and has almost no effect on cardiac function at therapeutic doses. Verapamil acts on both smooth muscle and heart muscle cells.

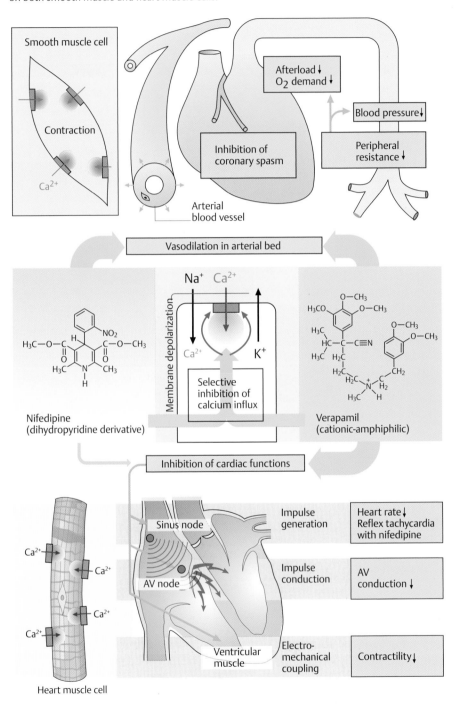

Table 20.1 summarizes the electrophysiological and hemodynamic effects of these agents.

Table 20.1 ▸ Summary of Electrophysiological and Hemodynamic Effects of Calcium Channel Blocker Agents								
	Electrophysiology				**Hemodynamics**			
	Sinus node conduction		AV node conduction					
Agent(s)	Direct effect	Indirect effect	Direct effect	Indirect effect	Contractility	Preload	Afterload	Oxygen consumption
Amlodipine Nifedipine Nicardipine	None	Increased	None	Increased	No change	No change	Decreased	Reduced
Diltiazem Verapamil	Decreased	Increased	Decreased	Increased	Decreased	No change	Decreased	Reduced
Abbreviation: AV, atrioventricular.								

Alpha$_1$-Adrenergic Receptor–blocking Agents

Prazosin, Terazosin, and Doxazosin

Mechanism of action. These agents act selectively on the postsynaptic α_1 receptor of vascular smooth muscle, causing vasodilation and lowering total peripheral resistance.

Uses
— Hypertension
— Congestive heart failure

Side effects. Orthostatic (postural) hypotension and reflex tachycardia are frequent, especially after the first dose.

Methyldopa

Mechanism of action. Methyldopa is metabolized to α-methylnorepinephrine (α-MNE), which can displace and deplete norepinephrine in storage sites. There is also an indirect reduction in renin release.

Uses
— Hypertension (The antihypertensive effect occurs via central nervous system [CNS] reduction of sympathetic outflow.)

Side effects
— Drowsiness
— Depression

Adrenergic Neuron Blockers

Reserpine

Mechanism of action. Reserpine depletes norepinephrine stores in the peripheral sympathetic nerve terminals and in the brain by preventing uptake and storage in neurosecretory granules. It appears to act by inhibiting transport and by binding of catecholamines in storage granules (see **Fig. 6.10**, page 62).

Uses
— Hypertension

Side effects. These are largely due to unopposed parasympathetic effects and include

— Bradycardia
— Nasal stuffiness
— Diarrhea, increased motility, and aggravation of peptic ulcers
— Excessive sedation, depression, extrapyramidal symptoms, and impotence

Guanethidine

Mechanism of action. Guanethidine has complex effects on the adrenergic neuron. It prevents norepinephrine release during nerve stimulation by blocking transmission of the action potential into the terminal nerve ending, as well as by causing the depletion of peripheral stores of norepinephrine and blocking its reuptake. It does not cross the blood–brain barrier; therefore, there are no CNS effects (see **Fig. 6.10**, page 62).

Pharmacokinetics
— Slow onset (2–3 days) with long duration of action (effects persist for about 1 week after the drug is stopped.)

Uses
— Hypertension

Side effects. Same as for reserpine.

Ganglionic blocking Agents

Trimethaphan

Mechanism of action. The hypotensive action of trimethaphan is primarily due to reduced vasomotor tone, decreased venous return, and lowered cardiac output.

Pharmacokinetics
— Given by a slow intravenous (IV) infusion

Uses
— Occasionally used for hypertensive crisis or in surgery to reduce blood pressure

Side effects. Potential side effects limit the usage of trimethaphan and may include

— Precipitous falls in blood pressure
— Histamine release from mast cells and basophils, which may lead to asthma

Alpha$_2$-Adrenergic Receptor Agonists

Clonidine

Mechanism of action. Clonidine causes stimulation of CNS α_2-adrenergic receptors, which in turn causes inhibition of sympathetic tone (see **Fig. 6.7**, page 58). Effects are long acting and are antagonized by yohimbine (*Pausinystalia yohimbe*), an alkaloid with stimulant and aphrodisiac properties.

Pharmacokinetics. Clonidine is very lipophilic; therefore, it can be administered orally or through a transdermal patch.

Uses
— Hypertension
— Migraine
— Menopausal flushing

Side effects
— Xerostomia (dry mouth)
— Sedation
— Fluid retention (use with a diuretic)

   Note: Withdrawal may precipitate hypertensive crisis, which may be treated with labetalol (a β-antagonist).

20.5   Direct Vasodilators

Agents that cause vasodilation will reduce blood pressure, but this stimulates counter-regulatory responses that are designed to maintain blood pressure (**Fig. 20.5**). Additional drugs (e.g., ACE inhibitors and β-blockers) are given to inhibit these responses.

Arterial Vasodilators

Arterial vasodilators all cause K+ channel activation, leading to hyperpolarization and vascular smooth muscle relaxation.

Hydralazine

Mechanism of action.   Hydralazine directly relaxes vascular smooth muscle and decreases peripheral resistance. It also causes reflex cardiac stimulation (increased cardiac output and tachycardia), which can be blocked with propranolol.

Pharmacokinetics
— Well absorbed after oral administration and generally well tolerated

Fig. 20.5 ► **Counterregulatory responses in hypotension due to vasodilators.**
Vasodilation causes a decrease in blood pressure. To counteract this, the body activates the sympathetic nervous system and the renin–angiotensin system. However, because these homeostatic mechanisms are undesired when using vasodilator drugs in hypertension, heart failure, and angina, additional drugs are given to block them.

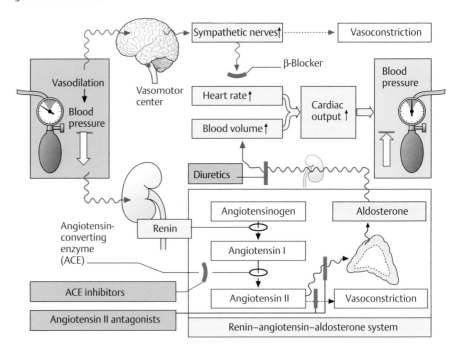

Uses
— Chronic hypertension
— Especially useful in acute hypertensive crisis (administered parenterally)

Side effects
— Headache
— Palpitations
— Gastrointestinal disturbances
— The most serious toxicity is a lupuslike syndrome occurring with long-term therapy. This side effect limits its chronic use and is reversible if the drug is stopped.

Minoxidil

Mechanism of action. The mechanism of action is the same as that for hydralazine, but minoxidil is longer acting.

Uses
— Severe and uncontrollable hypertension

Side effects
— Salt and water retention
— Hypertrichosis (excessive growth of hair)

Diazoxide

Diazoxide is a nondiuretic congener of the thiazide diuretic drugs.

Mechanism of action. The mechanism of action is unknown, but it exerts a direct effect on the arterioles to lower blood pressure.

Uses
— Acute hypertensive emergencies (given IV)

Side effects
— Hyperglycemia (inhibits insulin release from the beta cells of the pancreas)
— Hyperuricemia
— Amylase elevations and pancreatic necrosis

Arterial and Venous Vasodilators

Sodium Nitroprusside

Mechanism of action. This agent is a direct peripheral vasodilator that has long been considered obsolete, but has recently been revived.

Uses
— Acute hypertensive emergencies

  Note: Nitroprusside is not considered suitable for chronic management of hypertension.

Side effects. Nitroprusside is hazardous, as it can precipitate marked hypotension when administered as an IV dosage. It is also light sensitive, and its metabolite, thiocyanate, may cause psychotic syndrome.

Table 20.2 lists the antihypertensive agents and provides an at-a-glance reference to the parameters of blood pressure that they reduce and the mechanisms by which they do it.

Table 20.2 ▶ **Summary of Mechanisms of Antihypertensive Agents**		
Antihypertensive Agent(s)	**Parameter of BP Affected**	**Mechanism**
Diuretics	TPR	Initial decrease in CO, followed by sustained decrease in TPR (exact mechanism unclear)
ACE inhibitors	TPR	Indirect vasodilation by decreasing angiotensin II levels
Angiotensin II receptor antagonists	TPR	Indirect vasodilation by blocking angiotensin II receptor
Calcium channel blockers	TPR	Decrease influx of Ca^{2+} into vascular smooth muscle
β-blockers	CO, TPR	Decrease heart rate and force of contraction by sympathetic inhibition Decrease renin production, leading to decreased circulating angiotensin II
α_2-adrenergic receptor agonists	TPR	Stimulate presynaptic α_2-adrenergic receptors in brainstem to decrease sympathetic activity.
α_1-adrenergic receptor–blocking agents	TPR	Block α_1-receptor-mediated contraction of vascular smooth muscle
Adrenergic neuron blockers, ganglionic blockers	TPR	Depletes NE or prevents NE release
Direct vasodilators	TPR	Direct vasodilation of vascular smooth muscle

Abbreviations: ACE, angiotensin-converting enzyme; BP, blood pressure; CO, cardiac output; NE, norepinephrine; TPR, total peripheral resistance.

21 Drugs Used in the Treatment of Heart Failure

21.1 Heart Failure

Heart failure is a pathophysiological state in which cardiac output is inadequate to meet the demands of the body tissues. The basic cardiac dysfunction is decreased cardiac output. Heart failure is a complex condition in which a variety of primary pathologic events are blended with varying compensatory mechanisms to produce the commonly recognized spectrum of clinical symptoms and signs, including tachycardia, dyspnea (shortness of breath), decreased exercise tolerance, edema, and cardiomegaly. Drug treatment is not curative, but involves attempts to restore cardiac function.

Drug Management of Heart Failure

The following drug classes are utilized in the management of heart failure. Most drugs lead to improved cardiac function by decreasing both preload and afterload (**Fig. 21.1**). The positive inotropic agents act directly on the heart to increase contraction. The mechanism of the beneficial effect of the β-blockers in heart failure is not understood.

1. Diuretics
2. Angiotensin-converting enzyme (ACE) inhibitors
3. Angiotensin receptor antagonists
4. β-blockers
5. Positive inotropic agents
6. Direct vasodilators

Fig. 21.1 ▶ **Congestive heart failure (CHF).**
In CHF, the heart is failing as a pump; cardiac output is therefore insufficient to meet the metabolic demand for oxygen in the body. CHF also causes fluid congestion in the lungs and venous circulation. Compensatory mechanisms, such as the activation of the sympathetic system and the renin–angiotensin system, are designed to increase cardiac output on a short-term basis but eventually place further strain on the heart if the heart failure is chronic. Drug therapy in chronic CHF aims to inhibit these unhelpful compensatory mechanisms. (ACE, angiotensin-converting enzyme.)

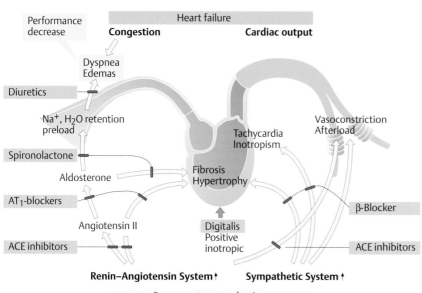

> **Etiology of heart failure**
>
> Heart failure can occur due to several etiologic factors, including intrinsic disease of the heart muscle (e.g., cardiomyopathy, ischemia, and infarction); chronic elevated preload (e.g., fluid overload and mitral regurgitation); chronic elevated afterload (e.g., aortic stenosis and hypertension); disorder of cardiac filling (e.g., cardiac tamponade); and when there is an inadequate heart rate, for example, following myocardial infarction (MI), β-blocker therapy, or negatively inotropic drug therapy (e.g., any antiarrhythmic drug).

> **Jugular venous pressure**
>
> The internal jugular vein passes medial to the clavicular head of the sternocleidomastoid muscle up behind the angle of the mandible. It is a reliable indicator of right atrial pressure. It is not normally visible or palpable but may become distended in right ventricular failure.

> **Preload**
>
> Up to a point, the heart pumps more when it is filled more during diastole. This is often labeled Starling's law of the heart or the Frank-Starling mechanism. The amount of filling is called preload. It is a reflection of forces in the vasculature acting to fill the ventricle. The amount of preload can be expressed in several ways, e.g., end diastolic volume, end diastolic pressure, or stretch (sarcomere length). It will be low in cases of hypovolemia or low systemic venous tone, and high in cases of fluid retention, many cases of heart failure, or excessive venous sympathetic stimulation. If the right ventricle is impaired, but not the left, right ventricular preload will tend to be high, while left ventricular preload will tend to be low.

Contractility

Contractility expresses the ability of the heart to contract at a given preload. Greater contractility manifests as greater systolic pressure or greater systolic ejection. At the cellular level, contractility reflects the amount of Ca^{2+} released from the sarcoplasmic reticulum with each heartbeat. The supply of Ca^{2+} in the sarcoplasmic reticulum is increased (positive inotropy) by anything that stimulates more Ca^{2+} to enter the cell through Ca^{2+} channels, or that stimulates the Ca^{2+}-ATPase (SERCA pump) to take up Ca^{2+} from the cytosolic space. Both effects increase the amount of Ca^{2+} stored in the sarcoplasmic reticulum between beats. Positive inotropic effectors include agents that cause a faster heart rate (more beats per minute allow more Ca^{2+} to enter per minute), sympathetic stimulation, drugs that are β-adrenergic agonists, and cardiac glycosides (e.g., digitalis) that reduce efflux of Ca^{2+} via Na^+/Ca^{2+} antiport. Negative inotropic effectors include β-adrenergic antagonists.

Afterload

Afterload is the pressure against which the ventricle works to eject blood during systole. At rest it is primarily a function of total peripheral resistance, i.e., it requires greater systolic pressure to eject blood in the face of high peripheral resistance. Afterload also depends on output of the heart, because pressure in the peripheral circulation is a function of the amount of blood ejected. For example, during exercise peripheral resistance is low, which by itself would decrease afterload, but afterload is actually somewhat elevated because the heart is ejecting so much blood that mean arterial pressure is increased.

21.2   Diuretics

Diuretics are first-line agents in heart failure therapy. They are used to resolve the signs and symptoms of volume overload, which are pulmonary and/or peripheral edema (**Fig. 21.2**). Once this goal has been achieved, diuretics are used to maintain a euvolemic state. The pharmacology of diuretics is discussed in detail in Chapter 19.

Fig. 21.2 ► **Mechanism of edema fluid mobilization by diuretics.**
Edema causes the accumulation of fluid, mostly in the interstitial space. Diuretics counteract this by increasing the renal excretion of Na^+ and water. This causes a reduction in plasma volume and the concentration of plasma proteins, which increases plasma colloid osmotic pressure and attracts water from the interstitium into the plasma.

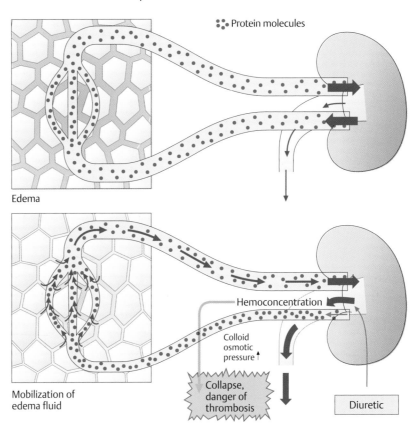

21.3   ACE Inhibitors and Angiotensin Receptor Antagonists

ACE inhibitors

ACE inhibitors are discussed in Chapter 20. Specific points in relation to heart failure are:

— ACE inhibitors, along with digitalis and diuretics, are now considered as first-line drugs for heart failure therapy.
— These agents acutely decrease systemic vascular resistance, venous tone, and mean blood pressure while producing a sustained increase in cardiac output.
— There is symptomatic improvement and reduced mortality in patients with heart failure.
— Exercise tolerance in patients with refractory heart failure is improved, and both salt and water retention are reduced.

Angiotensin Receptor Antagonists

Angiotensin receptor antagonists may be used in patients intolerant of ACE inhibitors or in combination with ACE inhibitors when a greater effect is required. These drugs are discussed in Chapter 20.

21.4   Beta-Blockers

Although administration of a β-blocker is seemingly paradoxical to improve cardiac function, several clinical trials have demonstrated that bisoprolol, carvedilol, and metoprolol have beneficial effects to improve cardiac function, decrease symptoms, and improve survival rates in chronic heart failure. Trials with other β-blockers have been negative. Bisoprolol and metoprolol are selective for the β_1 receptor (cardiac). Carvedilol blocks β_1, β_2, and α_1 receptors. The mechanism of this beneficial effect is unclear but may involve inhibition of pathologic changes of the myocardium that occur in heart failure or prevention of myocardial apoptosis. Beta-blockers are discussed in Chapter 20.

21.5   Positive Inotropic Agents

Digoxin

Digoxin, also known as digitalis, is a cardiac glycoside that was previously one of the mainstays in the treatment of heart failure. Its use is now reserved for when symptoms are not fully treated by standard therapies or in cases of severe heart failure while standard therapies are initiated. It can decrease symptoms and lower the rate of hospitalization for heart failure, but it does not decrease mortality.

Mechanism of action.   The therapeutic and toxic effects of digoxin are attributable to inhibition of Na^+-K^+-ATPase (the digitalis receptor) located on the outside of the myocardial cell membrane. Normally, this Na^+-K^+-ATPase pump is responsible for the exchange of these ions across the membrane. When the pump is inhibited, Na^+ accumulates intracellularly. Secondarily, the decreased Na^+ gradient affects Na^+-Ca^{2+} exchange, and Ca^{2+} accumulates inside the cell. Consequently, more intracytoplasmic Ca^{2+} (stored in the sarcoplasmic reticulum) is available for release and interaction with the contractile proteins during the excitation-contraction coupling process. At therapeutic doses of digoxin, there is an increase in contractile force. Toxicity to digitalis also relates to inhibition of the Na^+-K^+-ATPase pump. Inhibition of the Na^+-K^+-ATPase pump affects the K^+ gradient; this may lead to a significant reduction of intracellular K^+, predisposing the heart toward arrhythmias. Likewise, Ca^{2+} overload may contribute to serious arrhythmias.

Pharmacokinetics
— Digoxin can be given orally or IV

Effects
— The fundamental action of digoxin is to increase the force and velocity of cardiac contraction, resulting in a marked increase in cardiac output of the failing heart. The decrease in end-diastolic volume and pressure leads to a decrease in heart size, decreased venous pressure, and decreased edema.

— The second most important action of digitalis is to slow the heart rate (negative chronotropic action). The magnitude of slowing is dependent upon preexisting vagal or sympathetic tone. Both direct and indirect actions, mediated by the vagus nerve, contribute to the decrease in heart rate, decreasing the O_2 demand of the myocardium. The decreased sympathetic tone also increases renal blood flow and leads to diuresis and decreased edema.

Side effects.   Digoxin has a low therapeutic index, so toxicities are common and can be dangerous. They may include the following:

— *Cardiac arrhythmias:* as therapeutic concentrations are exceeded, the automaticity of secondary latent, ectopic pacemaker cells is increased. Premature ventricular contractions, ventricular tachycardia, and ventricular fibrillation are serious arrhythmias that occur in digitalis-toxic patients.
— Gastrointestinal effects are common and are among the earliest signs of toxicity. Anorexia, nausea, vomiting, and abdominal pain occur.
— Fatigue, headache, and drowsiness also are early signs of toxicity. More serious signs are disorientation, delirium, visual disturbances (photophobia, halos, and yellow vision), and, rarely, hallucinations or convulsions.

Treatment of toxicity.   Discontinue the drug, correct K^+ deficiency, and use digoxin antibodies (Fab fragments).

Drug interactions
— Digitalis toxicity is exacerbated most commonly by K^+ depletion with diuretics.
— Arrhythmias are enhanced by interaction with sympathomimetic agents.

21.6   Phosphodiesterase Inhibitors

Milrinone and Inamrinone

Mechanism of action.   Milrinone and inamrinone inhibit phosphodiesterase, leading to increased cyclic adenosine monophosphate (cAMP) in cardiac cells. This causes an increase in intracellular Ca^{2+} levels. These agents have positive inotropic effects and vasodilator activity.

Uses.   These agents are used infrequently. They are only given parenterally for short-term management of patients with heart failure that is refractory to digoxin, diuretics, and vasodilators. They are unacceptable for long-term use.

Side effects.   These include fever, nausea, vomiting, hypersensitivity reactions, hepatotoxicity, and thrombocytopenia. Milrinone is better tolerated.

21.7   Beta-Adrenergic Receptor Agonists

Dobutamine

Mechanism of action.   Dobutamine is a synthetic catecholamine that stimulates α_1 and β_1 receptors in both heart and blood vessels but selectively stimulates the cardiac β_1 receptors to produce its inotropic action.

Pharmacokinetics.   Dobutamine must be given by IV infusion.

Uses.   Dobutamine is used for short-term support in severe heart failure but is not used long-term, as it may cause arrhythmias and increase O_2 consumption.

21.8   Vasodilators

Direct Smooth Muscle Relaxants

Hydralazine, Isosorbide Dinitrate, Nitroprusside, and Nitroglycerin

See **Fig. 21.3** for an overview of the venous and arterial vasodilation of these agents.

Uses

The vasodilators hydralazine and isosorbide dinitrate added to an ACE inhibitor and a β-blocker have been effective in African American patients with more severe, class III and IV, heart failure.

Specific points in relation to heart failure

- Hydralazine is primarily an arteriolar vasodilator and may be beneficial in reducing afterload in congestive heart failure. Tolerance may develop to this drug. It may worsen fluid retention.
- Isosorbide dinitrate is an orally active agent similar in action to nitroglycerin and nitroprusside. It is combined with hydralazine in the treatment of heart failure.
- Nitroprusside is a potent relaxant for both veins and arteries. Its use is limited to short-term IV therapy. Its short half-life allows for titration and makes it beneficial in acute or severe refractory heart failure.
- Nitroglycerin is used for short-term IV treatment of severe heart failure. It dilates large-capacitance veins and reduces preload. Development of tolerance limits its therapeutic usefulness. See Chapter 22 for a more detailed discussion of nitroglycerin.

Fig. 21.3 ▶ **Vasodilators.**
Venous tone regulates the volume of blood returned to the heart and thus affects stroke volume and cardiac output. Arterial tone determines peripheral resistance. Vasodilator drugs may act preferentially on venous tone (nitrates) or on arterial tone (Ca^{2+} antagonists and hydralazine). They may also affect the tone of both (ACE inhibitors, α_1-antagonists, and sodium nitroprusside).

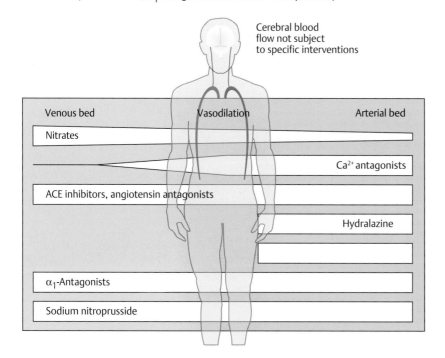

22   Antianginal Drugs

Coronary blood flow

The major right and left coronary arteries that serve the heart tissue are the first vessels to branch off the aorta. These arteries, when healthy, maintain coronary blood flow at levels appropriate to the needs of the heart muscle. When flow through a coronary artery is reduced to the point that the myocardium it supplies becomes hypoxic, angina pectoris develops. Some individuals have angina only on exertion; others have more severe restriction of blood flow and have anginal pain at rest. If the decrease in myocardial blood flow is severe and prolonged, irreversible changes occur in the muscle, and the result is an myocardial infarction (MI). Partially occluded coronary arteries can be constricted further by vasospasm, producing MI, or, most commonly, rupture of an atherosclerotic plaque triggers the formation of a coronary-occluding clot at the site of the plaque and leads to ischemia and MI.

Coronary artery bypass graft

Coronary artery bypass graft (CABG) is a surgical procedure performed to bypass atherosclerotic narrowings of the coronary arteries that are the cause of anginal pain. These narrowings can eventually occlude if untreated, leading to myocardial infarction (MI). There are two main coronary arteries, left and right, and these have several branches. A CABG is denoted as single, double, triple, and so on, depending on the number of arteries that are to be bypassed. The internal thoracic artery that supplies the anterior chest wall and breasts is usually harvested to use as the bypass artery.

Cardiac muscle metabolism

Cardiac muscle requires an abundant supply of oxygen-rich blood, because it depends almost exclusively on aerobic metabolism to supply the ATP for its contractions. Other tissues can vary their extraction of oxygen from blood and can survive on anaerobic metabolism. Cardiac tissue has a very high fractional extraction of oxygen and can only increase its uptake of oxygen by increasing coronary blood flow. At rest the heart uses oxidation of fatty acids for its ATP; only small quantities of glucose are utilized. When cardiac workload is increased, cardiac muscle removes lactic acid from coronary blood and oxidizes it directly.

22.1   Angina

Angina or angina pectoris is characterized by sudden, temporary, substernal pain that often radiates to the left shoulder and/or neck. It results from an imbalance of the supply of oxygenated blood to cardiac muscle and the oxygen demand of the tissue (**Fig. 22.1**). The primary goal in the treatment of angina is to restore the balance between oxygen supply and oxygen demand.

— Classic, typical, stable angina is induced by exercise or stress and is caused by atherosclerosis of the coronary arteries (**Fig. 22.2**).

— Variant or unstable angina is angina that is present at rest. It is due to coronary vasospasm.

Drug Management of Angina

1. Vasodilators
2. Beta-blockers
3. Calcium channel blockers

Fig. 22.1 ► **Oxygen supply to, and demand of, the myocardium.**
Oxygen supply to the myocardium occurs during diastole and is determined by the caliber of the coronary arteries and arterioles, as well as by preload. Oxygen demand occurs during systole and is determined by heart rate, contraction velocity, and afterload. Angina occurs when there is myocardial hypoxia due to inadequate myocardial blood flow (i.e., when oxygen demand exceeds supply). Therapy for angina therefore aims to restore balance, whether by increasing oxygen supply or decreasing oxygen demand.

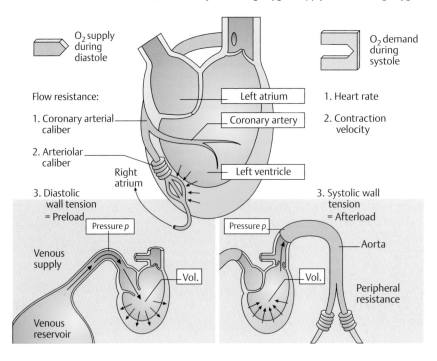

Fig. 22.2 ▶ **Pathogenesis of classic angina in coronary sclerosis.**
In a healthy person, the caliber of coronary arterioles determines myocardial oxygen supply and is adjusted automatically during exercise to meet the increased demand by increasing heart rate, contraction velocity, and afterload. In a patient with atherosclerosis of the coronary arteries, there is a dilation of arterioles at rest to compensate for the flow resistance caused by the atheroma, and myocardial oxygen supply is maintained. However, during exercise, further dilation cannot occur, leading to myocardial ischemia and pain.

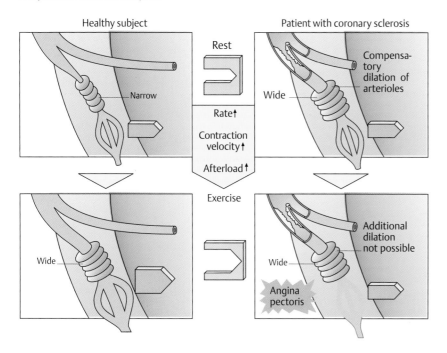

Myocardial infarction

Myocardial infarction (MI) is death of heart muscle. It is caused by complete occlusion of one or more coronary arteries by thrombosis. The pain of an MI is similar to that of angina but it is more severe and of longer duration. It is also accompanied by nausea, vomiting, diaphoresis (sweating), dyspnea (shortness of breath), and feeling "as if they are going to die." Common complications of MI include arrhythmias, heart failure, hypertension, and emboli formation. ECG analysis shows ST elevation, T wave inversion, and Q waves in the leads that "look at" the infarction. Cardiac enzymes are also measured and used as a basis for diagnosis of MI. Immediate treatment of an MI involves the use of thrombolytic drugs such as streptokinase (given as soon as possible after infarction) and aspirin, as well as morphine, and nitrates. Longer-term treatment involves the use of β-blockers and ACE inhibitors. Surgical treatment is the same as for angina.

Cardiac enzymes

Several enzymes are released when cardiac muscle cells are damaged: troponin I, creatine kinase, myoglobin, and lactate dehydrogenase. However, troponin I is the only one that is specific for cardiac muscle damage and is routinely measured to help diagnose MI.

22.2 Vasodilators

Organic Nitrates: Nitroglycerin, Isosorbide Dinitrate, Isosorbide Mononitrate, and Amyl Nitrite

Mechanism of action. Organic nitrates act like the endogenous compound nitric oxide (NO). They activate guanylate cyclase to increase cyclic guanosine monophosphate in smooth muscle. This leads to relaxation of vascular smooth muscle and both arterial and venous dilation (**Fig. 22.3**). By reducing preload and afterload, myocardial oxygen consumption is reduced. In the presence of a fixed stenosis, coronary blood flow is not altered. The decrease in mean blood pressure produces reflex activation of the sympathetic nervous system. Increases in heart rate and contractility partially reverse the decrease in oxygen consumption produced by arterial and venous vasodilation and can be blocked by β-adrenergic receptor antagonists. In patients with variant angina, the organic nitrates can prevent or reverse coronary artery spasm. Organic nitrates are effective for the treatment of classic and variant angina.

Pharmacokinetics
— Only isosorbide mononitrate is effective with oral administration.
— Nitroglycerin and isosorbide are given sublingually and are rapidly absorbed through the oral mucosa. Their therapeutic effects are observed within 2 to 4 minutes but last for only 1 to 2 hours.
— Nitrates are well absorbed through skin from ointments and sustained-release patches. The therapeutic effects of the ointment persist for 4 to 8 hours, and the sustained-release preparation can maintain stable blood levels of nitroglycerin for 24 hours. Usefulness is limited by rapid tolerance.

Fig. 22.3 ► **Vasodilators: nitrates.**
Nitrates cause vasodilation by acting like endogenous nitric oxide (NO), causing activation of guanylate cyclase and increased cyclic guanosine monophosphate (cGMP) levels in vascular smooth muscle cells. This vasodilation reduces cardiac work by reducing preload and afterload. Nitroglycerin and isosorbide dinitrate are both highly membrane permeable. (GTP, guanosine triphosphate; SH, sulfhydryl.)

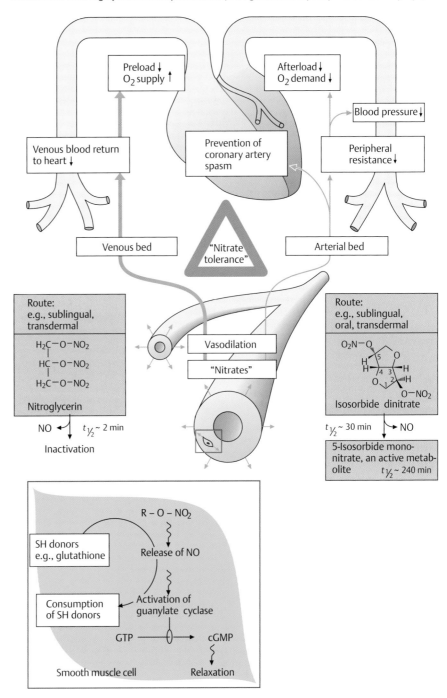

— Nitroglycerin may be given as an intravenous infusion in the treatment of myocardial infarction (MI).
— Amyl nitrite is volatile and is administered by inhalation.

Side effects
— Headache (Tolerance develops with repeated use.)
— Orthostatic (postural) hypotension

Tolerance.   The uninterrupted use of organic nitrates results in tolerance with subsequent doses of nitrates, producing little hemodynamic response. The use of dermal nitrates should not extend for more than 12 to 16 hours of any 24-hour period and must include a nitrate-free interval between doses.

22.3   Beta-Blockers

Beta-blockers are discussed in Chapter 20.

Specific points in relation to angina
— The β-adrenergic receptor antagonists are useful for the prophylaxis of effort-induced angina but are not effective for the acute termination of effort-induced angina or for the treatment of coronary artery spasm.
— When used in combination with organic nitrates, the drugs antagonize the increased sympathetic nervous system activity observed with the organic nitrates.

Table 22.1 compares the effects of nitrates and β-blockers on the heart.

Table 22.1 ▶ **Summary of Effects of Nitrates and β-blockers**					
Class of Drug	**Heart Rate**	**Contractility**	**Preload**	**Afterload**	**Oxygen Consumption**
Nitrates	Small increase	Small increase	Large decrease	Small decrease	Moderate decrease
β-Blockers	Large decrease	Large decrease	Small increase	Small increase	Moderate decrease

Note: The hemodynamic actions of the nitrates complement those of the β-blockers and are the basis for their concomitant use in the therapy of effort-induced angina.

22.4   Calcium Channel Blockers

Ca^{2+} channel blockers are discussed in Chapter 20.

Specific points in relation to angina
— In angina, calcium channel blockers act to increase coronary blood flow by dilating coronary vessels and decreasing myocardial oxygen demand by blocking Ca^{2+} channels on cardiac myocytes.

Table 22.2 provides a summary of the mechanisms by which antianginal drugs act.

Table 22.2 ► Summary of Mechanisms of Antianginal Drugs		
Drug Class	**Parameter Affected**	**Mechanism**
Nitrates	↓ preload and afterload	Activates guanylate cyclase to ↑ cGMP
	↓ myocardial O_2 consumption	
	↓ coronary artery spasm	
	↑ blood flow to ischemic areas of the heart	
β-blockers	↓ heart rate and contractility	Blocks sympathetic activation
	↓ myocardial O_2 consumption	
Calcium channel blockers	↑ coronary blood flow	Blocks L-type Ca^{2+} channels to dilate blood vessels and decrease contractility of cardiac muscles
	↓ myocardial O_2 consumption	
Abbreviation: cGMP, cyclic guanosine monophosphate.		

23 Antiarrhythmic Drugs

23.1 Electrophysiology of the Heart

Conduction System of the Heart

The sinoatrial (SA) node is the primary pacemaker of the heart, since it is able to spontaneously generate action potentials (inherent automaticity). These action potentials are conducted rapidly through the right atrial myocardium to the atrioventricular (AV) node, which delays the impulse before conducting it to the ventricles via the bundle of His and Purkinje fibers. This provides an orderly contraction sequence from apex to base for efficient ejection of blood from the ventricles (**Fig. 23.1**).

- The SA node spontaneously generates action potentials at a rate of ~80 to 100/min.
- The AV node also has inherent automaticity but at a slower rate than the SA node. If the SA node fails, the AV node will take over the pacemaker activity of the heart.
- The delay of the cardiac impulse at the AV node gives the contracting atria adequate time to empty their contents into the ventricles before ventricular contraction is initiated.

Note: The typical resting heart rate is 65 to 75 beats/min. This is due to vagal slowing of the heart below the intrinsic rate set by the SA node.

Fig. 23.1 ► **Cardiac conduction system.**
An impulse initiating cardiac contraction begins in the sinoatrial (SA) node. It travels through the atrial myocardium to the atrioventricular (AV) node. From the AV node, the impulse spreads to the ventricular myocardium via the bundle of His and Purkinje fibers. Contraction of the ventricular myocardium occurs from the inside to the outside from the apex to the base of the heart.

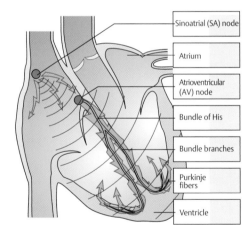

Sinoatrial (SA) node

Atrium

Atrioventricular (AV) node

Bundle of His

Bundle branches

Purkinje fibers

Ventricle

Cardiac Action Potentials

The ionic conductances that are a feature of action potential phases at the SA node, cardiac muscle, and branches of the conduction system are discussed in this section.

Action Potential Phases at the Sinoatrial Node

Refer to the action potential waveforms of slow response tissue in **Fig. 23.2**.

Phase 0

- This slow upstroke of the action potential shows membrane depolarization (it becomes less negative).
- It results from an increase in Ca^{2+} conductance, causing inward Ca^{2+} flow.

Fig. 23.2 ▸ **Membrane potential changes in cardiac muscle fibers.**
Slow response tissue includes the sinoatrial (SA) node and atrioventricular (AV) node. Fast response tissue includes the atrial and ventricular myocardium, the bundle of His, and Purkinje fibers. Slow and fast response tissues have distinct electrochemical properties. This causes them to react differently to antiarrhythmic drugs.

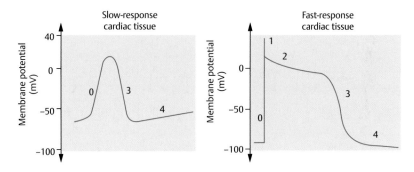

Phases 1 and 2

— These phases do not occur at the SA node.

Phase 3

— This is the repolarization phase.
— It results from an increase in K^+ conductance, which causes outward K^+ flow and repolarization of the membrane toward the K^+ equilibrium potential (the resting potential).

Phase 4

— The SA node does not have a stable resting membrane potential. During phase 4, it slowly depolarizes (which is responsible for its inherent automaticity).
— It results from an increase in Na^+ conductance, causing inward Na^+ flow and a decrease in K^+ conductance.

Note: The events at the AV node are similar to those at the SA node but slower. As a result, the AV node normally does not generate its own action potentials. This is because action potentials are conducted to the AV node more frequently than its own slow inherent rate of action potential generation.

Action Potential Phases at the Atrial and Ventricular Myocardium, Bundle of His, and Purkinje Fibers

Refer to the action potential waveforms of rapid response tissue in **Fig. 23.2**.

Phase 0

— This rapid upstroke of the action potential shows membrane depolarization (it becomes less negative).
— It results from an increase in Na^+ conductance, causing rapid inward Na^+ flow.
— This inward Na^+ flow stops after a few milliseconds due to inactivation of Na^+ channels.
— The maximum rate of voltage change during phase 0 (dV/dt) determines the conduction velocity.

Phase 1

— This is an early slight membrane repolarization (membrane becomes more negative).
— It results from rapid outward K^+ flow (due to a favorable electrochemical gradient) and a decrease in Na^+ conductance.

Phase 2

— This is the plateau of depolarization.
— In this phase, there is increased Ca^{2+} inward flow through L-type Ca^{2+} channels which approximately balances outward K^+ flow.
— Ca^{2+} entry during phase 2 is necessary for cardiac muscle contraction.

Phase 3

— This is the repolarization phase.
— It results from a decrease in Ca^{2+} conductance and an increase in K^+ conductance. The net effect of this is that there is a rapid outward K^+ flow, which repolarizes the membrane toward the K^+ equilibrium potential (the resting potential).

Phase 4

— This is the resting membrane potential.
— It is determined by high K^+ conductance, and its value is therefore close to the K^+ equilibrium potential (−96mV). At this potential, K^+ outflow and K^+ inflow are equal.

Measuring the Electrical Activity of the Heart: The Electrocardiogram

Recording an ECG

The *electrocardiogram* (ECG) is an overall representation of the electrical activity in the heart (**Fig. 23.3**). It is measured by recording voltages through surface electrodes, which "look" at the heart from different positions. A wave of depolarization moving toward a lead causes an upward deflection of the ECG. Analysis of the results of an ECG allows clinicians to diagnose a variety of cardiac disorders, including arrhythmias, ischemia, and the location of myocardial infarction (MI).

Interpretation of ECG Waves, Segments, and Intervals

Waves

— The P wave corresponds to atrial depolarization.
— The QRS complex corresponds to ventricular depolarization, which occurs from apex to base.
— The T wave corresponds to ventricular repolarization, which occurs from base to apex.

Note: Repolarization of the atria is masked by the QRS complex.

Excitation–contraction coupling in the heart

Contraction of cardiac muscle occurs when the excitation produced by an action potential is transmitted to cardiac myofibrils. Depolarization of the cardiac muscle cell membrane triggers an action potential that passes through T tubules. During phase 2 (plateau) of the action potential, there is increased Ca^{2+} conductance, causing inward Ca^{2+} flow. This inward Ca^{2+} flow initiates the release of Ca^{2+} from the sarcoplasmic reticulum (Ca^{2+}-induced Ca^{2+} release) which increases intracellular $[Ca^{2+}]$. Ca^{2+} binds to troponin C, and tropomysin moves out of its blocking position, allowing actin and myosin to form cross-bridges. The thick and thin filaments of actin and myosin slide past each other, resulting in cardiac muscle cell contraction. The contraction ends when Ca^{2+} ATPase facilitates the reuptake of Ca^{2+} into the sarcoplasmic reticulum, reducing the intracellular $[Ca^{2+}]$. The force of contraction of cardiac muscle cells is proportional to the amount of Ca^{2+} release, which varies depending on conditions.

Cardiac axis

The cardiac axis is the mean direction of electrical current flow through the ventricles during depolarization. It is calculated by analysis of the QRS complexes in the ECG leads. Many factors can alter the cardiac axis, including abnormal cardiac anatomy or position, myocardial infarction (MI), ischemia, pulmonary embolism, cardiomyopathy, and conduction abnormalities.

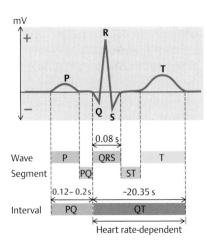

Fig. 23.3 ▶ **Electrocardiogram (ECG) curve.**
The ECG depicts electrical activity in the heart. The P wave corresponds to atrial depolarization. The QRS complex represents ventricular depolarization, and the T wave represents ventricular repolarization.

Segments

— The PQ segment is an isoelectric period between the P wave and the QRS complex. During this time, the wave of depolarization is traveling through the AV node into the bundle of His.
— The ST segment corresponds to the plateau phase of the cardiac action potential when all ventricular fibers are simultaneously depolarized.

Intervals

— The PQ interval corresponds to the conduction of the action potential through the AV node.
— The QT interval corresponds to ventricular depolarization and repolarization.

23.2 Arrhythmias

An *arrhythmia* is a disorder of the heart rate or rhythm. Arrhythmias may occur as a result of abnormal automaticity due to abnormal pacemaker sites within the atria or ventricles, known as *ectopic foci*. Under normal circumstances, their pacemaker activity is overridden by the pace set by the SA node; however, in cardiac disease states, they can cause additional beats, tachycardia (increased heart rate [>100 beat/min]), or bradycardia (decreased heart rate [< 60 beats/min]), depending on their site and the disease involved. Arrhythmias may also occur due to abnormal (reentry) conduction. This occurs when action potentials travel in a circuit within the heart rather than in one direction causing persistent excitation. Multiple reentry circuits within a chamber of the heart can lead to incoordination of cardiac muscle contraction known as *fibrillation*.

Table 23.1 provides a classification of arrhythmias.

Table 23.1 ▶ Classification of Cardiac Arrhythmias		
Arrhythmia	**Rhythm**	**Comment**
Atrial flutter	The atrial rhythm is both rapid and regular (300–400 beats/min).	One of every two (2:1 block) or three (3:1 block) atrial beats is conducted to the ventricle through the AV node. The ventricular heart rate (133–200 beats/min) is regular but too rapid to allow optimal ventricular filling during diastole.
Atrial fibrillation	The atrial rhythm is rapid (400–600 beats/min) and irregular. The ventricular rhythm is also rapid and irregular (100–150 beats/min).	The ventricular rate is slower than observed with atrial flutter.
Ventricular premature beats		These beats originate in the ventricles. They usually do not reduce cardiac output. Many patients with frequent premature ventricular beats may be bothered by palpitations.
Ventricular tachycardia	Rapid rhythm (200–400 beats/min) originating in the ventricles	Ventricular tachycardia can be self-terminating or sustained (lasting > 30 s). Patients with ventricular tachycardia and heart disease have a high probability of developing ventricular fibrillation. Ventricular tachycardia leading to ventricular fibrillation is the leading cause of death in the United States.
Ventricular fibrillation	Rapid rhythm (> 400 beats/min) originating in the ventricles	Ventricular fibrillation is invariably fatal unless electrical defibrillation is performed.
Abbreviation: AV, atrioventricular.		

Cardioversion

Cardioversion is a procedure in which an electrical shock is delivered to the heart via paddles or electrodes to convert an arrhythmia to a normal rhythm. It does this by causing all of the cardiac muscle cells to contract simultaneously. This brief interruption to the arrhythmia gives the SA nodes an opportunity to regain control over the pacing of the heart.

Valsalva maneuver

The Valsalva maneuver involves forceful expiration against a closed glottis, resulting in increased intrathoracic pressure that causes a reduction in venous return a reduction in cardiac output due to decreased preload (via the Starling mechanism), reduced heart rate and a fluctuation in aortic pressures (increased initially, then decreased). The Valsalva maneuver can be used to arrest episodes of supraventricular tachycardia and as a diagnostic aid to clinicians for some cardiac diseases (e.g., hypertrophic cardiomyopathy) that are worsened by the Valsalva. The Valsalva is also used by swimmers and people on aircraft to normalize ear pressures. A similar effect to the Valsalva maneuver is seen in people straining during a bowel movement. This is particularly dangerous for patients with pulmonary embolism.

23.3 Antiarrhythmic Drugs

Table 23.2 outlines a classification of antiarrhythmic agents that is based on the ion channel or receptor that they block and the effect they have on the action potential.

Table 23.2 ▸ **Classification of Antiarrhythmic Agents**		
Drug Class	**Mechanism of Action**	**Effect on Action Potential**
Class IA	Na^+ channel blockers	Slow phase 0, prolong action potential, slow conduction
Class IB	Na^+ channel blockers	Shorten phase 3, slow conduction
Class IC	Na^+ channel blockers	Markedly slow phase 0, slow conduction
Class II	β-blockers	Slow phase 4, slow automaticity, slow conduction
Class III	K^+ channel blockers	Prolong phase 3, slow conduction
Class IV	Ca^{2+} channel blockers (verapamil and diltiazem only)	Slow phase 0 to decrease automaticity, decrease amplitude and duration of phase 2

Class I Antiarrhythmic Drugs

All class I antiarrhythmic agents are local anesthetics that act to slow conduction in atrial and ventricular tissue. Their actions on the AV node are different for the individual agents. The effects of class I agents on channel opening, ionic conductances, and cardiac excitability are depicted in **Fig. 23.4.**

Class IA Agents: Quinidine, Procainamide, and Disopyramide

Mechanism of action. Class IA agents prolong the action potential duration and QT interval, thus slowing conduction. A prolonged QRS interval occurs at moderate and fast heart rates. All class IA drugs have anticholinergic actions. The drugs improve AV nodal conduction by antagonizing the actions of the vagus nerve on the AV node. They also directly depress AV nodal conduction. The net effect on AV nodal conduction is variable.

Uses

— Atrial fibrillation
— Atrial flutter
— Ventricular tachycardia
— Ventricular fibrillation

Note: These drugs should not be used alone for the treatment of atrial flutter or atrial fibrillation because the ventricular heart rate may dramatically increase, and the cardiac output may decrease. All three drugs depress myocardial contractility and can worsen existing heart failure.

Side effects

— May cause life-threatening arrhythmias (ventricular tachycardia or ventricular fibrillation) in patients treated for less serious arrhythmias. One life-threatening ventricular arrhythmia produced by both class 1A and class III agents is torsades de pointes.
— Heart failure due to negative inotropic effects
— Anticholinergic: dry eyes, dry mouth, and urinary retention
— Skin rash, muscle weakness, and arthralgia (joint pain)
— Cinchonism (ringing in the ears) and diarrhea (quinidine only [quinidine is the d-isomer of quinine])
— Acute lupus erythematosus (procainamide only)

▇ Torsades de pointes

Torsades de pointes is a rare form of ventricular tachycardia accompanied by distinctive ECG changes. It translates as "twisting of the points," which refers to the twisting of QRS complexes around the baseline electrical axis of the heart by at least 180 degrees. The QT interval is also prolonged. This arrhythmia can degenerate to ventricular fibrillation causing sudden death if untreated. Causes include therapy with class 1A and III antiarrhythmic agents, hypomagnesemia (low plasma Mg^{2+}), and hypokalemia (low plasma K^+).

Fig. 23.4 ▶ Effects of antiarrhythmic drugs of the Na⁺-channel blocking type.
Antiarrhythmics of the Na⁺ channel blocking type inhibit Na⁺ channel opening. This can result in a decreased rate of depolarization (phase 0), suppression of action potential (AP) generation, or an increase in the refractory period (phases 1–3).

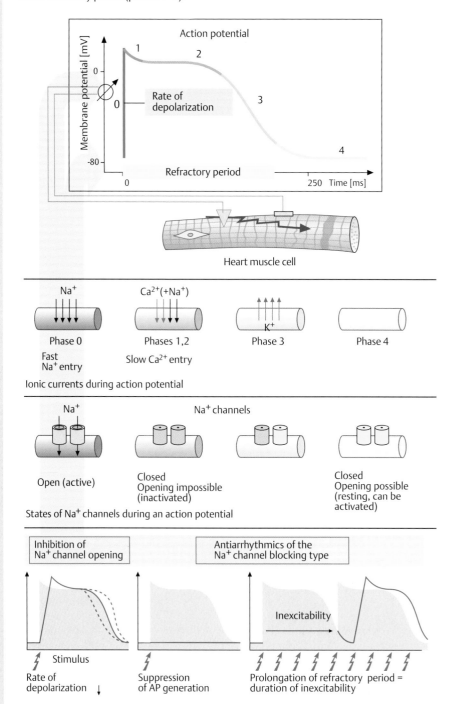

Class IB Agents: Lidocaine, Mexiletine, and Tocainide

Mechanism of action. Class IB agents shorten the action potential duration and the QT interval. Slow conduction and prolonged QRS interval occur at fast heart rates. Class IB drugs have little effect on AV nodal conduction or myocardial contractility.

Pharmacokinetics

— Lidocaine is rapidly metabolized in the liver. It has a short plasma half-life and is used as an intravenous (IV) infusion only in a hospital setting (**Fig. 23.5**).
— Tocainide and mexiletine are used orally for long-term therapy.

Uses

— Ventricular arrhythmias as an alternative to amiodarone (class III antiarrhythmic agent)

Side effects

— Central nervous system: act as local anesthetics in the brain
— Sedation at low doses
— Muscle twitching and vertigo with moderate dosages
— Convulsions at higher doses
— Agranulocytosis (acute low white blood cell count). This is a dangerous but uncommon side effect seen with tocainide.

Class IC Agents: Flecainide, Propafenone, and Moricizine

Mechanism of action. Class IC agents slow conduction, and prolonged QRS interval occurs at slow, moderate, and fast heart rates. These agents slow conduction in all cardiac tissues (including the AV node) and also depress cardiac contractility. They have no prominent effect on the duration of the action potential.

Fig. 23.5 ▶ **Antiarrhythmic drugs of the Na⁺-channel blocking type.**
Procaine and lidocaine are rapidly degraded in the body by cleavage (at the points indicated by arrows in the chemical structure box). These drugs must be given intravenously or by intravenous infusion. The orally administered drugs procainamide and mexiletine are not subject to such rapid degradation and are thus more likely to cause adverse effects. (CNS, central nervous system)

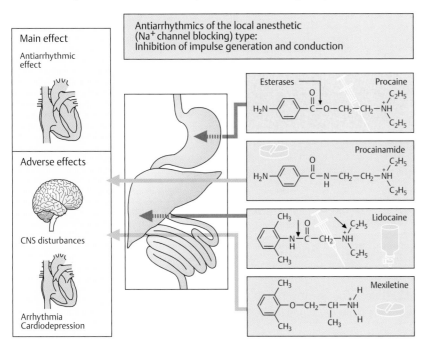

Uses

- Paroxysmal atrial flutter
- Paroxysmal atrial fibrillation
- Life-threatening ventricular arrhythmias

Side effects

- Heart failure (due to negative inotropic effects of all class IC drugs)
- Worsening of cardiac arrhythmias. These drugs may increase mortality when administered to patients surviving myocardial infarction (MI).
- Headache

Class II Antiarrhythmic Drugs

Beta-Adrenergic Receptor Antagonists: Propranolol and Esmolol

Mechanism of action. Class II β–adrenergic receptor antagonists slow phase 4 depolarization thus slowing automaticity, AV nodal conduction, and decreasing heart rate and contractility.

Uses. Class II agents are used to depress AV nodal conduction with atrial flutter-fibrillation and to prevent ventricular fibrillation during the first 2 years following myocardial infarction (MI).

Class III Antiarrhythmic Drugs

Amiodarone and Sotalol

Mechanism of action. The class III antiarrhythmic drugs prolong action potential duration without slowing conduction velocity.

Pharmacokinetics

- The half-life of amiodarone is ~30 days. There is a prolonged time to achieve efficacy with oral administration, and effects are prolonged after drug withdrawal.

Uses

- Treatment of recurrent ventricular tachycardia-fibrillation.

Note: Due to the high incidence of serious side effects, the class III drugs are restricted for life-threatening arrhythmias.

Side effects

- *Amiodarone:* corneal opacities, photosensitivity that produces a gray-blue skin rash, thyroid dysfunction (drug contains iodine atoms), peripheral neuropathy, and life-threatening pulmonary toxicity (pulmonary fibrosis and interstitial pneumonitis) that may not remit with drug withdrawal.
- *Sotalol:* all adverse effects seen with β-blockers and torsades de pointes

Class IV Antiarrhythmic Agents

Calcium Channel Blockers: Verapamil and Diltiazem

Mechanism of action. Class IV drugs inhibit calcium entry through L-type calcium channels in the myocardium and depress AV nodal transmission.

Note: Nifedipine and nicardipine, although excellent vasodilators and antianginal drugs, are poor inhibitors of AV nodal transmission and are ineffective as antiarrhythmic drugs.

Uses

- Treatment of atrial flutter-fibrillation
- Acute termination of AV nodal reentry

Side effects

- Sinus arrest or complete AV nodal blockade in the presence of β-adrenergic receptor blockade (verapamil)

Miscellaneous Antiarrhythmic Agents

Adenosine

Mechanism of action. Adenosine increases the vagal tone of the AV node and may directly depress AV nodal conduction.

Pharmacokinetics. Adenosine is administered as an IV bolus and has a plasma half-life of a few seconds (it is taken up by red blood cells). A repeat bolus can be given again within minutes if the first dose is ineffective.

Uses

- Acute termination of AV node reentry

Side effects

- Transient dyspnea
- Flushing

■ Nondrug therapies for arrhythmias

Surgical interventions have an important role in addition to or in place of drug therapy for arrhythmias. Catheter ablation of the source or conduction path of the arrhythmia by application of radiofrequency current applied through a large-tip electrode on a steerable catheter may be useful for supraventricular tachycardias, atrial arrhythmias, atrial fibrillation, and ventricular tachycardia. In patients with sinus node dysfunction or AV nodal block, or if heart block persists following an ablative procedure, implantation of a permanent pacemaker may be indicated. In ventricular fibrillation or ventricular tachycardia, implantation of a cardioverter defibrillator is superior to drug therapy in certain patient populations.

24 Drugs Acting on the Blood

Traumatic injury to blood vessels results in a series of events aimed at achieving hemostasis (cessation of bleeding), including vasoconstriction, platelet aggregation, and the deposition of fibrin (**Fig. 24.1**).

Platelet-mediated Hemostasis

Undamaged endothelium releases chemical mediators, such as prostacyclin and nitric oxide (NO). These are inhibitors of platelet aggregation. Prostacyclin acts by activating cyclic adensone monophosphate (cAMP). This, in turn, increases intracellular Ca^{2+} levels causing platelet inactivation and inhibition of platelet aggregation agents.

When there is physical damage to endothelium, platelets adhere to exposed subendothelial collagen fibers. This is bridged by von Willibrand factor (vWF) in the vascular epithelium interacting with glycoprotein 1b receptors on the surface of platelets. This adhesion activates platelets which release several substances: von Willibrand factor promotes adhesiveness and serotonin, platelet-derived growth factor (PDGF) and thromboxane A_2 promote vasoconstriction. Other mediators released by platelets enhance platelet activation and attract more platelets, e.g., adenosine diphosphate (ADP), platelet-activating factor (PAF), and thrombin. Activated platelets also change shape and glycoprotein IIb/IIIa (GPIIa/IIIb) receptors on their surface change their conformation which promotes the affinity of platelets for fibrinogen. Fibrinogen binding to GPIIa/IIIb on two separate platelets causes platelet cross-linking and further platelet aggregation.

Endothelial injury also stimulates the coagulation (clotting) cascade via the release of tissue factors and by mediators released by activated platelets. This results in the formation of thrombin (Factor IIa) which then catalyses the hydrolysis of fibrinogen to fibrin. Fibrin forms a meshwork within the platelet plug (aggregated platelets). Overall, a platelet-fibrin clot is produced that achieves hemostasis (**Figs. 24.1** and **24.2**).

> **Role of endothelial cells in preventing thrombus formation**
>
> Endothelial cells produce nitric oxide (NO) and prostacyclin, which inhibit platelets from adhering to undamaged, healthy endothelium. Diseases that impair endothelial function (e.g., elevated blood glucose, chronic hypertension, and smoking) therefore increase the tendency for platelets to adhere to epithelium and so predispose an individual to thrombosis.

Fig. 24.1 ▶ **Platelet-mediated hemostasis.**
Vascular injury and endothelial defects in vessel walls expose collagen and extracellular matrix. This causes the activation of platelets. Von Willebrand factor in vascular epithelium interacts with glycoprotein 1b in the platelet membrane to cause fast-flowing platelets to slow down at the site of an endothelial defect. The defect exposes collagen, which activates platelets and causes them to change shape and gain an affinity for fibrinogen. The platelets then become linked to each other via fibrinogen bridges, causing thrombus formation.

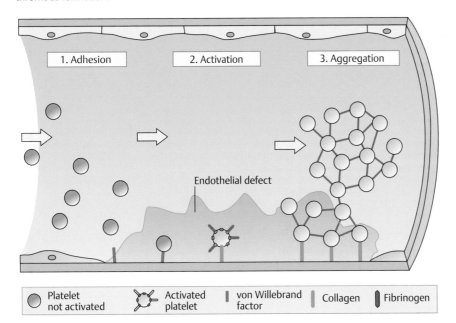

Fig. 24.2 ► **Aggregation of platelets by glycoprotein IIb/IIIa and fibrinogen.**
Glycoprotein IIb/IIIa in the platelet membrane change their conformation when platelets are activated by adhesion to collagen. This causes the platelets to gain an affinity for fibrinogen. Activated platelets release other substances, for example, serotonin and thromboxane A_2, which can activate other platelets. (ADP, adenosine diphosphate; PAF, platelet-activating factor.)

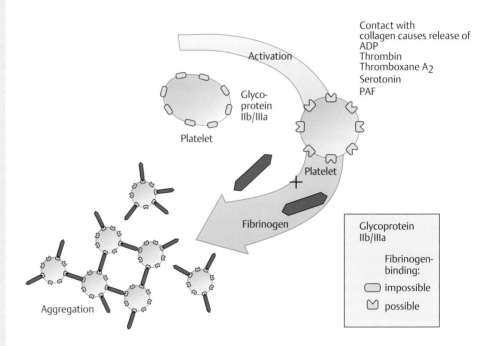

Thrombosis and Embolism

Thrombosis is the formation of an unwanted blood clot in a blood vessel or within the heart. It is an inappropriate response of the hemostatic process to alterations in the circulatory system, lesions in vascular walls, or other stimuli (**Fig. 24.2**).

Embolism occurs when thrombi are dislodged and are carried by the circulation to small vessels, where they may cause occlusions and tissue ischemia.

Thrombosis is treated by pharmacological agents designed to inhibit platelet function, inhibit fibrin deposition, or enhance fibrinolysis.

24.1 Antiplatelet Drugs

When platelets are stimulated to aggregate, arachidonic acid is liberated from platelet phospholipids and may be metabolized to thromboxane A_2 by the sequential actions of cyclooxygenase and thromboxane synthetase. As this occurs, platelet levels of cyclic adenosine monophosphate (cAMP) decrease, and adenosine diphosphate (ADP) is released. Both ADP and thromboxane A_2 are potent stimuli for platelet aggregation.

Aspirin

Aspirin is discussed in more detail in Chapter 33.

Mechanism of action. Aspirin acetylates platelet cyclooxygenase (COX-1) and irreversibly inhibits the enzyme (**Fig. 24.3**). This reduces the formation of thromboxane A_2.

Pharmacokinetics. Aspirin is usually given at a dose of 50 to 100 mg daily for its antithrombic effects.

Uses
- Prophylaxis or treatment of stroke or myocardial infarction (MI)
- Also used after vascular surgery, such as percutaneous coronary intervention, carotid endarterectomy or coronary artery bypass surgery, to prevent thrombosis

Side effects.   The major side effects of aspirin are gastrointestinal (GI) distress and bleeding.

Dipyridamole

Mechanism of action.   Dipyridamole inhibits platelet ADP release by increasing cAMP levels through two mechanisms: it increases adenosine concentrations in the blood, which stimulates adenylate cyclase to increase cAMP, and it is a phosphodiesterase inhibitor and slows cAMP catabolism to ADP. Dipyridamole also decreases the adhesion of platelets to artificial surfaces.

Uses.   This agent is available in combination with aspirin for prevention of cerebrovascular ischemia.

Side effects.   Dipyridamole produces vasodilation that may lead to flushing, headache, dizziness, and hypotension.

Clopidogrel and Ticlopidine

Mechanism of action.   Clopidogrel and ticlopidine inhibit ADP-induced platelet fibrinogen binding and subsequent platelet–platelet interactions (**Fig. 24.3**).

Uses
- Used in patients undergoing coronary stent placement to prevent thrombosis and restenosis
- Used for patients who have experienced or are at risk for cerebrovascular or cardiovascular thrombotic events (i.e., stroke or myocardial infarction) and is recommended for patients who cannot take aspirin

Fig. 24.3 ► Inhibitors of platelet aggregation.
Platelets attach to collagen via glycoprotein VI (GPVI) on platelet membranes. This activates them and causes them to secrete ADP and serotonin, as well as activating the enzyme cyclooxygenase (COX-1). COX-1 causes thromboxane A_2 to be produced from arachidonic acid. These substances activate glycoprotein IIb/IIIa (GPIIb/GPIIIa), which cause platelet aggregation via fibrinogen. Acetylsalicylic acid (ASA) inhibits COX-1, which prevents thromboxane formation. Clopidogrel is an ADP-receptor antagonist. Other agents (e.g., abciximab) block the binding of fibrinogen to GPIIb/GPIIIa. $P2Y_{12}$ is a subtype of purinergic receptor on platelets. TP, thromboxane prostanoid receptor.

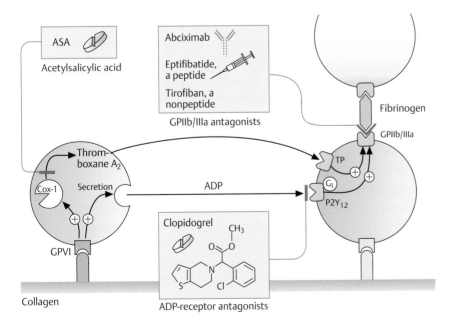

■ **Stroke**

Stroke is death of brain tissue due to either cerebral ischemia or intercerebral hemorrhage. Ischemic strokes are usually caused by thromboembolism but may rarely be caused by severe hypotension or vasculitis. Hemorrhagic strokes are usually due to rupture of an aneurysm. There are many risk factors for stroke including hypertension, diabetes, heart disease, peripheral vascular disesase, atrial fibrillation, and drugs (e.g., contraceptive steroids), and excess alcohol intake. Symptoms occur shortly after the cerebral event and relate to the area of brain affected. They may include difficulty speaking, understanding language, or walking; vision problems; contralateral paralysis or numbness; and headache. Treatment for ischemic stroke includes aspirin and t-PA anticoagulation. Hemorrhagic strokes require surgical removal of the clot and clipping or coiling of the aneurysm.

Side effects.   These drugs are generally well tolerated. Ticlopidine may produce agranulocytosis (acute low white blood cell count), and patients must be monitored for evidence of neutropenia.

Glycoprotein IIb/IIIa Receptor Antagonists

Abciximab, Eptifibatide, and Tirofiban

Abciximab is a monoclonal antibody, eptifibatide is a cyclic peptide, and tirofiban is a small molecule.

Mechanism of action.   This class of drugs prevents platelet aggregation by competing with fibrinogen and von Willebrand factor for occupancy of platelet receptors (**Figs. 24.2** and **24.3**).

Pharmacokinetics.   These agents are given intravenously (IV) for acute treatment or prophylaxis.

Uses

- Stent placement and coronary angioplasty (abciximab)
- Prevention of thrombosis in acute coronary syndrome (eptifibatide and tirofiban)

Side effects

- Bleeding at arterial sites
- Acute thrombocytopenia (low platelet count) may occur with abciximab

24.2   Anticoagulants

Heparin

Heparin is an endogenous sulfated mucopolysaccharide found in mast cells bound to histamine. The drug is commercially prepared from pork stomach and beef lung.

Mechanism of action.   Heparin combines with, and catalytically activates, a plasma cofactor named antithrombin III. This complex neutralizes several activated clotting factors, particularly factors IIa (thrombin) and Xa (**Figs. 24.4** and **24.5**). Heparin is active to a lesser extent against activated forms of factors VIII, IX, XI, and XII. It has no therapeutic effects other than the inhibition of clotting. Heparin causes the release of lipoprotein lipase from tissues, which hydrolyzes plasma triglycerides and has a "clearing" effect on turbid plasma.

Pharmacokinetics

- Heparin can be given IV or subcutaneously.
- Dosage is adjusted according to coagulation time (activated partial thromboplastin time) in therapy of acute thrombotic episodes.
- For prophylaxis, low doses of heparin are given, which cause little change in clotting time.

Uses

- Percutaneous coronary intervention
- Treatment and prevention of venous thromboembolism

Side effects

- Hemorrhage
- Thrombocytopenia. This may be mild and transient or severe if antiplatelet antibodies are formed.
- Osteoporosis. This occurs when long-term heparin therapy is necessary.
- Allergy. This probably develops to animal proteins in the solution.

▇ Heparin therapy in pregnancy

Heparins are used in the treatment of thromboembolic disease in pregnancy because they do not cross the placenta. Low-molecular-weight heparins are preferred because they have a lower risk of heparin-induced thrombocytopenia and osteoporosis.

▇ Heparin-associated osteoporosis

The exact mechanism of heparin-associated osteoporosis is unknown. It is thought that it may be due to the following: overactivation of osteoclasts by parathyroid hormone (PTH), reduced activity of osteoblasts, and/or increased bone resorption due to disruption of vitamin D metabolism and collagen activation. The fact that heparin has an affinity for Ca^{2+} leading to reduced Ca^{2+} in the blood and activation of PTH may support the first two theories.

▇ Heparin-induced hyperkalemia

Inhibition of aldosterone by heparin (including low-molecular-weight heparin) can result in hyperkalemia (low plasma K^+), especially with prolonged treatment. Patients with diabetes mellitus, chronic renal failure, acidosis, or raised plasma K^+ and those taking potassium-sparing diuretics are particularly at risk of hyperkalemia and should have their potassium levels monitored.

Fig. 24.4 ► Heparins: origin, structure, and mechanism of action.
Antithrombin III (ATIII) is a glycoprotein that can inactivate clotting factors. Heparin inhibits clotting by massively increasing the production of ATII. Different chain lengths of heparin are required to inactivate different clotting factors. The inactivation of thrombin (factor IIa) requires that heparin contact it and ATIII simultaneously; to inactivate factor Xa, contact between heparin and ATIII is sufficient. A serious complication of heparin usage is thrombocytopenia. This occurs when antibodies attach to heparin on platelets, causing platelet aggregation. This can lead to thromboembolism or hemorrhage. (MW, molecular weight; SC, subcutaneously.)

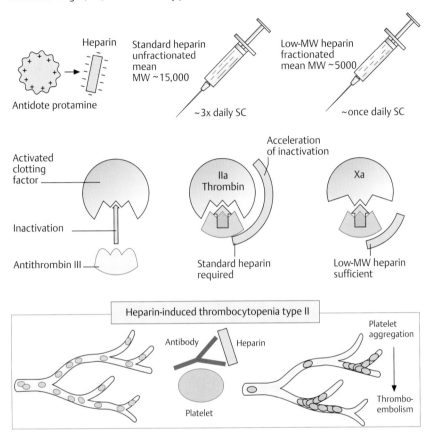

Thrombocytopenia

Thrombocytopenia is the term for a low platelet count. Causes include decreased production of platelets, e.g., due to leukemia or aplastic anemia, or increased breakdown of platelets, e.g., due to autoimmune disease, viruses, drugs (e.g., heparin and sulfa-containing antibiotics), thrombotic thrombocytopenic purpura (tTP), idiopathic thrombocytopenic purpura (ITP), and hypersplenism. Symptoms include nosebleeds, bruising, prolonged bleeding from cuts, and bleeding gums. Treatment may not be required for mild thrombocytopenia. Otherwise, treatment is aimed at the underlying cause.

Percutaneous coronary intervention

Percutaneous, meaning "through the skin," refers to procedures in which access to organs or tissues is achieved via needle puncture of the skin. Percutaneous coronary interventions include balloon angioplasty, implantation of stents, and rotational or laser atherectomy to clear atherosclerotic vessels.

Deep vein thrombosis

Deep vein thrombosis (DVT) is a blood clot (thrombosis) that most commonly occurs in the deep veins of the lower leg. It is precipitated by factors that cause abnormal blood clotting or venous circulation. Risk factors for developing DVT include immobility (e.g., sitting or lying for prolonged periods of time), surgery, obesity, pregnancy, malignancy, and estrogen-containing drugs. DVT is often asymptomatic, but it can present with swollen, hot, painful calves, with distended veins. There may also be increased resistance and pain on dorsiflexion of the foot (Homan sign). DVT is diagnosed by venograph or Doppler ultrasound and is treated by heparin, then warfarin anticoagulation. Deep vein thrombi may break off and cause a pulmonary embolism.

Antidote.   Protamine sulfate is an antidote for heparin and forms a 1:1 complex with the anticoagulant.

Enoxaparin

Mechanism of action.   Enoxaparin is a low-molecular-weight heparin that also binds antithrombin III, but the complex is less effective than the heparin-activated complex against thrombin. As a result, enoxaparin exerts an antithrombotic effect (primarily attributed to inhibition of clotting factor Xa) but has little effect on bleeding time.

Pharmacokinetics.   Enoxaparin is given by subcutaneous injection.

Uses
- Unstable angina
- Non-ST elevation myocardial infarction (NSTEMI)

Fig. 24.5 ► **Inhibition of clotting cascade in vivo.**
The clotting cascade requires the synthesis and activation of many clotting factors, so it can be inhibited at various steps. Coumarin anticoagulants decrease the synthesis of factors II, VII, IX, and X in the liver. Heparin and antithrombin III neutralize the protease activity of activated factors.

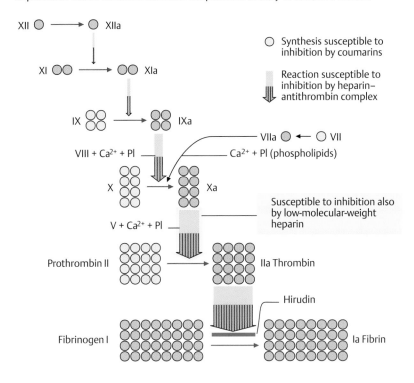

— Acute MI with ST elevation
— Percutaneous cardiac intervention

Note: These agents cannot be used interchangeably (unit for unit) with heparin or other low-molecular-weight heparin preparations.

Side effects
— May produce mild thrombocytopenia; thus, periodic platelet counts should be taken.

Contraindications
— Patients with major bleeding

Direct Thrombin Inhibitors

Bivalirudin, Lepirudin, and Argatroban

Mechanism of action. These agents inhibit clot-bound and circulating thrombin.

Pharmacokinetics. Given IV

Uses
— Bivalirudin can be used instead of heparin in patients undergoing coronary angioplasty.
— Lepirudin and argatroban are indicated for use in patients with heparin-induced thrombocytopenia.

Side effects. The main side effect of these agents is bleeding.

Warfarin

Mechanism of action. Warfarin is an coumarin oral anticoagulant drug that antagonizes the hepatic synthesis of the vitamin K–dependent clotting factors II (prothrombin), VII, IX, and X (**Figs. 24.5** and **24.6**).

■ Warfarin and International Normalized Ratio

Dosages of warfarin depend on the measurement of prothrombin time, reported as International Normalized Ratio (INR). This is usually measured daily in the early days of treatment and then at appropriate intervals thereafter. A normal INR is 1, and the target INR in oral anticoagulant therapy is different depending on the condition for which anticoagulation is required. For example, for treatment of DVT, an INR of 2.5 may suffice, whereas for patients with a prosthetic heart valve, a target INR of 3.5 is more appropriate.

Fig. 24.6 ► **Vitamin K antagonists of the coumarin type and vitamin K.**
Vitamin K promotes the carboxylation of glutamine residues on factors II, VII, IX, and X in the liver. Carboxyl groups are required for Ca^{2+}-mediated binding of factors to phospholipids. Coumarin anticoagulants (e.g., warfarin) act as "false" vitamin K molecules and prevent the regeneration of active vitamin K from vitamin K epoxide.

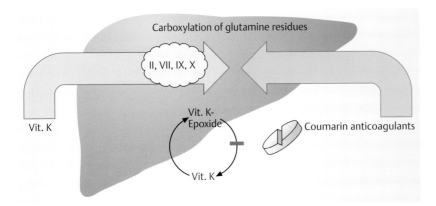

Pharmacokinetics

— Well absorbed after oral administration
— Highly bound to plasma proteins (> 90%)
— Metabolized in liver prior to excretion
— Onset of action of 2 to 3 days, during which time preexisting levels of clotting factors are diminished
— Highly variable effects are seen from patient to patient; dosage is adjusted on the basis of the prothrombin time (a standard clotting test).

Uses

— Long-term anticoagulant therapy
— Acute venous thromboembolism
— Atrial fibrillation (to reduce the risk of thromboembolic stroke)

Side effects

— Hemorrhage
— Teratogenesis, especially during the first trimester. This may be explained by the fact that other vitamin K–dependent functions are affected by warfarin administration.
— Liver and kidney toxicity are seen only with indanedione derivatives which limits the usefulness of this chemical class of anticoagulants.
— Drug interactions occur between the oral anticoagulants and many other drugs (**Fig. 24.7**).

Antidote. Phytonadione (vitamin K_1) is a warfarin antagonist that is used in warfarin poisoning.

■ **Clotting tests**

There are four tests used to gauge hemostatic activity:
1. *Quick test:* plasma is made incoagulable with a Ca^{2+} chelating agent (citrate, oxalate, or ethylenediaminetetraacetic acid [EDTA]). Excessive amounts of Ca^{2+} and tissue thrombokinase are then added. Clotting time is compared with normal values (70–125%).
2. *Partial thromboplastin time (PTT):* kephalin, kaolin, and Ca^{2+} are added to citrated plasma, and clotting time is measured (normal clotting time: 25–38 s).
3. *Prothrombin time (PT):* thrombin is added to citrated plasma (normal clotting time: 18–22 s).
4. *Bleeding time:* bleeding time is measured (e.g., prick in earlobe).
Note: Platelet counts are also extremely important in monitoring hemostatic activity.

Fig. 24.7 ► **Possible interactions of vitamin K antagonists and vitamin K.**
Dosages of coumarin anticoagulants must be balanced to protect against thrombosis while minimizing the risk of bleeding. Extrinsic factors, such as pharmacological interactions, may threaten this vitamin K/coumarin balance, so dosage adjustment will be necessary.

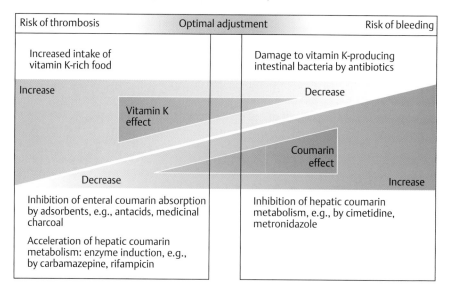

Pulmonary embolism

Pulmonary embolism (PE) is an obstruction in the pulmonary arterial system, usually caused by blood clots from the periphery, particularly the deep veins of the legs, which are transported to the lung. Symptoms include dyspnea (shortness of breath), chest pain exacerbated by taking a deep breath or coughing, cough +/– hemoptysis. PE decreases the area available for diffusion of gases (increases dead space) and so a ventilation/perfusion (V/Q) scan will show a mismatch. In severe cases pulmonary embolism can cause death due to hypoxia and cor pulmonale (right heart failure due to chronic pulmonary hypertension). Treatment involves the use of the anticoagulants heparin and warfarin or thrombolytics, e.g., streptokinase (not normally required). Surgical clot removal may be necessary for large pulmonary emboli.

Myocardial infarction and fibrinolysis

Thrombolytic drugs, such as streptokinase, have been shown to reduce mortality in patients having an acute myocardial infarction (MI). They need to be given within 12 hours of symptom onset but ideally within 1 hour. They should be used with caution if there is a risk of bleeding and are absolutely contraindicated if the patient has had a recent hemorrhage, trauma, or surgery, or has a known bleeding disorder.

Thrombolytic Drugs

Mechanism of action. These agents promote the dissolution of thrombi by stimulating the conversion of endogenous plasminogen to plasmin (fibrinolysin). Plasmin limits the growth of a clot and dissolves the fibrin meshwork as the endothelial injury heals (**Fig. 24.8**). Bleeding is the primary adverse effect of these drugs. Patients may also require anticoagulant therapy to prevent reocclusion of blood vessels.

Uses. These agents are used to degrade existing thrombi in cases of myocardial infarction (MI), stroke, or pulmonary embolism.

Streptokinase

Streptokinase is produced from cultures of β-hemolytic streptococci and is therefore antigenic but readily available.

Side effects. Allergic and febrile reactions are the most common nonhemorrhagic side effects.

Anistreplase

Anistreplase is an acylated plasminogen–streptokinase activator complex. It is activated after deacylation in the body. This combination is similar to streptokinase but has a longer duration of thrombolytic action.

Urokinase

Urokinase is obtained from human urine or kidney tissue culture and is not antigenic, but it is quite expensive.

Tissue Plasminogen Activators: Alteplase, Reteplase, and Tenecteplase

Mechanism of action. Tissue plasminogen activator (t-PA) is a human protein that specifically cleaves plasminogen, leading to the formation of plasmin. The activity of t-PA is accelerated in the presence of fibrin. Thus, it preferentially activates plasminogen bound to fibrin, which provides "clot-specific" thrombolytic activity.

– Alteplase is human t-PA produced by recombinant DNA methods.
– Reteplase and tenecteplase are bioengineered recombinant mutant forms of t-PA.

Fig. 24.8 ▶ **Fibrinolysis.**
Fibrinolysis occurs when plasminogen is activated to plasmin under the influence of factors such as kallikrein (a peptidase), urokinase, and tissue plasminogen activator (t-PA). Plasmin then acts on the fibrin meshwork to dissolve the clot into fibrinopeptides. Streptokinase and urokinase act as thrombolytic drugs by activating plasminogen. Some anticoagulant drugs (e.g., tranexamic acid), as well as endogenous substances (α_2-antiplasmin), act by inhibiting plasma-mediated fibrinolysis.

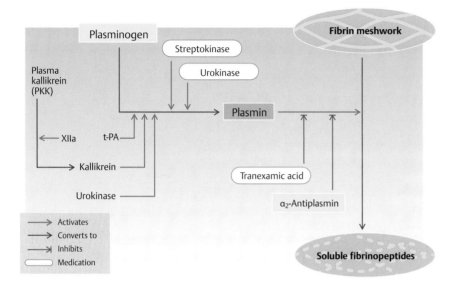

Pharmacokinetics

— Alteplase has a short plasma half-life (4–5 min) and requires a constant infusion to maintain a therapeutic level.
— The modifications of reteplase result in less fibrin binding, a longer half-life, and greater thrombolytic potency than t-PA. Tenecteplase also has a longer plasma half-life, but it has enhanced fibrin specificity.

Drugs Used in the Treatment of Bleeding

Aminocaproic Acid and Tranexamic Acid

Mechanism of action. These agents inhibit plasmin and plasminogen activator (**Fig. 24.8**).

Uses. They can be used to prevent bleeding in hemophiliacs undergoing dental extractions, as well as in hemorrhage secondary to aplastic anemia, hepatic cirrhosis, or nephrotic disease.

Desmopressin (Antidiuretic Hormone)

Desmopressin is also discussed on page 190.

Mechanism of action. Desmopressin stimulates the release of clotting factor VIII from the vascular endothelium.

Uses. Desmopressin is used preoperatively in hemophilic patients with low circulating levels of this factor.

Pentoxifylline

Mechanism of action

Pentoxifylline is a dimethylxanthine derivative that decreases blood viscosity and increases erythrocyte flexibility.

Uses. Pentoxifylline is indicated for muscle pain during exercise associated with occlusive arterial diseases of the limbs (intermittent claudication).

■ Hemophilia A and B

Hemophilia A is an autosomal recessive deficiency of factor VIII causing impairment of blood clotting. Symptoms depend on the severity of the factor VIII deficiency and include extensive nosebleeds, bruising, prolonged bleeding from cuts, bleeding gums, hemarthroses (bleeding into joints), muscle hematomas, and blood in the urine or stool. Hemarthroses may lead to arthritis and hematomas may cause nerve damage. Treatment involves the use of desmopressin and concentrated factor VIII replacement. NSAIDs and intramuscular injections should be avoided in these patients.

Hemophilia B (Christmas disease) is caused by a deficiency of factor IX. Clinically, it behaves the same as hemophilia A.

■ Von Willebrand disease

Von Willebrand disease is an autosomal dominant deficiency of a protein called Von Willebrand factor and factor VIII that is carried along with this. This causes reduced platelet adherence producing symptoms such as nosebleeds, bruising, prolonged bleeding from cuts, and bleeding gums. However, unlike hemophilia, hemarthroses and muscle hematomas are rare. Treatment is by concentrated Von Willebrand factor and factor VIII replacement, desmopressin, or antifibrinolytic drugs.

Iron deficiency anemia is referred to as a microcytic, hypochromic anemia because red blood cells are smaller and paler than usual when a blood smear is viewed through a microscope. Megaloblastic anemia is characterized by immature (megaloblastic) red blood cells that are macrocytic and hyperchromic. Flow cytometry is used in laboratories to measure red blood cell count; hemoglobin concentration; mean corpuscular volume (MCV), which reports the size of the red blood cell; and red blood cell distribution width (RDW), which measure the deviation of the volume of red blood cells. These can then be used to calculate the patient's hematocrit (percentage of the blood that is composed of red blood cells); mean corpuscular hemoglobin (MCH), which is the mean hemoglobin content of each red blood cell; and mean corpuscular hemoglobin concentration (MCHC), which is the mean hemoglobin content of a given volume of red blood cells. All of these measurements are used clinically to distinguish the different causes and the severity of anemia.

■ **Hematocrit**

The hematocrit is the percentage of blood volume that is red blood cells (RBCs). It is normally ~48% for men and ~38% for women. The hematocrit is elevated in polycythemia (a disorder in which the bone marrow produces excessive RBCs), and in diseases which cause hypoxia (e.g., chronic obstructive pulmonary disease [COPD]) as the body attempts to compensate by producing more RBCs. It can also be elevated in dehydration. The hematocrit is lowered in hemorrhage and iron-deficiency anemia.

■ **Signs and symptoms of anemia**

Anemia may be asymptomatic, or there may be any of the following signs and symptoms: fatigue, pallor (seen most readily by inspection of the conjunctiva or mucous membranes), dizziness, particularly upon standing (postural hypotension), headache, dyspnea (shortness of breath), coldness of the hands and feet, palpitations, and glossitis (swelling and soreness of the tongue). In severe cases, anemia can cause chest pain (angina due to hypoxia of cardiac muscle) and heart failure (as the heart has to work harder to oxygenate tissues). Iron deficiency anemia also commonly causes brittle nails, cracks at the corner of the mouth, and predilection to infection. Pernicious anemia causes neurologic symptoms, such as numbness, tingling, weakness, and impairment of coordination and memory.

24.3   Anemia and Antianemia Drugs (Hematinics)

Iron Deficiency Anemia

Iron deficiency anemia is a condition in which there is insufficient hemoglobin in red blood cells due to a lack of iron (which is an essential component of heme). Approximately two thirds of the iron content of the body (women: 2 g, men: 5 g) is bound to hemoglobin.

Iron deficiency anemia is usually caused by blood loss from menses in premenopausal women, but it can also be due to inadequate dietary intake of iron, gastrointestinal (GI) bleeding (e.g., from peptic ulcers, long-term use of nonsteroidal antiinflammatory drugs [NSAIDs], or certain GI cancers), from GI conditions that decrease the absorption of iron (e.g., Crohn disease), or by pregnancy (in which the need for iron is increased due to the increase in maternal blood volume and for fetal hemoglobin synthesis).

Drugs Used to Treat Iron Deficiency Anemia

Ferrous Sulfate

Pharmacokinetics

— See **Fig. 24.9** for absorption of iron and other pharmacokinetic factors.
— Ferrous sulfate is given orally, three or four times daily, preferably on an empty stomach to increase iron absorption.

Uses

— Drug of choice for iron deficiency anemia

Side effects.   Side effects involve GI symptoms, resulting from the direct toxic effect of iron. This may cause patient noncompliance and is the most common cause of therapeutic failure. This problem can usually be resolved by an adjustment in dosage.

Iron Dextran

Pharmacokinetics

— Iron dextran may be given by intramuscular or IV (preferred) injection.
— Parenterally administered iron is associated with several adverse effects and is indicated only when the need for iron cannot be met by oral administration.
— Dosages must be carefully calculated so that the body's storage capacity is not exceeded ("iron overload").

Antidote.   Deferoxamine mesylate is a specific chelating agent for iron. It may be administered orally or parenterally for treatment of acute iron poisoning or iron overload.

Megaloblastic Anemia

Megaloblastic anemia is a condition caused by inhibition of DNA synthesis in red blood cell production. It is caused by a lack of vitamin B_{12} and/or folic acid.

Folic acid is widely available in the diet, and deficiency due to dietary insufficiency alone is uncommon in the United States. Alcohol and some drugs (e.g., anticonvulsants) are folate antagonists and may exacerbate megaloblastic anemia caused by folate deficiency. Folic acid is necessary for the biosynthesis of thymidylate and subsequent formation of DNA. Orally administered folic acid is usually adequate for all folate-deficiency conditions.

The daily requirement for vitamin B_{12} is extremely low (2–5 µg), and because this vitamin is found in many foods of animal origin, a deficiency due to dietary insufficiency is rare. However, the absorption of vitamin B_{12} from the GI tract requires the presence of intrinsic factor, a protein secreted in the stomach. The absence of intrinsic factor, as in pernicious anemia, results in inadequate vitamin B_{12} absorption.

Fig. 24.9 ▶ Iron: possible routes of administration and fate in the organism.
Ferrous iron (Fe^{2+}) and heme are well absorbed in the small bowel, where they are oxidized and deposited as ferritin or transported in the plasma protein transferrin to erythroblasts for hemoglobin synthesis. Macrophages degrade erythrocytes, which liberate iron from hemoglobin. This iron can be stored as ferritin or recycled for erythropoiesis in bone marrow via transferrin. Iron is usually given orally for therapeutic replacement. When this is not possible, parenteral iron is given in the form of Fe^{3+} (ferric) complexes. This prevents free iron toxicity, as Fe^{3+} can bind to transferrin or be stored in macrophages.

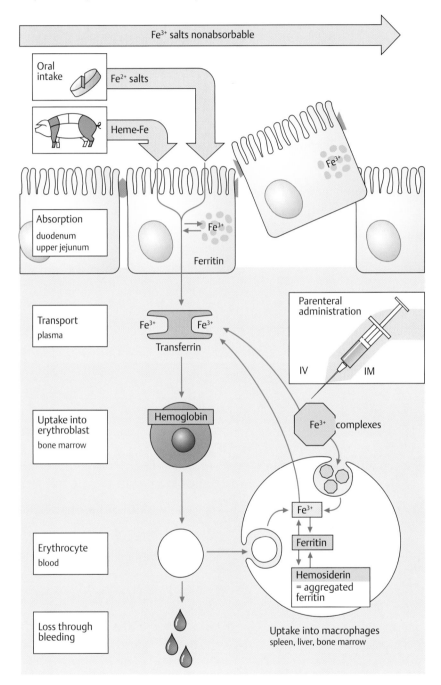

Hemochromatosis

Hemochromatosis is a condition in which there is failure of regulation of iron absorption in the bowel. This leads to excessive iron in the body, which then gets deposited in organs, such as the liver, heart, pancreas, and pituitary. Signs include fatigue, arthralgia (joint pain), changes in skin pigmentation, liver disease, cardiomyopathy, and diabetes. Management is by venesection until the patient is iron deficient.

■ Erythrocyte sedimentation rate

The erythrocyte sedimentation rate (ESR) is a nonspecific test that is a marker for conditions associated with acute and chronic inflammation. It does not provide a conclusive diagnosis but rather prompts the clinician to do further investigations. It measures the rate of sedimentation of red blood cells in anticoagulated blood over 1 hour. If certain proteins cover red cells, these will stick together and will fall faster. The ESR rises with age and anemia.

■ Folic acid and prevention of neural tube defects

Folic acid supplement taken before and during pregnancy can reduce the occurrence of neural tube defects, such as spina bifida. Dosages of folic acid are different depending on the couple's risk factors for neural tube defects.

■ Vitamin B$_{12}$ absorption

Vitamin B$_{12}$ absorption from the gastrointestinal tract involves several steps: B$_{12}$ is released from dietary proteins by gastric acid. It then binds to R proteins, which are secreted in saliva. In the duodenum, trypsin digests the R protein, liberating B$_{12}$ which then forms a complex with intrinsic factor (IF), a glycoprotein secreted by gastric parietal cells. This B$_{12}$-IF complex is resistant to the effects of trypsin and travels to the terminal ileum where it binds to specific receptors and is absorbed via receptor-mediated endocytosis.

Drugs Used to Treat Megaloblastic Anemia

Leucovorin (Folinic Acid)

Mechanism of action.   Folinic acid is a folic acid derivative with vitamin activity equal to folic acid. It does not require reduction by dihydrofolate reductase to be converted to tetrahydrofolate.

Uses

— Injected to "rescue" normal cells after high-dose methotrexate treatment in cancer chemotherapy
— Can also be given as a folate supplement if oral therapy is not feasible

Vitamin B$_{12}$

Mechanism of action.   Vitamin2 B$_{12}$ is required for the normal metabolism of folic acid, and a vitamin B$_{12}$ deficiency will cause a pernicious anemia (a type of megaloblastic anemia) because of diminished folate-dependent DNA synthesis. However, neurologic symptoms observed in pernicious anemia apparently develop from defective biosynthesis of myelin, which does not involve folic acid.

Pharmacokinetics.   See **Fig. 24.10** for the metabolism of vitamin B$_{12}$ and folate.
— Vitamin B$_{12}$ is given intramuscularly at monthly intervals for the rest of the patient's life.
— Oral vitamin B$_{12}$ preparations with intrinsic factor derived from animals give erratic and unreliable results.

Uses
— Pernicious anemia

Fig. 24.10 ▶ **Vitamin B$_{12}$ and folate metabolism.**
Vitamin B$_{12}$ is absorbed in the small intestine but requires intrinsic factor, produced by parietal cells in the stomach. It is transported in the blood by transcobalamin II to the liver for storage or to erythropoietic cells to facilitate the conversion of methyltetrahydrofolic acid to tetrahydrofolic acid (THF), which is important in DNA synthesis. Therapeutically, vitamin B$_{12}$ is given parenterally. Folic acid is also absorbed in the small intestine and is taken up into erythropoietic cells. Therapeutically, it can be administered orally.

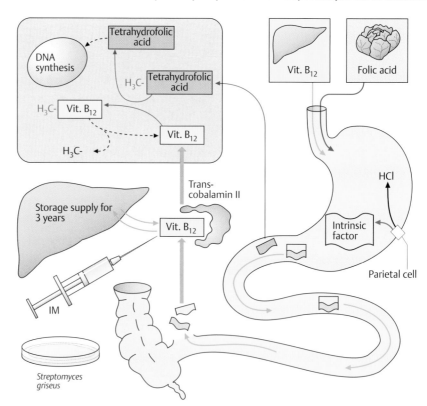

24.4 Hematopoietic Growth Factors

Filgrastim and Sargramostim

Granulocyte (G) and granulocyte-macrophage (GM) colony stimulating factors (CSF) are naturally occurring peptide growth factors. Filgrastim is a G-CSF; sargramostim, a GM-CSF.

Uses

— Stimulation of bone marrow growth after transplantation or cancer chemotherapy

Epoetin Alfa

Uses

— Anemia due to renal failure, bone marrow disease, cancer chemotherapy, or in patients with acquired immunodeficiency syndrome (AIDS) receiving AZT (zidovudine, formerly called azidothymidine).

Interleukin II (Opreleukin)

Mechanism of action. Interleukin II stimulates the formation of platelet progenitor cells.

Uses. Interleukin II is used to speed platelet recovery in patients undergoing chemotherapy with nonmyeloid malignancies.

■ Erythropoietin

Erythropoietin (epoetin α) is a renal hormone that regulates the production of red blood cells in the bone marrow. Patients with chronic renal failure develop anemia secondary to inadequate levels of erythropoietin. Human recombinant erythropoietin has been shown to be effective in treatment of anemia associated with uremia. There are no direct adverse effects of replacement therapy, although ~25% of patients experience hypertension during treatment (mechanism not understood).

25   Antihyperlipidemic Drugs

25.1   Lipids and Lipoproteins

Lipids (fats) are polar molecules made up of glycerol and fatty acids. Most dietary fats are triglycerides, which are made up of glycerol and three fatty acids. These are stored by the body and provide an energy source when required. Cholesterol is also ingested in smaller amounts. Cholesterol is an essential component of cell membranes. All lipids are insoluble in water and need to be coated in phospholipids, which contain apolipoproteins, to be absorbed in the circulation. These transport forms of lipids are designated as chylomicrons, low-density lipoproteins (LDLs), very-low-density lipoproteins (VLDLs), or high-density lipoproteins (HDLs), depending on their relative quantities of triglycerides and cholesterol, as well as the type of apolipoproteins in the phospholipid layer. Lipoprotein metabolism is shown in **Fig. 25.1**.

Dyslipidemia and Related Diseases

Dyslipidemia is a general term used to describe high levels of LDL cholesterol (LDL-C) or triglycerides, or low levels of HDL cholesterol (HDL-C). Dyslipidemias are major contributors to atherosclerosis and atherosclerosis-related conditions, such as coronary heart disease (CHD), ischemic cerebrovascular disease, and peripheral vascular disease. Genetic disorders and lifestyle may contribute to the dyslipidemias. Therapy for dyslipidemias is based on the blood levels of LDL-C, HDL-C, and triglycerides (found mainly in VLDL cholesterol).

> ### Lipoprotein levels
>
> The optimal level for LDL cholesterol is < 100 mg/dL. It is considered high when it is ≥ 160 mg/dL. HDL cholesterol should ideally be < 40 mg/dL. It is considered high if it is > 60 mg/dL. Total cholesterol should be < 200 mg/dL. It is considered high if it is > 240 mg/dL.

Fig. 25.1 ▶ **Lipoprotein metabolism.**
Enterocytes release absorbed lipids in the form of triglyceride-rich chylomicrons. These are acted upon by lipoprotein lipases in endothelial cells, producing fatty acids, which are stored in tissues. The remnants of chylomicrons are transported to liver cells, where they are a source of dietary cholesterol. The liver uses this and hepatically produced cholesterol to synthesize very-low-density lipoproteins (VLDLs) and bile acids. VLDLs are released into the blood and supply tissues with fatty acids. The low-density lipoprotein (LDL) remnants either return to the liver or supply cells with cholesterol. (HDL, high-density lipoprotein.)

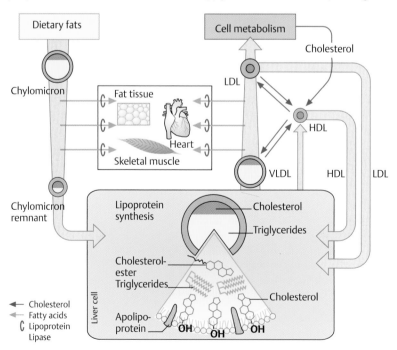

Antihyperlipidemic Therapy

Initial therapy is to institute lifestyle changes, including reduction of dietary intake of cholesterol and saturated fats and increased intake of soluble fiber and plant sterols. In addition, weight management and increased physical activity should be initiated. If these are insufficient to lower LDL-C to the desired level, drug therapy is indicated.

The National Cholesterol Education Program has established guidelines for initiation of drug therapy in dyslipidemias based on the blood levels of the lipoproteins after an overnight fast. The presence of other major risk factors, such as cigarette smoking, hypertension, low HDL-C (< 40 mg/dL), family history of premature CHD, and age, determine the level to which cholesterol should be lowered.

25.2 Antihyperlipidemic Drugs

Antihyperlipidemic drugs are used to treat hyperlipidemias or hyperlipoproteinemias and conditions characterized by elevated plasma levels of cholesterol or triglycerides, for example, type 2 diabetes, metabolic syndrome, and hypertriglyceridemia. Diabetics usually have high triglycerides, moderate elevations of total cholesterol and LDL-C, and low HDL-C.

Statins

The statins (3-hydroxy-3-methylglutaryl [HMG]–coenzyme A [CoA] inhibitors) have become the most widely prescribed drugs for lowering plasma cholesterol levels.

Atorvastatin, Fluvastatin, Lovastatin, Pravastatin, Rosuvastatin, and Simvastatin

Mechanism of action. The major mechanism of these agents is to competitively inhibit HMG-CoA reductase, the rate-limiting enzyme in cholesterol synthesis (**Fig. 25.2**). This causes significant reductions in LDL-C by causing an increased expression of LDL receptors on hepatocytes and increased removal of LDL from the blood (**Fig. 25.3**). Statins also reduce blood triglyceride levels.

Effects
— Lowers LDL and triglyceride levels
— Increases HDL levels

Uses
— First-line treatment for hypercholesterolemia
— Used prophylactically to prevent adverse vascular events in patients with diabetes mellitus or cardiovascular disease

Side effects. These include gastrointestinal (GI) upset in < 10% of patients, muscle weakness in combination with fibrates, and altered liver enzymes.

Contraindications
— Liver disease

Drug Interactions. The HMG-CoA reductase inhibitors increase warfarin levels so prothrombin times (expressed as International Normalized Ratio [INR, see page 288]) should be monitored.

Role of genetics in hyperlipidemic diseases

Genetic defects in the production of chylomicrons, lipoprotein lipase, the synthesis of LDL receptors, and overproduction of the lipids/lipoproteins can be familial causes for hyperlipidemic diseases.

Metabolic syndrome

Metabolic syndrome is a combination of medical disorders that increases the risk of developing atherosclerotic disease, for example, coronary heart disease, peripheral vascular disease, and stroke. It also increases the risk of developing type 2 diabetes. Its etiology is unknown, but weight, advancing age, lifestyle factors, and genetics are all known to be involved. Signs of metabolic syndrome include fasting hyperglycemia, hypertension, abdominal obesity, high levels of triglycerides, and low levels of HDL-C. Treatment primarily involves weight management and increasing exercise, then drug management for hypertension, diabetes, and to correct lipid levels as appropriate.

Rhabdomyolysis

Rhabdomyolysis is the rapid breakdown of skeletal muscle due to injury to muscle tissue. The muscle breakdown product, myoglobin, is harmful to the kidney and can precipitate acute kidney failure. Signs and symptoms include pain, tenderness, and swelling of the affected muscle, as well as nausea, vomiting, confusion, arrhythmias, coma, anuria, and later disseminated intravascular coagulation (DIC). This is a rare complication of treatment with statins and fibrates.

Fig. 25.2 ► **Accumulation and effect of HMG-CoA reductase inhibitors in the liver.**
The HMG-CoA reductase inhibitors mimic the normal enzyme substrate, which renders it unavailable for cholesterol synthesis in the liver. These drugs accumulate in the liver, as they have a high rate of presystemic elimination. This accumulation is advantageous because it concentrates the actions of these drugs where they are needed. The liver maintains its requirement for cholesterol by the uptake of LDL from the blood, thus lowering plasma cholesterol levels.

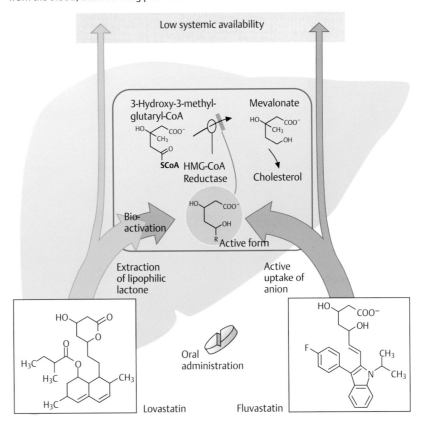

Fig. 25.3 ► **Regulation by cellular cholesterol concentration of HMG-CoA reductase and LDL receptors.**
In the presence of HMG-CoA reductase inhibitors, hepatocytes increase the production of LDL-receptor proteins. This allows LDL uptake from the blood to increase to provide the liver with its only source of cholesterol.

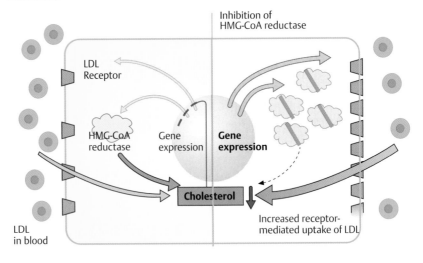

Bile Acid Sequestrants

Cholestyramine and Colestipol

Mechanism of action. These agents are insoluble resins that are not absorbed by the body, but that bind bile acids in the gut, thus preventing bile acids from being absorbed. This necessitates an increase in the hepatic conversion of cholesterol to bile acids, thereby reducing the cholesterol available through the enterohepatic circulation for production of plasma lipids. They also lower LDL and plasma cholesterol. **Figure 25.4** illustrates the effect of cholesterol-lowering drugs like cholestyramine on cholesterol metabolism in the liver.

Pharmacokinetics. Given orally, these drugs bind with bile acids in the intestine and produce an insoluble complex that is excreted in the feces.

Effects
— Decreases LDL levels
— May increase triglycerides, or they may remain unchanged
— Increases HDL levels

Uses. These agents are used alone for the treatment of hypercholesterolemia in patients 11 to 20 years of age. However, they are most often used as secondary agents if statin therapy does not reach its desired goal.

Side effects
— Nausea, constipation, steatorrhea (the presence of excess fat in feces), and deficiency of fat-soluble vitamins (A, D, E, K)
  Note: Compliance may be a problem due to the unpleasant taste of the drug.

Drug interactions. These agents may interfere with the absorption of other drugs given concurrently (e.g., warfarin); therefore, drugs should be taken ~1 to 2 hours before or several hours after taking bile acid sequestrants.

Fig. 25.4 ▶ **Cholesterol metabolism in liver cell and cholesterol-lowering drugs.**
Cholesterol-lowering drugs may act in the gut to reduce the absorption of dietary cholesterol, they may inhibit cholesterol synthesis in the liver, or they may act to increase the consumption of cholesterol.

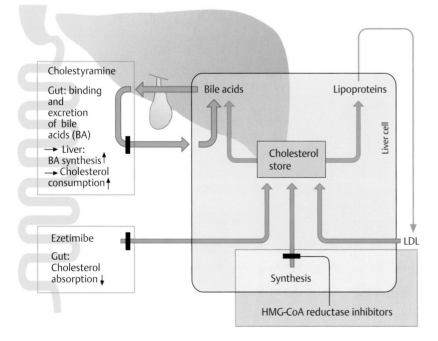

Ezetimibe

Mechanism of action. Ezetimibe inhibits cholesterol absorption in the small intestine.

Effects
— Lowers LDL-C levels by ~18%

Uses. It is used primarily as adjunctive therapy with statins.

Side effects
— May increase the hepatotoxicity and myopathy of statins

Nicotinic Acid (Niacin)

Niacin

Mechanisms of action
— Inhibition of hepatocyte diacylglycerol acyltransferase-2, a key enzyme for triacylglycerol synthesis, decreasing secretion of VLDL and LDL-C
— Decreased hepatic catabolism of apolipoprotein A-I increases the half-life and concentrations of HDL-C.
— Niacin also reduces vascular inflammatory genes involved in atherosclerosis.

Effects
— Decreases levels of LDL and triglycerides
— Increases HDL levels

Uses. Niacin is used to treat hypertriglyceridemias and hypercholesterolemia. It is especially useful in patients with both hypertriglyceridemia and low HDL-C levels.
  Note: Nicotinamide is not effective in lowering lipids, although it acts interchangeably with nicotinic acid as a vitamin.

Side effects
— Cutaneous flushing, burning, and itching are common, as is GI irritation, nausea, and vomiting. The niacin flush results from the stimulation of prostaglandins D_2 and E_2 from subcutaneous Langerhans cells by a G protein–coupled niacin receptor.
— Activation of peptic ulcers, abnormal elevation of liver enzyme levels, hyperglycemia, and hyperuricemia occur infrequently.

Contraindications
— Chronic liver disease
— Gout (see page 359)
— May be inappropriate for use in peptic ulcer disease, hyperuricemia, and diabetes

Fibrates

Gemfibrozil and Clofibrate

Mechanism of action. These drugs lower VLDLs and plasma triglycerides by stimulating lipoprotein lipase. They also lower cholesterol by inhibiting its synthesis and enhancing excretion in the bile.

Effects
— Decreases LDL and triglyceride levels
— Increases HDL levels

Uses

— Hypertriglyceridemia and hypercholesterolemia

Side effects.   Side effects include GI disturbances (nausea, diarrhea, and cramps), muscle weakness, and rash. Long-term use may increase the incidence of thromboembolism, angina, arrhythmias, or gallstones (see page 159).

Contraindications

— Pregnancy
— Impaired renal or hepatic function

Drug interactions.   These agents displace acidic drugs (e.g., warfarin and phenytoin) from plasma proteins; thus a reduced dose of anticoagulant (or other drug) is required.

Review Questions

1. A patient with edema is being treated with a drug that inhibits the absorption of bicarbonate ions from the glomerular filtrate. The effectiveness of this drug for long-term therapy is limited by drug-induced acidosis, which appears within the first weeks of therapy. With which of the following drugs is the patient being treated?

A. Metolazone
B. Ethacrynic acid
C. Amiloride
D. Acetazolamide
E. Spironolactone

2. Which of the following produces an acute increase in the urinary excretion of 20 to 30% of the filtered load of calcium and is therefore useful in treating symptomatic hypercalcemia, provided the plasma volume is maintained?

A. Furosemide
B. Chlorthalidone
C. Hydrochlorothiazide
D. Desmopressin
E. Mannitol

3. Which of the following may acutely reduce the glomerular filtration rate (GFR)?

A. Triamterene
B. Hydrochlorothiazide
C. Furosemide
D. Spironolactone
E. Mannitol

4. A 49-year-old man with high blood pressure tried to lower his blood pressure through diet and exercise. After 1 year, his blood pressure is slightly decreased, but it remains at 150/100 mm Hg. In the past year, he has been to your office once with a red, tender, and swollen first metatarsophalangeal joint at the base of the big toe. Which of the following drugs would have to be prescribed with caution in this patient?

A. Nifedipine
B. Labetalol
C. Prazosin
D. Chlorothiazide
E. Spironolactone

5. A 72-year-old man is being treated for congestive heart failure with a thiazide diuretic, an angiotensin-converting enzyme inhibitor, and a β-adrenergic receptor blocking agent. During a routine examination, serum electrolyte values were found to be the following: Na^+ = 135 mEq/L, Cl^- = 105 mEq/L, K^+ = 2.8 mEq/L, HCO_3^- = 24 mEq/L. The electrolyte values could be balanced by which of the following drugs?

A. Acetazolamide
B. Amiloride
C. Furosemide
D. Hydrochlorothiazide
E. Aldosterone

6. Which of the following is useful in the treatment of diabetes insipidus of pituitary origin?

A. Triamterene
B. Amiloride
C. Ethacrynic acid
D. Desmopressin
E. Furosemide

7. Which of the following is useful in the treatment of nephrogenic diabetes insipidus?

A. Triamterene
B. Hydrochlorothiazide
C. Furosemide
D. Desmopressin
E. Mannitol

8. A 70-year-old Caucasian woman is brought to the emergency room with heart palpitations and an erratic, irregular pulse. She is admitted to the hospital and diagnosed with hypertension complicated by paroxysmal atrial fibrillation. She had been taking a blood pressure medication but ran out of pills 1 week before the incident. Which of the following antihypertensive agents was she most likely taking?

A. Propranolol
B. Enalapril
C. Hydrochlorothiazide
D. Losartan
E. Clonidine

9. Which of the following antihypertensive drugs is contraindicated in patients with asthma?

A. Reserpine
B. Hydrochlorothiazide
C. Nifedipine
D. Verapamil
E. Propranolol

10. Which of the following antihypertensive drugs is less effective as monotherapy for African American patients?
A. Clonidine
B. Enalapril
C. Labetalol
D. Nifedipine
E. Prazosin

11. A 62-year-old woman is being treated for hypertension with captopril and hydrochlorothiazide. She has had a cough for the last 6 months that started ~2 months after she began antihypertensive therapy. Her blood pressure is well controlled. Chest radiograph (X-ray) and spirometry are normal. The cough is most likely a result of which of the following?
A. Pneumonia
B. The common cold
C. Poorly controlled blood pressure
D. A side effect of hydrochlorothiazide
E. A side effect of captopril

12. Given that the patient in question 11 has shown a favorable response to decreasing the function of angiotensin II, you decide to replace the drug with a drug that blocks the binding of angiotensin II to the angiotensin I–type angiotensin receptor. Which of the following drugs is prescribed?
A. Clonidine
B. Enalapril
C. Labetalol
D. Nifedipine
E. Losartan

13. A 48-year-old African American man has had a blood pressure of 160/90 mm Hg, 170/95 mm Hg, and 165/95 mm Hg on three monthly visits. The patient's hypertension is treated with nifedipine. How does this drug reduce hypertension?
A. By blocking α_2-adrenergic receptors
B. By inhibiting angiotensin-converting enzyme
C. By blocking β-adrenergic receptors
D. By blocking L-type calcium channels
E. By inhibiting sodium reabsorption in the loop of Henle

14. Abrupt cessation of antihypertensive therapy may cause a serious rebound hypertension with which of the following drugs?
A. Prazosin
B. Clonidine
C. Guanethidine
D. Enalapril
E. Reserpine

15. A 68-year-old man with asthma, long-standing hypertension, and diabetes mellitus who is receiving digoxin, hydrochlorothiazide, and 35 units of Neutral Protamine Hagedorn (NPH) insulin gradually develops congestive heart failure. Why would the addition of captopril to the patient's medication be potentially harmful?
A. It results in hypokalemia.
B. It blocks the subjective warning signs of hypoglycemia.
C. It aggravates the patient's asthmatic condition.
D. It may cause severe hypotension.
E. It activates the cytochrome P-450 enzymes that metabolize digoxin.

16. A 58-year old man is being treated for heart failure with a diuretic, an angiotensin-converting enzyme (ACE) inhibitor, and a β-adrenergic receptor blocking agent. He continues to experience dyspnea on exertion. The patient may benefit from the addition of a drug that inhibits which of the following proteins on the membrane of cardiac myocytes?
A. α_2-adrenergic receptors
B. Glucose transporter 1 (GLUT1)
C. $Na^+–K^+$–ATPase
D. L-type Ca^{2+} channels
E. Delayed rectifier K^+ channels

17. Digoxin is a cardiac glycoside used for the treatment of heart failure. The drug has a low therapeutic index, in part because it may affect the intracellular K^+ concentration of cardiac myocytes. What would be the expected effect of digoxin on intracellular K^+ levels?
A. It would lead to membrane hyperpolarization.
B. It would lead to membrane depolarization.
C. It would lead to no change in membrane potential.
D. It would decrease automaticity.
E. It would decrease contractility.

18. An elderly man comes to the emergency room with an acute myocardial infarction. He is in cardiogenic shock in which the cardiac output is very low, and there is a reflex vasoconstriction. He has tachycardia. Which of the following drugs would be most appropriate to administer?
A. Dobutamine
B. Isoproterenol
C. Bethanechol
D. Propranolol

19. Relief of pulmonary congestion after administration of nitroglycerin to a patient in congestive heart failure (CHF) is primarily due to
A. arteriolar dilation.
B. inotropic stimulation.
C. increased cardiac output.
D. increased venous capacitance.

20. A 62-year-old patient is experiencing chest pain on exertion. Effort-induced angina is diagnosed, and treatment is begun. Nitroglycerin and isosorbide dinitrate are given sublingually and are rapidly absorbed through the oral mucosa. Once in the bloodstream, they increase the level of which signaling molecule in smooth muscle?

A. Inositol triphosphate

B. Phospholipase Cß

C. RAF kinase

D. Cyclic guanosine monophosphate (cGMP)

E. Cyclooxygenase-3 (COX-3)

21. The patient in question 20 is prescribed another drug to take daily to prevent the effort-induced angina attacks. This drug is most likely which of the following?

A. Diltiazem

B. Nitroglycerin

C. Metoprolol

D. Isosorbide dinitrate

E. Verapamil

22. Organic nitrates may relieve angina by which of the following mechanisms?

A. Reduction of the heart rate

B. Reduction of myocardial contractility

C. Increase in the left ventricular residual volume

D. Reduction of ventricular wall stress

E. Increase in venous pressure

23. A common property of all class I antiarrhythmic drugs is

A. reduction of membrane responsiveness.

B. prolongation of the effective refractory period.

C. hyperpolarization of the membrane.

D. atropine-like effect.

24. A 58-year-old female patient with recurrent ventricular tachycardia requires treatment with an antiarrhythmic drug. She has a previous history of systemic lupus erythematosus (SLE). Which of the following drugs would be contraindicated in this patient?

A. Flecainide

B. Procainamide

C. Quinidine

D. Amiodarone

E. Verapamil

25. A 69-year-old man is taking mexiletine for prevention of ventricular arrhythmia. He has experienced some ataxia, paresthesias, and tremor 2 to 3 hours after taking the medicine. These effects result from mexiletine acting as which of the following?

A. Calcium channel blocker

B. β-blocker to decrease blood flow

C. Local anesthetic to affect neuronal conduction

D. Alcohol dehydrogenase inhibitor

E. Benzodiazepine receptor agonist

26. Following an acute myocardial infarction, a patient is given an antiarrhythmic drug to prevent supraventricular and ventricular arrhythmias. Administration of this drug will be continued for 2 to 3 years. Which of the following drugs was the patient given?

A. Phenylephrine

B. Isoproterenol

C. Norepinephrine

D. Nitroglycerin

E. Propranolol

27. A hospitalized patient is receiving heparin for prevention of deep vein thrombosis. One of the drugs the patient received during the procedure was eptifibatide. What is the action of this drug?

A. To inhibit platelet aggregation by reversibly binding to the platelet receptor glycoprotein

B. To block the glycoprotein IIb/IIIa receptor in human platelets

C. To inhibit the release of adenosine diphosphate (ADP) by increasing cyclic adenosine monophosphate (cAMP) levels

D. To acetylate platelet cyclooxygenase

E. To inhibit ADP-induced platelet fibrinogen binding

For questions 28–30.

A 44-year-old man has swelling and pain in his right leg, ankle, and foot. At first he thought he had a cramp, but then he noticed his calf had become red and warm. The swelling has not decreased after 3 days. He has chest pain but no shortness of breath. Blood pressure is 145/85 mm Hg, heart rate is 105 beats/min, and respiration is 30 breaths/min. Auscultation reveals a loud pulmonary heart sound. Arterial partial pressure of oxygen (pO_2) is slightly decreased. Pulmonary embolism is suspected, and the patient is admitted to the hospital. Heparin therapy is initiated. Two days later, the patient's activated partial thromboplastin time (aPTT) is found to be excessively prolonged.

28. Which of the following drugs could be used to restore the patient's aPTT to within an acceptable range?

A. Protamine

B. Warfarin

C. Vitamin K

D. Enoxaparin

E. Bivalirudin

29. In addition to monitoring aPTT, what other parameter should be monitored for patients receiving heparin?
- A. Platelet count
- B. Bone density
- C. Vitamin K levels
- D. Cytokine levels
- E. Vitamin C levels

30. A transition from heparin to warfarin anticoagulant therapy is initiated while the patient is in the hospital. After discharge of the patient from the hospital, warfarin anticoagulant therapy is continued. Following discharge, the patient decides to institute lifestyle changes, including diet and exercise. His dietary plan is to dramatically decrease his intake of meat to try to become a vegetarian. How would an increased consumption of green leafy vegetables (which contain vitamin K) be expected to alter the patient's International Normalized Ratio (INR)?
- A. It would be increased.
- B. It would be decreased.
- C. It would be unchanged.
- D. It would be doubled.
- E. It would be halved.

31. Which of the following decreases cholesterol synthesis by inhibition of 3-hydroxy-3-methylglutaryl (HMG) coenzyme A (CoA) reductase?
- A. Lovastatin
- B. Cholestyramine
- C. Nicotinic acid
- D. Clofibrate

32. A 56-year-old man has a total cholesterol of 245 mg/dL, low-density lipoprotein (LDL) = 160 mg/dL, high-density lipoprotein (HDL) = 60 mg/dL, and triglycerides = 107 mg/dL. He is 69 inches (5 ft 9 in, 175 cm) tall and weighs 160 lb (72.5 kg). His father had a heart attack at age 45, and his older brother has had coronary angioplasty. He was started on the initial recommended dose of lovastatin 6 months ago. The National Cholesterol Education Program goal for this patient is to reduce his LDL cholesterol to < 130 mg/dL. Which of the following would be most optimal for further lowering the patient's cholesterol?
- A. Increase the dose of lovastatin.
- B. Add a bile acid sequestrant.
- C. Add niacin.
- D. Add clofibrate.
- E. Lose more weight.

33. The main side effect of which of the following drugs is flushing of the skin?
- A. Lovastatin
- B. Cholestyramine
- C. Nicotinic acid
- D. Probucol

34. A 58-year-old Caucasian female patient has a total cholesterol of 299 mg/dL, low-density lipoprotein (LDL) = 240, high-density lipoprotein (HDL) = 30, and triglycerides = 928 mg/dL. She is 62 inches (5 ft 2 in, 157 cm) tall and weighs 220 lb (~100 kg). Which of the following drugs would be most effective for this patient?
- A. Nonselective β-blocker
- B. β_1 selective adrenergic receptor blocker
- C. Ezetimibe
- D. Gemfibrozil
- E. Verapamil

Answers and Explanations

1. **D** Acetazolamide is a carbonic anhydrase inhibitor that acts in the proximal convoluted tubule to reduce the absorption of bicarbonate ions from the glomerular filtrate. The effectiveness of its diuretic action decreases as plasma bicarbonate is depleted. This causes a metabolic acidosis (p. 185).
A Metolazone is a thiazide-like diuretic.
B Ethacrynic acid is a loop diuretic that inhibits the Na^+–K^+–$2Cl^-$ cotransporter in the thick ascending loop of Henle.
C Amiloride is a potassium-sparing diuretic used that directly interferes with sodium transport in the distal convoluted tubule.
E Spironolactone is a competitive antagonist to aldosterone and so inhibits the synthesis of Na+ channel proteins and Na+–K+-ATPases which promotes the reabsorption of Na+, Cl−, and water.

2. **A** Furosemide and the loop (or high-ceiling) diuretics increase calcium ion excretion into the urine and are therefore useful in treating symptomatic hypercalcemia (p. 185–187).
B, C Thiazide diuretics, such as chlorthalidone and hydrochlorothiazide, decrease calcium excretion.
D Desmopressin is the synthetic replacement for antidiuretic hormone (ADH), the hormone that reduces urine production.
E Mannitol is an osmotic diuretic that increases the solute load (solutes cannot be absorbed but bind to water), causing increased urine production.

3. **B** Thiazide diuretics, such as hydrochlorothiazide, may decrease the GFR in some patients. Thus, they may worsen existing mild renal failure (p. 187).
A, C–E The other drugs do not decrease the GFR.

4. **D** The foot inflammation in a male patient of this age indicates a gout attack. Thiazide diuretics, such as chlorothiazide, produce hyperuricemia (elevated blood uric acid level), which may precipitate further attacks (p. 187).

5. **B** The patient has hypokalemia (normal range 3.5–5.0 mEq/L). Amiloride is a potassium-sparing diuretic that is useful when given along with a thiazide to prevent potassium depletion (p. 188).
A Acetazolamide is a carbonic anhydrase inhibitor that will increase the excretion of bicarbonate.
C Furosemide is a loop diuretic that may worsen the hypokalemia.
D The patient is already taking hydrochlorothiazide, a thiazide diuretic.
E Aldosterone is an endogenous mineralocorticoid hormone that increases sodium reabsorption and potassium excretion.

6. **D** Diabetes insipidus of pituitary origin is the most common type of diabetes insipidus and is caused by a deficiency of arginine vasopressin (AVP). Desmopressin (1-deamino-8-d-arginine vasopressin) is a synthetic analogue of AVP used as replacement therapy for AVP (p. 190).
A, B Triamterene and amiloride are potassium sparing diuretics used in combination with a thiazide diuretic to treat hypertension.
C, E Ethacrynic acid and furosemide are loop diuretics used to treat chronic heart failure, pulmonary edema due to left ventricular failure, hypertension, acute oliguria, and hypercalcemia.

7. **B** Nephrogenic diabetes insipidus is caused by a defect in the tubules of the kidney, leading to an improper response to antidiuretic hormone (ADH) and overproduction of dilute urine. Thiazide diuretics, such as hydrochlorothiazide, exert a paradoxical effect to decrease the urine output of patients with nephrogenic diabetes insipidus (p. 189).
A Triamterene is a potassium-sparing diuretic used, in combination with a thiazide diuretic, to treat hypertension.
C Furosemide is a loop diuretic used to treat chronic heart failure, pulmonary edema due to left ventricular failure, hypertension, acute oliguria, and hypercalcemia.
D Desmopressin is the synthetic replacement for antidiuretic hormone (ADH), the hormone that reduces urine production.
E Mannitol is an osmotic diuretic that increases the solute load (solutes cannot be absorbed but bind to water), causing increased urine production.

8. **A** The patient's symptoms suggest that the antihypertensive drug she was taking may also have been preventing the atrial fibrillation.
A propranolol, a nonselective β-blocker, has both antihypertensive and antiarrhythmic effects (p. 195).
B Enalapril is an angiotensin converting enzyme (ACE) inhibitor that has antihypertensive but no antiarrhythmic effects.
C Hydrochlorothiazide is a thiazide diuretic that has antihypertensive but no antiarrhythmic effects.
D Losartan is an angiotensin II receptor antagonist that has antihypertensive but no antiarrhythmic effects.
E. Clonidine is an α_2-adrenergic receptor agonist that has antihypertensive but no antiarrhythmic effects.

9. **E** The nonselective β-adrenergic receptor blocking agents, such as propranolol, may worsen asthma by blocking the bronchodilation produced via β_2-adrenergic receptor activation (p. 196).
A Reserpine is an adrenergic neuron blocker that reduces blood pressure by depleting norepinephrine stores and by preventing its reuptake and storage. It will have no effect on asthma.
B Hydrochlorothiazide is a thiazide diuretic. It will have no effect on asthma.
C, D Nifedipine and verapamil are calcium-channel blockers. Nifedipine acts predominantly on vascular smooth muscle causing vasodilation and so reduces blood pressure. Verapamil also causes vasodilation of vascular smooth muscle but it also acts on cardiac muscle cells to reduce heart rate, force of contraction, and velocity of contraction. It is therefore also useful in the treatment of angina and some arrhythmias. Both nifedipine and verapamil have no effect on asthma.

10. **B** Angiotensin-converting enzyme (ACE) inhibitors, such as enalapril, are less effective in African American patients than in other patient groups unless combined with a thiazide diuretic (p. 194).
A, C–E The other drugs listed are not associated with this reduced effectiveness.

11. **E** The test results are negative for other causes for her cough, and cough is a common side effect of angiotensin-converting enzyme (ACE) inhibitors, such as captopril (p. 194).

12. **E** Losartan blocks the binding of angiotensin II to the angiotensin I–type angiotensin receptor. Its side effects are similar to those of captopril, but it does not produce cough (p. 194).
A–D The other drugs do not affect the angiotensin system directly.

13. **D** Nifedipine is a dihydropyridine calcium channel antagonist that acts by blocking L-type (long-lasting) calcium channels. This causes vasodilation of vascular smooth muscle and a reduction in blood pressure (p. 196).

14. B Clonidine stimulates α_2-adrenergic receptors in the medulla, which in turn decreases sympathetic tone and blood pressure. Persistent activation of α_2-adrenergic receptors leads to their downregulation. Upon cessation of clonidine, this decrease in α_2-adrenergic receptor function leads to a rebound in blood pressure that may last a day or two until the normal level of α_2-adrenergic receptors is restored (p. 200).

A Prazosin is an α_1-adrenergic receptor antagonist that reduces blood pressure by vasodilation of vascular smooth muscle. Orthostatic hypotension is common after the first dose.

C Guanethidine is an adrenergic neuron blocker that reduces blood pressure by preventing norepinephrine release, depleting norepinephrine stores, and blocking its reuptake.

D Enalapril is an angiotensin-converting enzyme inhibitor that reduces blood pressure by preventing the vasoconstrictive effects of angiotensin II on vascular smooth muscle.

E Reserpine is an adrenergic neuron blocker that reduces blood pressure by depleting norepinephrine stores and by preventing its reuptake and storage .

15. D Hypotension is a side effect of captopril, an angiotensin-converting enzyme inhibitor. This effect is amplified when it is combined with hydrochlorothiazide and is more frequently observed in patients with heart failure (p. 194).

A–C, E The other results are not normally associated with captopril.

16. C Because the patient is already being treated with a diuretic, an ACE inhibitor, and a β-blocker, a logical next choice would be digoxin. Both the therapeutic and toxic effects of digoxin are attributable to inhibition of Na$^+$-K$^+$–ATPase (the digitalis receptor) located on the outside of the myocardial cell membrane (p. 205).

A, B, D, E The other choices are not valid mechanisms for drugs that treat heart failure.

17. B As an inhibitor of Na$^+$– K$^+$–ATPase, which pumps Na$^+$ out of the cell and K$^+$ into the cell, digoxin would be expected to decrease the level of intracellular K$^+$. According to the Nernst equation, membrane potential is proportional to the level of K inside the cell/K outside the cell. Decreasing the K inside the cell will decrease membrane potential (i.e., depolarize the cell) (p. 205).

A, C–E The other effects listed are not typical of digoxin.

18. A Dobutamine is used for short-term support in severe heart failure. It acts by stimulating cardiac β_1 receptors to increase cardiac contractility. It is not used long term, as it may cause arrhythmias and increase oxygen consumption (p. 206).

B Isoproterenol is a nonselective β-adrenergic receptor agonist that increases heart rate and contractility. It is more likely than dobutamine to cause arrhythmias and increase oxygen consumption. It is used to improve cardiac output in patients with heart block.

C Bethanechol is a cholinergic muscarinic receptor agonist that would decrease, not improve, cardiac function.

D Propranolol is a nonselective β-adrenergic receptor blocker and would have a negative inotropic effect

E Phenylephrine is an α adrenoceptor agonist that would produce vasoconstriction, but reflex vasoconstriction is already present.

19. D In CHF, the main therapeutic actions of nitroglycerin are due to dilation of large capacitance veins (p. 207).

A Nitroglycerin will cause some arteriolar dilation but this is not its primary effect.

B,C Nitroglycerin does not increase cardiac contractility (inotropism) or increase cardiac output.

20. D Organic nitrates are converted to nitric oxide, which activates guanylate cyclase, increases intracellular cGMP concentrations, and causes vasodilation of venous and arterial blood vessels (p. 209).

21. C Metoprolol is a β-adrenergic receptor antagonist. It is useful for the prophylaxis of effort-induced angina but is not effective for the acute termination of effort-induced angina or for the treatment of coronary artery spasm (p. 211).

A, E The calcium channel blockers diltiazem and verapamil are more appropriate for variant or unstable angina due to coronary vasospasm.

B, D Nitroglycerin and isosorbide dinatrate are indicated for acute relief of an angina pectoris attack. They are given sublingually and rapidly absorbed through the oral mucosa. Therapeutic effects are observed within 2 to 4 minutes but last for only 1 to 2 hours.

22. D Organic nitrates act like the endogenous compound nitric oxide. They activate guanylate cyclase to increase the level of cyclic guanosine monophosphate (cGMP) in smooth muscle. This leads to relaxation of vascular smooth muscle and both arterial and venous dilation. This results in a decrease in ventricular preload and a reduction of ventricular wall stress (p. 209).

A–C The vasodilation produced by the organic nitrates may result in reflex increases in heart rate and contractility and a decrease in left ventricular residual volume.

E Organic nitrates will cause a decrease in venous pressure.

23. A By definition, class I antiarrhythmic action is Na$^+$ channel blockade, which reduces membrane excitability or responsiveness (p. 217).

24. B Acute lupus erythematosus has been observed with procainamide; thus, this drug is contraindicated in patients with a history of SLE (p. 217).

A, C–E None of the other drugs will precipitate lupus erythematosus.

25. C Class IB antiarrhythmic agents, such as mexiletine, are Na^+ channel blockers and act like local anesthetics, which is producing this patient's symptoms. The symptoms are most prominent as the drug levels peak at 2 to 3 hours after administration (p. 219).

26. E A β-adrenergic receptor antagonist, propranolol is a class II antiarrhythmic agent that is used to prevent ventricular fibrillation during the first 2 years following myocardial infarction (p. 220).

A Phenylephrine is an α adrenoceptor agonist.

B Isoproterenol is a nonselective β-adrenergic receptor agonist.

C Norepinephrine is the endogenous postganglionic sympathetic neurotransmitter with both α and β agonist activity.

D Nitroglycerin is indicated for acute relief of an angina pectoris attack.

27. B Eptifibatide is a cyclic peptide that blocks the glycoprotein IIb/IIIa receptor to prevent platelet aggregation (p. 226).

28. A Protamine sulfate is an antidote for heparin and forms a 1:1 complex with the anticoagulant. Administration of this drug will return the patient's aPTT to a normal range (p. 227).

B–E The other drugs have no effect on aPTT.

29. A Thrombocytopenia is one of the adverse effects that may be observed following heparin administration. It may be mild and transient, but it may become severe if antiplatelet antibodies are formed. Platelet counts should be performed to monitor for thrombocytopenia (p. 226).

B–E None of these have any relevance in heparin therapy.

30. B Warfarin is an oral anticoagulant drug that antagonizes the hepatic synthesis of the vitamin K-dependent clotting factors II (prothrombin), VII, IX, and X. It increases a patient's INR. Green leafy vegetables are a good source of vitamin K. Vitamin K is a warfarin antagonist. Thus, the expected result would be a decreased INR (pp. 228 and 229).

31. A Lovastatin competitively inhibits HMG-CoA reductase, the rate-limiting enzyme in cholesterol synthesis (p. 237).

B Cholestyramine is an insoluble resin that is not absorbed by the body, but binds bile acids in the gut, thus preventing bile acids from being absorbed. This necessitates an increase in the hepatic conversion of cholesterol to bile acids, thereby reducing the cholesterol available through the enterohepatic circulation for production of plasma lipids. This also lowers LDL and plasma cholesterol.

C Nicotinic acid (niacin) inhibits hepatocyte diacylglycerol acyltransferase-2, a key enzyme for triglyceride synthesis, decreasing the secretion of very low density lipoprotein (VLDL) and low density lipoprotein cholesterol (LDL-C). It also decreases the hepatic catabolism of apo A-I increases the half-life and concentrations of high density lipoprotein cholesterol (HDL-C).

D Clofibrate lowers very low density lipoproteins (VLDL) and plasma triglycerides by stimulating lipoprotein lipase. It also lowers cholesterol by inhibiting its synthesis and enhancing excretion in the bile.

32. A Because the patient was started on the initial recommended dose, the cholesterol-lowering response was not great enough, and adverse reactions to the drug are not reported, the next step should be to increase the dose (p. 237).

B Bile acid sequestrant may be added if the statin does not reach the desired goal, but an adequate dose of the statin should be tried first.

C Nicain is especially useful in patients with both hypertriglyceridemia and low HDL-C levels. This patient has normal triglycerides and borderline high HDL.

D Clofibrate is useful in hypertriglyceridemia and hypercholesterolemia.

E The patient's weight is near normal.

33. C Flushing of the skin is a side effect of nicotinic acid (niacin). It results from the stimulation of prostaglandins D_2 and E_2 by subcutaneous Langerhans cells by a G protein-coupled niacin receptor (p. 240).

A, B, D Flushing is not associated with lovastatin, cholestyramine, or probucol.

34. D Gemfibrozil is indicated for hypertriglyceridemia and hypercholesterolemia (p. 241).

A, B, E β-blockers and verapamil (a calcium channel blocker) do not lower cholesterol levels.

C Ezetimibe inhibits cholesterol absorption in the small intestine but it is not as effective at lowering cholesterol or triglyceride levels as gemfibrozil.

26   Drugs Acting on the Respiratory System

26.1   Asthma and Chronic Obstructive Pulmonary Disease

Asthma

Asthma is predominantly an inflammatory disease with associated bronchospasm, mucosal swelling, and increased mucus production. There is episodic bronchial obstruction causing wheezing, dyspnea, cough, and mucosal edema. In children, the only sign of asthma may be a persistent cough.

The etiology and immunopathogenesis of asthma are illustrated in **Figs. 26.1** and **26.2**. The role of inflammatory autocoids (e.g., histamine and leukotrienes) in relation to asthma is discussed in Chapter 32.

Chronic Obstructive Pulmonary Disease

Chronic obstructive pulmonary disease (COPD) is the term used to describe chronic obstructive bronchitis and emphysema, which always coexist, to varying degrees. The characteristic symptoms of COPD are persistent cough, sputum, dyspnea (shortness of breath), and wheezing.

Chronic bronchitis is defined clinically as sputum production on most days for 3 months of 2 consecutive years. Inflammation (most commonly caused by cigarette smoke) causes the bronchial tubes to thicken and scar and produce excess mucus. This mucus cannot be expectorated given that cilia are destroyed as part of the disease process. These factors combine to cause narrowing of the airway lumen and obstruction.

Emphysema occurs when the walls of the alveoli are progressively destroyed. This decreases the surface area of the alveoli for oxygen exchange with the blood and caused the small airways to collapse during expiration, trapping air in the lungs. This may be caused by cigarette smoke or α_1-antitrypsin deficiency.

Fig. 26.1 ▸ **Asthma: genetic predisposition and trigger factors.**
Bronchial hyperreactivity and the tendency to increased interleukin-4 (IL-4)–dependent immunoglobulin E (IgE) production may be inherited through genes on chromosome 5 in patients with allergic asthma. This type of asthma is commonly triggered by animal hair, dust mites, feathers, pollen, and mold. In nonallergic asthma, the bronchial hyperreactivity is caused by the inhalation of chemicals, cigarette smoke, viral infections, cold air, exercise, and stress. Drugs (e.g., aspirin) can also cause an attack.

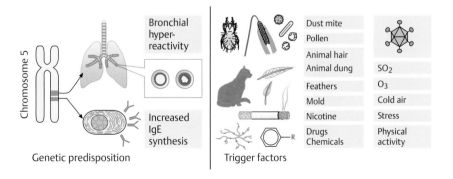

Drugs causing respiratory depression

Barbiturates, benzodiazepines, and opioids are all known to cause respiratory depression. Barbiturates and benzodiazepines act by facilitating the effects of GABA (the main inhibitory neurotransmitter in the CNS) at the α-subunit of the $GABA_A$ receptor. Opioids act at μ receptors throughout the body, the effects of which can be both excitatory and inhibitory. These drugs depress the response of the respiratory center in the medulla to hypercapnia ($\uparrow CO_2$) leading to respiratory depression.

Atopy and asthma

Atopy describes a hereditary predisposition for type I hypersensitivity reactions, which are mediated by IgE. Atopic conditions include asthma, eczema, hay fever, and generalized allergies (e.g., to certain foods and dust). Gastroesophageal reflux disease (GERD) is also known to have a strong association with asthma, although the cause of this is unclear (see page 260).

Nonsteroidal Antiinflammatory Drug–induced bronchospasm

A significant proportion of adults with asthma experience bronchospasm after taking aspirin and other nonsteroidal antiinflammatory drugs (NSAIDs). This can be serious and sometimes fatal. Aspirin and other NSAIDs are therefore contraindicated in patients with asthma who have a history of hypersensitivity reactions and should be used with caution in all asthmatics. Acetaminophen can be used by asthmatics to treat mild to moderate pain (see Chapter 33).

Drug delivery via an endotracheal tube

In an emergency situation, drugs are sometimes given via an endotracheal tube (e.g., epinephrine, naloxone, atropine, and lidocaine). They can exert local or systemic effects.

Alpha$_1$-antitrypsin deficiency

Alpha$_1$-antitrypsin is a glycoprotein protease inhibitor produced in the liver that plays a role in controlling inflammation and repairing tissues, as well as in blood coagulation. Deficiency of α_1-antitrypsin is a common inherited genetic disorder that causes uninhibited tissue breakdown by neutrophil elastase, mainly in the lungs (causing panacinar emphysema) and the liver.

Fig. 26.2 ▶ Asthma: immunopathogenesis.
Allergens attach to, and are taken up by, dendritic cells that lie in the ciliated respiratory epithelium. The interaction of the allergen (antigen), antigen presenting cells, and native T cells leads to the differentiation of the T cells to T-helper (TH_2) cells, which release cytokines. IL-4 activates B cells, which differentiate into plasma cells and release IgE that attaches to the surface of mast cells. The mast cells then degranulate when the allergens bridge two IgE molecules on their surface, especially when they are activated by IL-3. This cascade of events releases inflammatory mediators that are responsible for the bronchoconstriction/bronchospasm, mucosal swelling, and increased mucus production in allergic asthma. (ECP, eosinophil cationic protein; MBP, major basic protein; PAF, platelet-activating factor.)

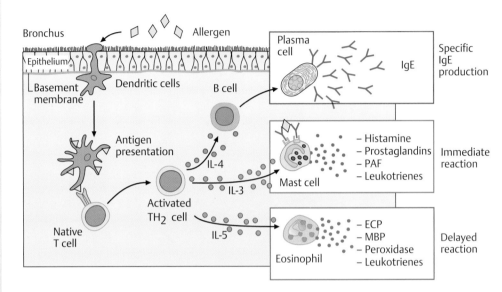

26.2 Treatment of Asthma and Chronic Obstructive Pulmonary Disease

Corticosteroids

Budesonide, Ciclesonide, Flunisolide, Fluticasone, Mometasone, Beclomethasone, and Triamcinolone

Mechanism of action. These antiinflammatory agents decrease bronchial hyperreactivity and the formation of mucus. They are the most effective antiasthmatic drugs available.

Pharmacokinetics
— These agents are inhaled through metered dose inhalers or dry powder inhalers. In severe persistent asthma, they may be given orally. In asthma emergencies (status asthmaticus), they may be given intravenously (IV).
— They should be used at the lowest dose that provides adequate control of symptoms.

Uses
— Moderate to severe asthma
— Corticosteroids are generally not used in COPD patients unless bronchodilation cannot be achieved with β_2-adrenergic receptor agonists and anticholinergic drugs.

Side effects
— Throat irritation and dysphonia (speech impairment and hoarseness) may limit compliance.
— Oral candidiasis (thrush) is possible as a result of inhibition of normal host defenses. The chances of developing thrush may be reduced by using spacer devices with the inhaler, rinsing the mouth after use of the inhaler, and/or decreasing the steroid dosing frequency.

— Endocrine effects have rarely been reported, but the growth of children should be monitored to ensure there is no suppression of the hypothalamic-pituitary axis (see Chapter 16).
— High doses inhaled or long-term systemic corticosteroid therapy for refractory asthma can lead to a Cushing-like response (see page 139).

Beta$_2$-Adrenergic Receptor Agonists

These agents are also discussed in Chapter 6.

Albuterol, Levalbuterol, Metaproterenol, Terbutaline, Salmeterol, and Formoterol

— *Short-acting:* Albuterol, Levalbuterol, Metaproterenol, Terbutaline
— *Long-acting:* Salmeterol, Formoterol

Mechanism of action. Beta$_2$-adrenergic receptor agonists relax bronchial smooth muscle, thereby reversing bronchoconstriction. They do not significantly decrease the bronchial hyperresponsiveness or the primary inflammatory reactions responsible for the persistence of asthma.

Uses

— Short-acting agents act rapidly to provide symptomatic relief of acute asthma symptoms.
— Long-acting agents are used to treat asthma that is not well controlled by corticosteroids alone.
— These drugs form the cornerstone of bronchodilation therapy in COPD, often in combination with an anticholinergic drug.

Side effects

— Tremor, anxiety, and restlessness

Anticholinergic Drugs

Ipratropium, Oxitropium, and Tiotropium

Mechanism of action. Anticholinergic drugs produce bronchodilation by blocking the bronchoconstrictive effects of acetylcholine acting on muscarinic receptors on bronchial smooth muscle. They have the further advantage of reducing mucus production by inhibiting vagal stimulation of goblet cells.

Uses. These drugs have limited efficacy in asthma but are useful add-ons to β$_2$ agonists in moderate to severe COPD.

Side effects

— Dry mouth, blurred vision, tachycardia, urinary retention, and constipation

Leukotriene Modifiers

Leukotrienes are potent bronchoconstrictors produced by cells involved in inflammatory responses, including mast cells and eosinophils (see Chapter 32).

Montelukast, Zafirlukast, and Zileuton

Mechanisms of action

— Montelukast and zafirlukast are leukotriene receptor antagonists (**Fig. 26.3**). They bind with high affinity to the cysteinyl leukotriene receptor 1 (cys-LT1) receptor, blocking the effects of the cysteinyl leukotrienes (LTC$_4$, LTD$_4$, and LTE$_4$).
— Zileuton is a leukotriene synthesis inhibitor. It inhibits the enzyme lipoxygenase and thus inhibits the formation of all lipoxygenase products, including the cys-LTs and non-cys-LTs (**Fig. 26.4**).

■ **Status asthmaticus**

Status asthmaticus is an acute, severe exacerbation of asthma characterized by a severe limitation of airflow and increased work of breathing, along with variable degrees of hypoxia (low tisssue O$_2$). Treatment includes oxygen therapy, IV fluids for hydration and to thin mucus secretions, nebulized albuterol and ipratropium, and parenteral corticosteroids. Treatment may also include intramuscular or subcutaneous epinephrine (never IV) to induce rapid bronchodilation.

■ **Respiration and acid–base balance**

The lungs, along with the kidneys, regulate acid–base balance. They do this by modulating the CO$_2$ concentration in the blood. A respiratory alkalosis occurs as a result of hyperventilation: CO$_2$ levels are reduced (as the patient is breathing out more CO$_2$), and pH is increased. Causes of this include stroke, meningitis, COPD ("pink puffers"), anxiety, and hyperthyroidism. A respiratory acidosis ($\uparrow$ CO$_2$; $\downarrow$ pH) is caused when CO$_2$ becomes trapped in the body due to a failure of respiration, which can be neuromuscular, physical, or respiratory (e.g., emphysema) in origin.

Fig. 26.3 ▶ **Atopy and antiallergy therapy.**
Atopy is thought to be linked to the differentiation of T-helper lymphocytes toward the TH_2 phenotype. Specific immunotherapy involves antigen injections that are intended to hyposensitize an individual by shifting T-helper cells toward TH_1. Monoclonal antibodies (e.g., omalizumab) inactivate IgE and prevent it from binding to mast cells. Cromolyn prevents the release of inflammatory mediators from mast cells. H_1 antihistamines and antileukotrienes block their respective inflammatory mediator at receptors. Glucocorticoids have significant antiallergic activity and act at various stages of the allergic response.

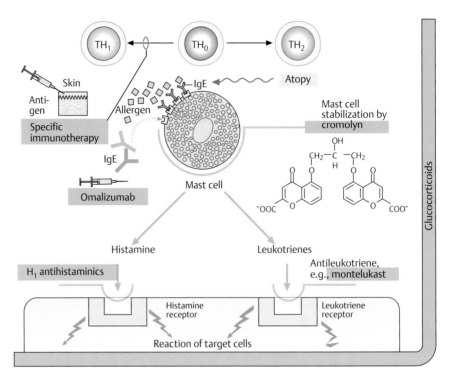

Fig. 26.4 ▶ **Leukotriene antagonists.**
Cysteine leukotriene synthesis can be blocked by inhibiting lipoxygenase, the enzyme responsible for converting arachidonic acid to leukotrienes. This can be achieved by drugs such as zileuton. Montelukast, on the other hand, blocks leukotriene receptors on target tissues.

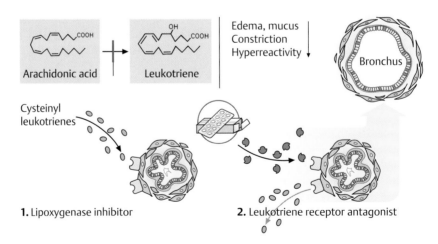

Pharmacokinetics. These drugs are administered orally and are well absorbed.

Uses
— Prophylaxis of asthma
— Allergic rhinitis (see page 254)

Side effects. Some patients experience headache with these drugs; otherwise, they are well tolerated.

Mast Cell Stabilizers

Cromolyn Sodium

Mechanism of action. Cromolyn sodium inhibits mast cell degranulation and other allergy mediators by blocking Ca^{2+} channels in the cell membrane. This causes a reduction of bronchial hyperresponsiveness.

Uses
— Prophylaxis of asthma. It is not a bronchodilator and is of no use in acute asthma. It is not as effective as corticosteroids, but it has an excellent safety profile.
— Allergic rhinitis

Side effects. The side effects associated with cromolyn sodium are minimal.

Methylxanthines

Theophylline

Mechanism of action. Theophylline has several molecular actions, although which is responsible for the therapeutic effect in asthma is not clear. Classically, theophylline was categorized as a phosphodiesterase inhibitor. It has also been shown to have activity as a prostaglandin antagonist, an inhibitor of Ca^{2+} transport, a stimulator of endogenous catecholamine release, a β-agonist, and an adenosine antagonist. All of these could contribute to its ability to relax the bronchial smooth muscle.

Pharmacokinetics
— Prolonged-release oral formulations are most commonly used.
— Monitoring of serum levels is essential because of large interindividual variability.

Uses. Theophylline is used infrequently in the maintenance therapy of moderate to severe asthma.

Side effects
— Life-threatening toxicity (seizures and cardiac arrhythmias) can occur at high doses without warning signs.
— Nausea, cramps, insomnia, and headache are common with loading doses.

Anti–immunoglobulin E Antibody

Omalizumab

Mechanism of action. Omalizumab is a recombinant humanized monoclonal antibody directed against IgE that binds free IgE. This prevents IgE from binding to mast cells and basophils, thereby inhibiting IgE-dependent hypersensitivity reactions to allergens.

Pharmacokinetics
— Given by subcutaneous injection, every 2 to 4 weeks

Uses. Omalizumab is generally reserved for use in patients with severe, persistent, IgE-mediated allergic asthma who are inadequately controlled with the other medications discussed above. It has also been proposed for use in other type I allergic reactions.

Alpha$_1$-Proteinase Inhibitors

Prolastin™, Zemaira™, and Aralast™

Note: There are no generic names for this type of drug.

Mechanism of action. These agents are α_1-antitrypsin products that are derived from the plasma of blood donors.

Pharmacokinetics
— Given IV on a weekly basis

Uses
— Indicated for patients with panacinar emphysema who have α_1-antitrypsin deficiency

26.3   Neonatal Respiratory Distress Syndrome

Neonatal respiratory distress syndrome (NRDS) is a hyaline membrane disease that is caused by a deficiency in surfactant.

Beractant and Colfosceril

Mechanism of action. Beractant is a modified bovine lung extract (a natural surfactant), and colfosceril is a synthetic surfactant.

Pharmacokinetics
— These agents are given by tracheal instillation.

Uses
— Used to modulate neonatal respiratory distress syndrome.

26.4   Treatment of Rhinitis

Rhinitis is inflammation of mucous membranes of the nasal cavity. Characteristic symptoms include sneezing, watery rhinorrhea, itching of the nose, eyes, ears, and throat, red and watering eyes, and nasal congestion. It can be caused by infection (usually viral) or allergy (**Fig. 26.5**).

Fig. 26.5 ▶ **Allergic rhinitis.**
Allergic rhinitis is triggered by the contact of an allergen with IgE-bearing mast cells in the nasal mucosa. The fact that mast cells have IgE attached suggests prior sensitization to the allergen. The mast cells release their mediators, causing sneezing, rhinorrhea, and contralateral hypersecretion in the unexposed nostril (due to a central reflex). The offending allergen can be identified by nasal allergen exposure or by a prick test.

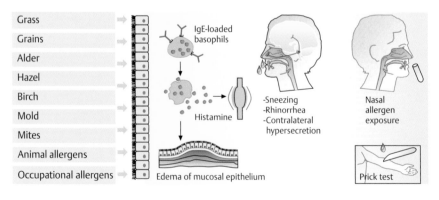

■ **Pulmonary surfactant**

Pulmonary surfactants are lipoproteins produced by alveolar cells (type II pneumocytes), starting at around 24 to 28 weeks' gestation. By week 35, most babies have developed an adequate amount. Surfactant acts to reduce the surface tension of the lung, thus increasing compliance (the ability of the lungs to stretch when pressure is applied) and preventing atelectasis (collapsing of the lung) at the end of expiration. Premature neonates born before lung maturation can be given steroids to promote type II pneumocyte differentiation and the production of surfactant.

■ **Test for fetal lung maturity**

Fetal lung maturity can be tested by extracting a sample of amniotic fluid and measuring the lecithin-sphingomyelin ratio (L/S ratio). A L/S ratio less than 2:1 indicates surfactant deficiency and therefore lung immaturity.

Decongestants

Phenylephrine, Oxymetazoline, Naphazoline, Pseudoephedrine, and Phenylephrine

— *Intranasal decongestants*: Phenylephrine, oxymetazoline, naphazoline
— *Oral decongestants:* Pseudoephedrine, phenylephrine

Mechanism of action. Decongestants are sympathomimetics that decrease nasal blood flow by activating α_1-adrenergic receptors (**Fig. 26.6**).

Pharmacokinetics. Intranasal agents have a more rapid onset of action and produce fewer systemic effects than oral agents, but oral agents have a longer duration of action.

Uses. Symptomatic treatment of rhinitis.

Side effects
— Oral decongestants can cause systemic effects, such as central nervous system (CNS) stimulation, tachycardia, hypertension, and urinary retention.
— Rebound nasal congestion may occur upon withdrawal of the drug if used for more than 5 days. This is more common with intranasal agents.

Fig. 26.6 ► **Medications used in rhinitis.**
Cromolyn and nedocromil inhibit mast cell degranulation of histamine and other allergy mediators by blocking Ca^{2+} channels in the cell membrane. Nedocromil also has an antiinflammatory effect by inhibiting chemotaxis and migration of inflammatory cells. Alpha sympathomimetics are given by nasal spray or drops to reduce nasal swelling and congestion.

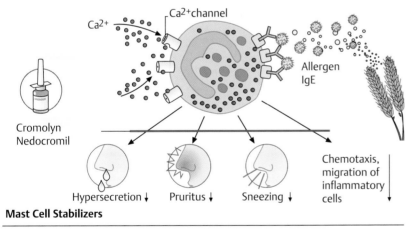

Mast Cell Stabilizers

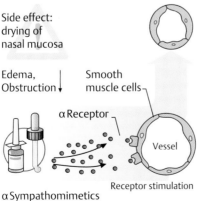

Contraindications
— Hypertension, coronary artery disease, or in patients on monoamine oxidase inhibitors (MAOIs) (see pages 87 and 88)

H₁ Antihistamines

Note: Only H_1 antihistamine agents that are used for allergic rhinitis are discussed here. See Chapter 32 for a full discussion of histamines and antihistamines.

Cetirizine, Loratadine, and Fexofenadine
— These are second-generation H_1 antihistamines.

Mechanism of action. H_1 antihistamines block H_1 receptors and prevent histamine-induced reactions (e.g., increased vascular permeability, smooth muscle contraction, mucus production, and pruritus [itching]). They also inhibit the "wheal and flare" response of the skin (**Fig. 26.7**).

Pharmacokinetics
— Usually given orally but may be given intranasally.
— These agents do not enter the brain as readily as first-generation H_1 antihistamines and so produce little, if any, sedation.

Uses
— First-line treatment for mild to moderate allergic rhinitis. In moderate to severe cases, intranasal corticosteroids are more effective than H_1 antihistamines.
— Also used for other allergy conditions

Side effects
— Mild sedation can occur with cetirizine at recommended doses and with loratadine in higher-than-recommended doses.
— Gastric effects: loss of appetite, constipation or diarrhea, nausea, and vomiting

Fig. 26.7 ► **Antihistamines for rhinitis.**
Antihistamines competitively inhibit histamine at its receptors. The newer second- and third-generation H_1 antihistamines (shown) are more effective and less sedative than older agents. They reduce hypersecretion, pruritis, and sneezing in patients with allergic rhinitis, allergic conjunctivitis, and urticaria (hives), but they do not have any effect on mucosal swelling.

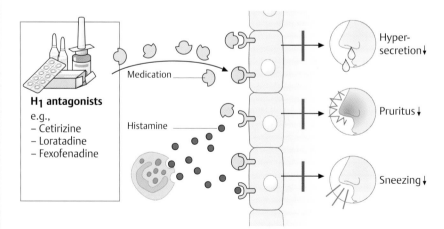

Mast Cell Stabilizers

Cromolyn Sodium and Nedocromil

Uses.   These agents are administered intranasally several times a day for the symptomatic treatment of allergic rhinitis (**Fig. 26.6**).

Intranasal Steroids

Beclomethasone and Flunisolide

Uses.   These agents are administered intranasally to provide a topical reduction of inflammation in allergic rhinitis. The reduction in systemic effects that is achieved by this method of delivery reduces the adverse effects associated with corticosteroid use (see page 154).

26.5   Treatment of Cough

Antitussive medication, such as opiates, the opiate analogue dextromethorphan, antihistamines, and decongestants may have beneficial effects in patients with an acute cough, depending on the cause. Persistent or chronic cough lasting more than 1 week may indicate an underlying infection (pertussis [whooping cough] or tuberculosis), a drug reaction (angiotensin-converting enzyme [ACE] inhibitors), another disorder (chronic bronchitis), or an environmental cause (smoke or occupational exposure).

The use and effectiveness of cough suppressants and over-the-counter cold medicines are controversial, especially in patients younger than 15 years. The risks of drug overdose, morbidity, and mortality may outweigh the benefits.

Opiates

Codeine and Dextromethorphan

Codeine is available in some over-the-counter cold remedies.

Dextromethorphan is an opiate analogue that is not analgesic or addictive; however, it is an antitussive (see Chapter 13).

Mechanism of action.   All opiates have central antitussive activity by acting on the cough center in the medulla to elevate the cough threshold.

Antihistamines and Decongestants

Diphenhydramine, Chlorpheniramine, Pseudoephedrine, and Phenylephrine

— *First-generation antihistamines*: Diphenhydramine and chlorpheniramine
— *Decongestants*: Pseudoephedrine and phenylephrine

Mechanism of action.   First-generation antihistamines possess anticholinergic drying activity and are used in combination with decongestants to decrease cough by decreasing postnasal drip, which stimulates the cough reflex.

26.6   Treatment of Excess Mucus Production

Expectorants

Expectorants facilitate the removal of fluids from the lungs.

Guaifenesin

Mechanism of action.   Guaifenesin increases the volume and reduces the viscosity of bronchial secretions. This may make it easier for coughing to remove the secretions, but the effectiveness to reduce cough is questionable.

Pharmacokinetics
— Given orally

Uses.   Although guaifenesin is found in over-the-counter medicines, its effectiveness in cough and colds is controversial. Its only approved use is to loosen phlegm in patients forming an abnormal amount of sputum (chronic bronchitis), but this usage is also of questionable efficacy.

Mucolytic Drugs

Mucolytic drugs decrease the viscosity of mucus.

Acetylcysteine

Mechanism of action.   Acetylcysteine has a free sulfhydryl group that opens the disulfide bonds in mucoproteins and lowers mucus viscosity.

Pharmacokinetics
— Given by inhalation or taken orally

Uses
— Acetylcysteine is used to decrease mucus viscosity in acute and chronic bronchopulmonary diseases, during surgery, in cystic fibrosis, and in diagnostic bronchial procedures.
— Acetylcysteine is also given orally to treat acetaminophen overdose (see page 356).

■ Cystic fibrosis

Cystic fibrosis is an autosomal recessive disease in which there is a defect in the epithelial transport protein CFTR (cystic fibrosis transmembrane conduction regulator) found in the lungs, pancreas, liver, genital tract, intestines, nasal mucosa, and sweat glands. This alters Cl^- transport in and out of cells and inhibits some Na^+ channels. In the lungs, Na^+ and water are absorbed from secretions that then become thick and sticky. In the pancreas, secretions are thick and sticky because duct cells cannot secrete Cl^- via the CFTR and water normally follows this ion movement. Sweat is salty because Cl^- is not being absorbed via the CFTR and so Na^+ also remains in the duct lumen. Symptoms include cough, wheezing, repeated lung and sinus infections, salty taste to the skin, steatorrhea (foul-smelling, greasy stools), poor weight gain and growth, meconium ileus (in newborns), and infertility in men. Complications of this disease include bronchiectasis (abnormal dilation of the large airways), deficiency of fat-soluble vitamins (A, D, E, K), diabetes, cirrhosis, gallstones, rectal prolapse, pancreatitis, osteoporosis, pneumothorax, cor pulmonale, and respiratory failure. Treatment involves daily physical therapy to help expectorate secretions from the lungs, antibiotics to treat lung infections, mucolytics, and bronchodilators.

27   Drugs Acting on the Gastrointestinal System

The gastrointestinal (GI) tract includes the mouth, stomach, small intestine (duodenum, jejunum, and ileum), large intestine (cecum and colon), rectum, anus, and its accompanying exocrine glands (the salivary glands, the pancreas, and the gallbladder).

Drugs affecting the GI system are used in the treatment of gastric acidity, peptic ulcers, and gastroesophageal reflux disease (GERD), bowel motility disorders (gastroparesis [delayed gastric emptying due to partial paralysis of the stomach muscles], constipation, and diarrhea), and for the treatment of nausea and vomiting.

27.1   Proton Pump Inhibitors

Omeprazole, Esomeprazole, Lansoprazole, Pantoprazole, and Rabeprazole

Mechanism of action.   Proton pump inhibitors inhibit the proton (H^+-K^+–ATPase) pump of the parietal cells in the stomach, thus inhibiting gastric acid (HCl) secretion into the lumen of the stomach (**Fig. 27.1**).

Fig. 27.1 ▶ **Drugs used to lower gastric acid production.**
Proton pump inhibitors block the H^+-K^+-ATPase pump on gastric parietal cells. H_2 receptor antagonists act to block histamine receptors on parietal cells. Both omeprazole and ranitidine ultimately lower gastric acid production. (ACh, acetylcholine; ECL, enterochromaffin-like cell.)

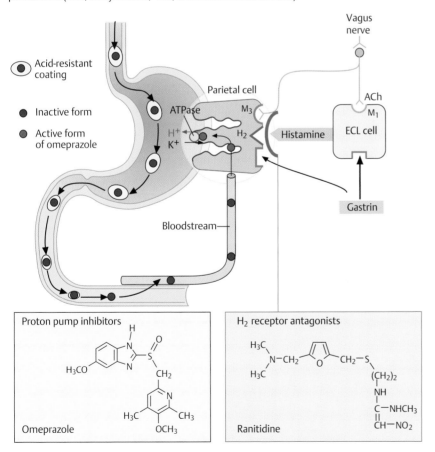

Uses
— Peptic ulcers
— GERD

Side effects.   There are minimal side effects. GI pain and diarrhea are the most common.

27.2   Gastric Antacids

Mechanism of action.   Gastric antacids (**Fig. 27.2**) partially neutralize gastric acid and inhibit pepsin (a proteolytic enzyme) activity both directly and by increasing pH, thus protecting the stomach mucosa. These agents must be taken frequently to maintain increased pH in the stomach.

— *Nonsystemic antacids* are compounds that are not absorbed into the systemic circulation. Their anionic group neutralizes the H^+ ions in gastric acid. This releases their cationic group which combines with HCO_3^- from the pancreas to form an insoluble basic compound that is excreted in feces. Thus these agents do not produce metabolic alkalosis.
— *Systemic antacids* are absorbed into the systemic circulation. They have a cationic group that does not form insoluble basic compounds with HCO_3^-. Thus the HCO_3^- can be absorbed producing a metabolic alkalosis.

Uses
— Peptic ulcers
— Acid indigestion
— Hyperchlorhydria (excess HCl in the stomach)

Nonsystemic Antacids

Calcium Carbonate

Side effects
— Ca^{2+} salts have an unpleasant chalky taste, and they precipitate in the GI tract to cause constipation. Rapid neutralization of gastric acid can also cause belching (CO_2 gas forms).
— Hypercalcemia can occur with chronic usage if large amounts of milk and dairy products are ingested ("milk–alkali syndrome").
— May cause a rebound acid secretion

Fig. 27.2 ▶ **Drugs used to neutralize gastric acid.**
Antacids have an anionic group that combines with H^+ in gastric acid, neutralizing it. The anion that is released in this reaction either remains in solution and is absorbed in the duodenum with HCO_3^- (from the pancreas) or it combines with HCO_3^- to form an insoluble precipitate that is excreted in feces.

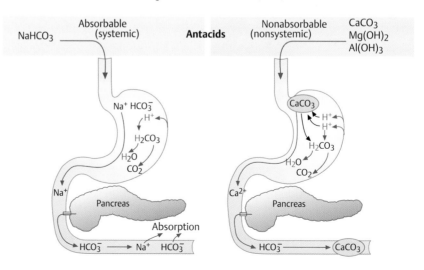

Magnesium Hydroxide (Milk of Magnesia)

Effects

- Mg^{2+} salts act as both antacids and laxative agents.
- The laxative effect is lessened by concomitant use with calcium carbonate or aluminum hydroxide; both tend to produce constipation.

Side effects. Some absorption and retention of Mg^{2+} (if renal function is impaired) could produce neurologic or cardiovascular toxicity.

Aluminum Hydroxide

Mechanism of action. Aluminum salts remain in the stomach for long periods and slowly react with stomach acid to form aluminum chloride. Aluminum hydroxide may inhibit the action of pepsin and stimulate stomach mucus secretion.

Side effects

- Constipation
- Osteomalacia (by interfering with PO_4^{3-} absorption)
- Decreased absorption of some drugs (e.g., tetracyclines and other antibiotics)

Note: Because some antacids have constipating effects and others laxative effects, a mixture of these salts are combined in over-the-counter and prescription preparations to negate and thus avoid these unwanted effects.

Systemic Antacids

Sodium Bicarbonate

Side effects. Sodium bicarbonate ($NaHCO_3$) is a highly soluble agent that rapidly neutralizes acid, producing lots of CO_2 and causing episodes of belching. Severe distention of the stomach by CO_2 gas may be dangerous if a gastric ulcer that could perforate is present.

27.3 Histamine (H_2) Receptor Antagonists

See Chapter 32 for a full discussion of histamine and antihistamines.

Cimetidine, Ranitidine, Famotidine, and Nizatidine

Mechanism of action. H_2 receptor antagonists act specifically to competitively block the H_2 histamine receptors of parietal cells (**Fig. 27.1**). They inhibit both basal and stimulated gastric acid secretion.

Pharmacokinetics. These drugs have a more rapid onset of action than the proton pump inhibitors and can be used for acute relief of symptoms.

- Ranitidine is several times more potent than cimetidine and thus requires less frequent dosing.
- Cimetidine inhibits cytochrome P-450 enzymes, possibly leading to drug interactions.

Uses

- Promotion of healing of peptic ulcers
- Prophylaxis of recurrent peptic ulcers
- GERD

Side effects. Headache, nausea, and skin rash

Peptic ulcers

An ulcer is a lesion extending through the mucosa and submucosa into deeper structures of the wall of the GI tract. Ulcers are the result of breakdown of the mucosal barrier (mucus and HCO_3^-) that normally protects the lining of the GI tract and/or increased secretion of H^+ or pepsin. There are two types of peptic ulcers: gastric ulcers and duodenal ulcers. Gastric ulcers are commonly found on the lesser curvature between the corpus and antrum of the stomach. They are often caused by *Helicobacter pylori* (*H. pylori*), a gram-negative spiral bacillus, which secretes cytotoxins that disrupt the mucosal barrier causing inflammation and destruction. *H. pylori* secretes high levels of membrane urease, which converts urea to NH_3. NH_3 neutralizes gastric acid around the bacterium, allowing it to survive in the acidic lumen of the stomach. Duodenal ulcers are the most common ulcers and are often associated with increased gastric H^+ secretion (but not necessarily). Doudenal ulcers also frequently occur due to *H. pylori* that inhibits somatostatin secretion leading to increased gastric H^+ secretion. There is also decreased HCO_3^- secretion in the duodenum, which impedes neutralization of the excess H^+ delivered from the stomach.

Zollinger–Ellison syndrome

Zollinger–Ellison syndrome is a condition caused by gastrin-secreting pancreatic adenomas that lead to multiple ulcers in the stomach and duodenum. These ulcers are frequently drug resistant and are accompanied by diarrhea and steatorrhea (as well as all of the usual peptic ulcers symptoms, e.g., burning abdominal discomfort, heartburn, nausea and vomiting, and weight loss). Tests for the condition will show raised serum gastrin and gastric acid levels. Treatment involves the use of proton pump inhibitors to heal the ulcers and surgical resection of the offending tumor if this is possible. If surgery is not an option, or if full resection is not possible, then chemotherapy may be employed to slow tumor growth. The 5-year survival rate is low (20%) if the tumor metastasizes (usually to the liver).

27.4   Mucosal Protective Agents

Sucralfate

Sucralfate is a complex of sulfated sucrose and polyaluminum hydroxide.

Mechanism of action.   Sucralfate is thought to accelerate the healing of duodenal ulcers by forming a protective barrier over the ulcer base. It forms an ulcer-adherent complex with the proteinaceous exudate at the ulcer site. It is also thought to protect ulcers from pepsin (**Fig. 27.3**). Sucralfate is not absorbed and does not inhibit acid secretion or neutralize acid.

Pharmacokinetics.   It may bind digoxin or tetracyclines, decreasing their absorption.

Uses
— Peptic ulcers

Side effects.   Constipation may occur.

Misoprostol

Mechanism of action.   Misoprostol is a prostaglandin derivative that acts to promote protective mucus secretion from epithelial cells in the stomach and inhibit gastric acid secretion for gastric parietal cells (**Fig. 27.4**).

Uses
— Peptic ulcers

Side effects
— Diarrhea and abdominal cramping

Bismuth Subsalicylate

Bismuth subsalicylate ($C_7H_5BiO_4$) is found in over-the-counter preparations such as Pepto-Bismol™, which is a suspension of trivalent bismuth and salicylate in magnesium aluminum silicate clay.

Fig. 27.3 ▶ **Chemical structure and protective effect of sucralfate.**
Sucralfate contains numerous aluminum hydroxide residues. When sucralfate is acted upon by gastric acid, it undergoes cross-linking and forms a paste that is able to adhere to the mucosal defect and exposed deeper layers. This coating of the ulcer protects it from acids and pepsin, allowing it to heal more rapidly.

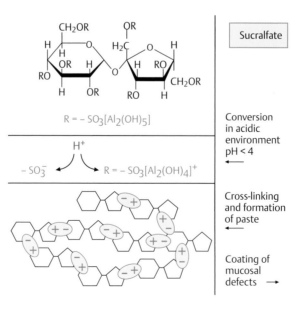

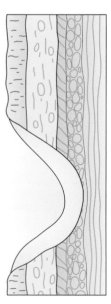

Fig. 27.4 ► **Chemical structure and protective effect of misoprostol.**
Locally released prostaglandins promote mucus production from surface epithelial cells and inhibit gastric acid secretion from parietal cells in the stomach. Misoprostol is a semisynthetic prostaglandin derivative and mimics these effects.

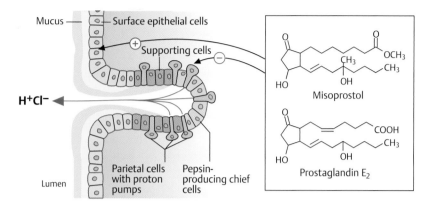

Mechanism of action. The mechanism of action is unclear.

Uses

- Heartburn
- Diarrhea
- It is included in combination drug regimens for *Helicobacter pylori*.

27.5 Drugs to Eradicate *Helicobacter pylori*

H. pylori is a gram-negative spiral bacillus that is found in the gastric epithelium of 70 to 90% of patients with peptic ulcers. It increases mucosal cell inflammation and destruction.

Treatment of *H. pylori*

Combination drug regimens are recommended for patients who test positive for *H. pylori*.

- *Triple therapy:* Proton pump inhibitor plus clarithromycin or metronidazole or tetracycline plus amoxicillin for 2 weeks
- *Quadruple therapy:* Proton pump inhibitor plus metronidazole plus bismuth plus tetracycline for 2 weeks

27.6 Drugs to Dissolve Gallstones

Ursodiol

Ursodiol is a naturally occurring bile acid found in high amounts in bear bile and in small amounts in human bile.

Mechanism of action. Ursodiol decreases secretion of cholesterol into bile by reducing cholesterol absorption and suppressing liver cholesterol synthesis. This alters bile composition and allows reabsorption of cholesterol-containing gallstones. Because reabsorption is slow, therapy must continue for at least 9 months.

Note: Ursodiol will not dissolve pigment stones or stones containing Ca^{2+}.

■ Diagnosis of *H. pylori* infection

H. pylori can be diagnosed by the carbon-13-urea breath test. This involves fasting for about 6 hours and then drinking a solution of ^{13}C-urea in water. Breath samples are then taken at intervals. If *H. pylori* is present, ^{13}C-urea is broken down to $^{13}CO_2$ by urease and will be measurable in the expired breath.

Pharmacokinetics

- Administered orally
- It is conjugated in the liver to glycine or taurine and excreted in the bile. Conjugated ursodiol undergoes extensive enterohepatic recirculation and has a long serum half-life. Thus, with long-term daily administration, ursodiol will eventually comprise 30 to 50% of the circulating bile acid pool.

Uses

- Treatment of gallstones
- It is also given prophylactically for the prevention of gallstones in obese patients undergoing rapid weight loss.

Side effects. Side effects associated with ursodiol are rare.

Contraindications

- Gallstones with a radiopaque component

> **Gallstones**
>
> The majority of gallstones (75%) are formed when the amount of cholesterol in bile exceeds the ability of bile salts and phospholipids to emulsify it, causing cholesterol to precipitate out of solution. Gallstones may also be caused by an increased amount of unconjugated bilirubin (often in the form of calcium bilirubinate) in the bile ("pigment stones"). Gallstones may be aymptomatic or they can cause obstruction of a duct causing severe pain, vomiting, and fever. Non-drug treatment includes lithotripsy (shock wave obliteration of gallstones that allow the stone fragments to be excreted) or surgical removal of the gallbladder (cholecystectomy).

27.7 Pancreatic Enzyme Replacements

Pancrelipase

Pancrelipase is the first pancreatic enzyme preparation approved by the U.S. Food and Drug Administration (FDA).

Mechanism of action. Pancrelipase is a combination of lipases, proteases, and amylases derived from porcine pancreas. It acts to replace the normal endogenous pancreatic enzymes.

Pharmacokinetics

- Enteric-coated microspheres in capsules withstand gastric acid and disintegrate at pH > 6.
- Administered with meals and snacks to treat malabsorption

Uses

- Chronic pancreatitis
- Cystic fibrosis (see page 258)
- Steatorrhea

> **Chronic pancreatitis**
>
> Chronic pancreatitis is ongoing inflammation of the pancreas. It is most commonly caused by alcohol abuse, but it may also occur with conditions such as gallstones, due to blockage of the pancreatic duct by the gallstone, or cystic fibrosis, due to blockage of the pancreatic duct by thick, viscous secretions. Typically, a patient with chronic pancreatitis has been ill for a prolonged period and has abdominal pain that radiates to the back, diabetes mellitus, steatorrhea (increased fat content of stools), and weight loss. Treatment involves pancreatic enzyme replacements, lifestyle changes, and surgery if necessary.

> **Steatorrhea**
>
> Steatorrhea is the production of feces that have a high content of fat. They are often oily and foul-smelling, and they tend to float. Steatorrhea occurs when fat digestion or absorption is impaired. This can occur due to pancreatic disease (e.g., cystic fibrosis, chronic pancreatitis) where there is a deficiency of pancreatic lipase that would normally digest fats. It may also occur in conditions that cause hypersecretion of gastrin (e.g., Zollinger-Ellison syndrome) where gastrin increases H^+ secretion which lowers duodenal pH, inactiviating pancreatic lipase. It may also occur due to liver disease which causes a deficiency of bile acids. Ileal resection will impair fat absorption due to impairment of bile recirculation to the liver. Treatment for steatorrhea due to pancreatic disease is pancreatic enzyme replacement (e.g., pancrelipase).

27.8 Antiemetic Drugs

Nausea and vomiting (emesis) are mechanisms to remove toxic or noxious substances after ingestion. However, they also may occur in response to motion, pregnancy, or disease. Vomiting is controlled by the vomiting center in the medulla, which receives inputs from the nearby chemoreceptor trigger zone (CTZ), the vestibular apparatus of the inner ear, the cerebral cortex, and the GI tract. **Table 27.1** summarizes the drugs that are most effective in treating different causes of nausea and vomiting and indicates their sites of action. Each class of drug includes a page reference to where these drugs are discussed in detail. The drugs that are not discussed in other sections are included below.

NK_1 Antagonists

Aprepitant

Mechanism of action. Aprepitant is a neurokinin-1-receptor (substance P) antagonist that blocks that action of neurokinin-1 in the brain.

Pharmacokinetics
— Given orally
— Extensively metabolized in the liver (via cytochrome P-450 3A4 [CYP3A4])

Uses
— Chemotherapy-induced nausea and vomiting

Side effects
— Constipation, diarrhea, and loss of appetite
— Headache, hiccups, and fatigue

Drug interactions. Interactions may occur due to induction of cytochrome P-450 enzymes in the liver.

Cannabinoid Agonists

Dronabinol

This agent is a derivative of marijuana.

Mechanism of action. Dronabinol acts on the vomiting center of the brain to prevent emesis, but the mechanism is unknown.

Pharmacokinetics
— Given orally

Uses
— Chemotherapy-induced emesis, which is unresponsive to other drugs

Side effects
— Sympathomimetic activity that leads to heart palpitations and tachycardia
— Marijuana-like central nervous system (CNS) effects, such as euphoria, somnolence, dizziness, and disturbances in thinking
— Abdominal pain, nausea, and vomiting
— Xerostomia (dry mouth) is very common.

Anticholinergic Drugs

Scopolamine

Mechanism of action. Scopolamine is a competitive antagonist at muscarinic receptors.

Pharmacokinetics. Scopolamine can be given via transdermal patch to reduce the side effects.

Uses
— Motion sickness
— Inner ear disease (vertigo)

Side effects. Side effects include dry mouth, blurred vision, urinary retention, palpitations, and headache.

Antihistamines

These agents are also discussed in Chapter 32.

Diphenhydramine and Dimenhydrinate

Mechanism of action. These agents act in the vestibular apparatus of the inner ear and the GI tract to prevent emesis, probably via their anticholinergic actions.

Vertigo

Vertigo is the illusion of movement (e.g., that the room is spinning). It is most commonly caused by disorders of the inner ear, such as Meniere disease (a syndrome characterized by vertigo, tinnitus, and deafness), vestibular neuronitis, lesions involving cranial nerve VIII, head injury causing vestibular damage, benign postural vertigo (vertigo occurs when certain positions are adopted or movements made), and by drugs (e.g., gentamicin, barbiturates, and alcohol). Other causes of vertigo are migraine, epilepsy, multiple sclerosis, and tumors. Treatment depends on the cause, but anticholinergic drugs and antihistamines are often used to prevent nausea and vomiting. Note that dizziness is a distinct entity from vertigo and is used to describe a feeling of lightheadedness or weakness.

The vomiting reflex

The vomiting reflex begins with a single retrograde peristaltic contraction beginning in the middle of the small intestine that propels intestinal contents through a relaxed gastroduodenal junction into the stomach. Inspiration occurs against a closed glottis, lowering intraesophageal pressure. The duodenum and antrum contract to prevent movement of chyme back into the small intestine. The abdominal muscles then forcibly contract (Valsalva maneuver), increasing intra-abdominal pressure which creates more pressure in the stomach than in the esophagus. This forces gastric contents into the esophagus. The larynx and hyoid bone are drawn forward, decreasing the tone of the upper esophageal sphincter (UES) leading to the gastric and esophageal contents being expelled via the oral cavity.

Uses

— Motion sickness
— Inner ear disease (vertigo)

Side effects

— Sedation and the usual anticholinergic side effects (listed above for scopolamine)

Dopamine Antagonists

Prochlorperazine and Thiethylperazine

Mechanism of action. These agents prevent vomiting by blocking D_2 dopamine receptors in the medullary chemoreceptor trigger zone.

Uses

— Medication-, toxin-, or metabolic-induced emesis

Side effects

— Anticholinergic: orthostatic (postural) hypotension, dry mouth, constipation, and blurred vision

Contraindications

— Parkinson disease

5-Hydroxytryptamine type 3 (5-HT$_3$) Antagonists

Ondansetron, Granisetron, Dolasetron, and Palonosetron

Mechanism of action. These agents block 5-HT$_3$ receptors in the CNS and GI tract. Activation of these receptors normally triggers vomiting.

Uses

— Chemotherapy- and radiation-induced emesis
— Postoperative emesis
— Pregnancy

Table 27.1 ▶ Summary of Drugs Used to Treat Different Causes of Nausea and Vomiting

Etiology of Nausea or Vomiting	Drug Class	Examples	Site of Action
Motion sickness Inner ear disease	Antihistamine (pp. 343 and 344)	Diphenhydramine, Dimenhydrinate	Vestibular, GI
	Anticholinergic (p. 52)	Scopolamine	CTZ, Vestibular, GI
Medication-, toxin-, or metabolic-induced vomiting	D_2 dopamine antagonist	Prochlorperazine, thiethylperazine	CTZ, GI
Chemotherapy- and radiation-induced vomiting Postoperative vomiting Pregnancy	5-HT$_3$ antagonist (p. 70)	Ondansetron, granisetron	CTZ, GI
Chemotherapy-induced nausea and vomiting	NK$_1$ antagonist	Aprepitant	GI
Chronic idiopathic nausea Functional vomiting Cyclic vomiting syndrome	Tricyclic antidepressant (p. 86)	Amitriptyline, nortriptyline	Cortex
Chemotherapy-induced vomiting unresponsive to other drugs	Cannabinoid agonist	Dronabinol	Vomiting center

Abbreviations: CTZ, chemoreceptor trigger zone; GI, gastrointestinal.

Side effects
- Constipation, diarrhea, headache, and fatigue

Tricyclic Antidepressants

Amitriptyline and Nortriptyline

Mechanism of action.   These agents act in the cortex of the brain to inhibit the reuptake of norepinephrine and serotonin (see Chapter 10).

Uses
- Chronic idiopathic nausea
- Functional vomiting
- Cyclic vomiting syndrome

27.9   Prokinetic (Gastric Motility Promoting) Drugs

Gastroparesis, also known as delayed gastric emptying, is a disorder in which the stomach takes too long to empty its contents. The most frequent cause is diabetes mellitus, but it can also be caused by smooth muscle or nervous system disorders and, in many cases, is idiopathic.

Metoclopramide

Mechanism of action.   Metoclopramide is a D_2 dopamine receptor antagonist that increases release of acetylcholine from nerve endings in the GI tract, leading to increased GI motility and rate of gastric emptying. It also increases lower esophageal tone.

Uses
- Gastroparesis
- Reflux esophagitis
- Antiemetic

Side effects
- Extrapyramidal side effects similar to those seen with typical antipsychotics, including parkinsonism, dystonia, and, with longer term use, tardive dyskinesia (see page 99)
- Sedation
- Prolactin secretion is increased.

Erythromycin

See pages 296 and 297 for a full discussion of this agent.

Mechanism of action.   Erythromycin stimulates motilin receptors and increases GI motility. Motilin is an endogenous peptide that produces contraction of the upper GI tract via motilin receptors on smooth muscle cells and enteric neurons.

Side effects.   Nausea, vomiting, and abdominal cramps

27.10   Laxative and Cathartic Drugs

Laxatives and cathartics are drugs that promote defecation. Laxatives promote the excretion of a soft, formed stool, and cathartics promote fluid evacuation. The uses and contraindications for these laxatives and cathartics are included in **Table 27.2.**

Table 27.2 ▶ Uses and Contraindications of Laxatives and Cathartics	
Uses	**Contraindications**
Radiologic exams of gastrointestinal tract Bowel surgery Proctologic exam Useful in patients with a hernia or cardiovascular disease (to avoid straining at stool) Anorectal disorders (e.g., hemorrhoids) Useful after anti-helmintic therapy or poisoning by drugs or foods	Colic (attacks of severe abdominal pain), nausea, and cramps Undiagnosed abdominal pain Patients with symptoms of appendicitis

Contact (Stimulant–Irritant) Cathartics

Mechanism of action. Contact cathartics increase intestinal motor activity (peristalsis) and stimulate water and electrolyte accumulation in the colon (**Fig. 27.5**).

Castor Oil

Castor oil is derived from the seeds of *Ricinus communis.*

Pharmacokinetics. Pancreatic lipases hydrolyze castor oil to the active irritant agent ricinoleic acid, which acts on the small intestine in 1 to 3 hours.

Side effects. Castor oil has a disagreeable taste and should not be used just prior to bedtime.

Diphenylmethanes

Bisacodyl

Pharmacokinetics. Bisacodyl given orally acts in 6 to 8 hours; thus, it is often given at bedtime to produce effects by morning. Rectal suppositories are effective within 1 hour.

Anthraquinones

Cascara, Aloe, and Senna

Pharmacokinetics. They act on the large intestine in 6 to 8 hours.

Side effects
— Electrolyte imbalance from excessive catharsis

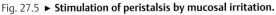

Fig. 27.5 ▶ **Stimulation of peristalsis by mucosal irritation.**
Irritant laxatives exert an irritant action on the intestinal mucosa. This causes less fluid to be absorbed than is secreted. This filling of the intestinal lumen stimulates reflex peristalsis. Peristalsis is also directly simulated by the irritant action.

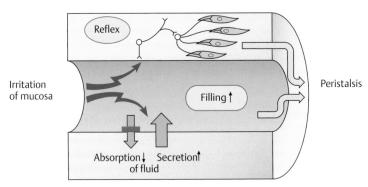

Saline (Osmotic) Cathartics

Mechanism of action. Saline cathartics act by causing water to be retained through an osmotic effect. Stretching of the bowel lumen by this increase in water stimulates peristalsis.

Magnesium Hydroxide, Sodium Phosphate, and Polyethylene Glycol

Pharmacokinetics
— Poorly and slowly absorbed from the GI tract
— Water retention indirectly increases peristalsis, with watery evacuation occurring in < 3 hours.
— Approximately 20% of magnesium is absorbed, but it is rapidly excreted if renal function is normal. Mg^{2+} intoxication can occur if renal function is impaired, resulting in weakness, nausea, vomiting, and respiratory depression.

Side effects
— Electrolyte imbalance
— Cerebral failure can occur with sodium phosphate.

Lactulose

Mechanism of action. Intestinal bacteria hydrolyze the drug, which leads to a more acid pH of the colon. This reduces the ability of bacteria to form ammonia.

Pharmacokinetics
— Given orally, but not absorbed

Uses. Lactulose is a specialized laxative for chronic liver disease or hepatic coma to decrease plasma levels of ammonia.

Stool Softeners

Mechanism of action. Stool softeners act by keeping feces soft so tenesmus (straining at stool) is avoided. There is no direct or reflex stimulation of peristalsis with these agents.

Docusate

Mechanism of action. Docusate produces stool softening by lowering surface tension to promote water penetration into feces.

Pharmacokinetics. Effects are seen within 1 to 2 days.

Uses. The main use of this agent is to limit straining, as it has minimal laxative effects.

Lubricant Laxatives

Mechanism of action. Lubricant laxatives act by retarding reabsorption of water.

Mineral Oil

Mineral oil is a mixture of liquid hydrocarbons obtained from petroleum.

Side effects
— Lipid pneumonia in elderly or debilitated patients if oil is aspirated
— Foreign-body reactions in mesenteric lymph nodes, liver, spleen, and intestinal mucosa may occur.
— Absorption of essential fat-soluble substances (vitamins A, D, and K, and carotene) may be blocked.

Bulk-forming Laxatives

Mechanism of action.   Bulk-forming laxatives act by absorbing and retaining water, causing fecal material to become hydrated and soft. They may also act to reflexively stimulate peristalsis (**Figs. 27.6** and **27.7**).

Bran (and Other Dietary Fiber), Methylcellulose, Sodium Carboxymethylcellulose, and Psyllium Preparations

These are naturally occurring or synthetic polysaccharides.

Pharmacokinetics
—   Action is within 1 to 3 days.
—   Some drug absorption may be reduced because of binding to these agents.

Side effects.   Intestinal obstruction has been reported.

> **Effects of fiber**
>
> In the stomach, fiber binds water which enlarges the particle size so that fiber passes the pyloric sphincter later, delaying gastric emptying. In the ileum and colon, in particular, the water-binding (swelling) capacity of fiber lowers transit time. Fiber may bind mineral and trace elements as well as fat-soluble vitamins, which may not allow them to be absorbed. The binding of steroids leads to an increased excretion of bile acids and cholesterol, which may be helpful in people with fat metabolism disorders. Glucose absorption is also delayed by high fiber intake, improving glucose control in diabetics. Stool volume is increased and the consistency of stool is softer with fiber intake. However, intestinal bacteria ferment the polysaccharides in fiber producing methane and CO_2. During fermenetation, short-chain fatty acids are produced that positively affect the composition of the intestinal flora and the intestinal pH. Finally, the binding of ammonia by fiber increases fecal nitrogen excretion thereby unburdening the liver and kidneys.

Fig. 27.6 ► **Bulk laxatives.**
Bulk laxatives are insoluble and nonabsorbable from the intestine. They absorb water and expand within the intestinal lumen; this stimulates peristalsis.

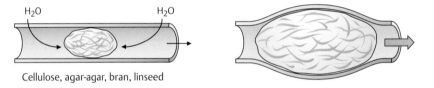

Cellulose, agar-agar, bran, linseed

Fig. 27.7 ► **Stimulation of peristalsis by an intraluminal bolus.**
Distention of the intestinal wall by fecal matter activates mechanoreceptors that induce a neuronally mediated ascending reflex contraction of intestinal smooth muscle (*red*) and a descending relaxation (*blue*). This propulsive movement of the intestinal musculature (peristalsis) allows fecal matter to move in the direction of the anus for evacuation.

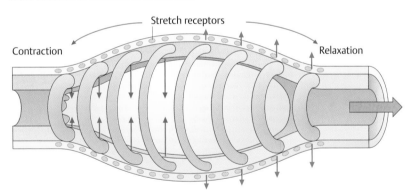

27.11   Antidiarrheal Agents

Antidiarrheal therapy aims to prevent the dehydration and electrolyte imbalance that can quickly occur in severe diarrhea, as well as preventing excessive bowel movements.

Note: Antibacterial agents are useful only if bacteria are the cause of the diarrhea (which is uncommon). They cause depletion of the normal intestinal bacterial flora, which, in turn, may cause proliferation of pathogenic bacteria, leading to diarrhea.

Adsorbents

Bismuth Subsalicylate, Kaolin, and Pectin

- Bismuth subsalicylate
- Kaolin (hydrated aluminum silicate)
- Pectin (a purified carbohydrate from acid extracts of apples or the rinds of citrus fruits)

Mechanism of action. These agents absorb bacterial toxins and fluid in the gut.

Pharmacokinetics

- Bismuth subsalicylate is given as chewable tablets or in an aqueous suspension.
- Kaolin is often given in a mixture with pectin.

Uses

- Diarrhea and dysentery

Side effects. These drugs are not absorbed, so they do not have systemic side effects. Constipation may occur.

Opioids

See Chapter 13 for a full discussion of these drugs.

Mechanism of action. These agents decrease propulsion and peristalsis. GI contents are delayed in passage, allowing time for feces to become desiccated. This further retards passage through the colon.

- Opioids are effective in acute diarrheal states, but they should not be used for enteric infections.
- Opium alkaloids are effective for controlling severe diarrhea or dysentery, but with chronic therapy, there is a risk of dependence.

Paregoric

Paregoric is a camphorated tincture of opium.

Uses

- Infantile diarrhea

Codeine and/or Morphine

These are purified opium alkaloids.

Pharmacokinetics. They exert a local action in the GI tract.

Diphenoxylate

Diphenoxylate is a congener of meperidine. It is often given in combination with atropine.

Side effects. High or chronic doses lead to euphoria and physical dependence.

Loperamide

Loperamide is a derivative of haloperidol that resembles meperidine.

This agent appears to be as effective as diphenoxylate, with few side effects reported.

Uses

- Prophylaxis and treatment of travelers' diarrhea
- Irritable bowel syndrome (IBS)

Antidiarrheal agents and their site of action are summarized in **Fig. 27.8.**

Irritable Bowel Syndrome (IBS)

IBS is a chronic idiopathic condition. Symptoms include abdominal pain, bloating, and cramps, which are associated with bowel habit alteration in the form of constipation or diarrhea. Treatment is guided by the symptoms and their severity. Mild IBS may respond to dietary changes. Drugs may be called for in patients with moderate to severe symptoms. Antispasmodics, such as hyoscyamine and dicyclomine, laxatives (docusate, bisacodyl, senna, or osmotic agents) and loperamide are standard. In severe cases with diarrhea, alosetron, a potent and selective antagonist of the 5-HT$_3$ receptor that decreases intestinal motility and pain may be used with caution, as it can lead to severe constipation. Note: IBS is not associated with pathophysiological changes in gut structure and is diagnosed only when all else has been excluded.

Fig. 27.8 ▶ Antidiarrheals and their site of action.
Bacteria can secrete toxins that inhibit the ability of enterocytes to absorb sodium chloride (NaCl) and water. They also stimulate fluid secretion into the intestinal lumen. Bacteria and viruses also cause mucosal inflammation, which further causes luminal fluid loss. This increase in luminal fluid stimulates peristalsis. Adsorbents bind to toxins and promote their evacuation. As a consequence, more salt and water are able to be reabsorbed. Opioids activate enteric nerves, resulting in inhibition of propulsion and peristalsis. Loperamide is pumped back into the body by the endothelial cells of the blood–brain barrier, so it does not produce the unwanted central nervous system (CNS) effects of morphine and diphenoxylate. Oral rehydration solutions contain glucose, which is absorbed into intestinal cells, drawing water along with it.

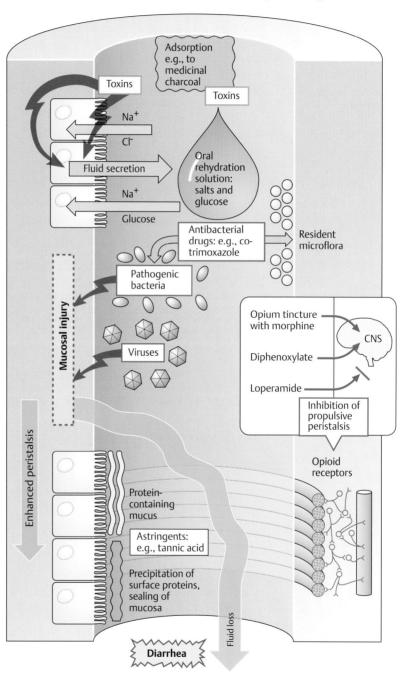

27.12   Drugs Used in Inflammatory Bowel Disease

There are two types of inflammatory bowel disease: Crohn disease and ulcerative colitis (**Fig. 27.9**). Crohn disease is a chronic inflammatory disease that can affect the entire GI tract but most commonly affects the terminal ileum and colon. It causes ulcers, fistulas (abnormal communications), and granulomata, producing symptoms such as fever, diarrhea, weight loss, and abdominal pain. Ulcerative colitis is a recurrent inflammatory disease of the colon and rectum that produces bloody diarrhea, weight loss, fever, and abdominal pain. The goal of therapy for inflammatory bowel diseases is to reduce the inflammatory response by using drugs such as steroids and sulfasalazine.

Fig. 27.9 ▶ **Crohn disease and ulcerative colitis.**
The typical pattern of Crohn disease is segmental inflammation that affects all layers of the intestinal wall, producing fistulae, abscesses, and perforation. Inflammatory conglomerate tumors develop in adjacent structures due to fistulae and abscess formation. Crohn disease is associated with human leukocyte antigens (HLA) DR1 and DQw5. Patients were often not breastfed for a long period as infants, and have a history of smoking and high intake of refined carbohydrates. In ulcerative colitis, there is relapsing and remitting inflammation of the colon, as well as superficial ulcerations that spread proximally. This leads to flattening of the intestinal mucosa and destruction of goblet cells. Hyperregeneration causes pseudopolyp production. Ulcerative colitis is thought to be autoimmune and is associated with immunoglobulin A (IgA) nephritis and autoimmune hepatitis, among other conditions.

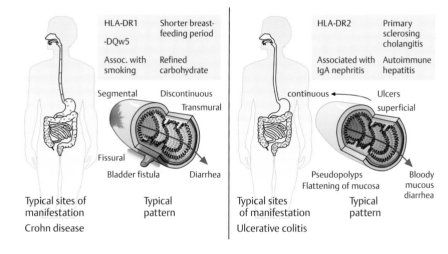

Aminosalicylates

Mesalamine, Balsalazide, Olsalazine, and Sulfasalazine

— Mesalamine is 5-aminosalicylic acid (5-ASA), the active moiety of all the aminosalicylates used to treat inflammatory bowel disease.
— Balsalazide, olsalazine, and sulfasalazine are prodrugs that are metabolized to 5-ASA.

Mechanism of action.   Five-aminosalicylate (5-ASA) acts within the intestinal tract (mainly the terminal ileum and colon) to inhibit prostaglandin and leukotriene synthesis thus reducing the inflammatory reaction (**Figs. 27.10** and **27.11**).

Uses
—Mild to moderate ulcerative colitis

Side effects
— Nausea, vomiting, diarrhea, headache, and abdominal pain
— Bone marrow suppression

Fig. 27.10 ▶ **Drug treatment of Crohn disease and ulcerative colitis.**
Acute attacks of Crohn disease and ulcerative colitis are treated with sulfasalazine and 5-aminosalicylic acid (5-ASA) (see also **Fig. 27.11**). Crohn disease also may involve treatment with steroids. These drugs inhibit prostaglandin and leukotriene synthesis and intervene late in the inflammatory cascade.

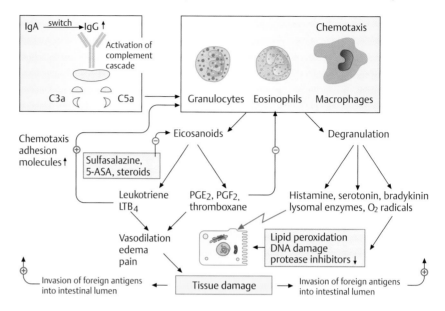

Fig. 27.11 ▶ **Sulfasalazine.**
Sulfasalazine is converted to its active forms sulfapyridine and 5-ASA by intestinal bacteria. These active forms inhibit the inflammatory reaction in intestinal mucosa.

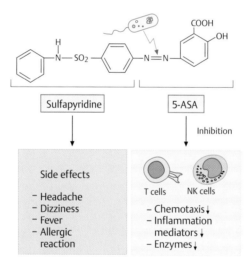

Tumor Necrosis Factor-α Inhibitors

Adalimumab, Certolizumab Pegol, and Infliximab

Mechanism of action.   These agents are monoclonal antibodies or antibody fragments that bind and neutralize tumor necrosis factor-α (TNF-α), a principal cytokine that mediates IBD.

Pharmacokinetics.   These drugs must be given by injection.

Uses
— Moderate to severe Crohn disease unresponsive to other therapies (adalimumab, certolizumab pegol, and infliximab)
— Moderate to severe ulcerative colitis not responsive to other drugs (infliximab)

Fig. 27.12 ► **Corticosteroids: effects and side effects.**
Corticosteroids act to decrease inflammation, and reduce connective tissue proliferation by the mechanisms shown. Short-term side effects are edema and weight gain. Gastric ulceration, hypertension, steroid-induced diabetes mellitus, and increased susceptibility to infections may also occur. Longer-term use may lead to more serious side effects, such as Cushing syndrome, skin atrophy, osteoporosis, and seizures. (IL-1, interleukin-1; IL-2, interleukin-2; MHC, major histocompatibility complex; TNF, tumor necrosis factor.)

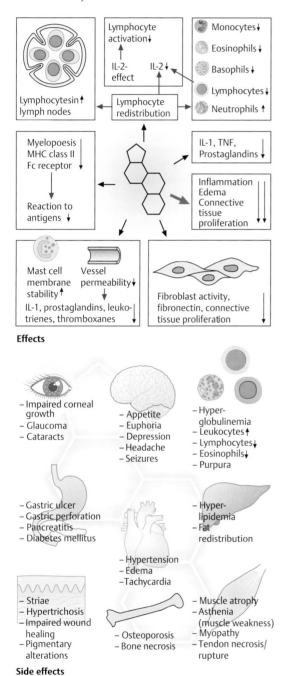

Effects

Side effects

Side effects
— Reactivation of tuberculosis
— Increased respiratory infections

Corticosteroids

These agents are also discussed in Chapters 16, 26, 32, and 34.

Prednisone and Budesonide

Uses.   Corticosteroids are effective in both ulcerative colitis and Crohn disease in inducing a remission in acute persistent disease. They are used systemically until adequate control of inflammation is achieved, then the dose is tapered and discontinued to avoid the side effects seen with long-term systemic steroid use (see page 154).

　　Figure 27.12 provides a summary of the effects and side effects of corticosteroids.

Immunosuppressants

These agents are also discussed in Chapter 34.

Cyclosporine

Mechanisms of action.   Cyclosporine decreases interleukin-2 (IL-2) synthesis in T-helper cells.

Uses.   These agents are sometimes used in patients unresponsive to steroids or in chronic cases of moderate to severe IBD, although they are not approved by the FDA for this purpose.

Antimetabolites

These agents are discussed further in Chapters 33 and 34.

Methotrexate, Azathioprine, and Mercaptopurine

Mechanisms of action
— Methotrexate inhibits dihydrofolate reductase, which reduces purine and pyrimidine synthesis in lymphocytes and so dampens the immune response (**Fig. 27.13**).

Fig. 27.13 ▶ **Antimetabolites.**
Methotrexate inhibits purine and thymidine synthesis. It does this by inhibiting the formation of tetrahydrofolate by binding to dihydrofolate reductase, the enzyme that catalyzes its formation from folate. Methotrexate also inhibits cell growth in rapidly proliferating tissues (e.g., bone marrow). Azathioprine is converted to 6-mercaptopurine, which is a false substrate for purine biosynthesis. It is also incorporated in DNA and RNA, where it acts as a "wrong" base and damages the cell.

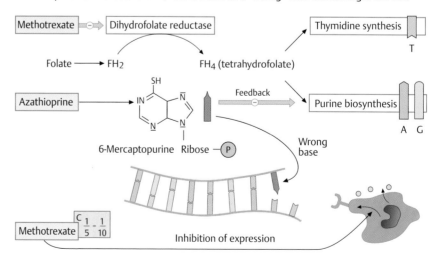

— Azathioprine is converted to 6-mercaptopurine. Mercaptopurine is a purine analogue that causes pseudofeedback inhibition of the first step in purine biosynthesis and inhibition of purine intraconversions.

Pharmacokinetics. The onset of action of these drugs takes several weeks.

Uses

— Moderate to severe inflammatory bowel disease (mainly Crohn disease)

Side effects

— Bone marrow depression

27.13 Appetite-suppressing and Appetite-enhancing Drugs

CNS-acting Appetite Suppressants

Amphetamine and Its Derivatives: Methylphenidate, Ephedrine, Phenylpropanolamine, and Phentermine

Mechanism of action. These sympathomimetic agents are effective in suppressing appetite; however, any weight lost while on the drug is rapidly regained upon cessation.

Uses. These agents are unsuitable for the treatment of obesity due to their CNS-stimulating and other side effects (see page 123).

Fenfluramine and Dexfenfluramine

Dexfenfluramine is the D-isomer of fenfluramine.

These agents were previously used as appetite suppressants, but they were shown to cause pulmonary hypertension and valvular heart disease, which led to their withdrawal from the market.

Sibutramine

Mechanism of action. Sibutramine is a serotonin and norepinephrine reuptake inhibitor.

Uses. Sibutramine is the only anorexiant currently approved for long-term use in patients with body mass index (BMI) > 30 or with diabetes and BMI > 27. It produces a weight loss of ~5 to 9% at 12 months.

Side effects. Headache, dry mouth, insomnia, and constipation. It also increases heart rate and blood pressure. Body weight increases when the medication is discontinued.

Peripherally Acting Weight-loss Medication

Orlistat

This agent is available over-the-counter.

Mechanism of action. Orlistat is an inhibitor of the pancreatic and gastric lipases that hydrolyze dietary fat into fatty acids and monoacylglycerols. This prevents ~30% of dietary fat from being absorbed. Orlistat produces a weight loss of ~9 to 10% in 12 months.

Pharmacokinetics. Not absorbed from the GI tract.

Side effects. No systemic side effects are seen; however, adverse GI effects are common and include flatulence, fecal urgency, fatty/oily stools, and increased frequency of defecation. These side effects can be minimized by decreasing dietary fat intake.

Appetite Enhancers

Megestrol

Megestrol is a synthetic form of progesterone.

Mechanism of action. The mechanism to affect the appetite is unknown.

Uses. Megestrol is used to enhance appetite in patients with human immunodeficiency virus/ acquired immunodeficiency syndrome (HIV/AIDS) and cancer.

Dronabinol

Dronabinol is synthetic δ-9-tetrahydrocannabinol, the main active ingredient in marijuana.

Mechanism of action. Dronabinol stimulates the appetite by acting on cannabinoid receptors in the CNS (see page 265).

Uses. In states where it is available, medicinal marijuana is used by patients with AIDS and cancer as an appetite enhancer and to prevent chemotherapy-induced nausea and vomiting.

Review Questions

1. Bronchodilation is best accomplished via
   A. activation of α_1-adrenergic receptors.
   B. activation of α_2-adrenergic receptors.
   C. activation of β_1-adrenergic receptors.
   D. activation of β_2-adrenergic receptors.
   E. activation of muscarinic receptors.

2. Which of the following agents is used for treatment of persistent asthma to decrease inflammation, decrease the formation of mucus, and decrease the hyperreactivity of bronchial smooth muscle?
   A. Inhaled corticosteroid
   B. Systemic corticosteroid
   C. Inhaled β_2-adrenergic selective agonist
   D. Systemic β_2-adrenergic selective agonist
   E. Systemic phosphodiesterase inhibitor

3. A patient with a history of asthma presents with severe respiratory distress and hypoxemia because of an acute, severe asthma attack. A β-adrenergic receptor agonist is administered immediately by inhalation. A systemic drug is then administered to treat the inflammatory component of the acute asthma. Which of the following was administered?
   A. Cromolyn
   B. A parenteral corticosteroid
   C. Oral theophylline
   D. An inhaled corticosteroid
   E. Antibiotics

4. A 12-year-old girl is being treated for asthma. The drug treatment has resulted in abdominal discomfort, difficulty sleeping, and a persistent headache. These are common side effects of which agent?
   A. Atropine
   B. Beclomethasone
   C. Cromolyn sodium
   D. Ipratropium
   E. Theophylline

5. Which of the following inhibits acid secretion by direct interaction with the H^+-K^+–ATPase in the parietal cell?
   A. Ursodiol
   B. Omeprazole
   C. Ranitidine
   D. Sucralfate
   E. Calcium carbonate

6. Prostaglandins present in the gastric mucosa are believed to
   A. increase capillary permeability when aspirin damages the gastric mucosal barrier to ion diffusion.
   B. block the binding of acetylcholine on parietal cell muscarinic receptors.
   C. inhibit parietal cell hydrochloric acid production.
   D. block the entry of calcium into the parietal cell.
   E. inhibit gastric bicarbonate secretion.

7. Which of the following is an H_2-histamine receptor antagonist?
   A. Cimetidine
   B. Ondansetron
   C. Lactulose
   D. Docusate
   E. Sodium bicarbonate

8. A 58–year-old woman has rheumatoid arthritis. The patient's symptoms have responded favorably to treatment with a nonsteroidal antiinflammatory agent. To decrease the potential of a gastric ulcer, the patient is instructed to take misoprostol simultaneously with the antiinflammatory agent. What is misoprostol?
   A. A prostaglandin E_1 analogue that inhibits gastric acid secretion
   B. An antacid that decreases the pH of gastric secretions
   C. A nonsteroidal antiinflammatory drug–binding agent that prevents absorption in the stomach
   D. An H_2-histamine receptor blocker that inhibits gastric acid secretion
   E. A proton pump inhibitor that inhibits gastric acid secretion

Answers and Explanations

1. **D** Activation of β_2-adrenergic receptors on bronchial smooth muscle produces smooth muscle relaxation and bronchodilation (p. 251).
   A α_1-adrenergic receptors may be present on the vasculature of the lung and regulate vasoconstriction.
   B α_2-adrenergic receptors may be found on presynaptic terminals of sympathetic neurons and regulate neurotransmitter release.
   C β_1-adrenergic receptors are found mainly in the heart. Activation of these receptors causes increased heart rate and force and velocity of contraction.
   D Activation of muscarinic cholinergic receptors causes bronchoconstriction.

2. **A** Decreased inflammation, decreased formation of mucus, and decreased hyperreactivity of bronchial smooth muscle are all effects of corticosteroids. They are administered by inhalation to minimize systemic side effects that would be seen if given systemically (B) (p. 250).
   C, D β_2 adrenergic receptor selective agonists do not produce these effects, but they do produce bronchodilation.
   E Theophylline is a systemic phosphodiesterase inhibitor that mainly produces bronchodilation, but it may also have some antiinflammatory actions. It does not decrease the formation of mucus or decrease hyperreactivity of bronchial smooth muscle.

3. **B** For acute, severe asthma attacks, parenteral steroids are used (p. 251).
   A, C Cromolyn, a mast cell stabilizer, and theophylline, a systemic phosphodiesterase inhibitor, are not used for acute asthma attacks.
   D Inhaled corticosteroids are used for the chronic treatment of asthma.
   E Antibiotics are not effective for treating asthma.

4. **E** These side effects are produced by theophylline, which is a systemic phosphodiesterase inhibitor (p. 253).
   A, D Atropine and ipratropium produce anticholinergic side effects, such as dry mouth, blurred vision, tachycardia, urinary retention, and constipation.
   B Beclomethasone may cause throat irritation, dysphonia, oral candidiasis, and growth disturbances in children (rarely).
   C Cromolyn sodium, a mast cell stabilizer, has minimal side effects.

5. **B** Omeprazole inhibits the proton pump (H^+-K^+–ATPase) of the parietal cells in the stomach, thereby inhibiting gastric acid secretion (p. 259).
   A Ursodiol decreases the secretion of cholesterol into bile by reducing cholesterol absorption and suppressing cholesterol synthesis in the liver. It is used to treat cholesterol-containing gallstones.
   C Ranitidine is an H_2-histamine receptor antagonist that blocks the H_2-histamine receptors of parietal cells, thereby inhibiting both basal and stimulated gastric acid secretion.
   D Sucralfate forms an ulcer-adherent complex with the proteinaceous exudate at the ulcer site.
   E Calcium carbonate is a nonsystemic antacid.

6. **C** Prostaglandins inhibit parietal cell hydrochloric acid production in the gastric mucosa. They also increase mucus production (p. 262).

7. **A** Cimetidine is an H_2-histamine receptor antagonist that blocks the H_2-histamine receptors of parietal cells, thereby inhibiting both basal and stimulated gastric acid secretion (p. 261).
   B Ondansetron is an anti-emetic drug that blocks 5-HT_3 receptors in the central nervous system and gastrointestinal tract.
   C Lactulose is a specialized laxative for chronic liver disease or hepatic coma as it decreases plasma levels of ammonia formed by intestinal bacteria.
   D Docusate is a stool softening agent that lowers surface tension and promotes water absorption into feces.
   E Sodium bicarbonate is a systemic antacid.

8. **A** Misoprostol is a prostaglandin derivative that has both cytoprotective and antisecretory actions. It does not act by any of the other listed mechanisms (p. 262).

28 Principles of Antimicrobial Therapy

Infectious diseases are caused by microbes or by microbial products. Antimicrobial drugs are intended to eliminate foreign organisms or abnormal cells from healthy tissues of the patient without comparable effects on the normal tissue cells of the host. This essential property of these drugs is called selective toxicity.

28.1 Classification of Antimicrobial Agents

Chemical Structure and Mechanism of Action

The main classification of antimicrobial agents is based on chemical structure (e.g., β-lactams and aminoglycosides) and mechanism of action (see **Table 28.1**).

Table 28.1 ▶ Mechanism of Action of Antimicrobial Agents	
Mechanism of Action	**Drugs**
Inhibition of bacterial cell wall synthesis	β-lactams: penicillins, cephalosporins, and carbapenems Others: cycloserine, vancomycin, and bacitracin
Reversible inhibition of protein synthesis by disrupting the function of 30S or 50S ribosomal subunits	Bacteriostatic: chloramphenicol, tetracyclines, erythromycin, clindamycin, streptogramins, and linezolid Bactericidal: aminoglycosides
Inhibition of nucleic acid metabolism by inhibiting RNA polymerase	Rifampin and rifabutin
Inhibition of nucleic acid metabolism by inhibiting DNA gyrase or topoisomerase	The quinolones
Inhibition of essential enzymes of folate metabolism (antimetabolites)	Trimethoprim and sulfonamides

Bacteriostatic or Bactericidal

Antimicrobial agents are also classified according to whether they are bacteriostatic or bactericidal (**Fig. 28.1**).

Fig. 28.1 ▶ **Bacteriostatic versus bactericidal antibacterial agents.**
Bacteria are able to multiply in vitro in a growth medium if conditions are favorable. If the growth medium contains an antibiotic, the bacteria may be killed (bactericidal effect), or the bacteria may survive but are unable to multiple (bacteriostatic effect).

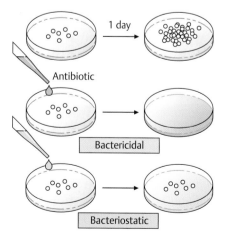

Anatomy of bacteria

Bacteria are single-cell organisms 0.3 to 5 μm in size and are typically spherical (cocci), straight (bacilli), curved, or spiral rods. They lack a nuclear membrane and have no true nucleus. The chromosome in bacteria is typically a single, closed circle DNA that is concentrated in a nucleoid region. Some bacteria possess smaller extrachromosomal pieces of DNA called plasmids. The cytoplasmic membrane is surrounded by a cell wall. The cell wall of gram-negative bacteria have an outer membrane that is absent in gram-positive bacteria.

Oxygen levels and bacterial growth

Different bacteria require different oxygen levels for optimal growth and cell division. There are obligate aerobes that require a high level of oxygen for growth, microaerophiles that require oxygen but at a reduced level, facultative anaerobes that can grow in the presence or absence of oxygen, aerotolerant anaerobes that can tolerate some oxygen, and obligate anaerobes that grow only in the absence of oxygen.

Superinfections

Antibiotic drugs alter the normal microbial population of the intestinal, upper respiratory, and genitourinary tracts. This alteration of the normal flora may lead to the development of a superinfection, which is defined as the appearance of a new infection during therapy of the primary infection. This phenomenon is relatively common and may be dangerous because the superinfecting microbes are frequently drug resistant. Superinfections are more likely to occur with broad-spectrum antibiotics and with longer treatment durations.

Gram staining

Gram staining is a laboratory test that allows bacteria to be classified in two groups, gram positive and gram negative, based on the composition of their cell walls. Gram-positive bacteria cell walls are rich in proteoglycan but have no lipopolysaccharide and stain purple, whereas gram-negative bacteria have little proteoglycan but are rich in lipopolysaccharide and stain pink. Gram staining is an important tool in helping to determine the species of bacteria responsible for infections so that the most appropriate antimicrobial agent is selected for treatment.

— *Bacteriostatic agents* primarily inhibit bacterial growth. Killing of the organism is then dependent upon host defense mechanisms. The disadvantage of these agents is that in the setting of inadequate host defense mechanisms, any partially inhibited organisms may survive, replicate, and produce recurrent disease when the antibiotic is discontinued.
— *Bactericidal agents* are capable of killing the bacteria and are preferable if the patient has neutropenia or immunosuppression.

Spectra of Antimicrobial Agents

Antimicrobial agents are further classified into spectra depending on the range of microorganisms on which they act:

— *Narrow-spectrum agents* are effective against a limited range of microorganisms.
— *Extended-spectrum agents* are principally effective against gram-positive bacteria, but they are also effective against a significant range of gram-negative bacteria.
— *Broad-spectrum agents* are effective against a wide range of microorganisms.

The use of broad-spectrum antibiotics should be limited, as they predispose patients to superinfection (the appearance of a new infection during treatment) by disrupting the body's natural bacterial flora.

28.2   Selection of Antimicrobial Agents

The selection of antimicrobial agents involves the consideration of many factors relating to the microorganisms involved, patient (host) factors, and pharmacology of the agents themselves.

Microorganism Factors

Species of Microorganism

Successful treatment of an infection requires knowledge of the pathogen(s) involved. Rapid tests are available to confirm the presence of some common infections prior to the initiation of antibiotic therapy. Examples include a dipstick test for the presence of bacteria in the urine and a throat swab for strep throat. Empiric therapy can then be initiated. In more severe infections, especially if the pathogen has shown antibiotic resistance, definitive identification of the infectious microorganism and its susceptibility to various antibiotics by laboratory testing is required.

Bacterial identification typically involves characterization by Gram staining, cell shape, and media requirements for growth. More advanced tests involve binding of specific antibodies and genetic analysis by polymerase chain reaction (PCR) or gene sequencing.

Susceptibility to Antimicrobial Agents

Bacterial strains, even of the same species, may vary widely in antibiotic sensitivity. Several tests are available for determination of bacterial sensitivity to antimicrobial agents to allow for optimal selection. The standard tests are disk diffusion tests and agar or broth dilution tests. Other quantitative tests are used to determine minimal inhibitory concentration (MIC) and minimal bactericidal concentration (MBC). The MIC is the concentration of an antibiotic necessary to inhibit microbial growth under standardized conditions; the MBC is the concentration of antibiotic required to kill the microorganism. The results of these tests can then be used to determine the antibiotic dose required.

Resistance to Antimicrobial Agent

Bacterial resistance to an antimicrobial agent may be intrinsic or acquired (**Fig. 28.2**). Acquired resistance can occur due to spontaneous mutations or by the transfer of drug-resistant genes.

Fig. 28.2 ▶ Bacterial resistance.
Some bacteria are naturally insensitive to antibacterial drugs and can grow and multiply in their presence. Other bacteria that are normally sensitive to antibacterial agents may develop mutant strains such that when an antibacterial agent is given, the sensitive bacteria are killed, but the mutant bacteria are able to multiply unimpeded.

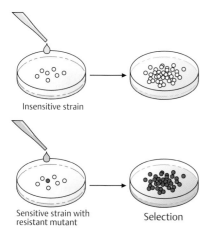

Insensitive strain

Sensitive strain with resistant mutant   Selection

Spontaneous mutations. Spontaneous DNA mutations are rare, occurring in one in 10^6 to one in 10^8 base pairs. The chance that a given mutation will lead to antibiotic resistance is even rarer. On the other hand, the fast replication rate of bacteria, as well as the large numbers of cells attained, increases the chance that a spontaneous mutation will lead to antibiotic resistance. The antibiotic provides selective pressure on the organisms, killing the nonmutant cells while the resistant mutants proliferate.

Transfer of drug-resistant genes. Bacteria are able to transfer genes that confer resistance to each other. This usually occurs via plasmids, which are small, circular, extrachromosomal pieces of DNA; or via transposons, which are small pieces of DNA that can hop from DNA molecule to DNA molecule. Once in a chromosome or plasmid, the transposons can be integrated stably. They then act by the four main mechanisms described in **Table 28.2** to achieve resistance.

Table 28.2 ▶ Mechanisms of Acquired Antibiotic Resistance	
Mechanism of Resistance	**Example**
Inactivation of the drug	Bacterial β-lactamases (penicillinases) inactivate penicillins and cephalosporins by cleaving the β-lactam ring of the drug.
Mutation of the target	Bacteria synthesize modified targets against which the drug has no effect (e.g., group B *Streptococcus*, which is frequently responsible for peripartum maternal and neonatal infections, can develop resistance to erythromycin via genes that modify the ribosomal target of the drug).
Prevention of the drug from entering the cell by decreasing permeability of the cell	Changes in porins in the outer cell membrane can reduce the amount of antibiotic that can enter the bacterium.
Actively transporting the drug out of the cell	The multidrug resistance pump exports a variety of foreign molecules, including some antibiotics, and imports protons in an exchange reaction.

■ **Disk diffusion test**

Sensitivity to various antibiotics can be determined with the disk diffusion method. Microorganisms are cultured over paper disks on an agar surface. The disks contain antibiotic drugs. After 18 to 24 hours of incubation, the size of the clear zone of inhibition around the disk is measured. The diameter of the zone depends on the activity of the drug against the test strain. Newer methods measure bacterial gene expression by the polymerase chain reaction (PCR) to identify specific pathogens.

■ **Broth dilution tests**

In dilution tests, the concentration of antibiotics is serially diluted in either solid agar or liquid broth containing a culture of the test microorganism. The lowest concentration of the agent that prevents growth after 18 to 24 hours of incubation is known as the minimal inhibitory concentration (MIC). Automated systems also use a broth dilution method. Bacterial growth is measured as the optical density of culture of the organism in liquid (broth) in various concentrations of drug. The MIC is the concentration at which the optical density remains below a threshold.

■ **Bacterial enzymes**

Enzymes are produced by many organisms and serve to promote or enhance the infection by breaking down tissues to produce foodstuffs and allowing the spread of the organism within tissue. Mucinase is produced by *Entamoeba histolytica* and acts to dissolve the protective mucoid coating on intestinal epithelial cells. Many clostridial organisms, including *Clostridium perfringens*, produce collagenase that dissolves collagen in connective tissue. The connective tissue between cells, hyaluronic acid, is degraded by many bacteria (e.g., streptococci, clostridia, and staphylococci) that produce hyaluronidase. Streptokinase and staphylokinase are examples of enzymes that break down blood clots. Other enzymes include phospholipase C, proteases, DNAase, lipases, and lysins.

■ **Bacterial toxins**

Many bacteria produce toxins that may cause damage to the host. Diseases such as diphtheria, tetanus, staphylococcal scalded skin syndrome, and cholera are caused by the production of a toxin at the site of the infection. Despite efforts to classify toxins, many are labeled by the site on which they act; for example, neurotoxins act on the nervous system, hemotoxins bring about the lysis of erythrocytes, hepatotoxins affect the liver, and enterotoxins act on the intestine. These differences in cell site are related to receptor specificity and ability of the toxin to bind to a host cell membrane receptor.

Exotoxins and endotoxins

Toxins that are released from the bacterial cell are termed *exotoxins* and can be released from both gram-positive and gram-negative bacteria. They can be single proteins or polymeric toxins composed of A and B subunits. The B component of subunit toxins bind to specific receptors on the host cell membrane, causing the release of the A or active subunit. Examples of A–B toxins include tetanus toxin, *Pseudomonas* exotoxin A, Shiga toxin, botulinum toxin, cholera toxin, and diphtheria toxin. The genes for exotoxin production may be located on the bacterial genome or encoded on a plasmid or lysogenic bacteriophage. In the gram-negative organism, part of the cell envelope is an endotoxin (lipopolysaccharide). Importantly, the toxic moiety of endotoxin is lipid A, which is released when the organism lyses. It binds to receptors on the cell membrane of B cells and macrophages, causing the release of interleukin-1 (IL-1), tumor necrosis factor-α (TNF-α), prostaglandins, and IL-6, which causes fever and hypoglycemia. Further, lipopolysaccharide activates the alternate complement pathway and causes the release of mediators from mast cells that increase vascular permeability, leading to hypertension and shock; lipopolysaccharide also causes platelets to be sticky and causes disseminated intravascular coagulation (DIC). In addition to the endotoxin, other cell wall components, including peptidoglycan, teichoic acids, and lipoteichoic acids, cause the induction of fever and are therefore pyrogenic.

Superantigens

In some instances, organisms produce superantigens that are capable of activating T cells by specific binding to the T cell and linkage to a class II major histocompatibility complex moiety on another cell type. Such linkage causes T-cell activation and the release of IL-1 and IL-2; the effect on T cells also can result in the loss of a T-cell response. Superantigens are produced by *Staphylococcus aureus* that results in toxic shock syndrome, *Streptococcus pyogenes* (erythrogenic toxins), and staphylococcal enterotoxins.

Antibiotics in abscesses

Antibiotics affect the growth and replication of bacteria; as such, they are most effective against actively growing bacterial cultures. When infection becomes more stagnant (e.g., in abscesses), antibiotics alone are often not sufficient, as they are unable to penetrate the capsule that forms around the abscess, and they tend to be less effective in low pH environments. In these cases, the abscess should be incised and drained to allow most of the pus to be evacuated and to promote better penetration of the antibiotic to any residual bacteria.

Resistance is more likely in cases of hospital-acquired infections because widespread antibiotic use in hospitals selects for resistant organisms. Furthermore, hospital strains are often resistant to multiple antibiotics. This resistance is usually due to the acquisition of plasmids carrying several genes that encode the enzymes that mediate resistance. Multidrug resistance (MDR) occurs when microorganisms develop resistance to multiple classes of antibiotics, either by use of the MDR pump or by acquiring various resistance genes.

Patient Factors

When selecting an antimicrobial agent, the mode of administration, dosing regimen, and patient's acute health status, as well as his or her overall health, need to be considered with regard to the factors listed in **Table 28.3.**

Table 28.3 ► **Patient Factors Affecting Selection of Antimicrobial Agents**	
Factor	**Explanation**
Renal disease	Drugs that are eliminated by the kidneys may accumulate in renal disease, causing toxicity. This may necessitate a dose reduction of any antibiotic given.
Hepatic disease	A dose reduction may also be necessary for antibiotics that are extensively metabolized and excreted by the liver. Some antibiotics are contraindicated in liver disease.
Pregnancy	All antibiotics are able to cross the placenta, so the risk of teratogenesis must be considered.
Lactation	The potential for a toxic accumulation of drug in the infant via breast milk must be considered.
Immune status	Patients with compromised immune systems (e.g., those undergoing cancer chemotherapy or with HIV) will generally require higher doses and longer courses of treatment.
Age	Older patients tend to have decreased renal function; infants have poorly developed drug detoxification mechanisms.

Abbreviation: HIV, human immunodeficiency virus.

Drug Factors

The pharmacokinetics of drugs has a bearing on antimicrobial selection. **Table 28.4** lists the factors that should be considered.

Table 28.4 ► **Drug Factors Affecting Selection of Antimicrobial Agents**	
Factor	**Explanation**
Site of infection	Access of the antimicrobial agent to the site of infection determines whether or not an adequate drug concentration can be achieved. — Drugs that are extensively bound to plasma proteins may not penetrate the site of infection to the same extent as those that show less protein binding. — If the infection involves the central nervous system, the drug must penetrate the blood–brain barrier (lipid-soluble and low-molecular-weight drugs).
Mode of administration	— Many agents are rapidly and completely absorbed after oral administration and can be given by mouth. Sometimes an initial injection will be followed by a course of oral therapy. — In patients with severe acute infections, drugs may be given intravenously or intramuscularly, so that effective therapeutic levels of antibiotics can reach the site of infection more rapidly.

28.3 Empiric Treatment of Infectious Diseases and Combination Therapy

Empiric Treatment

The selection of an antimicrobial agent for a patient who is diagnosed with an infectious disease can be empirical, that is, initiated with a drug that is most likely to treat the case at hand. The choice of an antibiotic with which to initiate empiric therapy is based on the most likely pathogen for a given infection and the susceptibility profile of the suspected pathogen. The site and severity of the infection, as well as patient factors also have an important bearing on the choice of agent. With empiric therapy, an otherwise healthy outpatient with a mild infection caused by a pathogen with known antibiotic susceptibility can be treated immediately, successfully, and without further testing. In more severe or prolonged infections, in patients who are hospitalized or have other illnesses, or when the causative pathogen exhibits antibiotic resistance, empiric factors may be used to initiate therapy without a delay. Once the infectious microorganism is identified by laboratory testing and its susceptibility to antibiotics determined, definitive therapy can be continued with a different agent if the empiric choice was not optimal.

Combination Therapy

In cases of superinfection or resistance, combinations of antibiotics may be warranted. The resultant antiinfective activity of two drugs may be
- *Indifferent* (the addition of the second drug makes no difference)
- *Additive* (the total effect of the two drugs is equal to the sum of the effect of each drug given individually)
- *Synergistic* (the effect of the two drugs given together is greater than the sum of the two drugs given individually). These interactions are the most important clinically, and several types can be exploited to achieve better therapeutic results. For example, two drugs may sequentially block a microbial metabolic pathway, one drug may enhance the entry of a second drug into bacteria or fungi, or one drug may prevent the inactivation of a second drug by microbial enzymes.
- *Antagonistic* (the effect of the drugs given together is less than the sum of the drugs given individually). Antagonism is rarely observed clinically, but it could occur if a bacteriostatic drug, which inhibits protein synthesis, is given with a bactericidal drug that depends on cell growth to be effective.

28.4 Prophylaxis of Infection with Antimicrobial Agents

Antibiotics may be used prophylactically to prevent infection in individuals exposed to contagious pathogens or to prevent recurrent infections. Because of the potential for the development of antibiotic resistance and the potential to cause superinfections, specific guidelines have been developed for the prophylactic uses of antibiotics. Prophylaxis is recommended for patients undergoing procedures that will cause bacteremia (e.g., dental, upper gastrointestinal, or respiratory tract procedures) for whom the complications of infection would be catastrophic.

This includes

- Patients with a history of bacterial endocarditis (see page 289)
- Patients with prosthetic heart valves
- Cardiac transplantation patients who have developed valve problems

Specific guidelines are also in place for surgical patients and for the treatment of wounds.

28.5   Reference Tables

Tables 28.5 and **28.6** have been included for reference when discussing the spectra of agents in the chapters that follow.

Table 28.5 ▸ Selected Examples of Gram-positive and Gram-negative Bacteria			
Gram-positive		**Gram-negative**	
Cocci	**Bacilli**	**Cocci**	**Bacilli**

Staphylococcus
   S. aureus
   S. epidermidis
Streptococcus
   S. pyogenes
   S. viridans
   S. pneumoniae
   S. sanguinis
   S. mitis
   S. bovis
Enterococcus
   E. faecalis
   E. mutans
	Bacillus
	   B. cereus
	   B. anthracis
	Listeria
	Actinomyces
	
	Clostridium
	   C. difficile
	   C. perfringens
	   C. tetani
	   C. botulinum
		Neisseria
		   N. gonorrhoeae
		   N. meningitides
			Enterobacteriaceae
			   Escherichia
			   Yersinia
			   Proteus
			   Serratia
			   Salmonella
			   Shigella
			   Morganella
			   Enterobacter
			   Citrobacter
			   Klebsiella
			Aeromonas
			Plesiomonas
			Campylobacter
			Legionella
			Vibrio
			Pseudomonas
			Helicobacter
			   H. pylori
			Bacteroides

Table 28.6 ▸ Miscellaneous Microorganisms

Mycobacterium
   M. tuberculosis
   M. leprae
Spirochetes
   Treponema
   Leptospira
   Borrelia

Mycoplasma
Chlamydia
Rickettsia

29 Antibacterial Drugs

Antibacterial agents act on the bacterial cell to disrupt the integrity of the cell structure or its metabolism (**Fig. 29.1**).

29.1 Inhibitors of Bacterial Cell Wall Synthesis

Antibacterial drugs that act as inhibitors of cell wall synthesis include the β-lactam antibiotics (listed in **Table 29.1** with their structures shown in **Fig. 29.2**), bacitracin, and vancomycin. These agents have a high degree of selective toxicity against bacteria because mammalian cells do not have cell walls. Another category of agents, β-lactamase inhibitors, has been included in this section, as they augment the action of β-lactam antibiotics.

Table 29.1 ▶ β-lactam Antibiotics	
β-lactam Antibiotics	**Individual Drugs**
Penicillins	*Narrow spectrum:* penicillin G, penicillin V *Extended spectrum:* amoxicillin, ampicillin, piperacillin, ticarcillin *Penicillinase-resistant:* naficillin, oxacillin, cloxacillin, dicloxacillin, methicillin
Cephalosporins	*First generation:* cefazolin, cephalexin *Second generation:* cefuroxime, cefaclor *Third generation:* cefotaxime, ceftriaxone, ceftazidime *Fourth generation:* cefepime, cefpirone
Others	Imipenem/cilastatin, aztreonam

Mechanism of action. The β-lactam antibiotics bind covalently to penicillin-binding proteins (PBPs) of bacterial cell membranes and inhibit their activity. One of the effects of this is that enzymes, such as transpeptidase, carboxypeptidase, and transglycosylase, are inhibited. Various strains of bacteria have different types of PBPs, which may account for their differential sensitivity to antibiotics. Incubation of susceptible bacteria with β-lactam antibiotics leads to morphological abnormalities and cell death. Cell lysis, when it occurs, may result from uncontrolled action of bacterial lytic enzymes (**Fig. 29.3**). These drugs are bactericidal.

Fig. 29.1 ▶ **Site of action of antibacterial agents.**
Antibacterial agents act at different sites in the bacterial cell to promote cell lysis or inhibition of growth.

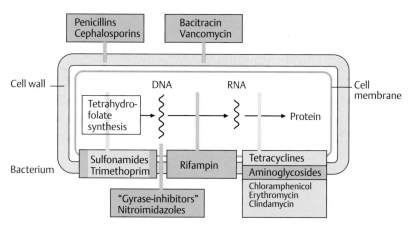

Structure of the bacterial cell wall

The peptidoglycan of the bacterial cell wall is composed of alternating units of polymers *N*-acetylglucosamine (NAG) and *N*-acetylmuramic acid (NAM). The polymers contain tetrapeptides that extend from the NAM residues. A pentaglycine bridge cross-links the tetrapeptides. In gram-positive bacteria, the cytoplasmic membrane is surrounded by a thick cell wall containing many layers of peptidoglycan and teichoic acids. In contrast, the cytoplasmic membrane of gram-negative bacteria is surrounded by a thin cell wall consisting of a few layers of peptidoglycan and an outer lipid bilayer containing polysaccharides and lipoproteins.

Gram-negative cell walls

The outer layer of gram-negative bacteria is a lipoprotein–lipopolysaccharide complex termed *lipopolysaccharide* or *endotoxin*. This component is composed of several polysaccharides linked to lipid A. The outermost portion of lipopolysaccharide is referred to as the *O antigen* and "flaps in the wind." The lipid A moiety is responsible for the toxic portion of lipopolysaccharide. An area referred to as the *periplasmic space* is located between the cell wall and cell membrane. The "space" contains several proteins, including those that inactivate antibiotics (e.g., β-lactamase). The outer membrane of the cell wall of gram-negative microbes is somewhat selective and is not as permeable to antibiotics as is the cell wall of gram-positive organisms. Hence, the former organisms have become more important in human medicine during the antibiotic era.

Penicillin-binding proteins

The penicillin-binding proteins (PBPs) are transpeptidases and similar enzymes involved in bacterial cell wall synthesis. They were named based on their ability to bind penicillin before their functional roles were discovered. A single type of bacterium may contain 3 to 10 different PBPs. PBPs are located in the cytoplasmic membrane and catalyze several reactions involved in cross-linking the peptidoglycan of the cell wall. The major activity is transpeptidase, but some also have carboxypeptidase and endopeptidase activity. They all have active sites that bind β-lactam antibiotics.

Hypersensitivity

Hypersensitivity results from immune responses against a normally innocuous antigen. These responses fall into two major categories.

1. *Immediate hypersensitivity:* Type I hypersensitivity is an allergic reaction to an antigen. It is mediated by IgE that attaches to mast cells and basophils, which degranulate upon subsequent exposure to the same antigen, releasing substances such as histamine, leukotrienes, and prostaglandins. These substances are responsible for allergy symptoms, e.g., tissue swelling and itching. Type II hypersensitivity produces antibodies that then bind to antigens on the surface of the patient's own cells. This activates an immune response against the antigen, e.g., via the complement cascade. Alternatively, cells to which antibodies attach are killed by natural killer cells and macrophages (cytotoxicity). Type III hypersensitivity reactions occur when antigens and antibodies bind forming immune complexes. Deposition of these immune complexes in tissues (e.g., joints blood vessels, renal glomeruli) produces inflammation.

2. *Delayed-type hypersensitivity:* Type IV hypersensitivity occurs 2 to 3 days after exposure to the antigen. In this case, the antigen forms a complex with type 1 or 2 major histocompatibility complex, (MHC), which then activates cytotoxic T cells (CD8+) and helper T cells (CD4+). T-helper cells secrete interferon gamma, which induces the release of cytokines and mediates the immune response. Cytotoxic T cells kill target cells.

Fig. 29.2 ▶ **Chemical structure of β-lactam antibiotics.**
The structural core of the β-lactam antibiotics is shown. The arrow points to the β-lactam ring that the compounds have in common. This is also the site at which resistant bacterial strains with β-lactamase activity can cleave the β-lactam ring and inactivate the antibiotics.

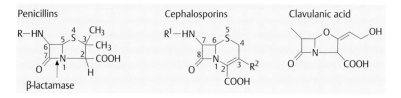

Fig. 29.3 ▶ **Penicillin G: structure, origin, and mechanism of action of penicillins.**
Bacteria possess a cell wall composed of peptidoglycan molecules cross-linked to form a lattice. The enzyme transpeptidase is responsible for this cross-linkage. Penicillins disrupt cell wall synthesis by inhibiting transpeptidase. When bacteria are in their growth and replication phase, penicillins are bactericidal. Hypersensitivity (type I) is the most common adverse effect of penicillins; however, they can be neurotoxic at very high doses due to gamma-aminobutyric acid (GABA) antagonism.

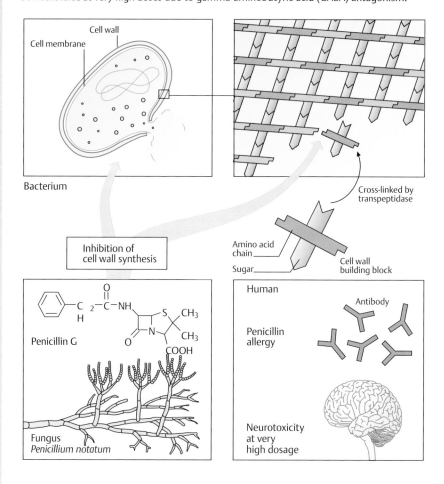

Penicillins

Side effects

- Hypersensitivity (allergic) reactions are the most common toxic complication. There is a small incidence (5 to 10%) of cross-reactivity among the penicillins and cephalosporins.
- Central nervous system (CNS) dysfunction (lethargy, confusion, and seizures) may occur with high blood and cerebrospinal fluid (CSF) levels.

Resistance.   Bacteria may acquire genes (usually via plasmids) to produce β-lactamase enzymes (e.g., penicillinase), which open the β-lactam ring and destroy the activity of the antibiotic (**Fig. 29.4**).

Natural Penicillins

Penicillin G and Penicillin V

Spectrum

- Narrow
- Both penicillin G and penicillin V are effective in mild to moderate streptococcal, staphylococcal, and pneumococcal infections, such as skin, ear, and respiratory infections.

Pharmacokinetics

- Penicillin G should be given parenterally because oral absorption is erratic due to instability in gastric acid.
- Penicillin G benzathine and penicillin G procaine are long-acting forms for intramuscular injection.
- Penicillin V is acid stable, so it is taken orally (**Fig. 29.5**).
- Neither penicillin G nor penicillin V penetrates cerebrospinal fluid (CSF).

Uses

- Endocarditis
- Skin infections
- Otitis media
- Strep throat
- Pneumonia
- Scarlet fever
- Syphilis

Side effects

- Hypersensitivity reactions
- Diarrhea, nausea, and vomiting can occur with penicillin V.

Penicillinase-resistant Penicillins

Methicillin, Oxacillin, Cloxacillin, Dicloxacillin, and Nafcillin

- *Parenteral agents:* Methicillin, oxacillin, nafcillin
- *Oral agents:* Oxacillin, cloxacillin, dicloxacillin, nafcillin

Spectrum

- Very narrow
- Effective against gram-positive organisms and they remain useful if the bacteria produce penicillinase (**Fig. 29.5**)

Uses

- Infection due to *Staphylococcus aureus* (penicillinase-producing)

    Note: These agents should not be used for penicillin G–susceptible organisms.

■ **Endocarditis**

Endocarditis is an infection of the endocardium of the heart. It occurs when bacteria from any source, e.g., dental procedures, periodontal tissues, gain entry to the blood and colonize the heart valves causing "vegetations." This is more likely to occur with damaged or artificial heart valves. Causative bacteria include *Streptococcus viridans*, *Enterococcus fecalis*, and *Staphylococcus aureus*. Symptoms include fever, changing heart murmur, fatigue, weight loss, night sweats, hematuria, and splenomegaly (enlarged spleen). Complications of endocarditis include stroke (from embolic vegetations), heart failure, renal failure, and abscesses. Treatment involves an extended course (4-6 weeks) of IV antibiotic therapy, the choice of which is directed by blood culture of the causative bacteria.

■ **Methicillin-resistant**
***Staphylococcus aureus* (MRSA)**

MRSA is an infection caused by *Staphylococcus aureus* exposure that is resistant to treatment by β-lactam antibiotics (e.g., methicillin, penicillin, and amoxicillin). It mostly occurs in hospitals (nosocomial) and other treatment centers. It tends to affect people with weakened immune systems. Staphylococcal infections, including MRSA, usually start with a boil on the skin, which can progress to form deep abscesses that enable the bacteria to penetrate into the bloodstream and bone. Treatment involves surgical drainage of abscesses and vancomycin therapy.

Fig. 29.4 ▶ **Disadvantages of penicillin G.**
Penicillin G is inactivated by gastric acid, which cleaves the β-lactam ring. This can be circumvented by parenteral administration of the drug. The β-lactam ring is also opened by β-lactamases (e.g., penicillinase), which are produced by some staphylococcal strains rendering them resistant to penicillins. Penicillin G has a narrow spectrum of action. It is active against many gram-positive bacteria, gram-negative cocci, and spirochetes but is inactive against many gram-negative pathogens.

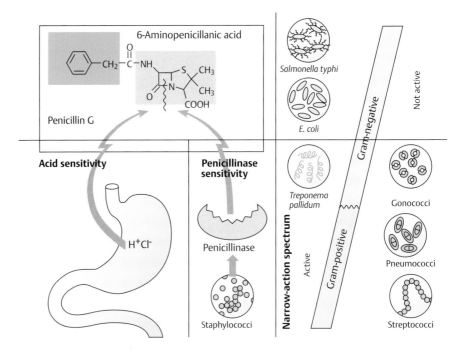

Extended-spectrum Penicillins

Ampicillin, Amoxicillin, and Ticarcillin

— *Amino penicillin agents:* Ampicillin and amoxicillin
— *"Antipseudomonal" penicillin agent:* Ticarcillin

Spectrum.   These are extended-spectrum agents.

— These agents are active against some important gram-positive (e.g., *Streptococcus pneumoniae*, enterococci, staphylococci) and gram-negative pathogens (e.g., *Haemophilus influenzae*, *Escherichia coli*, and *Proteus mirabilis*).
— Susceptible β-lactamase-producing strains of *Citrobacter, Enterobacter, E. coli, H. influenzae, Klebsiella, Pseudomonas, Serratia,* and *Staphylococcus* can be treated with ticarcillin/clavulanate.

Pharmacokinetics.   Normally, these agents do not penetrate CSF, but they may penetrate CSF if the meninges are inflamed.

— Ampicillin penetrates CSF in neonates with meningitis.

Fig. 29.5 ► **Derivatives of penicillin G.**
The derivatives of penicillin G have some advantages over their predecessor. Penicillin V has similar antibacterial properties to penicillin G but is stable in gastric acid and so can be given orally (as can the other derivatives shown). Oxicillin is one of the penicillins that are penicillinase resistant and is therefore useful in treating penicillinase-producing staphylococci infections. Amoxicillin has a broader spectrum of action than penicillin G, as it is active against more gram-negative pathogens.

	Acid	Penicillinase	Spectrum	Concentration needed to inhibit penicillin G-sensitive bacteria
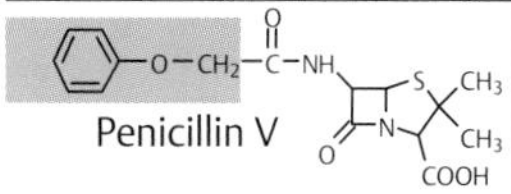 Penicillin V	Resistant	Sensitive	Narrow	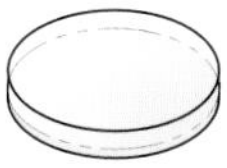
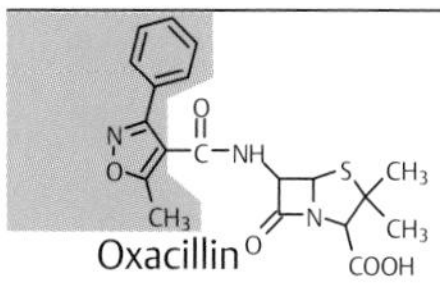 Oxacillin	Resistant	Resistant	Narrow	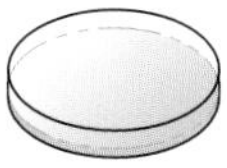
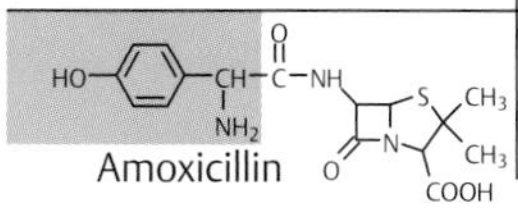 Amoxicillin	Resistant	Sensitive	Broad	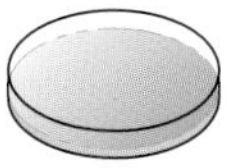

Uses. Ampicillin is used for treatment of the following:

— Endocarditis (staphylococci, streptococci, *E. coli*, *P. mirabilis*, and *Salmonella*). It is also used as a prophylactic agent in endocarditis. It is frequently used in combination with an aminoglycoside, such as gentamicin.
— Meningitis in newborns in combination with cefotaxime, with or without gentamicin
— Respiratory tract infections by susceptible *S. aureus* (including penicillinase-producing strains), *Streptococcus* (including *S. pneumoniae* and *S. pyogenes,* group A β-hemolytic streptococci), and *H. influenzae* (nonpenicillinase-producing strains only)
— Septicemia due to gram-positive organisms, such as streptococci, penicillin G–susceptible staphylococci, and enterococci

Amoxicillin is used for treatment of the following:

— Acute otitis media. If the illness is severe, or if the infection is being caused by β-lactamase-producing *H. influenzae* or *Moraxella catarrhalis*, amoxicillin is combined with clavulanate potassium (a β-lactamase inhibitor).
— Prophylaxis of bacterial endocarditis
— Primary treatment of *Helicobacter pylori* that causes gastric ulcers. Amoxicillin is part of clarithromycin-based triple therapy including clarithromycin and a proton pump inhibitor.

Ticarcillin is available in a fixed combination with clavulanic acid. This combination is used for treatment of the following:

— Infections of the lower respiratory tract, skin, bone, joints, urinary tract, peritoneum, and endometrium
— Septicemia

Note: These agents should not be used for the treatment of streptococcal or staphylococcal infections when a natural penicillin would be effective.

Otitis media

Otitis media is a bacterial or viral infection of the middle ear, usually in children. It tends to occur following an upper respiratory tract infection, e.g., the common cold, which causes congestion and swelling of the nasal passages, throat, and eustachian tubes. Blockage of the eustachian tubes causes fluid accumulation in the middle ear. Symptoms include ear pain, hearing deficits, purulent discharge from the ear, balance problems, headache, loss of appetite, vomiting, and diarrhea. Children may also tug or pull the ear, cry more than usual, and be more irritable. Otitis media is usually self-resolving in 1 to 2 weeks and so no treatment may be indicated. NSAIDs may be taken for ear pain. Amoxicillin is usually the antibiotic of choice when antibiotics are indicated.

Antibiotic penetration into cerebrospinal fluid

The ability of antibiotics to enter the brain depends on their plasma protein-binding properties, molecular size, lipid solubility, and degree of local inflammation. Penetration is greater for small, non-protein bound, lipid-soluble drugs. Drug penetration is also enhanced if the meninges are inflamed. Penicillin, amoxicillin, ampicillin, cefuroxime, ceftriaxone, cefotaxime, metronidazole, and vancomycin are useful in meningitis and brain abscesses.

Side effects.　Amoxicillin causes a maculopapular rash on the trunk of a small proportion of children who take it.

Contraindications.　People with infectious mononucleosis, cytomegalovirus, and acute lymphoblastic leukemia should not be given amoxicillin, as they are highly likely to develop a rash.

Piperacillin

Spectrum.　Piperacillin is an extended-spectrum agent.

— This agent is active against susceptible strains of *Pseudomonas, Proteus, E. coli, Enterobacter,* some streptococci, and some anaerobic bacteria.

Pharmacokinetics.　Piperacillin penetrates CSF, particularly when the meninges are inflamed, but it is not used for meningitis.

Uses

— Septicemia
— Acute and chronic respiratory tract infections
— Skin and soft tissue infections
— Urinary tract infections

Cephalosporins

This group of β-lactam antimicrobials includes the true cephalosporins (produced from *Cephalosporium* species) and cephamycins (produced from *Streptomyces* species). Cephamycins have greater resistance to β-lactamases and are classified into four "generations" based on their spectrum of antimicrobial activity, with each generation having increased activity against gram-negative bacteria. The newer agents also have improved pharmacokinetics, with half-lifes that allow a decrease in the frequency of dosing.

Side effects.　Cephalosporins are generally relatively free of severe adverse reactions. The most common adverse effects are hypersensitivity reactions, most commonly observed as a maculopapular rash after several days of therapy.

First-generation Cephalosporins

Cefazolin, Cephalothin, Cephapirin, Cephradine, Cephalexin, Cefadroxil, and Cephradine

— *Parenteral agents:* Cefazolin, cephalothin, cephapirin, and cephradine
— *Oral agents:* Cephalexin, cefadroxil, and cephradine

Mechanism of action

— Same as for penicillins

Spectrum

— First-generation cephalosporins are effective against many gram-positive cocci and useful for treating staphylococcal and streptococcal infections.
— These agents are all susceptible to β–lactamase inactivation and are not effective for infections due to enterococci or methicillin-resistant staphylococcus aureus (MRSA).

Pharmacokinetics

— Cefazolin has the longest half-life, reaches the highest plasma levels after injection, and is least irritating of the parenteral agents, making it the best choice for intramuscular injection.
— These agents do not penetrate CSF.

Uses

— Surgical prophylaxis
— Simple skin and soft tissue infections (parenteral cefazolin)
— Skin and urinary tract infections (oral cefadroxil)

Second-generation Cephalosporins

Cefuroxime, Cefamandole, Cefonicid, Cefoxitin, Cefotetan, Cefmetazole, Cefaclor, Cefuroxime Axetil, Cefpodoxime Proxetil, Cefprozil, and Loracarbef

— *Parenteral agents:* Cefuroxime, cefamandole, cefonicid, cefoxitin, cefotetan, and cefmetazole
— *Oral agents:* Cefaclor, cefuroxime axetil, cefpodoxime proxetil, cefprozil, and loracarbef

Spectrum

— The second-generation cephalosporins have a greater activity against gram-negative organisms, especially *H. influenzae*, while retaining some activity against gram-positive bacteria. They are also more resistant to β-lactamase. However, first-generation agents are preferred for most gram-positive indications, and third-generation agents are usually more active against gram-negative pathogens.
— Cefoxitin (a cephamycin) is probably the most notable drug of this class because of its activity against anaerobic bacteria.

Pharmacokinetics. Cefuroxime is the only second-generation agent that penetrates CSF.

Uses

— Upper and lower respiratory tract infections, sinusitis, and otitis media
— Urinary tract infections caused by *E. coli, Klebsiella,* and *Proteus*
— Surgical prophylaxis
— Mild intra-abdominal infections, for example, cholecystitis (cefoxitin)

Side effects

— Concurrent use of ethanol with cephalosporins that contain a methyltetrazolethiol side chain (cefamandole, cefotetan, cefmetazole, and cefoperazone) may result in a disulfiram-like reaction, including flushing, tachycardia, headache, sweating, thirst, nausea, and vomiting, due to inhibition of acetaldehyde metabolism.
— Competitive inhibition between the methyltetrazolethiol group and vitamin K–dependent carboxylase, which is responsible for converting clotting factors II, VII, IX, and X to their active forms, may lead to hypoprothrombinemia (low blood prothrombin levels). This problem may be averted by giving the patient a supplement of vitamin K.

Third-generation Cephalosporins

Cefotaxime, Ceftriaxone, Ceftazidime, Cefoperazone, Cefixime, Ceftizoxime, and Cefixime

— *Parenteral agents:* Cefotaxime, ceftriaxone, ceftazidime, cefoperazone, cefixime, and ceftizomine
— *Oral agent:* Cefixime

Spectrum

— Third-generation cephalosporins have further increased activity against gram-negative organisms, including *H. influenzae*; however, their potency against gram-positive microbes is generally inferior to first-generation agents. All third-generation cephalosporins are resistant to hydrolysis by β-lactamases. Their activity is variable against anaerobes, including *Bacteroides fragilis.*

— Ceftriaxone and cefotaxime have excellent activity against most strains of *S. pneumoniae*, including the vast majority of those resistant to penicillin.
— Ceftazidime has antipseudomonal activity.

Pharmacokinetics

— Penetration into CSF (ceftazidime and cefotaxime)
— Long half-life (ceftriaxone)
— Eliminated via biliary excretion (cefoperazone and ceftriaxone)

Uses

— Bacterial meningitis (ceftriaxone and cefotaxime)
— Community-acquired pneumonia protocol (ceftriaxone and cefotaxime)
— Treatment of *Pseudomonas* and all types of other gram-negative infections (ceftazidime).

Fourth-generation Cephalosporins

Cefepime

Spectrum.   Cefepime is an extended spectrum agent that is effective against the following:

— Gram-positive organisms, including MRSA
— Gram-negative organisms, including *Pseudomonas aeruginosa*
— Multiresistant gram-negative bacilli

It also exhibits significant activity against anaerobes and greater resistance to β-lactamases than third-generation cephalosporins.

Uses

— Infections caused by *P. aeruginosa,* including urinary tract infections, sepsis, and hospital-acquired pneumonia
— Used in combination with vancomycin for treatment of nosocomial meningitis

Other β-Lactam Antibiotics

Imipenem with Cilastatin

Mechanism of action.   Imipenem binds to all PBPs and is also an irreversible β-lactamase inhibitor. Cilastatin prevents renal enzymes from breaking down imipenem and prolongs its effects.

Spectrum.   Imipenem has the broadest spectrum of any β-lactam antibiotic.

Pharmacokinetics

— Imipenem is metabolized by a renal peptidase. To circumvent this, cilastatin, a specific inhibitor of the renal enzyme, is administered with imipenem. Cilastatin also prevents renal toxicity sometimes observed with imipenem alone. A 1:1 combination of imipenem:cilastatin is the only form available.
— Penetration into CSF is highly variable. It is not used for meningitis.

Uses

— Used to treat serious infections in which a mixture of gram-positive, gram-negative, and anaerobic bacteria may be involved

Resistance.   Resistance can develop to these agents, especially in *Pseudomonas* species.

Meningitis

Meningitis is inflammation of the meninges of the brain (pia mater and arachnoid), usually due to a viral infection but can also be caused by a bacterial or fungal infection. Symptoms include headache, stiff neck on passively moving chin toward chest, photophobia (sensitivity to light), irritability, drowsiness, vomiting, fever, seizures, and rashes (viral or meningococcal meningitis). Predisposing factors for meningitis include head injury (especially basal skull fracture), otitis media, sinusitis, mastoiditis, and a compromised immune system (e.g., carcinoma, AIDS, diabetes, splenectomy, immunosuppressant drugs). A lumbar puncture often provides a definitive diagnosis of meningitis. Blind treatment with a broad-spectrum antibiotic or prompt treatment with I.V. antibiotic(s) that are sensitive to the causative organism is required for bacterial meningitis. For viral meningitis, treatment includes bed rest and fluids but this normally resolves on its own in a week or two.

Side effects. Like other β-lactam antibiotics, imipenem has a low incidence of adverse reactions, but it may trigger seizures in epileptic patients and in patients with head trauma.

Aztreonam

Mechanism of action

— Same as for penicillins

Spectrum. Aztreonam is a narrow-spectrum agent with the following properties:

— Aztreonam is a potent antibiotic, with activity against only aerobic gram-negative bacteria. It is highly stable to β lactamases and does not induce β-lactamase enzymes.
— Limited cross-reactivity with other β-lactam antibiotics and so it is generally considered safe to administer to patients with a penicillin allergy.
— Aztreonam is synergistic with other β-lactam antibiotics and the aminoglycosides.

β-Lactamase Inhibitors

Many bacteria produce β-lactamase enzymes (e.g., penicillinase) that open the β-lactam ring and destroy the activity of the antibiotic. To combat this, β-lactamase inhibitors can be combined with β-lactam antibiotics (amoxicillin and ticarcillin) to further extend their usefulness. Many cephalosporins are resistant to β–lactamase enzymes.

Clavulanic Acid

Mechanism of action. Clavulanic acid is an irreversible inhibitor of many bacterial β-lactamases.

Sulbactam and Tazobactam

The properties of these drugs are similar to clavulanic acid.

— Sulbactam is marketed in combination with ampicillin.
— Tazobactam is marketed in combination with piperacillin.

Glycopeptide Antibiotic

Vancomycin

Mechanism of action. Vancomycin binds to the terminal D-alanine-D-alanyl peptide portion of the peptidoglycan precursor and inhibits bacterial cell wall synthesis. This is at a different step from β-lactam antibiotics. Bacterial autolysins subsequently cause cell wall lysis, so vancomycin is usually bactericidal.

Spectrum

— Active against gram-positive bacteria, including staphylococci, streptococci, and enterococci

Pharmacokinetics

— Vancomycin should not be given intramuscularly, as it causes tissue necrosis.
— When given intravenously, it must be administered slowly as a dilute solution to minimize thrombophlebitis, as well as flushing reactions associated with histamine release.
— Vancomycin is able to penetrate CSF in the presence of inflammation.

Uses. Vancomycin is indicated for susceptible pathogens in the bowel (even though it is not absorbed in the gastrointestinal [GI] tract), such as treatment of antibiotic-associated pseudomembranous colitis.

Antibiotic-associated pseudomembranous colitis

Pseudomembranous colitis is inflammation of the colon due to superinfection with *Clostridium difficile*, a gram-positive bacillus. It typically occurs following a course of antibiotic treatment in which the normal gut commensal bacteria are eradicated, allowing *C. difficile* to colonize the gut unimpeded. The most common antibiotics that cause this condition are the penicillins, cephalosporins, fluoroquinolone, and clindamycin. Symptoms of pseudomembranous colitis include diarrhea, fever, and abdominal pain. It is treated with metronidazole or vancomycin.

Necrotizing fasciitis is a rare infection that penetrates into deeper layers of the skin and subcutaneous tissue and is able to spread along fascial planes. It can be caused by a variety of bacteria, including group A streptococci, *S. aureus*, *Clostridium perfringens*, and *B. fragilis*. Signs and symptoms include intense pain, signs of inflammation (although these may be absent if the infection is in deep tissues), diarrhea, vomiting, and fever. The patient will look very ill. The skin will blister and undergo necrosis. Treatment for this condition involves giving antibiotics such as penicillin, vancomycin, or clindamycin early in the process, often before the diagnosis has been confirmed. Necrotic tissue will require surgical débridement or amputation.

■ Protein synthesis

The first stage in protein synthesis involves unzipping of the DNA double helix by RNA polymerase then transcription of DNA to mRNA (messenger RNA). This process occurs in the nucleus. mRNA (codon) migrates into the cytoplasm and attaches to a ribosome. Translation of mRNA into a protein occurs when transfer RNA (tRNA) and its accompanying amino acid bind to mRNA by forming complementary base pairs (anticodon). The amino acids join to form a polypeptide chain. Protein synthesis is stopped when a termination codon is translated, and the polypeptide chain is released from the ribosome.

Resistance
— Seldom develops to vancomycin

Other Inhibitors of Cell Wall Synthesis

Bacitracin

Mechanism of action.　Bacitracin is a polypeptide antibiotic that inhibits the formation of bacterial cell walls by blocking peptidoglycan chain formation and is usually bactericidal.

Spectrum
— Active against gram-positive organisms

Pharmacokinetics.　This agent is not absorbed after oral administration.

Uses
— The main use is for topical treatment of gram-positive infections on the skin or in the eye.
— Renal toxicity limits its usefulness to topical application, but it may be used in infants with staphylococcal pneumonia and empyema that are resistant to safer antibiotics.

Side effects
— Renal toxicity when given systemically

29.2　Inhibitors of Protein Synthesis

These agents exhibit selective toxicity for bacterial cells by binding to bacterial ribosomal subunits, which differ in structure from the mammalian ribosomal subunits. They inhibit bacterial protein synthesis.

Macrolide Antibiotics

Macrolide (large ring) antibiotics are characterized by the presence of a 14- or 15-member lactone ring. Erythromycin is the prototype of these antibiotics, but newer macrolides possess improved pharmacokinetic properties and modest changes in the antibacterial spectrum.

Mechanism of action.　Macrolides bind to the P site of the 50S bacterial ribosomal subunit. They block protein synthesis when a large amino acid or a polypeptide is in the P site (**Fig. 29.6**).

Erythromycin

Erythromycin is available as the base (unstable in acid), stearate, ethylsuccinate, or estolate salt.

Spectrum.　Erythromycin is a narrow-spectrum agent.

— Active against gram-positive bacteria (similar in spectrum to penicillin G), *Chlamydia,* and *Legionella* organisms

Pharmacokinetics
— The best absorption is obtained with the estolate salt.
— Erythromycin is distributed into total body water, but penetration into CSF is poor, even when the meninges are inflamed.
— Erythromycin is extensively metabolized in the liver; thus, dosage adjustments in renal failure are usually considered unnecessary.

Uses
— Mild to moderately severe infections of the upper and lower respiratory tract

Side effects

- Erythromycin is usually well tolerated, but many patients complain of gastric effects.
- Reversible intrahepatic obstructive jaundice may occur, especially with the estolate salt.
- Parenteral forms are highly irritating.

Resistance

- Develops rapidly

Clarithromycin

Clarithromycin is a hydroxylated derivative of erythromycin.

Spectrum.   Clarithromycin is a narrow-spectrum agent.

- Clarithromycin is somewhat more active against gram-positive pathogens, *Legionella,* and *Chlamydia* than erythromycin.

Pharmacokinetics

- Clarithromycin is much better absorbed after oral administration than erythromycin.
- No penetration into CSF

Uses

- Mainly used in triple therapy of *H. pylori* (see page 263)

Azithromycin

Azithromycin has a 15-member lactone ring.

Spectrum.   Azithromycin is a narrow-spectrum agent.

- Azithromycin is more active than erythromycin against several gram-negative pathogens.

Pharmacokinetics

- The most unusual property of azithromycin is its uptake into several tissues (lung, tonsil, and cervix), where it maintains high concentrations for prolonged periods.
- Azithromycin's long half-life allows once-daily oral administration.
- No penetration into CSF

Uses

- Urethritis or cervicitis (*Chlamydia trachomatis*)
- Treatment of coexisting chlamydial infection in patients being treated for gonorrhea, as well as urogenital chlamydial infections in pregnant women
- Chlamydial pneumonia in infants and chlamydial conjunctivitis in neonates (*C. trachomatis*)
- Legionnaires disease (*Legionella pneumophila*)
- *Mycobacterium avium-intracellulare* complex

Lincomycin and Clindamycin (7-Chlorolincomycin)

Mechanism of action.   These agents attach to the 50S ribosomal subunit at or near the erythromycin attachment site. They are chemically unlike but pharmacologically similar to erythromycin.

Spectrum.   Lincomycin and clindamycin are narrow-spectrum agents.

- Active against gram-positive bacteria
- Excellent activity against anaerobic bacteria

Pharmacokinetics

- Lincomycin is poorly absorbed after oral administration, whereas the oral absorption of clindamycin is excellent and is not affected by food.

■ **Jaundice**

Jaundice refers to the yellow pigmentation of the skin, sclerae, and mucous membranes due to raised plasma bilirubin.
- *Prehepatic (or hemolytic) jaundice.* Excess bilirubin (e.g., from hemolysis) or an inborn failure of bilirubin metabolism results in unconjugated bilirubin remaining in the bloodstream. Unconjugated bilirubin is water-insoluble and so does not appear in urine.
- *Hepatocellular (or hepatic) jaundice.* In hepatocellular jaundice, there is diminished hepatocyte function leading to an increased amount of both conjugated and unconjugated bilirubin. Diminished hepatocyte function may follow cirrhosis, autoimmune diseases, drug damage (e.g., acetaminophen, barbiturates), or viral infections (e.g., hepatitis A, B, C; Epstein-Barr virus).
- *Posthepatic (obstructive) jaundice.* This form of jaundice usually occurs following blockage of the common bile duct by gallstones. In this case, plasma conjugated bilirubin rises. Conjugated bilirubin is water-soluble and appears in urine (making it dark). At the same time, less conjugated bilirubin passes into the gut and is converted to stercobilin, therefore feces appear paler.

Fig. 29.6 ▶ Protein synthesis and modes of action of antibacterial drugs.
Protein synthesis involves the translation of genetic sequences in messenger RNA (mRNA), transcribed from DNA. Peptide synthesis occurs in the ribosome, where transfer RNA (tRNA) delivers amino acids to mRNA. Adjacent amino acids are linked into a peptide chain by the enzyme peptide synthetase. Tetracyclines inhibit the binding of amino acyl-tRNA complexes and have a bacteriostatic effect. They have a broad spectrum of action. Aminoglycosides induce the binding of wrong amino acyl-tRNA complexes, resulting in the synthesis of false proteins. These agents are bactericidal and act mainly against gram-negative pathogens. Chloramphenicol inhibits the enzyme peptide synthetase, which prevents growth of the peptide chain. It is bacteriostatic against a broad spectrum of pathogens. Macrolides prevent the ribosome from moving along the mRNA to "read" it. They are bacteriostatic against mainly gram-positive pathogens.

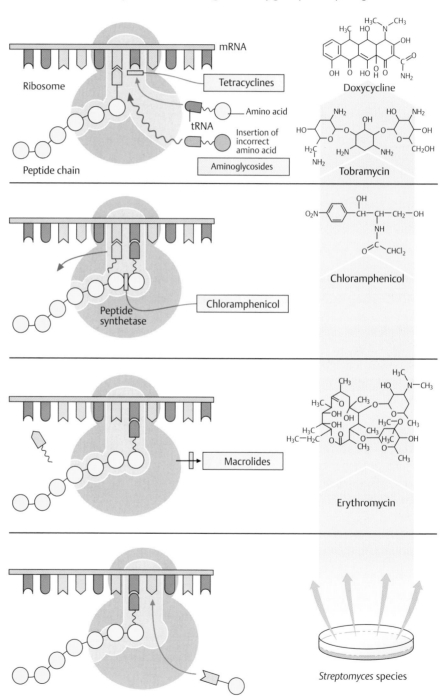

- These drugs are widely distributed in the body (but reach only low concentrations in CSF, even when the meninges are inflamed) and penetrate well into bone.
- Both drugs are metabolized extensively and excreted primarily in bile and feces.
- Clindamycin is a more potent antimicrobial agent than lincomycin.

Uses

- Lincomycin is seldom used clinically.
- Clindamycin is useful for therapy of anaerobic infections, including those caused by *B. fragilis*. It is potentially useful as a penicillin substitute but is more toxic than erythromycin.

Side effects

- Diarrhea is the most common adverse effect. Clindamycin is the antibiotic that most frequently causes antibiotic-associated pseudomembranous colitis (see call-out box on page 295).
- Skin rashes and reversible changes in hepatic enzymes in serum may also occur.

Tetracyclines

Tetracycline, Oxytetracycline, Doxycycline, Demeclocycline, Methacycline, and Minocycline

Mechanism of action. Tetracyclines preferentially bind to the 30S subunit of the microbial ribosome, interfere with binding of amino acyl-tRNA, and inhibit chain termination (**Fig. 29.6**). Tetracyclines are usually bacteriostatic.

Spectrum. Tetracyclines are broad-spectrum agents.

- Effective against gram-positive and gram-negative bacteria, *Rickettsia, Chlamydia,* spirochetes, and amebiasis

Pharmacokinetics

- Most tetracyclines are incompletely absorbed after oral administration. Absorption is further delayed by food, calcium salts, and aluminum salts (**Fig. 29.7**). An exception to this is the oral absorption of doxycycline, which is superior to other tetracyclines and is virtually unaffected by food.
- They are distributed in total body water.
- They are usually excreted in the urine; thus, renal function should be considered for dosage determinations. However, doxycycline is excreted primarily into the bile, and demeclocycline is metabolized in the liver.
- Tetracycline and oxytetracycline are rapidly eliminated.
- Demeclocycline and methacycline are more slowly eliminated.
- Doxycycline and minocycline are long acting.
- No penetration into CSF

Uses

- Rickettsial infections, chlamydial infections, sexually transmitted diseases, acne, and brucellosis
- Used as alternate therapy in penicillin-allergic patients

Side effects

- GI disturbances
- Superinfections
- Damage to developing teeth and bones, liver damage (particularly in pregnant women who receive the drug intravenously)

▪ Tetracycline staining of teeth

Tetracycline that is ingested is incorporated into developing enamel, causing intrinsic tooth discoloration. It appears as a yellow-brown band on the teeth that were forming at the time of the tetracycline therapy. It is not harmful to teeth but is unsightly and typically camouflaged by porcelain veneers.

▪ Cholera

Cholera is an infectious disease caused by *Vibrio cholerae,* a gram-negative bacteria. It is spread via the fecal–oral route. Vibrio cholerae toxin increases cAMP concentrations in intestinal mucosal cells, causing the opening of Cl^- channels and massive secretion of Cl^-. This results in the production of a profuse amount of watery diarrhea which, in turn, causes severe dehydration. This can lead to kidney failure, shock, coma, and death. Treatment requires rapid replacement of lost body fluids with oral or IV solutions containing salts and sugar. Tetracycline reduces fluid loss and diminishes transmission of the bacteria.

— Photosensitization (particularly with demeclocycline)
— Parenteral forms are irritating.

Aminoglycosides

Streptomycin, Neomycin, Kanamycin, Gentamicin, and Amikacin

— Amikacin is a derivative of kanamycin.

Mechanism of action.   All aminoglycosides inhibit bacterial protein synthesis. Streptomycin binds to a specific site on the 30S ribosomal subunit, but other aminoglycosides bind to sites on both the 30S and 50S ribosomal subunits. The antibacterial action is usually attributed to inhibition of protein synthesis, but disruption of cell membrane function caused by transport of the antibiotics across the bacterial cell membranes may also be involved (**Fig. 29.6**). Amikacin resists inactivation by many bacterial enzymes. These agents are bactericidal.

Spectrum.   Aminoglycosides are broad-spectrum agents.

— Active against gram-positive and gram-negative bacteria
— Because aminoglycosides are actively transported into a bacterial cell by an oxygen-dependent enzyme system, only aerobic bacteria are sensitive to these drugs.

Pharmacokinetics

— Aminoglycosides are not absorbed from the GI tract but are readily absorbed from intramuscular or subcutaneous sites (**Fig. 29.8**).
— They are distributed to extracellular water, but penetrate CSF poorly, even when the meninges are inflamed.

Fig. 29.7 ▶ **Aspects of the therapeutic use of tetracyclines and chloramphenicol.**
Tetracyclines are absorbed to varying degrees in the gastrointestinal (GI) tract. They tend to cause irritation to mucous membranes, and they alter the natural flora of the gut, which allows pathogenic bacteria to proliferate. These factors account for the GI upset that often accompanies tetracycline use. Tetracyclines also form insoluble complexes with cations, such as Ca^{2+} and Al^{3+}, which cause them to be unable to be absorbed, to be unable to exert their antibacterial effects, and to lose their irritant properties. Chloramphenicol is completely absorbed following oral administration and shows high penetrability into tissues, including through the blood–brain barrier. Its toxicity to bone marrow severely limits its use.

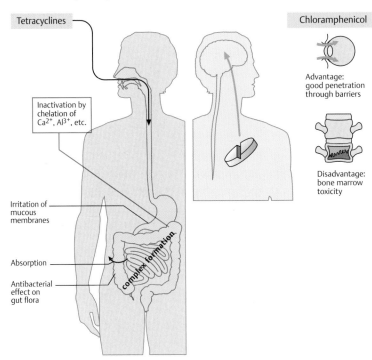

Tetracyclines

Chloramphenicol

Inactivation by chelation of Ca^{2+}, Al^{3+}, etc.

Advantage: good penetration through barriers

Disadvantage: bone marrow toxicity

Irritation of mucous membranes

Absorption

Antibacterial effect on gut flora

complex formation

— They are excreted in the urine after glomerular filtration of the parent compound.
— Neomycin is the most toxic agent.

Uses

— Tuberculosis (TB), bacterial endocarditis, plague, and tularemia (streptomycin)
— Gut sterilization (oral or topical neomycin)

Gentamicin, tobramycin, and netilmicin are essentially comparable agents for systemic use in serious infections. There may be slight differences in bacterial sensitivity or in their potential for renal or auditory toxicity.

Many infectious disease specialists feel that amikacin should be reserved for susceptible infections resistant to other aminoglycosides.

Kanamycin is an older agent that is seldom used.

Side effects

— Renal toxicity
— Ototoxicity (agents may damage both vestibular and auditory functions of the vestibulocochlear nerve)
— Allergic reactions occasionally occur.

Other Inhibitors of Protein Synthesis

Chloramphenicol

Mechanism of action. Chloramphenicol attaches at P sites of the 50S subunit of microbial ribosomes and inhibits functional attachment of the amino acyl end of amino acyl-tRNA to the 50S subunit. It is bacteriostatic.

Spectrum. Chloramphenicol is a broad-spectrum agent.

— Chloramphenicol is more effective than tetracyclines against typhoid fever and other *Salmonella* infections.
— There is good activity against many anaerobic bacteria and *Rickettsia*.

Pharmacokinetics

— Chloramphenicol is well absorbed after oral administration and is distributed into total body water. Its high lipid solubility results in excellent penetration into CSF, ocular fluids, and joint fluids (**Fig. 29.7**).
— It is rapidly excreted in urine, 10% as chloramphenicol and 90% as the glucuronide conjugate.

Uses. Chloramphenicol's broad spectrum and penetration into CSF makes it useful in meningitis, rickettsial infections, anaerobic infections, and *Salmonella* infections.

Side effects

— Irreversible aplastic anemia is a rare but serious effect. The risk of aplastic anemia limits its application to situations in which safer drugs are not likely to be effective.
— Reversible bone marrow depression
— "Gray baby" syndrome in neonates is due to deficient glucuronidation of the drug and its subsequent accumulation in the infant's body.
— Superinfection

Spectinomycin

This agent is chemically related to the aminoglycosides.

Notifiable diseases

Certain diseases must be reported by clinicians to the National Notifiable Diseases Surveillance System (NNDSS), operated by the Centers for Disease Control and Prevention (CDC). Examples of such diseases are human immunodeficiency virus/acquired immunodeficiency syndrome (HIV/AIDs), measles, mumps, pertussis, hepatitis C, meningococcal disease, typhoid fever, TB, polio, rubella, malaria, syphilis, and gonorrhea.

Fig. 29.8 ▶ **Aspects of the therapeutic use of aminoglycosides.**
Aminoglycosides consist of glycoside-linked amino sugars. They contain numerous hydroxyl and amino groups that can bind protons; hence, they are highly polar. This renders them unable to diffuse through membranes, and thus unable to be adsorbed enterally. This lack of absorption is used by giving neomycin orally to eradicate intestinal bacteria (e.g., prior to bowel surgery) or to reduce NH_3 formation by gut bacteria in hepatic coma. Otherwise, aminoglycosides are given by injection for serious infections. Aminoglycosides gain access to the bacterial interior via bacterial transport systems. In the kidney, they enter the proximal tubule via an uptake system for oligopeptides and cause damage to tubular cells. They can also cause damage to the vestibular apparatus and organ of Corti in the ear.

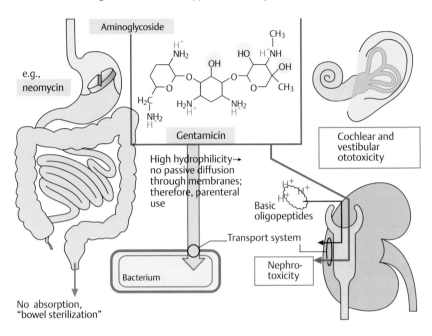

Mechanism of action.   Spectinomycin binds at the 30S subunit of the microbial ribosome, but at a site different from that of streptomycin. The drug seems to be bacteriostatic rather than bactericidal because of reversible binding.

Pharmacokinetics
— Spectinomycin is not absorbed orally and is given intramuscularly.
— No penetration into CSF

Uses
— Used exclusively for one-shot treatment of gonorrhea
— Ineffective against syphilis

29.3   Inhibitors of Nucleic Acid Metabolism

Gyrase Inhibitors: Fluoroquinolones (Quinolones)

Ciprofloxacin, Gemifloxacin, Levofloxacin, Moxifloxacin, Norfloxacin, and Ofloxacin

Fluoroquinolones are chemically derived from the urinary antiseptic nalidixic acid and are all fluorinated compounds.

Mechanism of action.   Fluoroquinolones inhibit bacterial DNA gyrase, an enzyme involved in DNA nicking and supercoiling, and are bactericidal drugs (**Fig. 29.9**).

Spectrum. Fluoroquinolones are broad-spectrum agents.

- Active against a wide variety of gram-negative bacteria, but gram-positive organisms are usually less susceptible
- Ciprofloxacin is highly active against *Pseudomonas* species.
- Anaerobic bacteria respond poorly to the fluoroquinolones.

Pharmacokinetics
- Well-absorbed after oral administration and widely distributed in the body, but highest concentrations accumulate in urine
- Renal excretion involves both glomerular filtration and active secretion.
- Fluoroquinolone metabolites have less antimicrobial activity than the parent drug.
- Their relatively long half-life allows twice-daily dosing.
- These agents penetrate CSF but are not approved for use in meningitis.

Uses
- Complicated infections of the genitourinary tract
- Abdominal, respiratory, skin, and soft tissue infections that are resistant to other agents
- Gram-negative bone infections
- Prophylaxis and treatment of anthrax

Side effects
- Fluoroquinolones are usually well tolerated.
- Irreversible damage to developing cartilage has been observed in studies with young animals; therefore, fluoroquinolones are not recommended for patients younger than 18 years or for use in pregnancy.

29.4 Inhibitors of Folate Metabolism (Antimetabolites)

Antimetabolites are substances that have structural similarity to substrates used in intermediary metabolism of the cell and that compete for enzymatic binding sites. Examples include purine and pyrimidine analogs used in cancer or antiviral chemotherapy, as well as the sulfonamide antibacterial drugs that are discussed in this section. The ultimate effects of these antimetabolites may be exerted on nucleic acids, proteins, and cell walls.

Sulfonamides (Sulfas)

Sulfacytine, Sulfadiazine, Sulfamethizole, Sulfisoxazole, and Sulfamethoxazole

Mechanism of action. Sulfonamides are structurally similar to *p*-aminobenzoic acid (PABA). They inhibit the synthesis of dihydrofolic acid in microbes that must synthesize dihydrofolic acid from PABA (**Fig. 29.10**). Dihydrofolic acid is then reduced to form tetrahydrofolic acid by dihydrofolate reductase. This is required for the synthesis of purines and pyrimidines and amino acids. They are bacteriostatic at concentrations achieved in most body tissues and fluids, but bactericidal concentrations may be found in the urine.

Spectrum. The sulfonamides are broad-spectrum agents.

- Effective against most gram-positive bacteria, many gram-negative bacteria, *Nocardia, Actinomyces, Chlamydia,* and *Plasmodium*

Pharmacokinetics
- Sulfonamides are readily absorbed after oral administration.
- Sodium salts may be given intravenously, but they are strongly alkaline and cause pain and tissue sloughing if extravasated (i.e., if the drug leaks into surrounding tissue).

Fig. 29.9 ► **Antibacterial drugs acting on DNA.**
Antibacterial drugs act on bacterial DNA, preventing the reading of the genetic information at the DNA template, thus damaging the regulatory center of cell metabolism. Gyrase (topoisomerase II) catalyzes the supercoiling of DNA strands. It does this by opening, underwinding, and closing the DNA strand such that the full loop need not be rotated. Gyrase inhibitors (green portion of ofloxacin formula) seem to act to prevent the resealing of opened strands. Metronidazole damages DNA by complex formation or strand breakage. Anaerobic bacteria are able to convert metronidazole to reactive metabolites that attack DNA; thus; it is effective only in this group of bacteria. Rifampin inhibits DNA-dependent RNA polymerase, the enzyme that catalyzes RNA transcription from the DNA template.

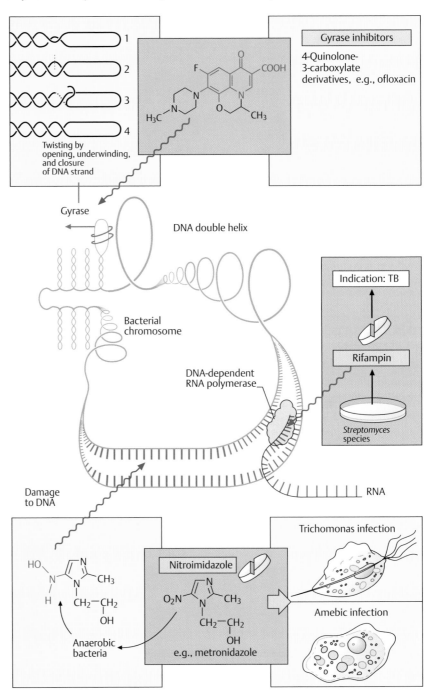

— Sulfonamides are 20 to 90% bound to plasma albumin, depending on the sulfonamide and its concentration. Free (unbound) drug is distributed to total body water.
— Sulfonamides are eliminated in the urine by glomerular filtration and tubular secretion.
— Metabolites include acetylated and glucuronide conjugates, along with oxidized products.
— Sulfacytine, sulfadiazine, sulfamethizole, and sulfisoxazole are short-acting sulfonamides that are rapidly absorbed and excreted into the urine, giving high urinary concentrations. They are usually given four times daily.
— Sulfamethoxazole is an intermediate-acting sulfonamide. Its longer half-life allows dosing at 8- to 12-hour intervals.
— No penetration into CSF

Uses

— Sulfonamides are used primarily in urinary tract infections, but they have been useful in tularemia, nocardia, actinomycosis, and resistant falciparum malaria.
— Burns (mafenide [not a true sulfonamide] and silver sulfadiazine)
— Trisulfapyrimidine: contains equal amounts of sulfadiazine, sulfamerazine, and sulfamethazine; an old "triple sulfa" formulation for additive antibacterial effects but less chance of crystalluria

Side effects

— Sulfonamides may precipitate in acidic urine and cause renal damage.
— Drug allergy
— Toxicity to the hematopoietic system (acute hemolytic anemia, thrombocytopenia, etc.)

Resistance.   Resistance has developed in many bacterial strains to sulfonamides.

29.5   Miscellaneous Antibacterial Drugs

Polymyxin B and Colistin

Mechanism of action.   These are polypeptide antibiotics that damage the bacterial cytoplasmic membrane and are bactericidal.

Spectrum.   Polymyxin B and colistin are primarily active against gram-negative organisms, particularly *Pseudomonas*.

Pharmacokinetics.   These agents do not penetrate CSF but can be used topically or intravenously for meningitis (inflamed meninges allow penetration).

Uses.   They may be used systemically in life-threatening infections resistant to safer antibiotics.
     Polymyxin is available in combination with neomycin and hydrocortisone for topical treatment of eye and ear infections.

Side effects.   Renal damage and various neurologic changes limit the usefulness of these drugs to topical applications.

Metronidazole

Mechanism of action.   Metronidazole has a cytotoxic effect on bacteria by damaging DNA, but the precise mechanism of action is unclear (**Fig. 29.9**).

Spectrum.   Active against amebic infections and many anaerobic bacteria, including *C. difficile* and *B. fragilis*.

Pharmacokinetics.   Well absorbed after oral administration

Side effects

— Neurologic effects, disulfiram-like inhibition of aldehyde dehydrogenase, Na$^+$ retention, and various GI symptoms

Anaerobic bacteria

The mucosal surfaces of the upper respiratory tract, GI tract, and genitourinary tract are colonized with a large number of anaerobic microbes. The infections are usually not transmissible and are polymicrobic, (they involve several different species). Infections with nonspore-forming anaerobes lead to necrosis and abscess formation and are chronic. Specific clinical syndromes include skin and soft tissue infections, gynecologic infections, respiratory tract infections, brain abscesses, bacteremia, and intra-abdominal infections.

Anaerobic infections

Clues for anaerobic infection are as follows:
— Clinical setting influence (i.e., infection following bowel surgery)
— Proximity to a mucosal surface
— Infectious discharge that is foul-smelling
— Presence of gas in tissue (palpable masses that move may be gas)
— Dead and necrotic tissue, or the presence of intestinal pseudomembrane
— Bite wound infections from humans or animals
— Malignancy-associated infections
— Presence of septic thrombophlebitis
— Infections that are slow to respond to antibiotics
— Presence of sulfur granules (actinomycosis)
— Laboratory cultures that are negative under aerobic culture
— Polymicrobial Gram stain assessment

Fig. 29.10 ► Inhibitors of tetrahydrofolate synthesis.
Bacteria, unlike humans, are able to synthesize dihydrofolic acid (DHF), which is converted to tetrahydrofolic acid (THF) by the enzyme dihydrofolate reductase. THF is then used to synthesize purines and thymidine. Sulfonamides structurally resemble *p*-aminobenzoic acid (PABA), a precursor in DHF synthesis. They act as a false substrate and so competitively inhibit the utilization of PABA, and hence DHF synthesis. Trimethoprim inhibits bacterial DHF-reductase. The human enzyme is less sensitive to this than the bacterial one, so it is relatively selectively toxic for bacteria. Co-trimoxazole is a combination of trimethoprim and sulfamethoxazole, so THF synthesis is inhibited on two fronts. Sulfasalazine, a drug used in inflammatory bowel disease (e.g., Crohn disease and ulcerative colitis), is cleaved by intestinal bacteria to mesalamine and sulfapyridine. Mesalamine exerts its antiinflammatory effects on the gut mucosa when present in high concentrations. Coupling to sulfonamide prevents premature absorption in the upper small bowel, but it can be absorbed following cleavage, and may exert typical adverse effects.

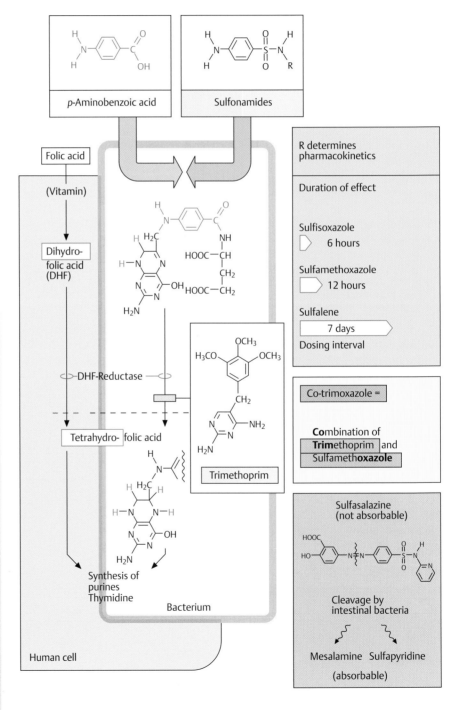

Fig. 29.11 ▶ **Drugs used to treat infections with mycobacteria (1. tuberculosis, 2. leprosy).**
Antitubercular drugs of choice are shown (1). Their mechanisms of action are unclear, but isoniazid
is converted to isonicotinic acid in the bacterium. This substance is unable to diffuse through cell
membranes and so accumulates intracellularly. Antileprotic drugs shown (2) are frequently combined with
rifampin. Dapsone inhibits dihydrofolate (DHF) synthesis. Clofazimine is a dye with bactericidal effects
against *M. leprae.* CNS, central nervous system.

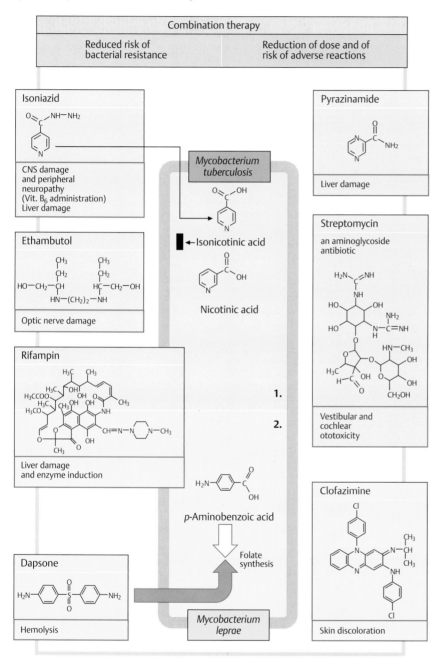

Table 29.2 provides a summary of common bacteria, the antimicrobial agents of choice to treat infections, and secondary agents that may be used if the primary agent is unsuccessful.

Table 29.2 ▶ Summary of the Treatment of Microorganisms		
Microorganisms	**Primary Antimicrobial Drugs**	**Secondary Antimicrobial Drugs**
Gram-positive cocci		
Staphylococcus aureus or *S. epidermidis*	Penicillinase-resistant penicillins: naficillin, oxacillin, cloxicillin, dicloxicillin, or methicillin	Vancomycin ± gentamicin
Enterococcus	Penicillin G + gentamicin	Vancomycin + gentamycin
Streptococcus	Penicillin G or penicillin V	Clindamycin or erythromycin
Penicillin-resistant *S. pneumonia*	Vancomycin + third-generation cephalosporin	
Gram-positive bacilli		
Bacillus cereus	Vancomycin	
Bacillus anthracis	Fluoroquinolone	
Listeria	Ampicillin ± gentamicin	
Clostridium difficile	Metronidazole or vancomycin	
Gram-negative cocci		
Neisseria gonorrhoeae	Ceftriaxone	
Neisseria meningitides	Penicillin G	
Gram-negative bacilli		
Enterobacteriaceae		
Escherichia	Third-generation cephalosporin	
Yersinia pestis	Streptomycin or tetracycline	
Proteus mirabilis	Ampicillin	
Proteus vulgaris	Third- or fourth-generation cephalosporin	
Salmonella	Ceftriaxone or a fluoroquinolone	
Shigella	Fluoroquinolone	
Enterobacter	Imipenem	
Klebsiella	Third- or fourth-generation cephalosporin	
Campylobacter jejuni	Erythromycin	
Legionella	Azithromycin or a fluoroquinolone ± rifampin	
Vibrio cholera	Tetracycline	
Helicobacter pylori	Amoxicillin + clarithromycin + omeprazole or tetracycline + metronidazole + bismuth subsalicylate	
Bacteroides	Metronidazole	
Miscellaneous		
Mycobacterium tuberculosis	Isoniazid + rifampin + pyrazinamide ± ethambutol	
Mycobacterium leprae	Dapsone + rifampin ± clofazimine	
Spirochetes		
Treponema pallidum	Penicillin G	
Leptospira	Penicillin G	
Borrelia burgdorferi	Doxycycline	
Mycoplasma	Macrolide or fluoroquinolone	
Chlamydia	Doxycycline	
Rickettsia	Doxycycline	

29.6   Antimycobacterial Drugs

Tuberculosis (TB) is an infection spread by inhalation of *Mycobacterium tuberculosis* that mainly affects the lungs. Most infected individuals have asymptomatic latent infections. Active TB occurs in ~10% of untreated individuals with latent infections, particularly in response to decreased immune function caused by stress, malnutrition, or other diseases. Most cases (75%) are pulmonary, with a chronic cough accompanied by malaise, anorexia, fever, chills, and night sweats. When the infection moves outside the lungs, it is denoted extrapulmonary TB.

Antimycobacterial drugs are used to treat TB, caused by *M. tuberculosis*; *M. avium-intracellulare* complex, caused by *M. avium-intracellulare*; and Hansen disease (leprosy), caused by *Mycobacterium leprae*. Therapy for active mycobacterial infections includes at least two drugs to prevent failure due to emergence of resistant strains and continues for at least 6 months.

Antituberculosis Drugs

Isoniazid (Isonicotine Hydrazine [INH])

Mechanism of action.   Isoniazid, or isonicotine hydrazine (INH), inhibits cell wall synthesis. It can be either tuberculostatic or tuberculocidal, depending on its concentration (**Fig. 29.11**).

Spectrum.   INH is effective only against mycobacteria.

Pharmacokinetics
— INH is readily absorbed after oral administration and is widely distributed in the body, including into CSF and tissues.
— Fast acetylators metabolize the drug more rapidly than slow acetylators.

Uses
— Used for prophylaxis as well as for treatment of active mycobacterial infections

Side effects
— INH reacts chemically with pyridoxal and causes peripheral neuritis (adults) and convulsions (children). However, co-administration of vitamin B_6 prevents these symptoms.
— Some patients may develop isoniazid-induced hepatitis during the first 3 months of therapy. Risk is higher in older patients. Ten to 20% of patients have asymptomatic minor elevations of transaminases that often resolve with continued therapy. Otherwise, INH is usually well-tolerated in most patients.

Ethambutol

Mechanism of action.   Ethambutol is a bacteriostatic agent that inhibits bacterial cell wall synthesis.

Pharmacokinetics
— Given orally

Uses
— Combination therapy of TB (*M. tuberculosis*) and *M. avium-intracellulare*

Side effects.   Ethambutol is usually well tolerated, but retrobulbar neuritis is seen occasionally at high doses.

Resistance
— Develops slowly

■ Retrobulbar neuritis

Retrobulbar neuritis is a form of optic neuritis in which the optic nerve becomes inflamed behind the eyeball. It is most commonly caused by drugs, multiple sclerosis, meningitis, syphilis, and tumors. Symptoms include pain on moving the eyes, blurred vision or loss of vision, and tenderness of the eye to pressure. This condition may resolve without the need for treatment, or prednisone may be required.

Rifampin

Mechanism of action.   Rifampin inhibits DNA-directed RNA synthesis. It may be bacteriostatic or bactericidal, depending on the concentration (**Fig. 29.2**).

Spectrum
— Active against *M. tuberculosis* and other microbes

Pharmacokinetics
— Orally effective

Resistance.   Resistance develops rapidly and limits its usefulness.

Uses
— Primarily used to treat TB
— Prevention of Haemophilus influenzae type B (HiB) infection

Side effects
— Gives a harmless orange color to body fluids, including contact lenses
— Induces most P-450 enzymes, which enhances elimination of warfarin, phenytoin, estrogen, and other drugs

Pyrazinamide

Mechanism of action.   The mechanism of action is uncertain.

Pharmacokinetics
— Orally effective

Uses
— TB

Side effects.   Patients must be monitored for signs of hepatotoxicity.
Table 29.3 lists the protocols for the treatment of TB.

Table 29.3 ▶ **Protocol for the Treatment of Tuberculosis**	
Treatment Type	**Antimicrobial Protocol**
Standard treatment	Combination therapy with isoniazid, rifampin, and pyrazinamide for 6 months
Prototype therapy for active TB	First 2 months: isoniazid, rifampin, pyrazinamide, and ethambutol (can be stopped if bacterial isolates test negative for resistance). This combination may be extended an additional 3 months if culture remains positive at end of first 2 months Next 4 months: isoniazid, rifampin
Prototype therapy for quiescent, previously untreated pulmonary TB (positive skin test with fibrotic upper lobe lesions)	Isoniazid alone for 1 year, or isoniazid, rifampin, and pyrazinamide for 3 months until cultures are negative and chest radiograph is stable

---

Antibiotics and the contraceptive pill

Antibiotics are thought to reduce the efficacy of the contraceptive pill, although the extent to which they do this is subject to debate. Rifampin and griseofulvin are known to induce hepatic enzymes and hasten the metabolism of the contraceptive pill. Other broad-spectrum antibiotics affect the absorption of estrogen from the gut by eradicating the bacterial flora responsible for this. Patients are advised to use barrier methods of contraception, in addition to using the contraceptive pill, while taking antibiotics and for 1 week after.

29.7   Antileprotic Drugs

Dapsone (Diaminophenylsulfone [DDS])

Mechanism of action.   Dapsone's mechanism of action is similar to that of sulfonamides. It is bactericidal.

Pharmacokinetics.   Its long half-life permits once-weekly administration.

Uses
- Leprosy
- DDS is sometimes used in the treatment of chloroquine-resistant malaria.

Side effects
- Hemolysis is a serious side effect.
- Exacerbation of lepromatous leprosy may occur.

Clofazimine

Mechanism of action.   Clofazimine's mechanism is uncertain. However, clofazimine has antiinflammatory properties combined with slow antibacterial effects.

Uses
- Leprosy

29.8   Antiseptics and Disinfectants

Urinary Antiseptics

Urinary antiseptics are defined as substances that can be given orally but provide significant antibacterial effects only in the urine.

Trimethoprim

Mechanism of action.   Trimethoprim causes selective inhibition of bacterial dihydrofolate reductase. It may be bacteriostatic or bactericidal.

Uses
- The only approved indication as a sole agent is for uncomplicated urinary tract infections caused by susceptible organisms.
- It is most often used in combination with sulfamethoxazole.

Nitrofurantoin

Mechanism of action.   This agent has bacteriostatic activity against several urinary tract pathogens. It appears to work by affecting the bacterial metabolism of the drug, which results in the formation of reactive metabolites that attack DNA.

Uses
- Urinary tract infections

Urinary tract infections

Urinary tract infections (UTIs) are common, especially in women due to the proximity of the urethra to the vagina (allowing easier spread of sexually transmitted infections and diseases) and due to the relative length of the urethra compared to men (men have longer urethras). UTIs present with any of the following symptoms: frequency of urination, urgency, strangury (frequent, painful expulsion of small amounts of urine despite urgency), hematuria (blood in the urine), cloudy urine, incontinence, fever with diarrhea and vomiting, and pain (usually suprapubic pain in women and anal pain in men). Trimethoprim with sulfamethoxazole is given to treat uncomplicated UTIs caused by susceptible bacteria (*E. coli*, *Staphylococci*, *Streptococci*, *Pseudomonas*, and *Proteus*). In addition, patients are advised to drink plenty of fluids and urinate often.

Side effects. Hypersensitivity reactions, nausea, and vomiting are limitations to its usefulness, but a crystalline form of nitrofurantoin has a reduced incidence of GI intolerance.

Resistance
— Rarely develops

External Antiseptics and Disinfectants

Germicides that are too toxic for internal use but that may be effective for removal of microbes from the skin (disinfectants) or surgical instruments (antiseptics) have important roles in medicine or dentistry. Some examples are included in **Table 29.4.**

Table 29.4 ▸ External Antiseptics and Disinfectants	
Class of Substance	**Examples**
Detergents	Anionic: ordinary soaps Cationic: benzalkonium chloride
Phenols (probably also act as detergents)	Phenol: hexylresorcinol Cresol: hexachlorophene
Alcohols	Ethanol and isopropyl alcohol
Halogens	Chlorine, chloramines, and iodine
Metals	Silver (used in combination with sulfadiazine) and mercury (thimerosal)
Oxidants	Hydrogen peroxide, permanganate, sodium peroxide, and perborate

30 Antiviral Drugs

Viruses are obligate intracellular parasites that have no energy-generating enzymes. They require the metabolic processes and activities of the host cell; thus, virus reproduction requires the virus particle to infect a cell and use the cytoplasmic machinery to synthesize the macromolecules necessary for assembly of new virus particles. They contain DNA or RNA, not both, and range in size from 20 nm (parvoviruses) to 300 nm (poxviruses); the largest virus approximates the size of the smallest bacterial cells (chlamydiae and mycoplasma). They are not susceptible to antibacterial agents.

Viral replication begins with attachment whereby specific ligands (antireceptors) on the virus recognize and bind to specific receptors on the host cell surface. This interaction is temperature and energy independent and is also related to the tropism of the virus, i.e., the specificity of the virus to a particular host tissue. For example, poliovirus receptors exist on anterior horn cells of the spinal cord but not on kidney cells. The virus then penetrates the host cell by endocytosis (e.g., polyomaviruses), direct fusion with the host cell membrane (e.g., HIV and measles), or receptor-mediated endocytosis (e.g., influenza and Epstein–Barr virus). Penetration is also temperature and energy dependent. Once inside the host cell, there is viral uncoating or dismantling, which is the removal of the viral nucleic acid from the capsid. The last stage in viral replication is genome expression. Viruses adapt host cell machinery to transcribe viral RNA from a viral DNA template, producing key proteins for new virus synthesis. Release of daughter viruses results in the spread of the virus, both within and outside the host (**Fig. 30.1**).

Antiviral drugs are used to treat susceptible viral infections, which include herpes simplex virus, varicella zoster virus, cytomegalovirus (CMV), influenza viruses, respiratory syncytial virus (RSV), hepatitis B, hepatitis C, and human immunodeficiency virus (HIV). Antiviral drugs target an essential viral enzyme or protein to inhibit a pathway unique to the virus but not the cell (**Fig. 30.1**).

Fig. 30.1 ▶ **Viral multiplication and mechanism of action of antiviral agents.**
Viruses can be destroyed by cytotoxic T lymphocytes, which are part of the specific immune response. These lymphocytes detect the virus via proteins on the viral membranes. They may also be inactivated by antibodies. Interferons are glycoproteins that are released from virus-infected cells. They stimulate the production of antiviral proteins in neighboring cells, which destroy or suppress viral DNA and thus prevent viral protein synthesis.

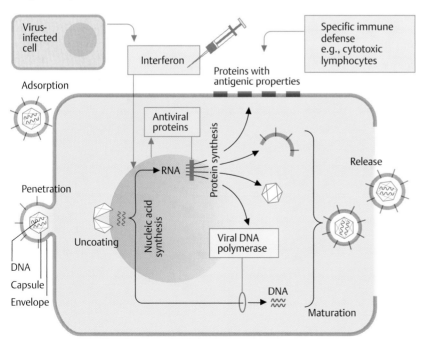

Table 30.1 is included for reference.

Table 30.1 ▶ Selected Viruses			
Family*	**Typical Example(s)**	**Nucleic Acid Polarity and Structure**	**Envelope**
DNA viruses			
Parvoviridae	Human parvovirus	ssDNA (+ or −)	No
Hepadnaviridae	Hepatitis B	dsDNA/ss portions	Yes
Papovaviridae	JC virus	dsDNA circular	No
Adenoviridae	Human adenovirus	dsDNA	No
Herpesviridae	Herpes simplex 1 (α) Herpes simplex 2 (α) CMV (β) Epstein–Barr (γ)	dsDNA	Yes
Poxviridae	Vaccinia virus	dsDNA closed ends	Yes
RNA viruses			
Togaviridae	Rubella virus	ssRNA (+)	Yes
Picornaviridae	Poliovirus	ssRNA (+)	No
Flaviviridae	Yellow fever virus (hepatitis C virus)	ssRNA (+)	Yes
Rhabdoviridae	Rabies virus	ssRNA (−)	Yes
Coronaviridae	Coronaviruses	ssRNA (+)	Yes
Paramyxoviridae	Measles virus	ssRNA ()	Yes
Orthomyxoviridae	Influenza virus	ssRNA (−) segments	Yes
Bunyaviridae	Encephalitis virus	ssRNA (− circular)	Yes
Arenaviridae	Lymphocytic choriomen	ssRNA (− circular)	Yes
Retroviridae	HIV	ssRNA (+ identical)	Yes
Reoviridae	Rotaviruses	dsRNA (segments)	No
Caliciviridae	Norwalk virus	ssRNA (+)	No
Filoviridae	Ebola, Marburg	ssRNA	Yes

Abbreviations: CMV, cytomegalovirus; ds, double-stranded; HIV, human immunodeficiency virus; ss, single-stranded.

30.1   Inhibitors of Nucleic Acid Synthesis

Most inhibitors of nucleic acid synthesis are nucleoside analogues that must be phosphorylated intracellularly to exert their antiviral effects. They act by inhibiting viral replication by acting as false nucleosides (**Fig. 30.2**).

Acyclovir, Famciclovir, Penciclovir, and Valacyclovir

Mechanism of action.   These agents inhibit DNA polymerase and, once incorporated into viral DNA, terminate chain elongation. They exhibit remarkable selective toxicity due to action on virus-specific thymidine kinase and viral DNA polymerase (**Fig. 30.3**).

Spectrum
— Herpes simplex virus (HSV) and varicella zoster virus

Pharmacokinetics.   Although oral bioavailablity of acyclovir is low, this compound is effective after oral administration, by injection, or topically applied. The other agents are available for oral administration and have longer half-lifes that require one or two doses daily.

Fig. 30.2 ▶ Chemical structure of virustatic antimetabolites.
Nucleosides consist of a base (e.g. thymine) and deoxyribose. Virustatic antimetabolites act as false nucleosides or sugars. In the body, they are incorporated into viral DNA and terminate replication. Acyclovir and ganciclovir also inhibit viral DNA polymerase.

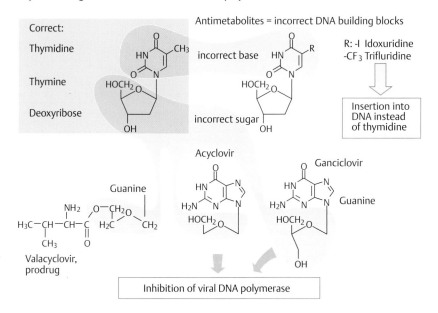

Fig. 30.3 ▶ Activation of acyclovir and inhibition of viral DNA synthesis.
In an infected cell, viral thymidine kinase performs the initial phosphorylation step then cellular kinases attach the remaining phosphate residues. This bioactivation of acyclovir occurs only in infected cells, which gives it high specificity and tolerability. Furthermore, the polar phosphate residues render acyclovir unable to diffuse across cell membranes and cause it to accumulate in infected cells. Acyclovir triphosphate is a preferred substrate of viral DNA polymerase and inhibits its activity. Following incorporation of acyclovir triphosphate into viral DNA, it induces strand breakage because it lacks the 3'-OH group of deoxyribose that is required for the attachment of additional nucleotides.

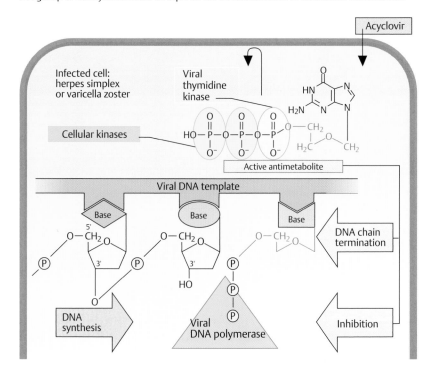

Herpes simplex virus

Herpes simplex virus (HSV) type 1 is the most common HSV infection and usually produces cold sores and other blisters around the mouth, lips, and face. These may be accompanied by fever, sore throat, and lymphadenopathy. It is spread via saliva. HSV type 2 is usually responsible for genital herpes and is sexually transmitted. Symptoms include blisters around the vagina, anus, buttocks, penis shaft/glans, or scrotum that may be accompanied by itching, pain, dysuria (difficult or painful urination), and fever. Complications of HSV infections include herpetic whitlow (vesicles develop on an infected digit), herpetic simplex keratitis (corneal ulcers), herpetic simplex meningitis (rarely occurs but is usually due to HSV type 2), and herpetic simplex encephalitis (usually HSV type 1). Treatment of HSV may include the use of antiviral medications, e.g., acyclovir, and analgesics. Herpes simplex encephalitis has a high risk of mortality and requires urgent care.

Herpes zoster (shingles)

Chickenpox is the primary infection with varicella zoster virus. Following the initial infection the virus remains dormant in the dorsal root ganglia. Reactivation of the virus causes shingles. Shingles starts with pain, tingling, or burning in a dermatomal distribution (often the ophthalamic division of the trigeminal nerve and lower thoracic dermatomes are affected). This is accompanied by fever and malaise. Later, a vesicular rash develops involving the same dermatome. Complications of shingles include post-herpetic neuralgia of the affected dermatome. This pain can range from mild to very severe and can persist for months or years. Treatment of shingles may involve the early use of antiviral medications, e.g., acyclovir, to shorten the course of the infection and to reduce pain and complications. Pain may also be treated with oxycodone (a narcotic analgesic), amitryptyline (a tricyclic antidepressant), gabapentin (an anticonvulsant), or lidocaine (a local anesthetic). Post-herpetic neuralgia can be treated with carbamazepine or phenytoin and prednisone. If these are unsuccessful, surgical ablation of the appropriate ganglion may be tried but this too is often unsuccessful and may leave the patient with numbness of the dermatome supplied.

Cytomegalovirus

Cytomegalovirus is an infection that is often asymptomatic and therefore goes unnoticed. It is spread by a variety of routes, e.g., saliva, blood, semen, urine, and breast milk. Like herpes simplex virus (HSV), it lies dormant after the initial infection and may become reactivated. Symptoms, if any, are similar to mononucleosis and include fever, fatigue, weakness, sore throat, swollen glands, muscle and joint aches, and a feeling of generally being unwell. Treatment with gancyclovir is generally reserved for immunocompromised patients.

Respiratory syncytial virus

Respiratory syncytial virus (RSV) is a virus that causes infections of the respiratory tract and lungs. It gains entry to the body through the eyes, nose, or mouth and is typically spread by droplets via coughing or sneezing or direct contact (e.g., shaking hands). Symptoms are usually mild and include congested or runny nose, cough, sore throat, headache, fever, and a generally feeling of being unwell. Treatment is usually limited to over-the-counter drugs, e.g., acetaminophen to reduce fever. Treatment with ribavirin is reserved for infants and children with severe RSV infections.

Uses
— Genital herpes
— Herpes simplex encephalitis
— Neonatal herpes
— Herpetic infections in immunocompromised patients

Ganciclovir and Valganciclovir

Mechanism of action.   The mechanism and structure are similar to acyclovir.

Spectrum.   Ganciclovir and valganciclovir are 100 times more active against CMV than is acyclovir.

Pharmacokinetics.   Ganciclovir is administered by intravenous (IV) infusion or as an intravitreal implant (for CMV retinitis). Valganciclovir is an orally active prodrug.

Uses
— Limited to treating CMV infection in immunocompromised patients

Side effects
— Bone marrow depression

Ribavirin

Ribavirin is a deoxyguanosine analogue that contains a fraudulent base.

Mechanism of action.   Ribavirin is phosphorylated to mono-, di-, and triphosphate forms that interfere with viral RNA polymerases.

Spectrum
— Effective against respiratory syncytial virus (RSV) and hepatitis C

Pharmacokinetics.   Ribavirin is administered by aerosol for RSV to prevent systemic toxicity. It is given orally for hepatitis C.

Uses.   For RSV, its use is limited to infants and children with severe lower respiratory tract infections. For hepatitis C, it is used in combination therapy with interferon alfa.

Toxicity
— Hemolytic anemia (if taken systemically)

Foscarnet

Foscarnet is a pyrophosphate analogue.

Mechanism of action.   Foscarnet inhibits viral DNA and RNA polymerases.

Spectrum
— CMV infections resistant to other drugs

Pharmacokinetics
Foscarnet is infused IV or by intravitreal injection (for retinitis).

Uses
— CMV infections resistant to other drugs or in patients with HIV

Toxicity
— Renal toxicity leading to electrolyte imbalances

Cidofovir

Cidofovir is a cytosine analogue.

Mechanism of action. Cidofovir interferes with viral DNA polymerases.

Spectrum
— CMV infections resistant to other drugs

Pharmacokinetics. Cidofovir is infused IV or by intravitreal injection.

Uses
— CMV retinitis in patients with acquired immunodeficiency syndrome (AIDS) after ganciclovir and foscarnet therapy have failed

Toxicity
— Renal toxicity and neutropenia

Fomivirsen

Fomivirsen is an antisense oligonucleotide.

Mechanism of action. Fomivirsen is a synthetic RNA with a sequence that is complementary to and binds to the messenger RNA (mRNA) of the immediate-early transcriptional unit (IE2) of human CMV. This inhibits translation of IE2 proteins necessary for CMV replication.

Spectrum. Fomivirsen was approved for intravitreal treatment of CMV retinitis in HIV-infected patients who could not tolerate or did not respond to other therapies, but it is no longer commercially available in the United States.

Trifluridine

Mechanism of action. Trifluridine is an analogue of thymidine that acts by inhibiting viral DNA polymerase.

Uses
— Herpes simplex keratitis (applied topically to the cornea of infected eyes)

Side effects
— Local stinging and irritation around the eyes

30.2 Viral M$_2$ Protein Blockers

Amantadine and Rimantadine

Mechanism of action. These agents are highly selective antiviral drugs that inhibit the growth of influenza A viruses by acting as ion channel blockers of the viral M$_2$ protein, thus preventing viral uncoating (**Fig. 30.4**).

Spectrum
— Influenza A

Pharmacokinetics. Completely absorbed from the gastrointestinal (GI) tract and excreted unchanged in the urine.

Uses
— Prophylaxis and treatment of influenza A virus infections

Side effects. Central nervous system side effects (nervousness, confusion, insomnia, lightheadedness, and hallucinations) are the most common.

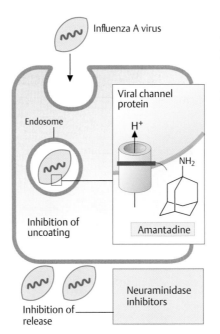

Fig. 30.4 ▶ **Prophylaxis for viral flu.**
Amantadine specifically prevents uncoating of influenza A viruses. Influenza A is endocytosed into cells, but they require protons, supplied by the endosome, to penetrate the virus and allow it to release its RNA. Amantadine prevents this influx of protons into the virus. Neuraminidase inhibitors are effective against influenza A and B. Normally, viral neuraminidase splits off N-acetylneuraminic (sialic) acid residues on the cellular cell surface coat, thereby enabling newly formed virus particles to be detached from the host cell.

Influenza

Influenza (or "flu") is a viral infection that affects the respiratory tract and lungs. The virus has three types: A, B, and C. It is spread by droplets that are either inhaled following coughing or sneezing or directly transferred from an infected person. Symptoms of flu may mimic the common cold initially with nasal congestion or runny nose, sneezing, and sore throat. However, these symptoms rapidly become worse and progress to include fever, chills and sweats, aching muscles, headache, fatigue, weakness, and a general feeling of being unwell. Complications include pneumonia, otitis media, sinusitis, and bronchitis. Treatment for influenza usually involves bed rest, fluids, and NSAIDs. However, antiviral medications such as oseltamivir and zanamivir may sometimes be used to shorten the course of the infection.

30.3　Selective Neuraminidase Inhibitors for Influenza A and B

Oseltamivir and Zanamivir

Mechanism of action. These agents are inhibitors of influenza neuraminidase. Without neuraminidase, the hemagglutinin of the virus binds to sialic acid, forming clumps and preventing virus release (**Fig. 30.4**).

Spectrum
— Influenza A and B

Pharmacokinetics. Oseltamivir is given orally. Zanamivir is inhaled.

Uses
— Used to reduce the severity and prevent the spread of influenza

Side effects
— Nausea and vomiting (oseltamivir)
— Cough, and nasal and throat symptoms (zanamivir)

30.4　Drugs for Hepatitis B and Hepatitis C

Interferon alfa

Several forms of interferon, including alfa-1, alfa-2a, and alfa-2b, are available.

Mechanism of action. Interferons are endogenous cytokine proteins that interfere with viral replication. They also activate immune responses.

Pharmacokinetics
— Injected subcutaneously
— Peginterferons, interferon formulated with polyethylene glycol, have longer half-lifes and can be given once weekly.

Uses
- Hepatitis B therapy
- Hepatitis C therapy when used in combination with ribavirin

Side effects. Flulike syndrome with headache, chills, fever, and muscle pain is common within hours of injection. Adverse effects on all systems may be observed with chronic use, including
- Alopecia, pruritis (itching), and rash
- Weight loss
- Bone marrow suppression
- GI upset
- Joint and muscle pain
- Dizziness, headache, and insomnia
- Anxiety, irritability, and depression

Adefovir Dipivoxil, Entecavir, Lamivudine, Telbivudine, and Tenofovir

Mechanism of action. These agents are nucleoside/nucleotide analogues that inhibit viral DNA polymerase.

Pharmacokinetics
- Orally effective

Side effects
- Asthenia and nephrotoxicity (adefovir dipivoxil [dose-dependent])
- Dizziness, fatigue, headache, and nausea (entecavir)
- Dizziness, headache, and nausea (lamivudine)
- Headache, cough, fatigue, flu, and increased serum creatine kinase level (telbivudine)
- Asthenia, rash, and GI upset (tenofovir)

Ribavirin

Mechanism of action. Ribavirin is a guanosine analogue that inhibits viral RNA polymerases.

Pharmacokinetics
- Orally effective

Uses
- Used in the therapy of hepatitis C in combination with interferon alfa

Side effects
- Hemolytic anemia
- Pruritis and rash
- Headache, fatigue, irritability, and insomnia
- Nausea

Table 30.2 summarizes the drugs used to treat non-HIV viral infections.

Hepatitis A, B, and C

Hepatitis is a viral infection that causes inflammation and dysfunction of the liver. The three main types are hepatitis A, B, and C (although D and E exist). Hepatitis A is spread by the fecal–oral route, often via contaminated food or water. Symptoms tend to appear one month following the initial infection and include nausea and vomiting, loss of appetite, fever, abdominal pain, muscle aches, fatigue, itching, and jaundice. Hepatitis A usually resolves with no treatment. Hepatitis B is spread via blood, semen, or saliva. Symptoms are the same as hepatitis A but itching and joint pain are more prominent. Chronic infection with hepatitis B may lead to cirrhosis and/or liver cancer. Antiviral drugs such as interferon alfa may be used to slow liver damage but treatment is usually limited to supportive measures. Hepatitis C is spread in the same manner as hepatitis B. It is typically asymptomatic initially and may remain so for many years. Symptoms, when they do occur, are the same as those listed for hepatitis A and B but are generally more mild. Like hepatitis B, chronic hepatitis C may lead to cirrhosis and liver cancer. Treatment may involve the use of interferon alfa. If hepatitis B or C lead to liver failure then liver transplantation may be indicated.

Table 30.2 ► Drugs Used to Treat Viral Infections (non-HIV)

Agents	Antiviral Activity
Amantadine/rimantadine	Influenza A
Neuraminidase inhibitors	Influenza A and B
Acyclovir and analogues	Herpes viruses
Ganciclovir and valganciclovir	CMV in HIV patients
Foscarnet	CMV, HSV (resistant)
Ribavirin	RSV, hepatitis C
Interferon	Hepatitis B, C; papillomavirus
Imiquimod, podoflox	Topical agents for papillomavirus

Abbreviations: CMV, cytomegalovirus; HIV, human immunodeficiency virus; HSV, herpes simplex virus; RSV, respiratory syncytial virus.

30.5   Management of HIV and AIDS

HIV is a retrovirus transmitted by free viral particles or infected immune cells (e.g., CD4 [T helper cells], macrophages, and dendritic cells) in blood, semen, vaginal fluid, preejaculate, and breast milk. It causes acquired immunodeficiency syndrome (AIDS). The goal of HIV/AIDS therapy is to increase CD4 cell counts, suppress viral load, and reconstitute the immune system.

Highly active antiretroviral therapy (HAART) is combination therapy used in the treatment of HIV/AIDS to decrease the development of resistance. It usually involves using three agents from two different classes.

Nucleoside Reverse Transcriptase Inhibitors

Mechanism of action.   Nucleoside reverse transcriptase inhibitors (NRTIs) are unnatural nucleoside analogues that decrease viral DNA synthesis by inhibiting viral reverse transcriptase (**Fig. 30.5**).

Abacavir (ABC), Didanosine (ddI), Emtricitabine (FTC), Lamivudine (3TC), Stavudine (d4T), Tenofovir, and Zidovudine (Azidothymidine, AZT),

— AZT is the first antiretroviral drug approved by the U.S. Food and Drug Administration for the treatment of HIV.

Pharmacokinetics

— Orally effective

Side effects.   Serious adverse effects for NRTIs include pancreatitis, fatty liver, lactic acidosis, and peripheral neuropathy. See **Table 30.3** for the side effects of individual agents.

Table 30.3 ▶ Side Effects of Nuceloside Reverse Transcriptase Inhibitor Drugs	
Agent	**Side Effects**
Abacavir (ABC)	Hypersensitivity, liver disease
Emtricitabine (FTC)	Nausea, vomiting, headache, fatigue
Lamivudine (3TC)	Nausea, vomiting, headache, fatigue
Stavudine (d4T)	Peripheral neuropathy, diarrhea, nausea, vomiting
Tenofovir	Rash, mild GI upset
Zidovudine (azidothymidine, AZT)	Asthenia (lack of energy and strength), headache, fatigue, insomnia, anorexia, constipation, nausea, vomiting

Abbreviations: GI, gastrointestinal; NRTI, nucleoside reverse transcriptase inhibitor.

Nonnucleoside Reverse Transcriptase Inhibitors

Mechanism of action.   Nonnucleoside reverse transcriptase inhibitors (NNRTIs) also interfere with viral DNA synthesis but bind near the active site of the viral reverse transcriptase to inhibit its activity (**Fig. 30.5**).

Side effects

— Hypersensitivity reactions and liver disease

Pharmacokinetics

— Orally effective
— These drugs are substrates of cytochrome P-450 enzymes and may induce or inhibit the metabolism of other drugs metabolized by the liver.

Fig. 30.5 ▶ AIDS drugs.

Inhibitors of reverse transcriptase are nucleosides containing an abnormal sugar moiety and require phosphorylation for activation. As triphosphates, they inhibit reverse transcriptase (RT) and induce strand breakage following incorporation into DNA. Nonnucleoside inhibitors inhibit RT without requiring prior activation. Protease inhibitors prevent polyprotein cleavage, which is necessary for the maturation of viral cells. Fusion inhibitors prevent the change in conformation of viral fusion proteins that allows them to attach to host CD4 cells. SC, subcutaneous.

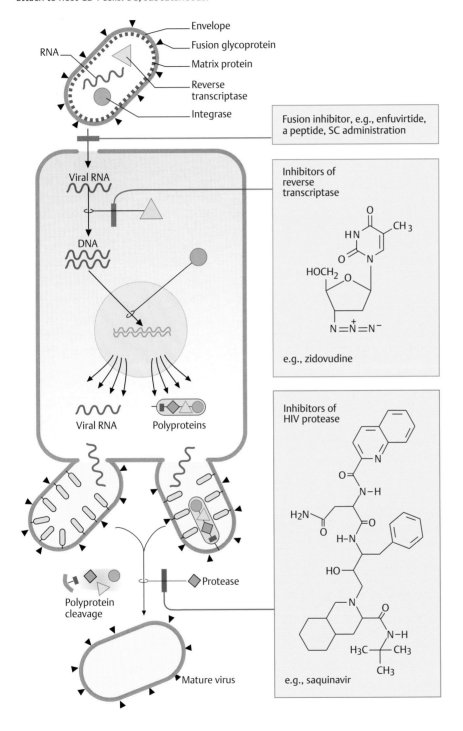

Replication of the HIV virus

There are several steps involved in the replication of the HIV virus:

1. Proteins (gp120 protein) on the surface of the HIV virus cell are fused to CD4+ receptors (glycoproteins) found on the surface of helper T cells, monocytes, and macrophages.
2. HIV RNA, reverse transcriptase, HIV integrase, and other viral proteins are released into the host cell.
3. Single-stranded viral RNA is transcribed to double-stranded DNA in the cytoplasm by the action of reverse transcriptase.
4. New viral DNA migrates into the nucleus and becomes spliced into host DNA by the action of HIV integrase.
5. DNA is transcribed into new viral RNA, which is then translated into viral proteins.
6. New viral RNA and proteins congregate near the cell membrane and become enclosed in the membrane, forming immature (not yet infective) HIV virus cells, which bud off from the host cell.
7. The virus is cleaved by proteases into its mature, infective form.

Delavirdine

Side effects. A rash develops on the upper body and arms within the first 1 to 3 weeks after taking the medication. This rash usually goes away within ~2 weeks. Other side effects include

— Severe skin rash accompanied by blisters, fever, joint or muscle pain, redness and swelling of the eyes, sores in the mouth, and swelling

— Serious kidney problems
— Anemia
— Liver
— Muscle problems

Efavirenz

Side effects

— Abnormal thinking, confusion, depression, hallucinations, memory loss, paranoid thinking, and thoughts of suicide
— Convulsions
— Liver complications
— Increase in cholesterol, fat accumulation, and fat redistribution

Etravirine

Side effects

— Mild to moderate rash sometimes occurs in the second week of therapy and generally resolves within 1 to 2 weeks of continued therapy.
— Serious side effects may include a severe skin rash with or without an accompanying fever, muscle or joint aches, blistering, oral lesions, facial swelling, and swelling and reddening of the eye.

Nevirapine

Side effects

— Severe skin rash, chills, fever, sore throat, and other flulike symptoms. These may be signs of liver disease.

Protease Inhibitors

Saquinavir, Ritonavir, Lopinavir, Indinavir, Nelfinavir, Amprenavir, Atazanavir, Tipranavir, and Darunavir

Mechanism of action. Protease inhibitors inhibit viral assembly and release from the host CD4 cells (**Fig. 30.5**).

Pharmacokinetics. These drugs are substrates for CYP3A4. Thus, they may inhibit the metabolism of other drugs that are CYP3A4 substrates.

Side effects. The general side effects of these drugs include the following:
— Changes in body fat distribution (central obesity, buffalo hump, gynecomastia)
— Increased bleeding in patients with hemophilia
— High sugar levels in the blood; onset or worsening of diabetes

The additional side effects of individual drugs are listed in **Table 30.4**.

Table 30.4 ▸ **Side Effects of Protease Inhibitor Drugs**	
Agent	**Side Effects**
Ritinavir	Inflammation of the pancreas, which can cause severe stomach pain, nausea, or vomiting; heart dysrhythmias (this may happen when ritonavir is used alone or when used with other drugs that affect the heart)
Lopinavir	Disease of the pancreas; dizziness, lightheadedness, fainting, or sensation of abnormal heartbeats
Indinavir	Kidney stones
Amprenavir	Severe rash
Atazanavir	Yellowing of the eyes or skin; change in heart rhythm; diarrhea, infection, nausea, and blood in the urine
Tipranavir	Increased cholesterol and triglyceride levels; serious liver problems; bleeding in the brain; rash
Darunavir	Inflammation of the liver and abnormal liver function tests (liver injury, specifically drug-induced hepatitis, may occur when darunavir and ritonavir are taken together); severe skin rash; fever; abnormally high cholesterol and triglyceride levels; hypersensitivity; metabolic disturbances

Entry (Fusion) Inhibitor

Enfuvirtide

Mechanism of action. Enfuvirtide binds to the transmembrane glycoprotein subunit (gp41) of the viral envelope and prevents the fusion of viral envelope and cell membrane (**Fig. 30.5**).

Chemokine coreceptor antagonist

Maraviroc

Mechanism of action. Maraviroc blocks certain strains of HIV from binding to chemokine receptor type 5 (CCR5) thus preventing the virus from entering target cells. This agent can only be used when the virus is CCR5-tropic. If the patient's virus is chemokine receptor type 4 (CCR4)-tropic or has a mixed population, as seen in later stages of the disease, maraviroc will not be effective.

Integrase Inhibitor

Raltegravir

Mechanism of action. Raltegravir inhibits the viral integrase that mediates the integration of the newly synthesized viral DNA into host cell DNA.

Highly Active Antiretroviral Therapy (HAART)

HAART is combination therapy used in the treatment of HIV/AIDS to decrease the development of resistance. It usually involves using three agents from two different classes.

31   Antifungal and Antiparasitic Drugs

A human fungal infection, termed a *mycosis,* is related to either true fungal agents that possess virulence factors capable of avoiding the host defense or opportunistic fungi that thrive in a compromised immune system. Fungi are eukaryotic, but their cell membrane contains ergosterol instead of cholesterol that is present in the mammalian cell membrane. It is this unique cell membrane that allows for the selective toxicity of antifungal agents. The cell wall of fungi contains chitin and complex polysaccharides.

31.1   Drugs Used in the Treatment of Fungal Infections

Polyene Antifungals

Mechanism of action.   Polyene antifungals are named for large numbers of unsaturated bonds in their chemical structures. These drugs permeate into ergosterol-rich membranes (characteristic of fungi), where they produce a detergent-like effect (**Fig. 31.1**).

Nystatin

Pharmacokinetics
— Nystatin is available in tablets and suspensions for topical application. It is not absorbed after oral administration.
— It is highly toxic and is not used parenterally.

Uses
— *Candida* infections of the mouth or the gastrointestinal (GI) tract

Amphotericin B

Pharmacokinetics.   This agent is ineffective after oral administration; therefore, it is given intravenously (IV).

Spectrum.   Amphotericin B has a broad antifungal spectrum and is useful for most systemic fungal infections.

Uses
— Serious systemic fungal infections (use limited by toxicity)

Side effects
— Renal toxicity

Imidazole Antifungal Agents

Mechanism of action.   Imidazole antifungal agents interfere with cytochrome P-450–dependent biosynthesis of ergosterol, causing disorganization of the fungal cell membrane (**Fig. 31.1**). These agents have a broad spectrum of activity against pathogenic fungi. They may also inhibit several cytochrome P-450–dependent drug oxidations in patients, leading to drug interactions.

Miconazole and Clotrimazole

Pharmacokinetics
— Topical use only

Uses
— Superficial tinea (ringworm) infections and vulvovaginal candidiasis
— Treatment of oral and esophageal candidiasis; prophylaxis against oral candidiasis in immunosuppressed patients (clotrimazole lozenges)

Pathogenic fungal forms

Pathogenic fungi are able to grow in two forms: filamentous and yeasts, depending on the growth conditions. Filamentous, or mold, forms grow as branching, threadlike filaments called hyphae. Several hyphae are collectively referred to as a mycelium. The hyphae may be septate, that is, divided by partitions, or coenocytic, with no partitions but a multinucleate hyphal structure. Yeasts grow as single cells that are ovoid or spherical and divide by budding or, rarely, by binary fission like bacteria. The ability to switch from one form to another is termed *dimorphism* and, with some fungi, correlates to a switch from free living to infectious organism.

Fungal reproduction

Fungi generally are capable of reproduction by asexual or sexual means. Asexual reproduction usually refers to the formation of spores, which show resistance to environmental conditions. Spores may be thallospores, which are produced from cells of the body of the fungus, or conidia, which are produced from specialized structures. Sexual reproduction occurs when two haploid nuclei come together in a single cell. The nuclei are combined to become diploid. Meiosis occurs and results in genetic exchange. Division then results in four haploid progeny nuclei.

Fig. 31.1 ▶ Antifungal drugs.

Imidazole derivatives inhibit the synthesis of ergosterol, an integral component of fungal cell membranes. Polyene antibiotics insert themselves into fungal cell membranes and cause the formation of hydrophilic channels. Flucytosine is an antimetabolite that is converted to 5-fluorouracil in candidal fungi by fungal cytosine deaminase. It is then incorporated into fungal DNA, causing disruption of DNA and RNA synthesis. Caspofungin inhibits fungal cell wall synthesis. Griseofulvin is active only against dermatophytes. It seems to inhibit fungal mitosis by acting as a spindle poison.

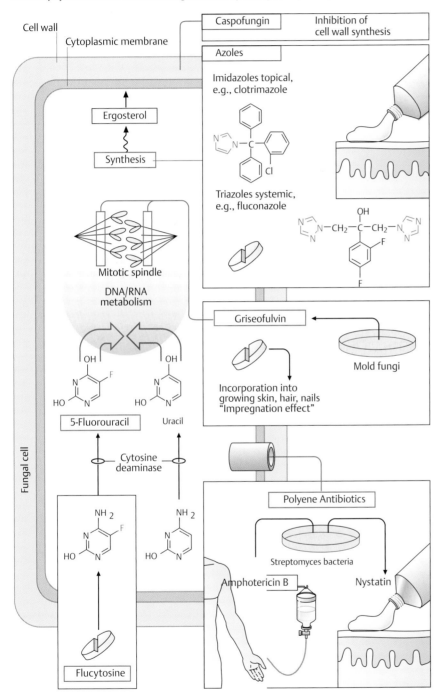

Side effects.   Vaginal preparations may cause vaginal or stomach discomfort.

Ketoconazole

Pharmacokinetics.   Ketoconazole has erratic oral absorption. It is dependent on GI pH.

Uses.   Use has declined due to erratic absorption, toxicity, and availability of other agents.

Side effects
— Fatal hepatic toxicity; adverse cardiac events when taken with terfenadine, astemizole, or cisapride

Tetrazole Antifungal Agents

Mechanism of action.   The tetrazole drugs are chemically related to imidazoles and also act by inhibiting ergosterol biosynthesis by fungal cytochrome P-450 enzymes.

Fluconazole

Pharmacokinetics
— Eliminated in the urine; dosage modifications are necessary in cases of renal insufficiency
— Can penetrate into cerebrospinal fluid (CSF)

Uses.   Useful for a variety of systemic fungal infections, including
— Candidiasis
— Cryptococcosis
— Especially useful for cryptococcal meningitis (due to CSF penetration)

Itraconazole

Pharmacokinetics
— Unlike fluconazole, itraconazole is cleared by hepatic metabolism.

Uses
— Similar to fluconazole in its properties and indications

Other Antifungals

Flucytosine

Mechanism of action.   Fungi metabolize the drug to its active form, 5-fluorouracil (**Fig. 31.1**), which inhibits fungal DNA and RNA synthesis.

Pharmacokinetics
— Orally effective

Uses
— Systemic *Candida* or *Cryptococcus* infections, often in combination with amphotericin B

Side effects.   Patients must be monitored carefully for hematologic, renal, and hepatic function.

Griseofulvin

Mechanism of action.   Griseofulvin inhibits fungal cell mitosis.

Pharmacokinetics
— Given orally

Uses
— Used when itraconazole and terbinafine are contraindicated (e.g., hypersensitivity or liver disease)
— Persistent ringworm (tinea) infections, but prolonged administration is required

Side effects
- May include GI disturbances, central nervous system (CNS) abnormalities, and skin rashes

Terbinafine

Mechanism of action. This agent inhibits squalene epoxidase, a key enzyme in sterol biosynthesis.

Pharmacokinetics
- Given orally or topically

Uses
- Onychomycosis (nail infections) that are difficult to treat with other agents

Side effects
- After oral administration: hypersensitivity rash; increased liver enzymes; rare cases of liver failure

Echinocandins

Caspofungin, Micafungin, and Anidulafungin

Mechanism of action. These agents block the synthesis of β (1,3)-D-glucan, a polysaccharide component of the cell wall in many pathogenic fungi.

Spectrum
- Fungicidal against *Candida* and *Aspergillus* species

Uses
- Fluconazole-resistant candidiasis, aspergillosis

Side effects. These agents are generally well tolerated, but side effects may include
- Fever
- Elevated liver enzymes
- Anemia
- Occasional maculopapular rash

31.2 Drugs Used in the Treatment of Protozoan Infections

Amebicidal Drugs (*Entamoeba histolytica*)

Entamoeba histolytica is an intestinal protozoan. Most infections are asymptomatic but may lead to clinical syndromes ranging from dysentery to abscesses of the liver or other organs.

Metronidazole

Mechanism of action. Metronidazole has a direct amebicidal effect and acts by inhibiting a unique electron transfer system of a variety of anaerobic organisms.

Pharmacokinetics
- Orally effective

Uses
- Systemic and intestinal forms of amebiasis except for asymptomatic cyst carriers
- Useful for trichomoniasis and giardiasis

Side effects
- Nausea, vomiting, and headache
- Seizures

— Ataxia
— Leucopenia
— Alcohol intolerance (disulfiram-like reaction [see page 121]) has been reported.

Contraindications
— Pregnancy

Iodoquinol (Diiodohydroxyquinoline)

Spectrum.   Iodoquinol is directly amebicidal to trophozoites and cysts.

Uses
— Used only for intestinal amebiasis

Side effects
— GI disturbances
— Neurotoxic effects: headache in the short term; peripheral neuropathy with higher doses in the longer term
— Thyroid enlargement

Paromomycin

Paromomycin is a poorly absorbed aminoglycoside antibiotic.

Spectrum.   In addition to eliminating intestinal bacteria, paromomycin directly kills trophozoites and intestinal cestodes.

Uses
— Mild intestinal disease

The occurrence of protozoan infections in the United States is relatively rare, but it can be seen in immigrants or those returning from travel overseas. Protozoan organisms, the diseases they cause, and the drugs of choice are included in **Table 31.1.**

Table 31.1 ► Treatment of Protozoan Infections		
Organism	**Disease**	**Drug(s) of Choice**
Entamoeba histolytica	Amebiasis	Metronidazole (pages 304 and 326)
Cryptosporidium parvum	Cryptosporidiosis	Nitazoxanide
Giardia lamblia (Giardia duodenalis)	Giardiasis	Metronidazole (1), quinacrine (2)
Leishmania braziliensis, Leishmania mexicana, and other species	Leishmaniasis	Sodium stibogluconate
Pneumocystis jiroveci	Pneumocystosis	Trimethoprim + sulfamethoxazole (1) (pages 302–304, 310, and 330)
Trichomonas vaginalis	Trichomoniasis (a sexually transmitted protozoan infection)	Metronidazole (pages 304 and 326)
Toxoplasma gondii	Toxoplasmosis	Pyrimethamine + sulfadiazine (pages 303 and 331–332)
Trypanosoma	South American trypanosomiasis (Chagas disease)	Nifurtimox
	African sleeping sickness	Early stage: pentamidine (1), suramin (2) Late stage: melarsoprol (an organic arsenical)

1, first-line agent; 2, second-line agent.
Note: Page references in parentheses indicate sites of fuller discussions of these agents.

Antimalarial Drugs

Malaria is one of the most common protozoan infections. It is caused by *Plasmodium* species that are transferred into the bloodstream via the bite of infected mosquitoes. Symptoms include interspersed bouts of fever and chills. The disease is most commonly found in tropical and subtropical climates.

The *Plasmodium* species involved include

— *P. vivax, P. ovale,* and *P. malariae,* which have erythrocytic and tissue (exoerythrocytic) cycles
— *P. falciparum,* which has no tissue cycle

Chloroquine

Mechanisms of action.   Growth of malarial parasites in host erythrocytes requires digestion of hemoglobin in their acidic food vacuoles. This produces heme, which is normally crystallized to a nontoxic form. Free heme is highly reactive and toxic to the parasite. Chloroquine accumulates in the digestive vacuoles and prevents detoxification of heme, leading to increased free heme and parasite death. Chloroquine also has an antiinflammatory effect (**Fig. 31.2**).

Spectrum.   Chloroquine kills erythrocytic forms of *P. falciparum* but is not effective on liver forms.

Pharmacokinetics
— It is rapidly and almost completely absorbed after oral administration.
— It accumulates in the liver (which suggested its use for hepatic amebiasis) and is slowly excreted.

Uses
— Malaria prophylaxis and treatment
— Rheumatoid arthritis (see p. 356)

Side effects
— Toxicity is dose related, ranging from GI distress, rashes, and headache to ocular toxicity (retinopathy and corneal deposits, which suggest a "bull's-eye") and CNS hyperexcitability.
— Methemoglobinemia and hemolytic anemia can occur in individuals with a genetic deficiency of glucose-6-phosphate dehydrogenase (G6PD) deficiency (see page 27).

Primaquine

Mechanism of action.   The mechanism of action of primaquine is unclear.

Spectrum.   Primaquine can destroy exoerythrocytic, liver-lurking forms and is gametocidal.

Pharmacokinetics
— Rapidly absorbed after oral administration and metabolized to active forms by the liver

Side effects
— Mild toxicity includes anorexia, nausea, vomiting, and cramps.
— In individuals with G6PD deficiency, methemoglobinemia and hemolytic anemia can occur.

Quinine

Mechanism of action.   Quinine is thought to act similarly to chloroquine (**Fig. 31.2**).

Spectrum
— Effective against erythrocytic forms and not on liver forms

Uses.   Quinine is a traditional agent now largely replaced by newer drugs, but it is still useful in drug-resistant strains of *P. falciparum.*

Methemoglobinemia

Methemoglobinemia is a condition in which there are higher levels of methemoglobin in the blood than normal. It occurs when the ferrous ion (Fe^{2+}) is oxidized to the ferric state (Fe^{3+}) in red blood cells when they are exposed to exogenous oxidizing drugs and their metabolites. Methemoglobin does not bind oxygen, so people with this condition will show signs of hypoxia, including dyspnea (shortness of breath), dizziness, cyanosis, fatigue, and mental changes. It is treated by giving oxygen therapy and methylene blue, which is a substance that is able to reduce iron in hemoglobin to its normal, oxygen-carrying state.

Fig. 31.2 ▶ **Malaria: stages of the plasmodial life cycle in the human, therapeutic options.**
A mosquito carrying malaria feeds on human blood and injects a parasite in the form of sporozoites
into the bloodstream. The sporozoites travel to the liver and invade liver cells. Sporozoites mature into
forms known as schzionts, which divide to form haploid twins called merozoites. Merozoites exit the
liver and enter the bloodstream, where they invade erythrocytes and undergo asexual replication.
Some merozoites develop into sexual forms of the parasite, called male and female gametocytes, that
circulate in the bloodstream. When a mosquito bites an infected human, it ingests the gametocytes,
which eventually form sporozoites. Different antimalarials selectively kill different developmental forms
of parasites. Chloroquine and quinine accumulate within the acidic vacuoles of blood schizonts and
inhibit the polymerization of heme released from digested hemoglobin. Free heme is toxic to schizonts.
Pyrimethamine and proguanil inhibit dihydrofolate reductase, and sulfadoxine inhibits the synthesis of
dihydrofolic acid. Atoraquone suppresses the synthesis of pyrimidine bases, probably by interfering with
mitochondrial electron transport.

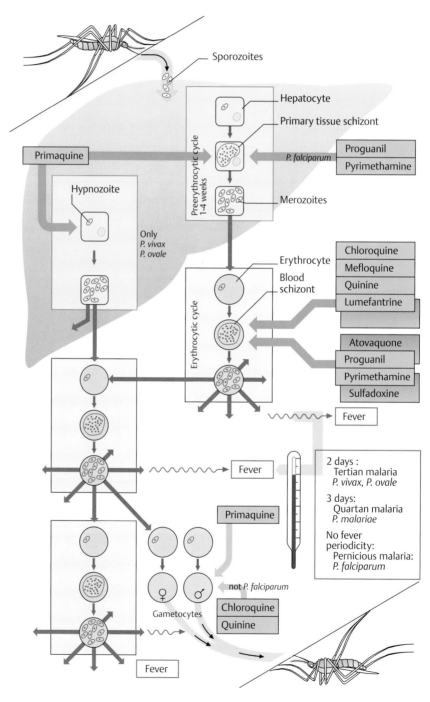

Side effects
— Cinchonism (headache, tinnitus, and diplopia)
— Allergic skin rashes
— Hypotension
— Skeletal muscle weakness
— Renal damage
— It can cause intravascular hemolysis in sensitized individuals and also methemoglobinemia and hemolytic anemia in individuals with G6PD deficiency.

Note: All quinine antimalarials ("quines") possess this genetically determined toxicity.

Mefloquine

Mechanisms of action
— Similar to chloroquine

Spectrum
— Effective against erythrocytic forms and not on liver forms

Pharmacokinetics
— Mefloquine has a long half-life (10–14 days) and is taken as a single dose to treat mild to moderate malaria and once per week as prophylaxis.

Uses
— Used when chloroquine resistance is likely
— Mild to moderate malaria (not for severe cases)
— Malaria prophylaxis

Side effects
— GI distress is the most common.

Atovaquone/Proguanil

Mechanisms of action
— Atovaquone inhibits mitochondrial electron transport of *Plasmodium.*
— Proguanil inhibits dihydrofolate reductase of *Plasmodium.*

Spectrum
— Effective against erythrocytic and exoerythrocytic forms

Pharmacokinetics
— Effective orally
— Three doses daily to treat malaria
— Daily as prophylaxis

Uses
— Used for chloroquine-resistant malaria
— Malaria prophylaxis

Side effects
— GI distress is the most common.
— Serum liver enzyme levels increased

Dihydrofolate Reductase Inhibitors

Pyrimethamine, Chloroguanide, and Trimethoprim

Mechanism of action. These agents act slowly by inhibiting dihydrofolic acid reductase and preventing the production of tetrahydrofolic acid (**Fig. 31.2**).

Spectrum.   Erythrocytic and exoerythrocytic forms are inhibited.

Pharmacokinetics
— Pyrimethamine is the most potent and has the longest duration of action.
— Chloroguanide is a prodrug (the active metabolite is cycloguanil) and has the shortest action.

Uses.   Use of these agents is limited primarily to treatment of chloroquine-resistant *P. falciparum*, but many strains are now resistant to dihydrofolate reductase inhibitors as well.

Side effects.   These agents can cause weak inhibition of human dihydrofolic acid reductase, which results in megaloblastic anemia. Folinic acid will remedy the anemia without interfering with the chemotherapy.

Resistance.   Resistance to one drug usually confers resistance to the others.

31.3   Drugs Used in the Treatment of Metazoan Infections

Treatment of Nematode Infections (Roundworm)

Mebendazole

Mechanism of action.   Mebendazole binds to and inhibits tubulin synthesis; it also inhibits glucose uptake and larval development.

Pharmacokinetics
— Largely unabsorbed

Side effects.   Side effects are uncommon and include occasional abdominal distress and diarrhea.

Contraindications
— Pregnancy and allergy

Pyrantel

Mechanism of action.   Pyrantel is a noncompetitive, depolarizing neuromuscular blocking agent that causes worm paralysis.

Side effects.   Some mild and transient GI, CNS, skin, and hepatic reactions may occur.

Thiabendazole

Mechanism of action.   Thiabendazole inhibits the mitochondrial fumarate reductase of helminths.

Pharmacokinetics
— Rapidly absorbed

Uses
— Cutaneous larvae migrans (a common tropical skin disease caused by the larvae of various nematode parasites)

Side effects.   Side effects are mild and transient and include
— Vomiting, nausea, lethargy, and dizziness. These symptoms are reduced by giving thiabendazole after meals.
— Hepatotoxic higher doses diminish mental alertness.

Piperazine

Mechanism of action.   Piperazine produces competitive block of acetylcholine on worm muscle. Worms are paralyzed and eliminated alive.

Side effects
— Mild, transient GI effects and rash

Ivermectin

Mechanism of action.   Ivermectin paralyzes worms by actions on gamma-aminobutyric acid (GABA) synapses in the periphery.

Treatment of Cestode Infections (Flatworm)

Praziquantel

Mechanism of action.   Praziquantel increases the permeability of cell membranes to Ca^{2+}, causing spastic paralysis of worm muscle followed by disintegration of its tegument.

Spectrum
— Broad

Pharmacokinetics
— Well absorbed and well tolerated

Uses
— Effective for a variety of cestode and trematode infections

Side effects.   No major adverse effects have been reported.

Review Questions

1. Bacteria are able to transfer genes that confer resistance to each other. This usually occurs via which of the following?
   A. Liposomes
   B. DNA gyrase
   C. Plasmids
   D. Proteins
   E. Nuclear fusion

2. A 13-year-old male patient has a sore throat but no cough. His pharynx, soft palate, and tonsils are red and edematous, with tonsillar exudate. His cervical lymph nodes are tender. There is no evidence of airway compromise. Before beginning drug treatment, which of the following should be assessed?
   A. Sensitivity of the infecting organism to antibiotics
   B. The ability to obtain intravenous access
   C. Whether the patient is allergic to penicillin
   D. Previous use of the antibiotic clindamycin
   E. White blood cell count

3. A patient diagnosed as having pneumococcal (*Streptococcus pneumoniae*) pneumonia has received an intramuscular injection of an antibiotic in the clinic. The patient has received penicillins before without having an allergic reaction. For continued oral therapy on an outpatient basis, which of the following would be the most appropriate therapy?
   A. Erythromycin
   B. Cefazolin
   C. Amoxicillin
   D. Penicillin V
   E. Piperacillin

4. Broad-spectrum ampicillin is different from penicillin G in that it
   A. has a lower Michaelis constant (K_m) for the transpeptidases of many gram-negative bacteria.
   B. covalently inactivates the transpeptidases of many gram-negative bacteria.
   C. is inactive against gram-positive organisms.
   D. cannot show synergism with an aminoglycoside.
   E. penetrates better through the outer membranes of many gram-negative bacteria.

5. A 15-day-old male infant has a fever and has been crying nonstop overnight. He vomited after breastfeeding. He was born by vaginal delivery after an uncomplicated pregnancy to a healthy mother with no history of infectious diseases. The infant's nasopharynx was inflamed, and mild nuchal rigidity was noticed. The infant's white blood count is elevated, and a urinalysis is normal. Gram stain of the cerebrospinal fluid reveals small gram-positive bacilli. Which of the following would be the best empiric therapy for this patient?
   A. Penicillin G
   B. Ampicillin
   C. Gentamicin
   D. Miconazole
   E. Metronidazole

6. A 64-year-old man has severe abdominal pain and tenderness, as well as a fever. He is nauseous and has been vomiting. Bowel sounds are absent. A computed tomography (CT) scan of the abdomen reveals the presence of colonic diverticula and extramural air. He is admitted to the hospital and started on intravenous fluids and intravenous piperacillin and tazobactam. Why is piperacillin preferred over cefazolin for treating this patient?
   A. Piperacillin is more tolerable when given intravenously.
   B. Cefazolin cannot be given intravenously.
   C. Piperacillin is less expensive.
   D. Piperacillin has greater activity against gram-negative anaerobes.
   E. Piperacillin has a longer duration of action.

7. Which antibiotic inhibits terminal cross-linking of cell wall glycopeptides?
   A. Streptomycin
   B. Cephalosporin
   C. Chloramphenicol
   D. Sulfamethoxazole
   E. Lincomycin

8. A 62–year-old man presents with dyspnea, angina and dizziness on exertion. An echocardiogram reveals a calcified aortic valve with a restricted opening and diminished flow. Valve replacement surgery is recommended. Thirty minutes prior to the start of surgery, the patient receives a dose of cefazolin given intravenously. Why is cefazolin preferable to other agents for this patient?

  A. First-generation cephalosporins have superior activity against gram-positive organisms.
  B. The patient is likely to be allergic to penicillin.
  C. Cefazolin is resistant to β-lactamases.
  D. Cefazolin is cheaper than a third-generation cephalosporin.
  E. Cefazolin is the only cephalosporin that can be given intravenously.

9. A patient with penicillin-resistant *Streptococcus pneumoniae* requires an antibiotic for effective therapy. Which of the following agents would be the best choice?

  A. Cephalosporins
  B. Penicillin
  C. Isopropyl alcohol
  D. Glycerin

10. An 82-year-old man who has been living at home has developed a fever with a productive cough and is having difficulty breathing. He reports having alternately sweats and chills and being tired. Auscultation reveals bronchial breath sounds and rales. Sputum culture shows penicillin-resistant *Streptococcus pneumoniae*. He is admitted to the hospital. Which of the following would be recommended therapy for this patient?

  A. Amikacin
  B. Cefotaxime
  C. Doxycycline
  D. Cephalexin
  E. Ampicillin

11. A 64-year-old man has severe abdominal pain and tenderness, as well as a fever. He is nauseous and has been vomiting. Bowel sounds are absent. A computed tomography (CT) scan of the abdomen reveals the presence of colonic diverticula and extramural air. He is admitted to the hospital and started on intravenous fluids and intravenous piperacillin and tazobactam. Why is tazobactam included in this patient's treatment?

  A. To counteract the side effects of piperacillin
  B. To increase the half-life of piperacillin
  C. To inhibit the breakdown of piperacillin by bacterial penicillinases
  D. To enhance the excretion of toxic metabolites of piperacillin
  E. To buffer the pH of piperacillin to prevent metabolic acidosis

12. When their sensitivity has been tested in the laboratory, staphylococcal strains that are clinically resistant to vancomycin have been found to have minimal inhibitory concentrations (MICs) that are the same as vancomycin susceptible strains, but the resistant strains have very high minimal bactericidal concentrations (MBCs). These data indicate that the vancomycin resistance of these strains is most likely due to which of the following?

  A. Altered penicillin-binding proteins
  B. Reduced accumulation of vancomycin
  C. Increased efflux of vancomycin
  D. Decreased ability of vancomycin to block peptidoglycan synthesis
  E. Decreased dependency of the bacterium on folic acid

13. A 38-year-old bank branch manager noticed a small pimple on her left finger that increased in size in a span of 3 hours. She reports to a medical clinic that drains it and does a bacterial culture of the fluid. Empiric antibiotic therapy is started with a cephalosporin. The culture indicates the presence of methicillin-resistant *Staphylococcus aureus* (MRSA). The patient's antibiotic is changed to vancomycin. What is the reason for changing the patient's antibiotic?

  A. Vancomycin is the most potent cephalosporin that can be given orally.
  B. Vancomycin is less likely to produce diarrhea than a cephalosporin.
  C. Vancomycin inhibits bacterial cell wall synthesis at a different step from β-lactam antibiotics.
  D. Vancomycin is less expensive than the cephalosporin she was taking.

14. A relatively high incidence of pseudomembranous colitis occurs with

  A. clindamycin
  B. sulfonamides
  C. nitrofurantoin
  D. tobramycin
  E. nalidixic acid

15. An antibiotic-resistant plasmid enters a *Pseudomonas aeruginosa* cell. This plasmid carries a β-lactamase gene and an aminoglycoside phosphotransferase gene. Which one of the following would be an effective antimicrobial agent against this cell?

  A. Tetracycline
  B. Gentamicin
  C. Neomycin
  D. Ampicillin
  E. Cephalothin

16. A woman presents with urethritis. A culture has revealed the organism to be *Neisseria gonorrhoeae,* which was sensitive to penicillin G, ampicillin, spectinomycin, tetracycline, and erythromycin. The patient is 4 months pregnant and has previously had a severe hypersensitivity reaction to oxacillin. Which of the following drugs would be indicated for this patient?

A. Spectinomycin
B. Tetracycline
C. Erythromycin
D. Ampicillin
E. A cephalosporin

17. Which of the following may cause erosion of cartilage?

A. Ciprofloxacin
B. Cefazolin
C. Gentamicin
D. Penicillin G
E. Chloramphenicol

18. A 29-year-old woman has dysuria, increased frequency of urination, and urgency to urinate. A urine sample is yellow and cloudy. Dipstick urinalysis gives a pH of 5.0 and is positive for leukocyte esterases, nitrites, and blood. What is the rationale for prescribing for this pateint a combination drug containing sulfamethoxazole and trimethoprim?

A. Neither drug alone has an antibacterial action.
B. The combination has a synergistic antibacterial effect.
C. Trimethoprim prevents the development of sulfa drug allergies.
D. Sulfamethoxazole traps trimethoprim in the urine.
E. Sulfamethoxazole has a short half-life, and trimethoprim has a longer duration of action.

19. A 24-year-old woman with a history of epilepsy presents with a cough, weight loss, and night sweats. Her chest radiograph (X-ray) shows cavitary lesions in the upper left lobe of her lung. A sputum smear reveals many acid-fast bacilli. She is admitted to the hospital, put in a negative pressure room, and placed on a combination of isoniazid, rifampin, pyrazinamide, ethambutol, and vitamin B_6. What would be the reason for including B_6 in her regimen?

A. To increase bacterial uptake of the drugs
B. To prevent central nervous system effects of isoniazid
C. To inhibit gastrointestinal side effects of the drugs
D. To inhibit bacterial resistance
E. To decrease the night sweats

20. What is the usual dose-limiting adverse effect of the antitubercular drug ethambutol?

A. Hepatotoxicity
B. Bone marrow depression
C. Loss of visual acuity
D. Central nervous system toxicity
E. Nephrotoxicity

21. Hand disinfectant dispensers are commonly found in hospitals, doctors' offices, and many public places. Which of the following ingredients is active against vegetative bacteria, *Mycobacterium tuberculosis,* many fungi and lipophilic viruses?

A. Cephalosporins
B. Penicillin
C. Isopropyl alcohol
D. Glycerin
E. Isoniazid

22. A 63-year-old man had a sharp, burning, intermittent pain in his left lower back for 3 days. He has now developed a rash in the area that was painful. The rash consists of rose-colored macules with clusters of vesicles and is restricted to a band along his back. There are no symptoms suggesting genitourinary or gastrointestinal involvement. Which of the following agents might be useful for treating this patient's symptoms?

A. Acyclovir
B. Amantadine
C. Penicillin V
D. Cefazolin
E. Rifampin

23. Which of the following, when administered to susceptible individuals, will reduce the incidence and/or severity of influenza types A and B disease?

A. Trifluridine
B. Ribavirin
C. Oseltamivir
D. Interferon-alfa
E. Gancyclovir

24. A 28-year-old man has a fever, headache, and chills, accompanied by joint and muscle aches and pains. Because seasonal influenza has been prevalent in the area, he is given zanamivir for inhalation. How does this drug prevent virus particle aggregation and release?

A. Inhibits influenza neuraminidase
B. Inhibits influenza DNA polymerase
C. Acts as an ion channel blocker of the influenza M_2 protein
D. Inhibits influenza reverse transcriptase
E. Inhibits influenza protease

25. Ribavirin inhibits the replication of which of the following viruses?
- **A.** Rubella viruses
- **B.** Adenoviruses
- **C.** Respiratory syncytial virus
- **D.** Human immunodeficiency virus
- **E.** Cytomegalovirus

26. Which of the following is most likely to impair renal function?
- **A.** Flucytosine
- **B.** Griseofulvin
- **C.** Amphotericin B
- **D.** Ketoconazole
- **E.** Terbinafine

27. Which one of the following is the drug of choice in acute amebic dysentery?
- **A.** Chloroquine
- **B.** Iodoquinol
- **C.** Dehydroemetine
- **D.** Metronidazole
- **E.** Diloxanide furoate

28. Which of the following is administered for 2 weeks after patients leave an endemic malarial area to eradicate hepatic forms of the parasite?
- **A.** Mefloquine
- **B.** Chloroquine
- **C.** Quinine
- **D.** Primaquine
- **E.** Pyrimethamine

29. A 29-year-old woman being treated for cystitis with a combination drug containing sulfamethoxazole and trimethoprim has a vaginal discharge with itching. Although her dysuria has improved, she now has a thick, curdlike, white discharge from her vagina. There is no cervical discharge or tenderness, and the uterus and adnexa are normal. Which of the following agents may be useful for treatment of this patient?
- **A.** Topical miconazole
- **B.** Oral penicillin
- **C.** Oral metronidazole
- **D.** Oral terbinafine
- **E.** Topical terbinafine

30. A woman who was born in the United States travels frequently to Pakistan to visit friends and relatives. Her last visit there was 9 months ago. She has had a fever with sweating, malaise, joint pain, and severe headache. Thin-film Giemsa-stained blood smear shows *Plasmodium vivax* schizonts. The patient is given a drug that accumulates within the acidic vacuoles of blood schizonts and inhibits the polymerization of heme released from digested hemoglobin. Which of the following drugs was she given?
- **A.** Atoraquone
- **B.** Chloroquine
- **C.** Pyrimethamine
- **D.** Proguanil
- **E.** Pyrantel

Answers and Explanations

1. **C** Transfer of drug-resistant genes usually occurs via plasmids (p. 283).

2. **C** The symptoms are indicative of a group A β-hemolytic streptococcus infection. Penicillin is the antibiotic of choice for group A β-hemolytic streptococcal pharyngitis. Thus, the patient must be evaluated for penicillin allergy prior to beginning therapy. Obtaining a comprehensive patient history is the most practical way to reveal a penicillin allergy (p. 289).

3. **D** Penicillin is effective primarily against gram-positive organisms (e.g., streptococci). Penicillin V is acid stable, so it can be taken orally (p. 289).
A Erythromycin is a second-line agent for *S. pneumoniae.*
B Cefazolin is also effective against many gram-positive cocci, but it is not effective orally.
C Amoxicillin is an extended spectrum penicillin and is active against *S. pneumoniae,* but it should not be used for the treatment of streptococcal infections when a natural penicillin would be effective.
E Piperacillin is also an extended spectrum agent, but it is not effective orally and is not being recommended for the treatment of streptococcal infections when a natural penicillin would be effective.

4. **E** Ampicillin is an "extended spectrum" penicillin. It differs from penicillin G, which is effective primarily against gram-positive organisms, by also being active against some gram-negative organisms, that is, by being able to more easily penetrate the gram-negative bacteria (p. 290).

5. **B** The most common causes of meningitis in neonates are *Listeria* and group B *Streptococcus.* The symptoms with either bacteria are similar. When the disease presents 2 to 3 weeks postpartum, it is most likely to result from exposure to *Listeria* during or shortly after delivery. Treatment of *Listeria* meningitis is with ampicillin plus or minus gentamicin because of the resistance of *Listeria* to cephalosporins, which are commonly chosen as empiric therapy for streptococcal meningitis in children (p. 291).

6. **D** The patient has diverticulitis. Piperacillin has greater activity than cefazolin against gram-negative anaerobes likely to be involved in the inflammation (p. 292).

7. **B** Cephalosporins inhibit bacterial cell wall synthesis in a manner similar to that of penicillin (p. 292).
A, C Streptomycin, chloramphenicol, and lincomycin inhibit bacterial protein synthesis.
D Sulfamethoxazole, a sulfonamide, is structurally similar to p-aminobenzoic acid (PABA). It blocks folic acid synthesis in microbes that must synthesize folic acid from PABA

8. **A** Cefazolin is a first-generation cephalosporin that has superior activity against gram-positive organisms. In this case, it is being used to prevent infection, particularly endocarditis, during the surgery (p. 292).

9. **A** Third-generation cephalosporins have a further increased activity against gram-negative organisms. The parenteral third-generation cephalosporins ceftriaxone and cefotaxime have excellent activity against most strains of *S. pneumoniae,* including the vast majority of those resistant to penicillin (p. 293).
B−E The other agents listed would not be effective.

10. **B.** Cefotaxime, a third-generation cephalosporin, has excellent activity against most strains of *S. pneumoniae,* including the vast majority of those resistant to penicillin, and is given by injection (p. 293).
A Amikacin is an aminoglycoside antibiotic that is primarily used for the treatment of serious bacterial infections.
C, D Doxycycline, a tetracycline, and cephalexin, a first-generation cephalosporin, are not indicated for this patient.
E Because the patient's infection is penicillin-resistant, ampicillin would not be appropriate.

11. **C** Tazobactam is a β-lactamase inhibitor that prevents the breakdown of piperacillin (p. 295).

12. **D** Vancomycin's effectiveness depends on its ability to inhibit bacterial cell wall synthesis. Resistance is most likely due to a decreased ability of vancomycin to block peptidoglycan synthesis (p. 295).
A Because vancomycin acts at a different step from β-lactam antibiotics, it does not depend on penicillin-binding proteins.
B, C The fact that the MICs are the same indicates that the amount of vancomycin in the cells is the same; thus there is not a reduced accumulation or increased efflux of vancomycin.
E Vancomycin does not act through the folic acid pathway.

13. **C** Methicillin-resistant *Staphylococcus aureus* (MRSA) is a *Staphylococcus aureus* infection that is resistant to treatment by β-lactam antibiotics e.g., methicillin, penicillin, amoxicillin, and some cephalosporins. Thus, the patient is changed to vancomycin, a drug that is not a β-lactam antibiotic (p. 289).

14. **A** Clindamycin, like many antibacterial agents, alters the normal flora of the colon, which may lead to overgrowth of *Clostridium difficile.* Proliferation of drug-resistant *C. difficile* produces two toxins that may cause pseudomembranous colitis. The antibiotics that most commonly produce pseudomembranous colitis are ampicillin and clindamycin. The disease is treated by discontinuing ampicillin or clindamycin and giving either metronidazole or vancomycin (p. 299).
B−E The other agents listed typically do not produce pseudomembranous colitis.

15. **A** β-lactam and aminoglycoside antibiotics would be ineffective against this cell. Tetracycline is the only agent listed that is not a β-lactam or aminoglycoside (p. 299).
B, C Gentamicin and neomycin are aminoglycosides.
D, E Ampicillin and cephalothin are β-lactam antibiotics.

16. **A** Spectinomycin is used for treatment of gonorrhea (p. 302).
B, E Tetracycline and erythromycin are not for use in pregnant women.
D, E The patient is allergic to penicillins, such as ampicillin, and is also likely to be allergic to cephalosporins.

17. **A** Ciprofloxacin is a fluoroquinolone antibiotic. Fluoroquinolones are associated with an increased risk of erosion of cartilage (p. 303).
B−E The other drugs are not typically associated with cartilage damage.

18. B The combination is used because the drugs exert synergistic antibacterial activity. Sulfamethoxazole inhibits bacterial folic acid synthesis by competing with para-aminobenzoic acid, and trimethoprim inhibits dihydrofolate reductase, thus blocking two consecutive steps in the synthesis of nucleic acids and proteins essential to bacteria (pp. 303 and 311).

A Each drug alone does have some antibacterial activity.

C Trimethoprim does not prevent the development of sulfa drug allergies.

D, E Sulfamethoxazole does not trap trimethoprim in the urine, and the half-lives of the drugs are about equal.

19. B Isoniazid reacts chemically with pyridoxal and can cause neuropathy and convulsions. This is usually not a problem in patients receiving adequate vitamin B_6 in the diet, but this patient has a history of seizures. Thus, coadministration of vitamin B_6 is used to avoid potential adverse neurologic effects (p. 309).

20. C Ethambutol is usually well tolerated, but retrobulbar neuritis (a visual field defect) is seen occasionally at high doses (p. 309).

A, B, D, E, The other conditions are not associated with ethambutol administration.

21. C Isopropyl alcohol is the active antimicrobial agent in many hand disinfectants (p. 312).

A, B, E Cephalosporins, penicillin, and isoniazid are systemic antibiotics not found in hand disinfectants.

D Glycerin is found in soaps and lotions and is used to attract moisture.

22. A The symptoms are indicative of a herpes zoster flare-up, or shingles. Acyclovir is an antiviral drug that is effective in the treatment of herpes (p. 314).

A Amantadine is an antiviral drug used in the prophylaxis and treatment of influenza A.

C Penicillin V is a β-lactam antibiotic that is effective in mild to moderate streptococcal, staphylococcal and pneumococcal infections, such as skin, ear, and respiratory infections.

D Cefazolin is a first generation cephalosporin that is effective against many gram-positive cocci.

E Rifampin is active against tuberculosis and other microbes.

23. C Oseltamivir is an inhibitor of influenza neuraminidase and acts on both influenza types A and B. Without neuraminidase, the hemagglutinin of the virus binds to sialic acid, forming clumps and preventing virus release (p. 318).

A Trifluridine is effective against herpes simplex keratitis.

B Ribavirin is effective against respiratory syncytial virus and hepatitis C.

D Interferon-alfa is used to treat hepatitis B and hepatitis C (in combination with ribavirin).

E Gancyclovir is used to treat cytomegalovirus infection in immunocompromised patients

24. A Zanamivir inhibits influenza neuraminidase. Without neuraminidase, the hemagglutinin of the virus binds to sialic acid, forming clumps and preventing virus release (p. 318).

25. B Ribavirin is administered by aerosol to treat lower respiratory tract infections caused by respiratory syncytial virus (p. 319).

26. C Of the drugs listed, amphotericin B is the one most likely to have renal side effects (p. 324).

A Flucytosine is most likely to have hematological side effects.

B Griseofulvin may cause gastrointestinal disturbances, central nervous system abnormalities, and skin rashes.

D Ketoconazole may cause fatal hepatic toxicity, and adverse cardiac events when taken with terfenadine, astemizole, or cisapride.

E Terbinafine may cause a hypersensitivity rash, increased liver enzymes or liver failure (rarely).

27. D Metronidazole is used to treat systemic and intestinal forms of amebiasis (p. 327).

A Chloroquine is an antimalarial agent.

B Iodoquinol is only used for intestinal amebiasis.

C Dehydroemetine is an investigational drug available from the U.S. Centers for Disease Control and Prevention.

E Diloxanide is an antiprotozoal drug not currently available in the United States.

28. D Primaquine can destroy exoerythrocytic, liver-lurking forms of the parasite and is gametocidal (p. 329).

A Mefloquine is effective against erythrocytic forms and not on liver forms of the parasite.

B,C Chloroquine and quinine kill erythrocytic forms but are not effective on liver forms of the parasite.

E Pyrimethamine inhibits erythrocytic and exoerythrocytic forms of the parasite.

29. A The patient has vulvovaginal candidiasis. Alteration of the normal flora by the systemic antibiotics likely contributed to the emergence of the *Candida* infection. Usually a topical antifungal agent such as miconazole is effective (p. 324).

B, C Penicillin and metronidazole are antibiotics agents that are unsuitable for fungal infections.

D, E Terbinafine is used to treat onychomycosis (nail infections).

30. B Chloroquine accumulates within the acidic vacuoles of blood schizonts and inhibits the polymerization of heme released from digested hemoglobin (p. 329).

32   Autocoids and Related Drugs

Autocoids are biological factors synthesized and released locally that play a role in vasoconstriction, vasodilation, and inflammation. These include serotonin, bradykinin, histamine, and eicosanoids.

32.1 Serotonin and Related Drugs

Serotonin

Serotonin is also discussed in Chapter 10.

Synthesis.   Serotonin (5-hydroxytryptamine [5-HT]) is synthesized from tryptophan by tryptophan hydroxylase.

Location.   High concentrations of serotonin are found in enterochromaffin cells of the gastrointestinal (GI) tract. They are also found in platelets and in the central nervous system (CNS).

Metabolism.   Metabolism is by oxidative deamination via monoamine oxidase.

Receptors.   Serotonin receptors are found in the CNS and GI tract and on smooth muscle. They are grouped into four major groups: $5\text{-}HT_1$, $5\text{-}HT_2$, $5\text{-}HT_3$, and $5\text{-}HT_{4\text{-}7}$. Each of these families has numerous members.

- The $5\text{-}HT_1$ (G_i), $5\text{-}HT_2$ (G_q), and $5\text{-}HT_{4\text{-}7}$ (G_s) receptor families are G-protein coupled receptors.
- The $5\text{-}HT_3$ receptor is a ligand-gated ion channel.

Effects

- *CNS:* ascending systems are involved in the promotion of sleep, in determining mood, and in mental illness (through interactions in limbic areas); descending systems may be involved in modulating pain perception.
- *GI tract:* increases contractility of the gut
- *Smooth muscle:* vasoconstriction

Serotonin Agonist Drugs: Triptans

Sumatriptan, Zolmitriptan, Naratriptan, Riatriptan, Eletriptan, Frovatriptan, and Almotriptan

Mechanism of action.   These agents are selective $5\text{-}HT_{1B/1D}$ receptor agonists. Their mechanism to decrease migraine may result from the ability of these drugs to

- Directly produce constriction of pial and dural blood vessels
- Inhibit the release of vasodilator and proinflammatory peptides (calcitonin gene-related peptide [cGRP], substance P, and vasoactive intestinal peptide [VIP])
- Activate presynaptic inhibitory serotonin receptors of trigeminal nerve afferents innervating intracranial vessels

Pharmacokinetics

- Administered by subcutaneous injection, as a nasal spray, or orally
- Agents vary in speed of onset and duration of action.
- Effective at any time during the attack but more effective if given earlier (during the aura preceding migraine onset)
- Also help to relieve nausea and vomiting, which accompany the attack

---

Carcinoid tumors and serotonin syndrome

Carcinoid tumors are neuroendocrine tumors of the GI tract, urogenital tract, or the pulmonary bronchioles. Carcinoid tumors can contain and secrete numerous autocoids, including prostaglandins and serotonin, causing symptoms such as flushing and diarrhea. Cardiac diseases due to fibrosis of the endocardium and valves, as well as asthmalike symptoms, are also common. Flushing may be precipitated by stress, alcohol, certain foods, and drugs, particularly selective serotonin reuptake inhibitors (SSRIs), so these should be avoided. Heart failure, wheezing, and diarrhea are treated, respectively, with diuretics, bronchodilators, and with antidiarrheal agents, such as loperamide and diphenoxylate. If patients remain symptomatic, serotonin receptor antagonists, antihistamines, and somatostatin analogues are the drugs of choice. $5\text{-}HT_3$ receptor antagonists (ondansetron, tropisetron, dolasetron, granisetron, palonosetron, ramosetron, alosetron, and cilansetron) can control diarrhea and nausea and occasionally ameliorate the flushing. A combination of histamine H_1 and H_2 receptor antagonists (diphenhydramine and cimetidine or ranitidine) may control flushing in patients with upper GI or pulmonary carcinoids. Synthetic analog of somatostatin (octreotide and lanreotide) are the most widely used agents to control the symptoms of patients with carcinoid syndrome.

Uses
- Acute migraine
- Cluster headaches

Side effects
- Chest pain, flushing, nausea, weakness, and dizziness
- In rare cases, serious cardiac events (coronary artery vasospasm, transient myocardial ischemia, myocardial infarction, ventricular tachycardia, and fibrillation) and hypertensive episodes have occurred.

Contraindications
- Coronary, cerebrovascular, or other arterial disease; uncontrolled hypertension

Drug interactions
- Hypertensive crisis (see page 88) may occur if patient has used monoamine oxidase inhibitors (MAOIs) within 2 weeks.
- Serotonin syndrome (see page 89) may occur if these agents are combined with selective serotonin reuptake inhibitors (SSRIs).

Mixed Serotonin Drugs: Ergot Alkaloid Derivatives

Ergot alkaloids are also discussed in Chapter 17.

Ergotamine

Mechanism of action. Ergotamine causes intense vasoconstriction. It also has partial agonist or antagonist activity against serotonergic, dopaminergic, and α-adrenergic receptors.

Pharmacokinetics
- Variable absorption after oral administration
- May be given via sublingual, rectal, and intramuscular routes
- Caffeine enhances both the absorption and the peripheral action of ergotamine.
- Limitations have been placed on the total dose of ergotamine that can be taken per attack and per week to prevent ergot poisoning.

Uses
- Acute migraine

Side effects
- Nausea, vomiting, weakness, and paresthesias

Toxicity. The most serious toxic effects result from sustained vasoconstriction, which can lead to brain or cardiac ischemia.

Contraindications
- Pregnancy.

Dihydroergotamine Mesylate

Dihydroergotamine mesylate is an ergot alkaloid derivative.

Pharmacokinetics
- Given by intramuscular injection, subcutaneous injection, or nasal spray

Uses
- Acute migraine

Note: Dihydroergotamine mesylate is less effective than ergotamine but has a lower incidence of vomiting when injected.

▮ Migraine

Migraines are characterized by a severe, unilateral throbbing headache, which is often preceded by an aura (usually visual), and may be accompanied by nausea, vomiting, and photophobia. They are caused by the dilation of blood vessels in the pia mater and dura mater surrounding the brain. This triggers the release of neuropeptides, such as calcitonin gene-related peptide (cGRP) and substance P from parasympathetic nerve fibers approximating these vessels, and excites nociceptive fibers, which travel in the trigeminal nerve back to the brain. The involvement of 5-HT in migraine is suggested by the finding that blockade of 5-HT receptors can prevent or stop migraine attacks. Treatment of acute migraine includes triptans and ergot alkaloid derivatives. Drugs used for migraine prophylaxis include the β-blockers, anticonvulsants, and antidepressants, although the mechanisms of action of these agents in migraine are not understood.

▮ Cluster headaches

Cluster headaches (migrainous neuralgia) are severe, unilateral, nonpulsatile, periorbital headaches that occur frequently throughout the day for several weeks, followed by a pain-free period that can last several months. Like migraine headaches, cluster headaches have an unknown etiology but appear to result from changes in brain blood flow. Drugs that are effective in terminating migraine are usually effective in terminating cluster headaches, including the triptans and dihydroergotamine. Approximately 50 to 70% of cluster headaches can be terminated by inhalation of 100% oxygen.

Table 32.1 lists other serotonin agonists, and antagonists, noting their uses and where they have been discussed in other chapters.

Table 32.1 ▶ Serotonin Agents and Uses			
Serotonin Agents	**Receptor Subtype**	**Uses(s)**	**Chapter/Page Reference(s)**
Agonists			
Triptans	5-HT$_{1D}$	Migraine	Chapter 32/340, 341
Partial agonist			
Buspirone	5-HT$_{1A}$	Anxiety	Chapter 9/85
Antagonists			
Ondansetron, dolasetron, and palonosetron	5-HT$_3$	Nausea and vomiting	Chapter 27/266
Trazadone	5-HT$_{2A}$	Antidepressant	Chapter 10/88
Clozapine and other atypical antipsychotic agents	5-HT$_{2A}$	Antipsychotic	Chapter 12/100, 101
Reuptake Inhibtors			
Fluoxetine and other SSRIs*	-	Antidepressant	Chapter 10/89

* These agents are thought to act by decreasing neuronal serotonin uptake.
Abbreviations: 5-HT, 5-hydroxytryptamine; SSRI, selective serotonin reuptake inhibitor.

Sepsis

Sepsis is a potentially life-threatening condition in which there is a widespread inflammatory state caused by the release of inflammatory mediators, including cytokines and kinins. These inflammatory mediators are released in response to infection and cause damage to the endothelium of blood vessels, which allows them to leak fluid. This causes tissue edema, hypotension, and hypoperfusion of organs. It also activates the clotting cascade, which leads to disseminated intravascular coagulation (DIC). The hypoperfusion of organs (from hypotension or DIC) may result in multiple organ failure and death.

Disseminated intravascular coagulation

DIC is a pathologic activation of coagulation mechanisms. Events such as malignancy, infection, trauma, and obstetric complications trigger the release of kinins, which leads to the formation of small blood clots in blood vessels, which in turn consumes clotting factors and platelets (hence, DIC is known as a consumption coagulopathy). The fibrin strands in these blood clots also hemolyze passing red blood cells. Patients with DIC are acutely ill and show signs of shock. There is bleeding at any site in the body, including any old venipuncture sites or wounds. The patient may also have renal failure. Treatment mainly involves treating the underlying cause of the DIC, but other supportive measures, such as the administration of fresh frozen plasma, platelets, and blood, may be needed.

32.2 Bradykinin and Related Drugs

Bradykinin

Synthesis. Bradykinin is formed from the α_2 globulin precursor bradykininogen by the plasma enzyme kallikrein. Kallikrein is activated by kinins, trypsin, plasmin, factor XIIa, and pepsin.

Location. Bradykinin is found in plasma and tissues.

Metabolism. Bradykinin exists in plasma in an inactive form and has a half-life of ~15 seconds. A single passage through the pulmonary vascular bed destroys 80 to 90% of the kinins. The principal catabolizing enzymes in the lung are kininase I (carboxypeptidase) and kininase II (angiotensin-converting enzyme).

Receptors. There are three types of bradykinin receptors: B$_1$, B$_2$, and B$_3$. B$_2$ receptors mediate the majority of bradykinin effects, including vasodilation, stimulation of pain, smooth muscle contraction, and increased capillary permeability.

Effects
— *Cardiovascular:* bradykinin is a potent vasodilator (10 times more potent than histamine). It causes vasodilation of blood vessels in the muscle, kidney, viscera, heart, and brain. Plasma kinins increase capillary permeability, which leads to edema.
— *Renal function and blood pressure:* bradykinin may be involved in the local regulation of renal function. The kinin system may be activated to blunt the effects of pressor agents.
— *Smooth muscle:* bradykinin is a potent constrictor of uterine, bronchiolar, and GI smooth muscle.
— *Nerve endings:* bradykinin is a potent inducer of pain.
— *Inflammation:* kinins mimic the manifestations of inflammation.

Bradykinin Antagonists and Kallikrein Inhibitors

Bradykinin antagonists and kallikrein inhibitors are currently being developed. Initial trials suggest that they may be useful in the treatment of cold symptoms caused by rhinovirus, burn pain, and allergic asthma.

32.3 Histamine and Related Drugs

Histamine

Synthesis. Histamine is synthesized from histidine by histidine decarboxylase.

Location. Histamine is found in basophils within blood, in mast cells in tissues, and in some neurons. It is also found in high concentrations in the skin, mucosa of the bronchi, and intestinal mucosa.

Metabolism. The breakdown of histamine involves two main pathways:

— Ring methylation, which is catalyzed by histamine-*N*-methyltransferase, followed by oxidative deanimation by monoamine oxidase
— Oxidative deamination, which is catalyzed by diamineoxidase

 The metabolites are excreted in urine.

Receptors

— H_1 receptors are coupled to G_q, leading to activation of phospholipase C and the phosphatidylinositol (PIP2) signaling pathway. H_1 receptors mediate bronchoconstriction, contraction of the gut, and vascular dilation.
— H_2 receptors are coupled to G_s, activate adenylate cyclase, and stimulate cyclic adenosine monophosphate (cAMP) production. H_2 receptors are present in gastric parietal cells. They mediate gastric secretion and vascular dilation.
— H_3 and H_4 receptors have also been identified, but there are no therapeutic agents that selectively interact with these receptors. H_3 receptors are found mainly in the CNS, whereas H_4 receptors are found in bone marrow and white blood cells.

Release. Tissue release and production of histamine are stimulated by damage to cells and tissues (**Fig. 32.1**). Antigen-antibody reactions, snake venoms, and drugs (e.g., curare and morphine) can also liberate histamine from tissue stores.

Effects

— *Cardiovascular system* (effects are mediated by both H_1 and H_2 receptors): dilation of small blood vessels results in flushing and decreased systemic pressure. Increased capillary permeability results in edema.
— *CNS:* histamine acts as a neurotransmitter.
— *Smooth muscle:* with the exception of vascular smooth muscle (which is relaxed), most other smooth muscle is stimulated to constrict by histamine. Constrictor effects (H_1) are most prominent in the bronchi and uterus. Responses of intestinal muscle vary, and there are few effects on the bladder, gallbladder, ureter, or iris.
— *Glands:* histamine stimulates secretions via H_2 receptors from the salivary, bronchial, and gastric glands.

Nitric oxide

Nitric oxide (NO) is a transmitter substance that is synthesized as required from arginine under the influence of the enzyme NO synthase. NO synthase is activated by Ca^{2+}/ calmodulin in neurons and endothelial cells. NO diffuses into neighboring cells, where it activates guanylate cyclase. This, in turn, activates protein kinase G, which blocks the nuclear IP_3 receptor. This cascade of events results in decreased cytosolic Ca^{2+} concentration, and vasodilation. Histamine promotes vasodilation by causing the vascular endothelium to release NO.

Histamine and allergy

Allergy (also known as hypersensitivity [type I]) is an immune reaction to an allergen (e.g., pollen, dust, or insect stings) that would not elicit such a response in most people. When an allergen is encountered for the first time, it stimulates the production of immunoglobulin E (IgE). IgE attaches to mast cells and sensitizes these cells to this allergen, so that when it is next encountered, mast cells are stimulated to produce histamine and other inflammatory mediators (e.g., prostaglandins, interleukins, cytokines, and leukotrienes). The inflammatory mediators released are then responsible for producing all of the classic signs of allergy, such as rhinorrhea (runny nose), itch, swelling, and difficulty breathing. Anaphylactic shock is a severe type I hypersensitivity reaction characterized by generalized vasodilation, marked fall in blood pressure, and severe bronchoconstriction. Mediators other than histamine are also involved in the anaphylactic response, so the most effective treatment is epinephrine (given intramuscularly). Antihistamines and glucocorticoids decrease the magnitude of the late-occurring response (e.g., hives or itching).

Fig. 32.1 ► **Histamine.**
Histamine is formed by tissue mast cells and basophils. Its release is stimulated by immunoglobulin E (IgE) complexes (type 1 hypersensitivity), activated complement, burns, inflammation, and some drugs. Its release is inhibited by epinephrine, prostaglandin E_2, and feedback inhibition from histamine itself. The effects of histamine via its different receptors are shown.

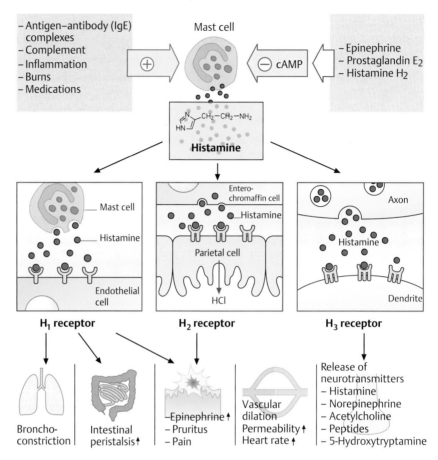

— *Nerve endings:* histamine stimulates nerve endings via H_1 receptors, causing pain and pruritus (itching).
— *Inflammation:* intradermally injected histamine elicits the following triple response: a localized red spot forms followed by a brighter red flush or flare extending ~1 cm beyond the original red spot, then a wheal that develops in 1 to 2 minutes.

H_1 Antihistamines

Diphenhydramine, Promethazine, Chlorpheniramine, Loratadine, Fexofenadine, and Cetirizine

— *First-generation H_1 antihistamines:* Diphenhydramine, promethazine, and chlorpheniramine. These agents have significant sedative, anticholinergic, and antiemetic effects.
— *Second-generation H_1 antihistamines:* Loratadine, fexofenadine, and cetirizine. These agents are nonsedating antihistamines.

Mechanism of action. H_1 antihistamines block H_1 receptors and prevent histamine-induced reactions, for example, increased vascular permeability, smooth muscle contraction, mucus production, and pruritus. They also inhibit the "wheal and flare" response of the skin.

Pharmacokinetics
— These agents are well absorbed following oral administration.
— They are widely distributed and extensively metabolized. They induce hepatic microsomal enzymes and may facilitate their own metabolism.
— First-generation agents can penetrate into the CNS, whereas second-generation agents show poor CNS penetration.
— Metabolites are eliminated in the urine (they are frequently eliminated more rapidly by children).

Effects
— *Smooth muscle:* these agents antagonize the constrictor action of histamine on respiratory and vascular smooth muscle. They also antagonize the changes in capillary permeability produced by histamine that results in edema.
— *CNS:* CNS depression is common with first-generation agents, characterized by sedation and decreased alertness. Paradoxical restlessness, nervousness, and insomnia are occasionally observed. These agents may possess antiemetic effects and are effective against motion sickness.
— *Autonomic nervous system:* anticholinergic effects
— *Allergic reactions:* antagonizes normal hypersensitivity symptoms
— *Local anesthetics* (promethazine): this effect is thought to be due to Na^+ channel blockage in nervous tissue.

Uses
— Used for symptomatic relief of allergic rhinitis, allergic conjunctivitis, and the common cold
— Over-the-counter sedative drugs (diphenhydramine)
— Motion sickness, vertigo, and emesis (dimenhydrinate, meclizine, prochlorperazine, promethazine)
— Appetite suppressants

Side effects
— Sedation is the most common adverse effect and often is responsible for poor compliance.
— Loss of appetite, constipation or diarrhea, nausea, and vomiting
— Anticholinergic effects: dry mouth, cough, palpitations, and headache
— Allergic dermatitis (with topical application)

Toxicity. Initially, there are central excitatory effects, including hallucinations, excitement, ataxia, and convulsions. This can progress to coma, respiratory collapse, and death within 1 to 2 hours. Treatment is supportive, i.e., it involves treatment to prevent, control, or relieve side effects and complications.

Gastric acid and histamine

Histamine is one of the main regulators of gastric acid secretion. It is released from enterochromaffin-like cells in response to stimulation by the vagus nerve and gastrin (a hormone). Once released, histamine acts on parietal cells to increase the activity of H^+-K^+-ATPase (the proton pump), which pumps H^+ ions out of parietal cells in exchange for K^+. The H^+ ions cause an osmotic gradient across the membrane, resulting in an outward diffusion of water. The water then combines with H^+ and Cl^- ions to form gastric acid. (See call-out boxes on page 260 in Chapter 27.)

H_2 Antihistamines

These agents are also discussed in Chapter 27.

Cimetidine, Ranitidine, Famotidine, and Nizatidine

Mechanism of action. H_2 antihistamines are competitive antagonists at the H_2 receptor that inhibit gastric acid secretions elicited by histamine.

Pharmacokinetics
— Well absorbed orally and eliminated in the urine
— Cimetidine inhibits cytochrome P-450 in the liver, which metabolizes many drugs, thus potentiating the effects of such drugs.

Uses
— Treatment of peptic ulcers
— Treatment of gastroesophageal reflux disease (GERD)

Side effects. These include diarrhea, nausea and vomiting, dizziness, headaches, and skin rashes. Cimetidine may also cause loss of libido, impotence, and gynecomastia.

Inhibitors of Histamine-and Leukotriene Release from Mast Cells

Cromolyn Sodium and Nedocromil Sodium

These drugs are also discussed in Chapter 26.

Mechanism of action. These agents inhibit mast cell degranulation of histamine and other inflammatory mediators. They also reduce bronchial hyperresponsiveness.

Uses
— Used prophylactically for asthma
— Seasonal allergic rhinitis

Side effects. Side effects are minimal.

Other Histamine-Related Drug: Anti-IgE Antibody

Omalizumab

Mechanism of action. Omalizumab is a recombinant humanized monoclonal antibody directed against IgE. It binds to free IgE, thus preventing activation of mast cells and basophils.

Uses. IgE-mediated allergic asthma and has been proposed for use in other type I allergic reactions.

Table 32.2 summarizes the effects of serotonin, bradykinin, and histamine.

Table 32.2 ▸ Summary of Effects of Serotonin, Bradykinin, and Histamine			
System	Serotonin	Bradykinin	Histamine
Smooth muscle:			
Vascular	Direct vasoconstriction and endothelial-mediated dilation	Vasodilation	Vasodilation
Bronchial	Mild contraction	Contraction	Contraction
Uterine	Contraction	Contraction	Contraction
Gastrointestinal	Contraction	Contraction	Contraction
Inflammation	Mediator	Mediator	Mediator
Platelet aggregation	Enhances	Inhibits	Enhances
Gastrointestinal system	Stimulates smooth muscle to increase peristalsis		Stimulates gastric acid secretion
Cardiovascular system	Direct vasoconstriction of pulmonary and lung vessels Endothelial-mediated vasodilation in heart and skeletal muscle	Vasodilation, lowering blood pressure	Vasodilation, lowering blood pressure Increases capillary permeability, leading to edema
Central nervous system	Ascending systems: – Sleep – Determining mood Descending systems: – Modulating perception of pain		Acts as a neurotransmitter
Peripheral nervous system	Sensitizes sensory nerve endings, causing pain and itching	Sensitizes sensory nerve endings to pain	Sensitizes sensory nerve endings, causing pain and itching

32.4 Eicosanoids and Related Drugs

Eicosanoids

Eicosanoids (*eicosa* = Greek for 20) are a group of autocoids derived from the 20-carbon fatty acid, arachidonic acid, and include the prostaglandins, prostacyclins, thromboxanes, and leukotrienes.

Synthesis. Eicosanoids are generated from cell membrane phospholipids. Phospholipase A_2 is activated by hormones or other stimuli to form arachidonate, which is then metabolized by cyclooxygenases (COX-1, COX-2, and COX-3) to form prostaglandin H_2 (PGH_2). Alternatively, arachidonate is metabolized by lipoxygenase to form the leukotrienes. PGH_2 is further converted to prostacyclin, other prostaglandins, and thromboxanes (**Fig. 32.2**). The eicosanoids bind to specific G protein-coupled receptors.

Fig. 32.2 ► **Eicosanoid synthesis.**
Arachidonic acid, a polyunsaturated fatty acid found in membrane phospholipids, is the starting material for eicosanoids. The arachidonate moiety is released from the phospholipids by the action of the enzyme phospholipase A_2 (1). Phospholipase A_2 is activated by hormones and other signals (via G proteins), and it is inactivated by steroids. Arachidonic acids may then form prostaglandin H_2 (PGH$_2$) when acted upon by cyclooxygenase (COX) (2). PGH$_2$ is the parent substance for prostacyclins, prostaglandins, and thromboxanes. In a different pathway, PGH$_2$ may be acted upon by lipoxygenase (3), forming hydro- and hydroperoxy fatty acids, which then form leukotrienes. Aspirin (acetylsalicylic acid) and related nonsteroidal antiinflammatory drugs (NSAIDs) inhibit the cyclooxygenase activity of prostaglandin synthase, so the formation of most eicosanoids is blocked. This explains their analgesic, antipyretic, and antirheumatic effects.

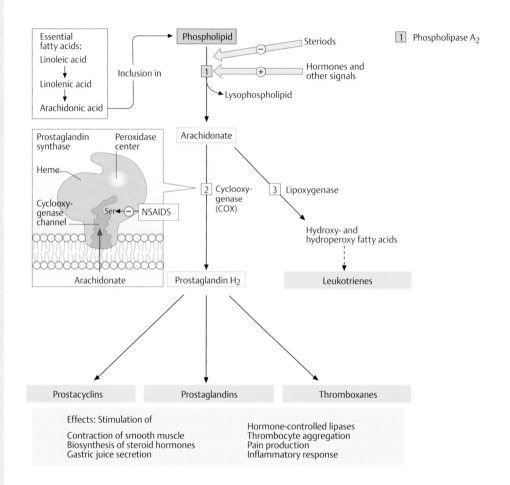

Effects. The major effects of prostaglandin, prostacyclin, and thromboxanes are summarized in **Table 32.3**.

Table 32.3 ▶ Actions of Prostaglandins (PGs), Prostacycline, and Thromboxanes				
System	PGEs	PGFs	Prostacycline	Thromboxanes

Smooth muscle:
  Vascular
  Bronchial
  Uterine
  Gastrointestinal
	Vasodilation
	Relaxation
	Contraction
	Contraction
		Vasoconstriction
		Contraction
		Contraction
		Contraction
			Dilation	Constriction
				Contraction

Inflammation	Mediator	Mediator	Mediator	Mediator
Platelet aggregation	Inhibits		Inhibits	Stimulates
Gastric acid secretion	Decreases		Decreases	
Central nervous system	Fever and sedation			
Peripheral nervous system	Sensitizes nerve endings to pain		Sensitizes nerve endings to pain	
Kidneys	Increased renal blood flow, renin secretion, and natriuresis			

Prostaglandin Agonists

Alprostadil

Mechanism of action. Alprostadil is a prostaglandin E_1 analogue that relaxes vascular smooth muscle, causing vasodilation.

Uses
— Maintaining the patency of ductus arteriosus in neonates who are dependent on the patent ductus for survival while they are awaiting surgery to repair the congenital heart defect. It is administered intravenously (IV).
— Treatment of erectile dysfunction in patients not responding to other therapies (behavioral therapy, vacuum constriction devices, or selective phosphodiesterase type 5 inhibitors). It is administered by intracavernosal injection or intraurethral suppository.

Side effects. No side effects have been noted.

Bimatoprost, Latanoprost, and Travoprost

Mechanism of action. These agents are prostaglandin $F_{2\alpha}$ analogue agonists.

Uses
— Ocular hypertension or open-angle glaucoma. These agents are believed to reduce intraocular pressure by increasing uveoscleral outflow. They are administered as eyedrops.
— Hypotrichosis (reduced amount of hair) of the eyelashes (bimatoprost)

Dinoprostone and Carboprost Tromethamine

Mechanism of action
— Dinoprostone is a synthetic form of PGE_2.
— Carboprost tromethamine is a synthetic form of 15-methyl $PGF_{2\alpha}$.

Ductus arteriosus

Prostaglandin E (PGE_2) is responsible for keeping the ductus arteriosus open during fetal development. The ductus arteriosus is the vascular connection between the pulmonary artery and aorta that allows blood to bypass the fetus's lungs in utero. It begins to close shortly after birth. If it fails to close, the condition is known as patent ductus arteriosus. This can be closed surgically or by using indomethicin, a nonsteroidal antiinflammatory drug (NSAID), which inhibits prostaglandin synthesis.

Prostaglandins in sperm

Sperm is rich in prostaglandins. Prostaglandins help to soften and ripen the cervix, which is why sexual intercourse is advocated as a natural way to induce labor around the time of the due date.

Uses
— Abortifacients (second trimester)
— Induction of labor at term

Misoprostol

Mechanism of action.   Misoprostol is a synthetic PGE_1 methyl ester.

Uses
— Abortifacient (in combination with mifepristone [see page 165]
— Prophylaxis of NSAID-induced gastric ulcers (as it is a potent inhibitor of gastric secretion of acid)

Contraindications.   Do not administer any of the above synthetic prostaglandin agents to pregnant women, as they can cause abortion, premature birth, or birth defects.

Prostaglandin Antagonists: Nonsteroidal Antiinflammatory Drugs

Aspirin (Acetylsalicylic Acid)

Mechanism of action.   NSAIDs (including aspirin) block the synthesis of prostaglandins by inhibiting cyclooxygenase and the formation of both PGG_2 and PGH_2, the precursors of all other prostaglandins. This mechanism is discussed in more detail in Chapter 33.

Prostaglandin Antagonists: Corticosteroids

Prednisone

Mechanism of action.   Corticosteroids block the synthesis of prostaglandins by inhibiting the enzyme phospholipase A_2, which blocks the conversion of membrane phospholipids into arachidonic acid, the precursor of all of the eicosanoids.

32.5   Leukotrienes and Related Drugs

Leukotrienes

Synthesis.   See eicosanoid synthesis.

Location.   Leukotrienes are produced in cells involved in inflammatory responses: mast cells, basophils, and eosinophils.

Effects
— Leukotrienes are involved in the development of the inflammatory responses by promoting endothelial cell adherence of inflammatory mediators, leukocyte chemotaxis (movement in response to the influence of chemical stimulation), and chemokine (a family of chemotactic cytokines) production at the site of inflammation.
— Leukotrienes are potent bronchoconstrictors.

Leukotriene Modifier Agents

These agents are discussed in Chapter 26 for the treatment of asthma.

33 Analgesic, Antipyretic, and Antiinflammatory Drugs

Inflammation is usually the result of a noxious stimulus that results in the destruction of or injury to tissue. Inflammation functions to remove noxious agents from the site of injury, to repair damage, and to return tissue function to normal. The clinical features of inflammation are swelling, redness, heat, and pain.

33.1 Nonsteroidal Antiinflammatory Drugs

Nonsteroidal antiinflammatory drugs (NSAIDs) are analgesic, antipyretic, and antiinflammatory drugs, thus named to distinguish them from the glucocorticosteroids, which also possess antiinflammatory properties. This class of drugs includes some commonly used over-the-counter agents, as well as many prescription-only agents.

Mechanism of action

— *Antiinflammatory:* NSAIDs inhibit the cyclooxygenase enzymes COX-1 and COX-2 (**Fig. 33.1**). These enzymes catalyze the formation of prostaglandin H_2, which is the precursor for prostaglandin, prostacyclin, and thromboxane synthesis. COX-1 is present in most tissues, and in the gastrointestinal (GI) tract it maintains the normal lining of the stomach. It is also involved in kidney and platelet function. COX-2 is induced by inflammation. COX-2 inhibition is thought to lead to the analgesic, antipyretic, and antiinflammatory effects of aspirin and the other NSAIDs.
  — Aspirin inhibits the cyclooxygenase enzymes by acetylating a single serine residue. This is an irreversible covalent modification that inactivates both COX-1 and COX-2. Other NSAIDs are competitive inhibitors of the cyclooxygenases.
— *Analgesic:* NSAID analgesic effects occur as a result of decreased prostaglandin formation.
— *Antipyretic:* Antipyretic effects are the result of decreasing prostaglandins in the temperature control center in the hypothalamus.

Uses

— Mild to moderate pain (e.g., dental, muscle, joint, and postoperative)
— Inflammation and accompanying pain associated with diseases, such as rheumatoid arthritis (high doses)
— Reduction of fever
— Aspirin is also used for the treatment and prophylaxis of thrombosis (low doses). It is widely used to prevent myocardial infarction (MI), stroke, and peripheral vascular thrombosis. It is also used after angioplasty, placement of stents, or bypass surgery to prevent thrombosis and re-stenosis.

Side effects. Many of the adverse effects of aspirin and the other NSAIDs result from inhibition of COX-1 (**Fig. 33.2**). These include
— Acute renal failure
— Skin rash or hypersensitivity reactions, which require immediate discontinuation of the drug
— Gastric distress, occult gastric bleeding, and acute hemorrhage. These effects may be worsened with concomitant use of ethanol and selective serotonin reuptake inhibitors (SSRIs).
— Bronchospasm in NSAID-sensitive asthmatics (see p. 249)

▬ Inflammatory mediators

Cytokines, which are secreted primarily by activated macrophages, are important mediators of inflammation. The most important inflammatory mediators are interleukin-1 (IL-1), interleukin-6 (IL-6), and tumor necrosis factor-α (TNF-α). Local effects include induction of adhesion molecule expression on vascular endothelium (promoting cell adherence), increased vascular permeability (promoting influx of serum components), and activation of lymphocytes. Systemic effects include increased leukocyte production, fever, and induction of acute phase response. Other important cytokines include interleukin-8 (IL-8), a potent chemotactic factor for recruitment of neutrophils, basophils, and T cells, and interleukin-12 (IL-12), which activates NK cells and promotes differentiation of T cells into T helper (TH) cells.

▬ Set point temperature and temperature regulation

The preoptic region and adjacent anterior nuclei of the hypothalamus contain a thermostat for establishing the set point temperature. The set point temperature (~37°C) is the body core temperature that the system attempts to maintain. If core temperature falls below the set point, then the following mechanisms may be induced by the posterior hypothalamus: somatic nervous system activation induces shivering generating heat by causing ATP hydrolysis in the contractile apparatus of skeletal muscle; thyroid hormones may be released generating heat by increasing the activity of Na^+-K^+–ATPase; and sympathetic nervous system activation causes vasoconstriction of blood vessels to the skin resulting in heat conservation. If core temperature rises above the set point, then the following mechanisms may be induced by the anterior hypothalamus: sympathetic cholinergic activation of sweat glands (via muscarinic receptors) increases heat loss by evaporation of water from the skin; and lowered sympathetic adrenergic activity causes dilation of blood vessels to the skin resulting in heat loss by convection and radiation.

Fever and antipyretic drugs

Fever is produced by endogenous pyrogens (e.g., interleukin-1) released by infective bacteria. These pyrogens act on the anterior hypothalamus to increase prostaglandin synthesis, which in turn stimulates the thermoregulatory center to reset the new set point to a higher temperature. Because body temperature is cooler than the new set point, body temperature increases (heat production and conservation of heat) until it stabilizes at the new, elevated set point temperature. After the fever breaks and the new set point returns to 37° C, the patient vasodilates and sweats to lose heat until body temperature returns to normal. Aspirin (and other NSAIDs) and acetaminophen are effective in suppressing fever because they inhibit cyclooxygenase and therefore prostaglandin synthesis. In doing so, they lower the set point temperature and will cause activation of the heat loss mechanisms. Steroids may also be used to reduce fever by blocking the release of arachidonic acid (the precursor of prostaglandins) from membrane phospholipids.

Fig. 33.1 ▶ **Nonsteroidal antiinflammatory drugs (NSAIDs).**
NSAIDs inhibit prostaglandin metabolism by inhibiting both forms of the enzyme cyclooxygenase (COX-1 and COX-2). Cyclooxygenase catalyzes the formation of prostaglandin H_2 which is the most important step in prostaglandin production. The normal physiological effects of COX-1 and COX-2 are shown. Because NSAIDs block these actions, they have an antiinflammatory effect (wanted), but they also block the physiological effects of COX-1, which are the main cause of NSAID side effects. Glucocorticoids also inhibit prostaglandin (and leukotriene) production by inhibiting phospholipase A_2 and COX-2 (indirectly).

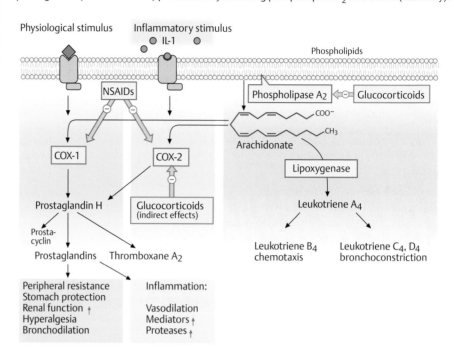

Fig. 33.2 ▶ **Adverse effects of NSAIDs.**
NSAID-induced inhibition of COX enzymes leads to decreased production of prostaglandins from arachidonic acid. This leads to gastric mucosal damage and its sequelae and nephropathy. COX-2 inhibitors show a lower incidence of gastropathy. Inhibition of this side of the arachidonic acid metabolic pathway may lead to increased leukotriene production, depending on arachidonic acid availability. This proinflammatory mediator can cause asthma and bronchoconstriction.

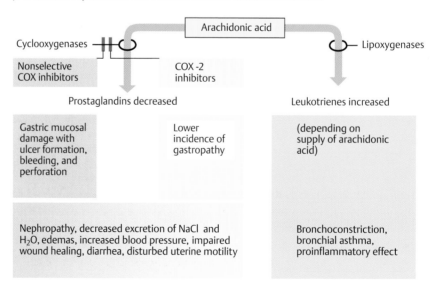

Contraindications

- Gastric ulcers (gastric irritation may aggravate ulcers)
- Asthma (NSAIDs can induce bronchospasm in asthmatics)
- Influenza-like illnesses in children or teenagers (up to 19 years of age). There is an increased risk of developing Reye syndrome in children with influenza or chickenpox.
- Pregnancy (third trimester). NSAIDs may cause premature closure of the ductus arteriosus.

The relative strength of the antiinflammatory, analgesic, and antipyretic actions varies slightly among different NSAID agents. The major difference is in pharmacokinetics. Individual patients may show different therapeutic responses and adverse reactions to the different agents. The unique features of specific NSAID agents are discussed in the following section.

Salicylates

Aspirin (Acetylsalicylic Acid)

Pharmacokinetics

- Well absorbed following oral administration
- Rapidly metabolized by plasma esterases to salicylic acid and acetic acid
- Salicylate ion is highly bound (80–90%) to plasma proteins
- Conjugation in the liver is the primary route of metabolism.
- Metabolites are excreted in the urine.

Effects

- *Cardiovascular system:* at low doses, aspirin inhibits platelet COX-1 and prevents thrombosis. Aspirin does not affect blood pressure.
- *Blood:* increased bleeding time due to inhibition of platelet aggregation
- *Kidney:* no nephrotoxicity
- *Liver:* there may be dose-dependent alterations in liver function with salicylate use. These changes usually are subclinical and reversible.

Contraindications/Precautions

- Influenza-like illnesses or chickenpox in children or teenagers (up to 19 years of age), as there is an increased risk of developing Reye syndrome.
- Asthma and nasal polyps, as there is an increased likelihood of hypersensitivity reaction
- Bleeding disorders such as hemophilia, as aspirin may increase bleeding
- Alcohol use (three or more drinks/day) or peptic ulcer, as there is an increased risk of GI bleeding
- Decreased hepatic function

Toxicity

- Acute toxicity may occur in children and teenagers (Reye syndrome) and is life-threatening.
- Overdose progressively leads to tinnitus, hyperventilation, respiratory alkalosis, fever, metabolic acidosis, shock, coma, and death. Treatment is gastric lavage for acute cases, alkaline diuresis with sodium bicarbonate to increase excretion, and supportive measures.

Salicylic Acid Salts and Derivatives

Mesalamine, Olsalazine, and Sulfasalazine

Mechanism of action.   These agents do not irreversibly inhibit COX enzymes and are much less effective than aspirin as COX inhibitors. They also do not inhibit platelet aggregation.

Reye syndrome

Reye syndrome is a rare disorder that affects all organs of the body, but liver and brain involvement is the most serious. It initially presents following a viral infection. Signs and symptoms progress from vomiting, lethargy, hyperventilation, and confusion to severe mental state changes, coma, respiratory failure, multiple organ failure, and death. Treatment is supportive and includes mechanical ventilation (if necessary), insulin (to increase glucose metabolism), corticosteroids (to reduce brain swelling), and diuretics (to increase fluid loss).

Pharmacokinetics. These agents are taken orally or rectally.

Uses
- Ulcerative colitis (local effect on the GI tract)
- Crohn disease
- Rheumatoid arthritis (sulfasalazine)

Side effects
- Less frequent and minor compared with aspirin

Other Salicylates

Choline Magnesium Salicylate, Salsalate, and Diflunisal

Salsalate is the salicylate ester of salicylic acid; in vivo, the drug is hydrolyzed to two molecules of salicylate.

Diflunisal is a salicylic acid derivative but is not metabolized to salicylate.

Pharmacokinetics
- Given orally but also found in over-the-counter creams, gels, and patches for topical use

Uses
- Treatment of fever, pain, and arthritis in patients who cannot tolerate or are unresponsive to aspirin or other NSAIDs

Acetic Acids

Indomethacin

Mechanism of action. Similar to aspirin.

Uses
- Indomethacin has been the agent of choice for gout; however, there is no evidence it is superior to other NSAIDs for acute gout.
- To accelerate closure of patent ductus arteriosus (see p. 349)

Side effects. A very high percentage (35–50%) of patients receiving usual therapeutic doses of indomethacin experience untoward symptoms, and ~20% must discontinue its use because of the side effects.
- The most frequent central nervous system (CNS) effect (indeed, the most common side effect) is severe frontal headache, occurring in 25 to 50% of patients who take the drug for long periods. Dizziness, vertigo, lightheadedness, and mental confusion may occur. Seizures have been reported, as have severe depression, psychosis, hallucinations, and suicide.
- GI complaints are common and can be serious. Diarrhea may occur and sometimes is associated with ulcerative lesions of the bowel. Acute pancreatitis has been reported, as have rare but potentially fatal cases of hepatitis.
- Neutropenia, thrombocytopenia, and, rarely, aplastic anemia
  Note: Most adverse effects are dose-related.

Contraindications
- Underlying peptic ulcer disease
  Note: Caution is advised when administering indomethacin to elderly patients or to those with underlying epilepsy, psychiatric disorders, or Parkinson disease because they are at greater risk for the development of serious CNS adverse effects.

Thrombocytopenia

Thrombocytopenia is a condition in which the platelet count is low. It can be caused by the decreased production of platelets, such as in bone marrow failure, and from the destruction or consumption of platelets, for example, in disseminated intravascular coagulation (DIC), hypersplenism, and viral infections, and from drugs (e.g., indomethacin). There may be no signs and symptoms of thrombocytopenia, and it may be diagnosed incidentally when the patient's blood count is measured, or there may be signs such as spontaneous bleeding from mucous membranes (e.g., gums and nose), easy and excessive bruising, and petichiae (superficial bleeding into the skin). The underlying cause should be treated if necessary.

Table 33.1 summarizes other NSAIDs.

Table 33.1 ▶ Summary of Other NSAIDs	
Drugs	**Comments**
Diclofenac, etodolac, ketorolac, sulindac, tolmetin	These NSAIDs have greater potency against COX-2, have some COX-2 selectivity, and have less antiinflammatory activity than other NSAIDs
	They are similar to indomethacin
Ibuprofen, fenoprofen, flurbiprofen, ketoprofen, naproxen, oxaprozin	Propionic acid derivatives that differ mainly in pharmacokinetics.
Piroxicam, meloxicam	Major advantage is long duration of action
Nabumetone	Unique structure but similar activity to other NSAIDs

COX-2 Selective Inhibitor

Celecoxib

Mechanism of action. Celecoxib is a selective COX-2 inhibitor and as such inhibits the production of vascular prostaglandins, which are inhibitors of platelet aggregation and vasodilators. Unlike the nonselective NSAIDS, which inhibit both COX-1 and COX-2, celecoxib does not reduce the endogenous production of thromboxane A_2, a potent activator of platelet aggregation and a vasoconstrictor. Thus inhibition of prostacyclin without inhibition of thromboxane A_2 creates a prothrombotic state. However, the fact that it does not inhibit COX-1 leads to fewer GI side effects because it does not inhibit prostaglandins in the GI tract which maintain the normal lining of the stomach.

Side effects. Adverse cardiovascular and cerebrovascular events are more likely due to the prothrombotic state.

Note: Rofecoxib and valdecoxib have been withdrawn from the market because of the increased risk of cardiovascular events. Although celecoxib also carries such risks, it remains available, and its benefits (i.e., the reduced GI side effects) may outweigh the risks in properly selected and informed patients.

33.2 Other Analgesic-Antipyretic Drugs

Acetaminophen is excluded from the NSAID group of drugs because it does not have significant antiinflammatory activity, although it is analgesic and antipyretic.

Acetaminophen

Mechanism of action. Acetaminophen is a weak inhibitor of cyclooxygenases. Its mechanism of action is not well understood.

Pharmacokinetics
— Well absorbed following oral administration
— The primary route of metabolism is conjugation in the liver.
— Elimination is by filtration and active proximal tubular secretion into the urine.

Effects
— *Antipyretic effects:* comparable to aspirin
— *Analgesic effects:* comparable to aspirin
— *Cardiovascular system:* no effects at therapeutic doses
— *Respiratory system:* no effects at therapeutic doses
— *Blood:* no antiplatelet effects
— Acetaminophen has no significant antiinflammatory properties, which may be accounted for by the fact that it has greater activity against CNS cyclooxygenases than those in the periphery.

Uses

- Mild to moderate pain and pyrexia in patients for whom aspirin is contraindicated
- Analgesic of choice in pregnancy

    Note: Acetaminophen does not cause Reye syndrome and may be used in children.

Toxicity.   Acetaminophen has a high therapeutic index, requiring ≥ 6 g to be ingested for toxicity to occur. Hepatotoxicity is the most serious toxic effect, which is caused by the accumulation of N-acetyl-p-benzo-quinone imine (NAPQI), a toxic compound produced in small amounts during the metabolism of acetaminophen. Normally, it is immediately detoxified in the liver by conjugation with glutathione. In cases of acetaminophen overdose, glutathione may be depleted, and NAPQI may accumulate and damage the liver. Concurrent ethanol use may worsen the hepatic effect. Treat with acetylcysteine, which both replenish glutathione stores and may conjugate directly with NAPQI by serving as a glutathione substitute (only effective within 10 to 24 hours of overdose).

33.3   Drugs Used in the Treatment of Rheumatoid Arthritis

Rheumatoid arthritis (RA) is a chronic inflammatory disorder that is mainly characterized by inflammation of the synovium of joints, especially the small joints of the hands and feet. This causes all of the signs of inflammation: pain, swelling, stiffness, redness, and loss of function. The synovium thickens as the disease progresses, and inflammatory mediators erode bone and cartilage, causing deformation of the joints. There is also a systemic component to RA that is thought to be mainly due to vasculitis (inflammation of blood vessels). Weight loss, fever, and malaise are often present, and there may be cardiovascular and respiratory disease, as well as problems with the skin and eyes.

Disease-modifying Antirheumatic Drugs

Disease-modifying antirheumatic drugs (DMARDs) are commonly used with NSAIDs for the treatment of RA (**Fig. 33.3**). Corticosteroids may be used in conjunction with these agents.

Methotrexate

This agent is discussed in detail in Chapter 27.

Mechanism of action.   Methotrexate is a folic acid analogue that competitively inhibits dihydrofolate reductase, the enzyme that normally converts folate to tetrahydrofolate. This is needed for purine and thymidine synthesis.

    Note: The mechanism of action in RA is unknown.

Pharmacokinetics

- Administered orally for the treatment of RA
- Fifty percent is bound to plasma proteins (displaced by salicylates, sulfonamides, etc.).
- Excreted unchanged in urine (caution in patients with renal damage)

Uses.   Methotrexate is generally the DMARD of choice for the treatment of RA.

Side effects.   Side effects include oral and GI ulceration, bone marrow depression (dose-limiting toxicity), hepatic damage, and renal damage.

Hydroxychloroquine

Mechanism of action.   The mechanism for RA is unknown.

Pharmacokinetics

- Administered alone (in mild cases) or in combination with other antiinflammatory agents
- Clinical improvement may require 3 to 6 months of therapy.

■ Pathogenesis of rheumatoid arthritis

In RA, the immune system pathologically reacts to insults on the body by trigger factors, which may be genetic, environmental, infection, or trauma. The initial noxious stimulus causes inflammation of synovial membranes. The antigens released in this process are taken up by antigen presenting cells, and this in turn, activates lymphocytes and macrophages. The macrophages release further proinflammatory mediators, including cytokines and TNFα. Cytokines activate COX-2 and induce prostaglandin synthesis. This inflammatory response leads to a viscous circle of lymphocyte and macrophage activation. Synovial fibroblasts also proliferate during this time and release destructive enzymes. These enzymes are responsible for the characteristic inflamed pannus tissue of RA, which progressively invades joint cartilage and bone, cumulating in ankylosis and connective tissue scar formation. This causes loss of joint motion (Fig. 33.3).

■ Purines

Purines are a group of extremely biochemically significant organic compounds. The nucleic acids adenine and guanine, which comprise 50% of our DNA and RNA, are derived from purines, as well as several other important substances, for example, adenosine triphosphate (ATP), guanosine triphosphate (GTP), cyclic adenosine monophosphate (cAMP), the reduced form of nicotinamide adenine dinucleotide (NADH), and coenzyme A.

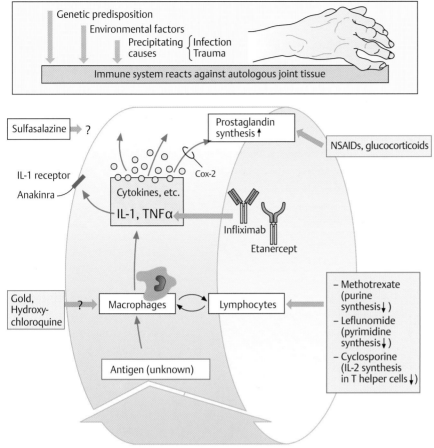

Fig. 33.3 ▶ Rheumatoid arthritis.
Refer to call-out box on p. 355 for the pathogenesis of rheumatoid arthritis. NSAIDs (COX inhibitors) and glucocorticoids inhibit prostaglandin synthesis, which provides acute relief from the inflammatory symptoms. Disease-modifying agents slow disease progression. Methotrexate and leflunomide reduce purine and pyrimidine synthesis in lymphocytes, which prevents them from replicating (due to inhibition of DNA and RNA synthesis). Cyclosporine decreases interleukin-2 (IL-2) synthesis in T helper cells. The antibodies infliximab and adalimumab and the fusion protein etanercept intercept tumor necrosis factor-α (TNFα) molecules (which are proinflammatory cytokines) and prevent them from interacting with membrane receptors on target cells. Anakinra is an analog of endogenous IL-1 antagonists. The mechanism of action of sulfasalazine is unknown.

Side effects. Serious ocular toxicity is associated with this agent but is rare at doses used for RA.

Sulfasalazine

Mechanism of action. Sulfasalazine is a prodrug that is metabolized to 5-aminosalicylate (5-ASA). 5-ASA acts within the intestinal tract (mainly the terminal ileum and colon) to inhibit prostaglandin and leukotriene synthesis, thus reducing the inflammatory reaction (see Chapter 27).

The mechanism of action of sulfasalazine in RA is unknown.

Uses
— Mild cases of RA

Side effects
— Nausea, vomiting, diarrhea, headache, and abdominal pain
— Bone marrow suppression

Gold Salts

Mechanism of action.   Gold salts have antiinflammatory properties and inhibit prostaglandin synthesis. They have no analgesic or antipyretic effects.

Uses
— Used infrequently for the treatment of inflammatory conditions
— May induce remission of RA, but the duration is highly variable. The mechanism by which they induce remission is unknown.

Side effects
— Mucocutaneous lesions, blood dyscrasias, and anaphylactoid reactions

Leflunomide

Mechanism of action.   Leflunomide is an inhibitor of pyrimidine synthesis. Its mechanism to relieve symptoms of RA is unclear, but it may inhibit the proliferation of T cells to reduce inflammation.

Pharmacokinetics
— Orally effective

Uses
— Initial monotherapy for RA instead of methotrexate, or added to methotrexate for patients who have not responded

Effects
— Reduces symptoms and improves function

Side effects
— Diarrhea occurs frequently.
— Reversible alopecia and skin rash are common.
— Hypertension
— Hepatotoxicity

Contraindications
— Pregnancy

Tumor Necrosis Factor-α (TNF-α) Inhibitors

These agents are also discussed in Chapter 34.

Etanercept, Infliximab, and Adalimumab

— Etanercept is a soluble recombinant TNF receptor: Fc fusion protein.
— Infliximab is a chimeric monoclonal antibody that binds to TNF-α.
— Adalimumab is a human monoclonal antibody to TNF.

Mechanism of action.   These agents bind to TNF-α, a proinflammatory cytokine, and prevent it from attaching to its receptor (**Fig. 33.4**).

Pharmacokinetics
— Etanercept and adalimumab are administered subcutaneously.
— Infliximab requires IV administration.

Uses.   Use of a TNF inhibitor concurrently with methotrexate is more effective for treating RA than either one alone. These drugs provide symptomatic relief in 60% of patients, but they are not curative.

Fig. 33.4 ▶ **TNF-α and inhibitors.**
TNF-α receptor activation produces a number of effects that can worsen rheumatoid arthritis (RA). TNF levels are elevated in the synovial fluid of patients with RA. Infliximab is a chimeric monoclonal antibody to TNF-α. Etanercept is a soluble recombinant TNF receptor:Fc fusion protein. Both of these drugs bind to TNF-α and prevent it from interacting with its receptor. Adalimumab (not shown) is a human monoclonal antibody to TNF-α that works like infliximab.

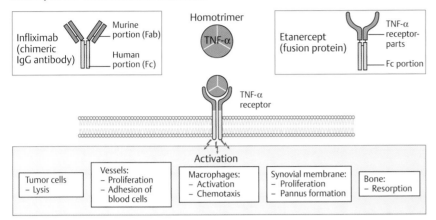

Side effects

— Minor irritation at injection sites is the most common side effect of etanercept and adalimumab.
— Increased susceptibility to bacterial and fungal infections. Serious and fatal infections have occurred.

IL-1 Antagonist

Anakinra

Anakinra is a recombinant form of the human interleukin-1 receptor antagonist IL-1 Ra.

Mechanism of action. Anakinra blocks the actions of endogenous IL-1, thereby decreasing IL-1-mediated inflammatory responses. It has shown moderate effectiveness.

Pharmacokinetics
— Given by daily subcutaneous injection

Side effects. Side effects of anakinra are the same as TNF-α inhibitors: injection site reactions and increased susceptibility to infections.

33.4 Drugs Used in the Treatment of Gout

Gout is an arthropathy caused by hyperuricemia and the deposition of uric acid crystals in the joints. It may be precipitated by trauma, surgery, starvation, infection, or diuretic therapy. It often occurs in the metatarsophalangeal joint of the great toe (hallux). Symptoms include severe pain, redness, and swelling of the affected joints. The therapy of gout involves treatment of the acute attack with colchicine and NSAIDs, and chronic treatment of the hyperuricemia.

Treatment of Acute Gout

Colchicine

Mechanism of action. Colchicine inhibits mitotic activity, neutrophil migration, and phagocytic activity in inflamed tissue (**Fig. 33.5**).

Fig. 33.5 ▶ Gout and its therapy.

Gout results from increased levels of uric acid (an end product of purine degradation). Uric acid tends to crystallize in the metatarsophalangeal joints and provides a strong stimulus for neutrophils and macrophages. Neutrophils are attracted (1) and phagocytose (2) the uric acid crystals. Neutrophils release proinflammatory cytokines (3). Macrophages also phagocytose the crystals and release lysosomal enzymes that promote inflammation. This results in an acute and very painful attack of gout (4). Colchicine and NSAIDs are used to treat acute attacks of gout. Colchicine binds to microtubular proteins and impairs their function, causing inter alia arrest of mitosis at metaphase ("spindle poison"). Its acute antigout activity is due to inhibition of neutrophil and macrophage reactions. Allopurinol is a uricostatic agent that, along with its accumulating metabolite, oxypurinol, inhibits xanthine oxidase, which catalyzes the formation of uric acid from hypoxanthine via xanthine. Uricosurics promote the renal excretion of uric acid by saturating the organic acid transport system in the renal proximal tubules, making it unavailable for uric acid resorption.

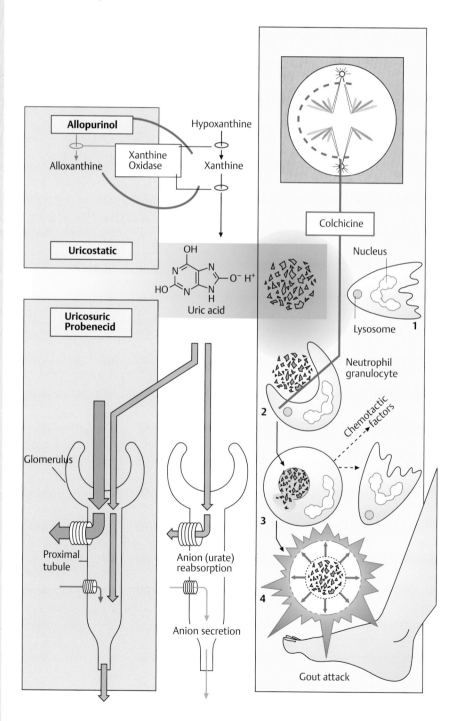

Side effects.   GI irritation, bone marrow depression, myopathy, and alopecia with long-term use.

Indomethacin and Other NSAIDs

Indomethacin (p. 353) has been the traditional NSAID used for acute gout attacks, but there is no evidence that it is superior to other NSAIDS. Ibuprofen, naproxen, and celecoxib may be just as effective.

Treatment of Chronic Gout

Probenecid and Sulfinpyrazone

Mechanism of action.   These agents block the proximal tubular reabsorption of uric acid.

Pharmacokinetics
— Rapidly absorbed orally

Side effects.
— GI irritation and allergic reactions

Contraindications.   Aspirin can impair the excretion of uric acid from the kidneys at the usual over-the-counter doses; however, low-dose aspirin taken for heart attack or stroke prevention should not significantly alter the uric acid level.

Allopurinol

Mechanism of action.   Allopurinol reduces the synthesis of uric acid by inhibiting xanthine oxidase, which is the enzyme that catalyzes the formation of uric acid from hypoxanthine via xanthine.

Side effects.   GI irritation, allergic reactions, and blood dyscrasias

Review Questions

1. A 42-year-old woman has been experiencing severe, unilateral throbbing headaches. The headaches are frequently preceded by flashing shapes of light in her vision. The headaches are accompanied by nausea, vomiting, and sensitivity to light. Which of the following might be suitable for treating this patient's headaches?
   A. Selective 5-HT_3 receptor antagonists
   B. Selective D_2 receptor antagonists
   C. Selective 5-$HT_{1B/1D}$ receptor agonists
   D. Selective calcium channel antagonists
   E. Selective H_1 receptor antagonists

2. A 62-year-old woman has been experiencing an increased frequency of migraine headaches. She has also been experiencing dyspnea on exertion and mild peripheral edema. Which of the following would be contraindicated for migraine prophylaxis for this patient?
   A. Acetaminophen
   B. Amitriptyline
   C. Aspirin
   D. Propranolol
   E. Valproate

3. Loratadine differs from most older H_1 antihistamines in that it
   A. inhibits gastric acid secretion.
   B. has few central nervous system (CNS) side effects, such as sedation.
   C. has a much shorter duration of action.
   D. does not have gastrointestinal (GI) side effects.
   E. has no tendency to induce impotence and gynecomastia in men.

4. Gynecomastia and impotence in men may occur with prolonged administration of which of the following?
   A. Diphenhydramine
   B. Cimetidine
   C. Ranitidine
   D. Loratadine
   E. Cromolyn sodium

5. A 25-year-old Hispanic woman complains of itchy, watery eyes and an itchy, runny nose. The symptoms occur in the spring and summer and become worse if she mows the lawn. Which of the following might be useful for treatment of this patient's symptoms?
   A. Diphenhydramine
   B. Ranitidine
   C. Amantadine
   D. Chlorpromazine

6. A 36-year-old man has epigastric pain he describes as burning. Which of the following drugs would be most useful to relieve the pain this patient is experiencing?
   A. Diphenhydramine
   B. Ranitidine
   C. Amantadine
   D. Chlorpromazine

7. A 58-year-old man with rheumatoid arthritis is taking antiinflammatory doses of diclofenac. The drug is available in a combination with an analog of prostaglandin E_1 (PGE_1). What is the purpose of adding a PGE_1 analogue to diclofenac?
   A. To provide a synergistic antiinflammatory effect
   B. To prevent the breakdown of diclofenac in the gastrointestinal tract
   C. To prolong the duration of action of diclofenac
   D. To prevent diclofenac from causing nephritis
   E. To protect the stomach lining from potential damage by diclofenac

8. Which of the following promote platelet aggregation?
   A. Prostaglandins
   B. Thromboxanes
   C. Prostacyclins
   D. Leukotrienes
   E. Bradykinin

9. Which of the following inhibits platelet aggregation by acetylating platelet cyclooxygenase?
   A. Aspirin
   B. Acetaminophen
   C. Celecoxib
   D. Indomethacin
   E. Ibuprofen

10. A 5-month-old infant has been crying, has a decreased appetite, and has a fever of 39°C (102°F). Which of the following antipyretics should be used?
    A. Aspirin
    B. Acetaminophen
    C. Salicylate
    D. Indomethacin
    E. Ibuprofen

11. A 48-year-old man attempts to commit suicide by taking an overdose of acetaminophen after consuming several shots of vodka. He is brought to the emergency room, and acetylcysteine is administered intravenously. What is the purpose of including acetylcysteine in the treatment regimen?
    A. To prevent cardiac failure
    B. To increase urine flow
    C. To block absorption of acetaminophen from the gastrointestinal tract
    D. To enhance metabolism of ethanol
    E. To prevent liver damage

12. A patient has mild osteoarthritis (i.e., the disease is not progressing rapidly). Her pain is no longer effectively managed with aspirin, except by doses that cause unacceptable tinnitus. Which of the following would be the best course of action for treating this patient?
    A. Stop all medications for 4 weeks, then try aspirin again.
    B. Treat with acetaminophen.
    C. Treat with morphine.
    D. Treat with naproxen.
    E. Treat with an antiinflammatory steroid.

13. Which of the following increases urinary excretion of uric acid?
    A. Probenecid
    B. Colchicine
    C. Acetaminophen
    D. Allopurinol

14. A 56-year-old man has pain, swelling, and redness in the first metatarsophalangeal joint of his right foot that began 2 days ago. He has a history of previous gout attacks. To treat the patient's symptoms, a drug may be given that does which of the following?
    A. Decreases the production of uric acid
    B. Increases the excretion of uric acid
    C. Lowers the concentration of serum uric acid
    D. Inhibits the migration of leukocytes and interrupts the inflammatory response to uric acid by reducing phagocytosis

15. Which of the following drugs is the best choice to treat severe chronic gout in the presence of impaired renal function?
    A. Naproxen
    B. Sulfinpyrazone
    C. Allopurinol
    D. Probenecid
    E. Acetaminophen

Answers and Explanations

1. **C** These are migraine symptoms that can be treated with triptans, which are selective 5-HT$_{1B/1D}$ receptor agonists (p. 340).
   A Selective 5-HT$_3$ receptor antagonists are used to prevent nausea.
   B Selective D$_2$ receptor antagonists are antipsychotics.
   D Selective calcium channel antagonists are used to treat hypertension.
   E Selective H$_1$ receptor antagonists are used to treat allergies.

2. **D** Although propranolol is used to treat migraines, it is a β-adrenergic receptor blocking agent that may have adverse effects in a patient with heart failure and/or difficulty breathing (p. 341).
   A, C Acetaminophen and aspirin are for acute treatment of pain not for prophylaxis.
   B, E Amitriptyline and valproate are used for migraine prophylaxis.

3. **B** The main difference between loratadine and the first-generation antihistamines, such as diphenhydramine and chlorpheniramine, is that loratadine does not cross the blood-brain barrier. Thus, it has fewer CNS side effects (p. 344).
   A Neither first- nor second-generation H$_1$ antihistamines inhibit gastric acid secretion; that is an H$_2$-mediated effect.
   C The duration of action of loratadine is longer than that of the H$_1$ agents.
   D Loratadine may have GI side effects.
   E None of the H$_1$ agents have a tendency to induce impotence and gynecomastia in men. These are rare side effects of cimetidine.

4. **B** These side effects have been reported with cimetidine, an H$_2$ receptor blocker, but not with the other agents listed (p. 346).

5. **A** The patient is experiencing symptoms of allergic rhinitis. Diphenhydramine is a first-generation H_1 antihistamine useful for alleviating these symptoms (p. 345).

B Ranitidine is an H_2 antihistamine used in the treatment of peptic ulcers or gastroesophageal disease.

C Amantadine is an antiviral agent.

D Chlorpromazine is an antipsychotic agent.

6. **B** The patient is having heartburn from gastroesophageal reflux, which can be treated with an H_2 antihistamine such as ranitidine which inhibits gastric acid secretions (p. 346).

A Diphenhydramine is an H_1 antihistamine that has no effect on gastric acid production.

C Amantadine is an antiviral agent.

D Chlorpromazine is an antipsychotic agent.

7. **E** Misoprostol is a synthetic PGE_1 methyl ester analogue agonist that is a potent inhibitor of gastric acid secretion. It is used for prophylaxis of gastric ulcers induced by nonsteroidal antiinflammatory agents (p. 350).

8. **B** Thromboxanes stimulate platelet aggregation (p. 349).

A, C, E Prostaglandins, prostacyclins and bradykinin inhibit platelet aggregation.

D Leukotrienes do not promote platelet aggregation.

9. **A** Aspirin inhibits the cyclooxygenase enzymes by acetylating a single serine residue. This is an irreversible covalent modification that inactivates both cyclooxygenase-1 and -2 (COX-1 and COX-2). Inhibition of platelet COX-1 prevents thrombosis (p. 351).

B Celecoxib is a COX-2 selective inhibitor

C Acetaminophen is a weak inhibitor of COX.

D, E Indomethacin and ibuprofen are competitive inhibitors of the cyclooxygenases.

10. **B** Although most of the nonsteroidal antiinflammatory drugs have some antipyretic action, aspirin is usually the antipyretic of choice. In patients younger than 19 years of age, however, aspirin and other salicylates are contraindicated in cases of fever associated with viral illness, due to an association of Reye syndrome with aspirin use in such cases. Acetaminophen is recommended to reduce fever in these cases (p. 356).

11. **E** Acetylcysteine protects against hepatic injury from the acetaminophen overdose (p. 356).

A-D The other choices are not applicable.

12. **D** Although aspirin and acetaminophen can be used as initial treatment for osteoarthritis pain, an agent such as naproxen with greater analgesic activity is often required (p. 355).

A, B In general, aspirin and acetaminophen have equal analgesic activity.

C Morphine is for severe pain and has numerous side effects.

E Long-term use of antiinflammatory steroids is not recommended due to side effects.

13. **A** Probenecid blocks the proximal tubular reabsorption of uric acid, thus increasing its excretion (p. 361).

B Colchicine inhibits mitotic activity, neutrophil migration, and phagocytic activity in inflamed tissue. It does not affect production, excretion, or serum levels of uric acid.

C Acetaminophen is an analgesic and antipyretic.

D Allopurinol reduces the synthesis of uric acid by inhibiting xanthine oxidase.

14. **D** The therapy of gout involves treatment of the acute attack with nonsteroidal antiinflammatory drugs (NSAIDs) or colchicine. Colchicine inhibits mitotic activity, neutrophil migration, and phagocytic activity in inflamed tissue. NSAIDs inhibit cyclooxygenase to reduce inflammation (p. 359).

A-C Drugs that affect uric acid production, excretion, and/or serum concentration are not effective for acute attacks but are used to treat chronic gout.

15. **C** Allopurinol is the correct choice because it reduces the synthesis of uric acid (p. 361).

A Naproxen is a nonsteroidal antiinflammatory agent that may be used to treat symptoms of an acute attack of gout.

B, D Sulfinpyrazone and probenecid block the proximal tubular reabsorption of uric acid and would be less effective in cases of impaired renal function.

E Acetaminophen is an analgesic but not an antiinflammatory agent, so it is generally not used in treating chronic gout.

34 Cancer Chemotherapy and Immunosuppressants

34.1 General Principles of Cancer Chemotherapy

Cell Cycle

An understanding of the cell cycle is essential for the effective use of anticancer agents (**Fig. 34.1**). Most anticancer drugs kill dividing cells (they are proliferation dependent); thus, tumors with a high cell turnover are most susceptible (certain leukemias and lymphomas, small proliferating tumors, "recruited" tumor cells, and micrometastases). The killing of tumor cells follows first-order kinetics. To produce a cure, therapy must continue until the final tumor cell has been eradicated. Agents that act preferentially on tumor cells in a given phase of the cell cycle are called *cell cycle specific*. Agents that act during several stages of the cell cycle are called *cell cycle nonspecific*.

Anticancer Drugs

Several neoplastic diseases can be cured with drugs alone or with a combination of drugs and other treatment modalities. Examples of these neoplastic diseases include choriocarcinoma, Hodgkin disease, acute lymphocytic leukemia, Burkitt lymphoma, and testicular carcinoma. Adjuvant chemotherapy in combination with surgery and/or radiotherapy has increased survival rates for several solid tumors; however, the most prevalent forms of human cancer respond poorly or not at all to chemotherapy.

Drug treatment regimens for cancer usually involve combinations of agents given intermittently. Combining drugs with different mechanisms of action can produce larger therapeutic effects with fewer side effects. Intermittent therapy allows the patient to recover from drug toxicities, such as bone marrow suppression, between courses.

Fig. 34.1 ▶ **Cell cycle.**
The cell cycle describes the cellular events that take place, cumulating in cell division. It is divided into four phases: G_1, S, G_2, and M. Fully differentiated cells are in the G_0 stage when further cell division does not usually occur (hence, it is not part of the cell cycle). However, cells in the G_0 phase can reenter the G_1 phase if acted upon by certain mitotic signals (e.g., tumor viruses and cytokines). In the G_1 phase, the cell is growing and accumulating proteins and RNA. The restriction point in the G_1 phase is a control point that ensures that everything is ready for DNA synthesis, which occurs in the S phase. In the G_2 phase, the cell is preparing for mitosis, which occurs in the M phase, producing two daughter cells.

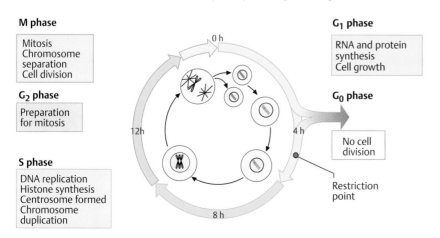

M phase
Mitosis
Chromosome separation
Cell division

G₂ phase
Preparation for mitosis

S phase
DNA replication
Histone synthesis
Centrosome formed
Chromosome duplication

G₁ phase
RNA and protein synthesis
Cell growth

G₀ phase
No cell division

Restriction point

0 h
12h
4 h
8 h

Tumor development

Tumors develop when the normal regulation of the balance between cell proliferation (mitosis) and programmed cell death (apoptosis) is lost. Tumor initiation is the process by which normal cells are changed so that they are able to form tumors. This involves DNA damage of multiple genes (6–10). Substances that cause cancer can be tumor initiators. Tumor promotion is the process by which existing tumors are stimulated to grow. Tumor promoters are not able to cause tumors to form, but increase the frequency of tumor formation in tissue previously exposed to the tumor initiator.

Chemical carcinogenesis

Many chemicals that are present as industrial or environmental pollutants, dietary components, combustion by-products, or therapeutic agents may increase the risk of cancer development. Genotoxic carcinogens are thought to initiate tumorigenesis by interacting with DNA. Chemicals may be inherently genotoxic, but many chemical carcinogens are metabolized to highly reactive metabolites, which in turn damage DNA. Alternatively, chemicals could act by altering DNA replication or repair. Epigenetic carcinogens do not appear to interact directly with DNA, but instead appear to augment neoplastic growth by poorly defined mechanisms. This class of carcinogens includes various hormones (e.g., estrogen and diethylstilbestrol), immunosuppressive drugs (e.g., azathioprine), solid-state carcinogens (e.g., asbestos), and promoting agents (agents that increase tumor development when given after a genotoxic chemical).

Cancer critical genes

The two main types of genes that are now recognized as playing a role in cancer are oncogenes and tumor suppressor genes. Most oncogenes are mutations of normal genes called *proto-oncogenes*. The mutant proteins coded by oncogenes (oncoproteins) are overactive and allow cells to proliferate when they should not. The protein products of tumor suppressor genes are normal genes that slow down cell division, repair DNA mistakes, and tells when to undergo apoptosis (programmed cell death). These genes are deleted or inactivated in cancer cells, allowing unregulated proliferation.

P53 gene

P53 is a tumor suppressor gene that codes for a transcription factor that regulates the expression of other genes and arrests the cell cycle. It is the most frequently mutated gene in human cancers. Mutations in *p53* have been associated with carcinogenesis at multiple sites within the body.

Tumor markers

Tumor markers are substances that can be detected in the peripheral blood and are derived from neoplastic populations, but lack functional hormonal or other physiologic activity. They include carcinoembryonic antigen (CEA), seen in colon, gastric, pancreatic, and breast carcinoma; prostate-specific antigen (PSA), seen in prostate carcinoma; cancer antigen 125 (CA-125), seen in ovarian carcinoma; alpha fetoprotein (AFP), seen in hepatocellular carcinoma and germ cell neoplasms, especially yolk sac carcinoma; and human chorionic gonadotropin (hCG), seen in choriocarcinoma testicular germ cell neoplasms. In general, serum tumor markers are characterized by low sensitivity and low specificity. Nonetheless, they are employed routinely for several purposes, including screening, monitoring therapy, and detection of recurrences.

Radiotherapy and its systemic effects

Radiotherapy involves the use of focused ionizing radiation to treat malignant cancer cells by damaging their DNA. It can be curative, used as an adjuvant therapy, or employed in palliative therapy to limit disease progression or to provide symptomatic relief. The systemic effects of radiation include several syndromes. Hematopoietic syndrome (200–500 rads) is development of a pancytopenia within a few weeks of exposure. Bleeding and infection are the major complications. Gastrointestinal (GI) syndrome (500–1000 rads) reflects injury to the GI epithelium, resulting in the development of nausea, vomiting, and severe diarrhea within several days of exposure. This may lead to severe metabolic disturbances, vascular collapse, sepsis, and death. Cerebral syndrome (> 2500 rads) is caused by vascular endothelial damage, resulting in cerebral edema, convulsions, coma, and death within hours of exposure.

Local effects of radiotherapy

Depending on the tissues involved, acute radiation injury may manifest as an acute dermatitis, pneumonitis, and/or enteritis. Chronic changes reflect organ ischemia due to vasculopathy (endothelium is highly radiation sensitive). Neoplasms (primarily sarcomas) may develop even after an interval of 10 years or more. Acutely, blood vessels may dilate, thrombose, or rupture. Over time, however, reactive endothelial cell proliferation and mural scarring may lead to narrowing or even obliteration of the vessel lumens, causing tissue ischemia. The chronic effects of radiation injury, therefore, include interstitial fibrosis of various tissues and strictures of hollow organs.

Toxicity of Anticancer Drugs

Anticancer drugs generally have low therapeutic indices and potentially lethal toxicities. Many of the toxic effects of anticancer drugs are due to cytotoxic effects on normal tissues that have high proportions of dividing cells (**Fig. 34.2**).
— Anticancer drugs frequently produce nausea and vomiting, which can be ameliorated with phenothiazines or cannabinoids.
— The release of nucleic acid breakdown products following a very large cell kill from anticancer drugs can result in hyperuricemia and renal damage. Hyperuricemia is prevented with allopurinol (see Chapter 33 for details of this drug).
— Many anticancer drugs are mutagenic and carcinogenic.

Combination Therapy

When selecting a combination of anticancer drugs, they should ideally have the following attributes:
— They should be effective when used alone.
— They should have different mechanisms of action.

Fig. 34.2 ▶ **Chemotherapy of tumors: principle and adverse effects.**
Chemotherapeutic agents lack specificity and thus affect both malignant and endogenous cells. Because cytostatic agents act on proliferating or dividing (mitotic) cells, rapidly dividing malignant cells are preferentially injured (growth is retarded, and apoptosis is initiated). Endogenous tissues with a high mitotic rate (hair and epithelial cells) are also injured. In bone marrow, inhibition of mitosis causes neutropenia (producing a lowered resistance to infection), thrombocytopenia (producing an increased bleeding tendency), and anemia (producing fatigue, shortness of breath, dizziness, etc.). Infertility is also common due to suppression of spermatogenesis and follicle maturation. Healthy tissues and those with a low mitotic rate are largely unaffected by cytostatic agents.

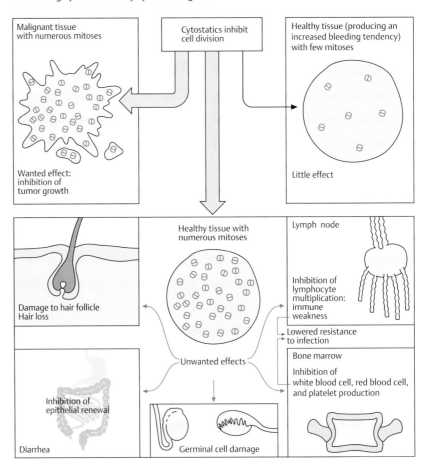

- They should have minimally overlapping toxicities.
- There should be no cross-resistance.

This means that doses close to the regular doses for each drug as a single agent can be used to optimize the cytotoxic effects without additive toxicity. Drug resistance is the greatest obstacle to successful chemotherapy.

Drug Resistance

When tumor cells lack sensitivity to a drug, the drug resistance is termed *primary* or *natural.* Acquired drug resistance occurs when tumor cells undergo genotypic and phenotypic changes during therapy that render them insensitive to the drug (**Fig. 34.3**).

The Goldie–Coldman hypothesis states that the probability of tumor containing a cell resistant to a specific drug is related to both tumor size and mutation frequency. Even the smallest detectable cancer would be expected to contain at least one drug-resistant cell. Drug exposure then provides the selection pressure for growth of a resistant cell population. Drug resistance may be to a single or multiple drugs. Common mechanisms include decreased drug uptake, increased drug metabolism, and increased drug efflux from the cell. Increased drug efflux results from increased expression of P-glycoprotein and multidrug resistance protein and leads to multidrug resistance.

Fig. 34.3 ▶ **Mechanisms of cytostatic resistance.**
The initial success of cytostatic agents can be followed by diminution of effect because of the emergence of resistant tumor cells. Genotypic and phenotypic changes may lead to reduced uptake of the drug into cancer cells, increased efflux of the drug from cells, diminished activation of prodrugs, and increased DNA repair.

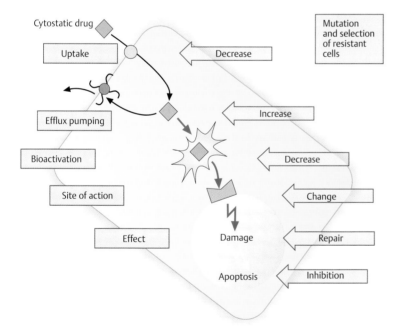

34.2   Cancer Chemotherapy Drugs

Alkylating Agents

Mechanism of action.   Alkylating agents bind covalently to guanine nucleotides of DNA and cross-link DNA strands. This prevents DNA replication and transcription to produce cytotoxicity (**Fig. 34.4**). They are proliferation dependent but cell cycle nonspecific.

Benign versus malignant neoplasms

The distinction between benign and malignant tumors is based on their microscopic appearance, which predicts clinical behavior. It reflects the degree of cellular differentiation, the extent to which neoplastic cells resemble their mature counterparts. Benign neoplasms are well differentiated (i.e., closely resemble mature cells of origin); hence, features such as gland formation are retained. Malignant cells, however, exhibit incomplete or lack of differentiation (anaplasia), and thus resemble stem cells. Anaplasia is characterized by cellular and nuclear pleomorphism (due to alterations in the cell cytoskeleton), increased nuclear/cytoplasmic ratio, increased nuclear chromatin density and bizarre mitoses (due to chromosomal aneuploidy), and loss of cellular orientation. Rate of growth tends to parallel the degree of differentiation of the neoplastic cells, as well as the cell turnover rate of the cell of origin. Thus, benign neoplasms have slow growth. Malignant neoplasms are characterized by a wide range of growth rates. Neoplasms derived from rapidly cycling populations (e.g., bone marrow and GI tract) grow much more rapidly than slowly proliferating tissues (e.g., prostate and salivary gland).

Fig. 34.4 ▶ Cytostatics: alkylating agents and cytostatic antibiotics (1), inhibitors of tetrahydrofolate synthesis (2), and antimetabolites (3).
Mitosis is preceded by protein synthesis (RNA synthesis) and chromosomal replication (DNA synthesis). Existing DNA (*gray*) acts as a template for new DNA (*blue*). Alkylating agents (1) form covalent bonds with DNA, cross-linking it, and thus rendering it impossible to "unzip" and replicate. DNA strand breakage may also occur with some cytostatic antibiotics and topoisomerase inhibitors. Methotrexate is an antimetabolite (2) that inhibits dihydrofolate reductase, suppressing the production of purine and thymine nucleotides. Other antimetabolites (3) are purine and pyrimidine analogues that inhibit DNA/RNA synthesis or lead to the production of incorrect nucleic acids.

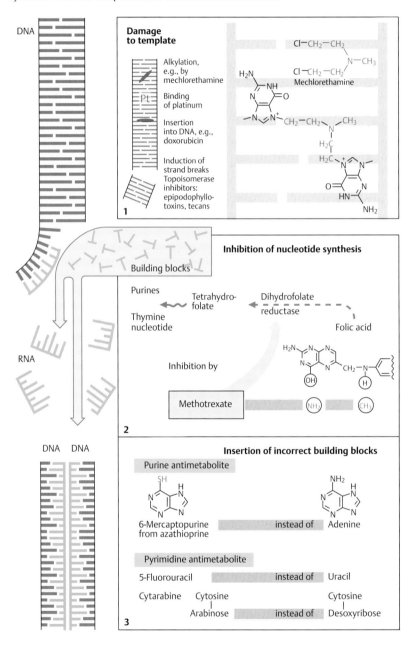

Resistance.   High rates of DNA repair may be a cause of resistance.

Mechlorethamine

Mechlorethamine was the first anticancer drug to be used clinically, but it has largely been replaced by drugs that are better tolerated.

Pharmacokinetics
— Administered intravenously (IV)
— Highly reactive (the active drug has a very short half-life)
— A potent vesicant (i.e., it can cause chemical burns, resulting in large water blisters on contact with skin)

Uses.   Mechlorethamine's main use is in the mechlorethamine, oncovin, procarbazine, and prednisone (MOPP) regimen for treatment of Hodgkin disease.

Side effects
— Bone marrow depression (leading to leucopenia and thrombocytopenia) is dose-limiting.
— Severe nausea and vomiting may occur.

Cyclophosphamide and Ifosfamide

Cyclophosphamide is the most widely used alkylating agent. Ifosfamide is an analogue of cyclophosphamide.

Pharmacokinetics
— Effective orally or IV
— Require cytochrome P-450−mediated metabolism for activation
— Nonvesicant

Uses
— Leukemia, lymphoma, ovarian cancer, breast cancer, and for solid tumors in children (cyclophosphamide in combination with other drugs)
— Prevention of organ rejection after transplantation (cyclophosphamide)
— Immune disorders, such as Wegener granulomatosis, rheumatoid arthritis, and systemic lupus erythematosus (cyclophosphamide)
— Ifosfamide is approved as third-line therapy for testicular cancer, but it can also be used to treat the diseases for which cyclophosphamide is indicated.

Side effects
— Bone marrow depression is dose-limiting.
— Alopecia and immunosuppression are prominent.
— Renal excretion of metabolites causes hemorrhagic cystitis. This can be prevented with adequate prophylactic hydration.
— Isofosfamide has greater myelosuppressant, renal, and neurologic side effects.

Carmustine and Lomustine

These drugs have a nitrosoureas structure.

Pharmacokinetics
— These agents are highly lipophilic and cross the blood−brain barrier.
— Carmustine is given IV, and lomustine is given orally.

Uses
— Central nervous system (CNS) malignancies
— Hodgkin disease

Side effects.   Bone marrow depression is delayed and may be prolonged.

◼ Hodgkin disease

Hodgkin disease is a type of lymphoma (tumor of lymphocytes). On histological examination, there are characteristic cells (Reed−Sternberg cells) that have mirror image nuclei. Patients present with enlarged, painless lymph nodes in the neck or axillae, as well as fever, weight loss, night sweats, and general malaise (in 25%). Treatment depends on the stage of the disease but may involve radiotherapy and/or chemotherapy. This is one of the more treatable forms of cancer, with survival rates of up to 90% if detected early.

◼ Chemotherapy wafer implants

Chemotherapy wafer implants are a new way of administering chemotherapy for certain brain tumors (gliomas and glioblastoma multiforme). Brain surgery is performed to remove all or most of the tumor, and the wafer is placed in the resulting space, where the drug (carmustine) slowly leaches out and treats the tumor locally. All of the usual chemotherapy side effects are still seen with this method of drug delivery.

Cisplatin, Carboplatin, and Oxaliplatin

Mechanism of action. Each of these agents consists of a complex of inorganic platinum ions. They act by forming DNA cross-links, which prevents DNA replication and transcription.

Pharmacokinetics
— Administered IV
— Bind to plasma proteins (90%)
— Concentrate in the liver, kidneys, intestines, and ovaries
— Excreted in the urine

Uses. Solid tumors, especially testicular, ovarian, and bladder cancer.

Side effects
— Renal damage (dose-limiting). This can be decreased by prehydration and concomitant mannitol diuresis.
— Moderate bone marrow depression, ototoxicity (damage to the inner ear by a toxin), hypomagnesemia, and hypocalcemia

Busulfan

Pharmacokinetics
— Given orally

Uses
— Chronic granulocytic leukemia

Side effects
— Bone marrow depression is selective for granulocytes (neutrophils, basophils, and eosinophils).
— Leukopenia (decreased number of white blood cells) and skin pigmentation may occur.

Procarbazine

Mechanism of action. Procarbazine's mechanism of action is unclear.

Pharmacokinetics
— Administered orally
— It must undergo metabolic activation.
— It is not cross-resistant with other alkylating agents.

Side effects
— Bone marrow depression is dose-limiting.
— CNS depression may occur (synergistic with phenothiazines and barbiturates).

Antimetabolites

Mechanism of action. These drugs include purine, pyrimidine, and folate analogues that act primarily by inhibiting DNA synthesis. They inhibit cells in the S phase (except fluorouracil, which has no clear-cut phase specificity) and may be incorporated into DNA and RNA. These drugs are converted by the cells to lethal metabolites (**Fig. 34.4**).

Methotrexate

Methotrexate is also discussed in Chapters 27 and 33.

Mechanism of action. Methotrexate is a folic acid analogue that competitively inhibits dihydrofolate reductase, the enzyme that normally converts folate to tetrahydrofolate, which is needed for purine and thymidine synthesis. This results in reduced DNA, RNA, and protein synthesis (**Fig. 34.4**).

Bone marrow function

There are two types of bone marrow: red and yellow. Red bone marrow contains myeloid tissue and produces red blood cells, most white blood cells, and platelets. Yellow bone marrow is largely made up of fat cells. At birth, all bone marrow is red, but in adults, it has been reduced by approximately half and is generally found in the flat bones, such as the hip, skull, vertebrae, and sternum, along with the cancellous ends of the long bones.

Pharmacokinetics
- Administered orally, IV, or intrathecally
- It is poorly transported across the blood–brain barrier unless given in high concentrations or administered intrathecally.
- Fifty percent is bound to plasma proteins (displaced by salicylates, sulfonamides, etc.).
- Excreted unchanged in urine (so it should be used with caution in patients with renal damage)

Uses
- Drug of choice for gestational choriocarcinoma
- Acute lymphocytic leukemia (in children)
- Burkitt lymphoma
- Breast cancer
- Psoriasis
- Rheumatoid arthritis
- Inflammatory bowel disease
  Note: It is sometimes used in very high doses with leucovorin, an active form of folate, to prevent damage to normal cells.

Side effects
- Bone marrow depression (dose-limiting toxicity)
- Oral and GI ulceration
- Hepatic damage
- Renal damage (due to precipitation of crystallized metabolites in the kidney)

Mercaptopurine

Mechanisms of action. Mercaptopurine is a purine analogue that causes pseudofeedback inhibition of the first step in purine biosynthesis and inhibition of purine interconversions. This leads to the insertion of the incorrect bases into DNA (**Fig. 34.4**).

Pharmacokinetics
- Administered orally
- Metabolism to inactive products is inhibited by allopurinol.

Uses
- Acute lymphoid leukemia

Side effects. Side effects include bone marrow depression (major toxicity) and liver damage.

Thioguanine

Thioguanine has similar pharmacological properties to mercaptopurine except that allopurinol does not interfere with its inactivation.

Fluorouracil

Mechanism of action. Fluorouracil is a pyrimidine analogue that is converted to 5-fluodeoxyuridine monophosphate, causing inhibition of thymidylate synthesis. DNA synthesis is therefore reduced due to a lack of thymidine. It also forms 5-fluodeoxyuridine triphosphate, which is incorporated into RNA and blocks translation. There is no cell cycle phase specificity.
- Leucovorin is also used in combination with fluorouracil. While it protects normal cells from damage by methotrexate, leucovorin potentiates the effectiveness of fluorouracil, presumably by providing active folate as a cofactor for the interaction of fluorouracil with thymidylate synthase.

Pharmacokinetics

— Administered IV
— Able to enter the cerebrospinal fluid (CSF)
— Rapidly metabolized in the liver

Uses

— Breast, pancreatic, colorectal, and gastric cancer

Side effects

— Oral and GI ulcers
— Bone marrow depression (dose-limiting toxicity)
— Neurologic defects (cerebellar)
— Hyperpigmentation
— Alopecia

Capecitabine

Mechanism of action.   Capecitabine is a prodrug for fluorouracil and therefore acts similarly.

Uses

— Advanced colon and breast cancer

Fludarabine and Cladribine

Mechanism of action.   These agents are purine analogue antagonists that cause a reduction in DNA synthesis.

Uses

— Chronic lymphocytic leukemia and some non–Hodgkin lymphomas (fludarabine)
— Hairy cell leukemia (cladribine)

Cytarabine and Gemcitabine

Mechanism of action.   Cytarabine and gemcitabine are metabolized to cytidine analogues that block DNA synthesis by inhibiting DNA polymerases and by becoming incorporated into DNA, preventing further elongation of the DNA.

Pharmacokinetics

— Administered IV
— Rapidly deaminated in the liver, plasma, and other tissues

Uses

— Acute lymphoid leukemia, acute myeloid leukemia, chronic myeloid leukemia, and meningeal leukemia (cytarabine)
— Advanced pancreatic, breast, ovarian, and non–small cell lung cancers (gemcitabine)

Side effects

— Bone marrow depression (major toxicity)
— Oral ulceration
— Liver dysfunction

Antibiotics

Antibiotic treatment of infections is discussed in Chapter 29. The agents discussed in this section are used to treat cancer. They act by binding to DNA (noncovalently by intercalation) and altering its function. They are cycle nonspecific (**Fig. 34.4**).

■ Tumor grading

Grade refers to a microscopic pathologic determination of tumor aggressiveness based on the degree of differentiation of the neoplastic cells and the number of mitoses. Most tumors are graded from 1 (low grade, well differentiated) through 3 (high grade, undifferentiated). Some malignant neoplasms progress to a higher grade over time as less differentiated clones of cells become dominant. Criteria for grading include mitotic rate, nuclear pleomorphism, and architectural features (e.g., preservation of gland formation).

■ Tumor staging

Stage refers to a clinical and pathologic determination of tumor extent based on the size of the neoplasm, the presence or absence of regional lymph node metastases, and the presence or absence of distant metastases. This is the basis of the tumor size, node involvement, metastasis (TNM) staging system. Tumors are staged numerically from 0 through IV as follows:
0: in situ
I: small, organ confined
II: large or regional node metastases
III: invasion of adjacent organs
IV: distant metastases
In general, stage has greater prognostic value than grade.

Dactinomycin (Actinomycin D)

Mechanisms of action. Dactinomycin intercalates between G-C pairs in double-stranded DNA and inhibits DNA-directed RNA synthesis. It is equally cytotoxic to proliferating and stationary cells.

Pharmacokinetics
— Administered IV (can cause local inflammation and phlebitis)

Side effects. Side effects include bone marrow depression (toxicity is dose limiting), oral and GI ulceration, and alopecia.

Doxorubicin

Mechanisms of action
— Inhibition of DNA and RNA synthesis due to intercalation
— DNA fragmentation from reactive oxygen species
— Inhibition of DNA topoisomerase II
— Interaction with cell membranes, causing a broad spectrum of antitumor activity

Pharmacokinetics
— Administered IV (extravasation leads to severe local reaction and necrosis)
— Extensively metabolized in the liver and excreted into the bile (decreased dose in the presence of hepatic dysfunction)
— Drug and metabolites color urine red.

Uses. Doxorubicin has a broad spectrum of activity and is used in the following cancers:
— Acute lymphoid leukemia, chronic lymphoid leukemia, and acute myeloid leukemia
— Breast, stomach, bone, thyroid, kidney, liver, and pancreatic cancers

Side effects
— Bone marrow depression is their major toxicity (except for bleomycin). This is dose-limiting.
— Cardiotoxicity (refractory congestive heart failure). This is due to avid uptake by and oxidative damage to heart muscle. The damage caused is potentially irreversible and can be delayed many months. It is related to the total dose administered.
— Alopecia, stomatitis (inflammation of the mucosa of the mouth), fever, and chills

Daunorubicin

Daunorubicin is similar to doxorubicin but has a narrower spectrum of activity.

Idarubicin

Idarubicin is an analogue of daunorubicin used in combination with therapy for acute lymphoid leukemia.

Bleomycin

Mechanism of action. Bleomycin is a mixture of complex glycopeptides that causes strand scission of DNA by producing reactive oxygen species. It is unusual in that it produces very little bone marrow depression.

Pharmacokinetics
— Administered IV
— Enzymatically inactivated in several tissues (toxicity occurs in tissues with low inactivating activity, i.e., lungs and skin)
— Fifty percent is excreted unchanged in the urine.

Uses
— Hodgkin and non–Hodgkin lymphomas
— Testicular cancer
— Squamous cell carcinomas of the head, neck, nasopharynx, penis, vulva, and cervix

Side effects
— Pulmonary toxicity (pneumonitis and fibrosis) is dose-limiting.
— The more common toxic effects involve the skin and mucous membranes.
— Alopecia and stomatitis

Topoisomerase Inhibitors

Etoposide and Teniposide

Mechanism of action.   These agents inhibit topoisomerase II, which acts on single-stranded DNA to cause strand breakage (**Fig. 34.4**).

Uses
— Small cell lung cancer, testicular carcinoma, acute nonlymphocytic leukemia, and malignant lymphoma (etoposide)
— First-line therapy for neuroblastoma and retinoblastoma in combination with other agents
— Refractory leukemias (teniposide)

Side effects
— Nausea and vomiting (short term)
— Alopecia and myelosuppression (longer term)

Irinotecan and Topotecan

Mechanism of action.   Irinotecan and topotecan inhibit topoisomerase I, which acts on double-stranded DNA to induce strand breakage.

Uses
— Metastatic colorectal cancer (irinotecan)
— Ovarian and small cell lung cancers (topotecan)

Side effects.   Side effects are the same as for etoposide and teniposide.

Antimitotics

Mechanism of action.   Antimitotic agents bind to tubulin, inhibiting mitotic spindles and arresting cell development in the M phase of the cell cycle.

The vinca alkaloids vincristine and vinblastine are structurally similar but have different activities and toxicities and show no cross-resistance.

Pharmacokinetics
— Administered IV (extravasation and subsequent local reactions may occur)
— Excreted into bile (use with caution in patients with obstructive jaundice)

Vincristine

Uses
— Acute leukemia
— Hodgkin disease
— Nephroblastoma (Wilms tumor)
— Rhabdomyosarcoma

Topoisomerase

DNA is arranged as in a double helix formation, which is then supercoiled or knotted in chromosomes. This is a very stable and efficient way to store our genetic information. To avoid having to uncoil and unwind entire lengths of DNA, topoisomerase enzymes bind to DNA and cut the phosphate backbone, thus allowing specific sections to uncoil and unwind for transcription and replication to occur. They reconnect the DNA strands when the process is finished.

Nephroblastoma (Wilms tumor)

Nephroblastoma (Wilms tumor) is a malignant renal tumor composed of mixed embryonal cell elements. Increased mature elements and decreased anaplastic cells are indicative of the best prognosis. Signs and symptoms include painless hematuria, abdominal pain, an enlarged abdomen, and a palpable abdominal mass. Computed tomography scans or magnetic resonance imaging of the abdomen is diagnostic for a mass. Hematuria is seen with urinalysis. Treatment includes surgery (nephrectomy), radiation therapy, and chemotherapy. The prognosis for 2-year survival (with favorable histology) is 95% for stage I, II, and III tumors and 50% for stage IV tumors.

Side effects
— Neurologic toxicities are dose-limiting. Suppression of the Achilles tendon reflex and paresthesias appear first, followed by other peripheral neuropathies, neuritic pain, constipation, and disorders of cranial nerve function.
— Alopecia
— Mild bone marrow depression (vincristine is considered to be marrow-sparing compared with other agents)

Vinblastine

Uses
— Some lymphomas and solid tumors

Side effects
— Bone marrow depression (dose-limiting)
— Neuropathy is less frequent and less serious than with vincristine
— Alopecia, stomatitis, and peripheral neuropathy

Vinorelbine

Vinorelbine is a semisynthetic derivative of vinblastine.

Pharmacokinetics
— Given orally

Uses
— Non-small cell lung cancer

Side effects.   They are similar to vinblastine.

Taxanes

Paclitaxel and Docetaxel

Mechanism of action.   These drugs promote the assembly of microtubules from tubulin dimers and stabilize microtubules by preventing depolymerization. This prevents reorganization of the microtubule network for mitosis.

Uses
— Breast cancer
— Lung cancer
— Ovarian cancer

Side effects
— Bone marrow suppression
— Moderate nausea and vomiting
— Alopecia
— Sensory neuropathy
— Hypersensitivity to the drug

Monoclonal Antibodies

Mechanism of action.   Monoclonal antibodies bind specifically to proteins on cancer cells, resulting in inhibition of growth and antibody-dependent cellular cytotoxicity. Labeling the antibodies with radioactive isotopes allows the bound antibody to specifically deliver the radioactivity to target cells.

Pharmacokinetics.   These agents must be given IV.

Achilles tendon reflex

The Achilles tendon reflex is plantar (downward) flexion extension of the foot resulting from contraction of the calf muscles following a sharp blow to the Achilles tendon. This reflex is suppressed by vincristine.

Rituximab

Mechanism of action.   Rituximab binds to CD20, which is found on pre-B and mature B lymphocytes. It is also expressed on > 90% of B cell non–Hodgkin lymphomas, but not expressed on hematopoietic stem cells, pro-B cells, normal plasma cells, or other normal tissues.

Pharmacokinetics
— Given by slow IV infusion to prevent adverse reactions

Uses
— B-cell lymphoma
— Chronic lymphoblastic leukemia

Side effects
— Changes in blood pressure
— GI upset: nausea and vomiting
— Neurologic effects including weakness, dizziness, headache, and sensory neuropathy
— Fever and shivering

Tositumomab and Iodine 131 Tositumomab

Mechanism of action.   Tositumomab and iodine 131 tositumomab bind to CD20.

Uses
— B-cell lymphoma

Side effects
— Diarrhea

Indium 111 Ibritumomab and Yttrium 90 Ibritumomab Tiuxetan

Mechanism of action.   Indium 111 ibritumomab and yttrium 90 ibritumomab tiuxetan bind to CD20.

Uses
— B-cell lymphoma

Side effects
— Severe allergic reactions have been observed.
— Severe hematological reactions, including anemia, leukopenia, thrombocytopenia, and bone marrow suppression
— Nausea and vomiting
— Weakness, dizziness, headache, and sensory neuropathy
— Fever and shivering

Alemtuzumab

Mechanism of action.   Alemtuzumab binds to CD52, which is present on the surface of essentially all B and T lymphocytes, a majority of monocytes, macrophages, and NK cells, and a subpopulation of granulocytes.

Uses
— B-cell chronic lymphocytic leukemia
— T-cell lymphoma

Side effects
— Changes in blood pressure
— Severe hematological reactions, including anemia, leukopenia, thrombocytopenia, and bone marrow suppression
— Diarrhea, nausea, and vomiting

— Weakness, dizziness, and headache
— Fever and shivering
— Infection and viremia

Trastuzumab

Mechanism of action.   Trastuzumab binds to HER2/neu (ErbB-2) protein, which is overexpressed in 25 to 30% of primary breast cancers.

Uses
— Breast cancer

Side effects
— Edema
— Rash
— Diarrhea, nausea, and vomiting
— Weakness, dizziness, headache, and backache or muscle pain
— Fever and shivering
— Cough, dyspnea, rhinitis, and pharyngitis

Cetuximab

Mechanism of action.   Cetuximab binds to epidermal growth factor receptor (EGFR), which has been detected in many human cancers, including those of the colon and rectum.

Uses
— Colorectal cancer
— Head and neck cancers

Side effects
— Rash
— Hypomagnesemia
— Constipation, diarrhea, nausea, and vomiting
— Fatigue, pain, headache, and insomnia
— Fever and shivering
— Cough, dyspnea, and pharyngitis

Bevacizumab

Mechanism of action.   Bevacizumab binds to vascular endothelial growth factor (VEGF) prevents the proliferation of endothelial cells and formation of new blood vessels, thus starving tumors of their blood supply.

Uses
— Colorectal cancer
— Lung cancer
— Breast cancer
— Pancreatic cancer

Side effects
— Hypertension
— Alopecia
— Hypokalemia
— Constipation, diarrhea, nausea, anorexia, and stomatitis
— Fatigue, pain, headache, and sensory neuropathy
— Epistaxis
— Hemorrhage

Gemtuzumab Ozogamicin

Mechanism of action.   Gemtuzumab ozogamicin binds to CD33 expressed on hematopoietic cells. The receptor is then internalized. Upon internalization, the ozogamicin portion of the molecule is released inside the lysosomes of the myeloid cell and binds to DNA to cause cell death.

Uses
— Acute myeloid leukemia

Side effects
— Shivering, nausea, fever, and bone marrow suppression

Table 34.1 provides a summary of the monoclonal antibody agents, the antigen on cancer cells that they bind to, and their uses.

Table 34.1 ▶ **Summary of Monoclonal Antibodies**		
Agent	**Antigen**	**Uses**
Rituximab	CD20	B-cell lymphoma and chronic lymphoblastic leukemia
Tositumomab and iodine 131 tositumomab	CD20	B-cell lymphoma
Indium 111 ibritumomab and yttrium 90 ibritumomab tiuxetan	CD20	B-cell lymphoma
Alemtuzumab	CD52	B-cell CLL and T-cell lymphoma
Trastuzumab	HER2/neu (ErbB-2)	Breast cancer
Cetuximab	EGFR (ErbB-1)	Colorectal, head and neck
Bevacizumab	VEGF	Colorectal, lung, breast, pancreatic
Gemtuzumab ozogamicin	CD33	Acute myeloid leukemia

Abbreviations: CLL, chronic lymphocytic leukemia; EGFR, epidermal growth factor receptor; VEGF, vascular endothelial growth factor.

Tyrosine Kinase Inhibitors

Tyrosine kinase inhibitors target receptor tyrosine kinases on the membranes of cancer cells, inhibiting their activity and thus decreasing cancer cell growth.

Imatinib

Mechanism of action.   Imatinib is a selective inhibitor of the tyrosine kinase activity of the bcr-abl protein, which is the product of the Philadelphia chromosome. It is present in virtually all patients with chronic myelogenous leukemia and some patients with acute lymphoblastic leukemia (**Fig. 34.5**).

Pharmacokinetics
— Given orally

Uses
— Chronic myelogenous leukemia
— Acute lymphoblastic leukemia

Side effects
— Edema, nausea, and vomiting

Dasatinib

Mechanism of action.   Dasatinib is a tyrosine kinase inhibitor active against bcr-abl and Src family kinases. Dasatinib is more potent than imatinib, and it inhibits mutated forms of bcr-abl that are resistant to imatinib.

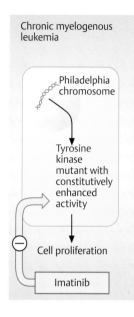

Fig. 34.5 ▶ **Targeting of the chemotherapeutic drug imatinib.** Targeted treatment of cancer can occur when cancer cells display metabolic properties that are different from those of healthy cells. Patients with chronic myelogenous leukemia almost always possess the Philadelphia chromosome. This recombinant gene encodes a tyrosine kinase mutant with unregulated, enhanced activity, causing cell proliferation. Imatinab specifically inhibits this mutant tyrosine kinase, thus inhibiting cell proliferation.

Uses
— Acute lymphoblastic leukemia and chronic myelogenous leukemia that is resistant to imatinib

Gefitinib and Erlotinib

Mechanism of action.   Gefitinib and erlotinib are selective EGFR tyrosine kinase inhibitors. They block EGFR-mediated signal transduction pathways involved in tumor growth.

Uses
— Non−small cell lung cancer in patients with advanced forms who have failed both platinum and docetaxel-based chemotherapies
— Pancreatic cancer (erlotinib)

Side effects
— Rash
— Diarrhea, nausea, and vomiting

Sorafenib

Mechanism of action.   Sorafenib is a multiple kinase inhibitor that blocks the receptor tyrosine kinases VEGFR (vascular endothelial growth factor receptor) and PDGFR (platelet-derived growth factor receptor) and the Raf serine/threonine kinases along the RAF/MEK/ERK pathway.

Uses
— Liver and kidney cancers

Side effects
— Hypertension
— Alopecia, rash, and chemotherapy-induced acral erythema (hand-foot syndrome)
— Abdominal pain, diarrhea, nausea, and anorexia
— Headache and fatigue
— Hemorrhage

Sunitinib

Mechanism of action.   Sunitinib is a multitargeting tyrosine kinase inhibitor that decreases tumor cell proliferation and angiogenesis.

Uses
- Advanced stomach and kidney cancers

Side effects
- Hypertension and heart failure
- Abdominal pain, constipation, diarrhea, nausea, anorexia, and stomatitis
- Anemia, leukopenia, lymphocytopenia, and hemorrhage
- Yellow discoloration of skin, hand-foot syndrome, and dry skin

Bortezomib

Mechanism of action. Bortezomib is an inhibitor of the 26S proteasome, a protease important for intracellular degradation of proteins involved in cell cycle control and cellular apoptosis. Disruption of the degradation of these proteins results in disruption of cell proliferation and increases cell death.

Uses
- Patients with multiple myeloma who have not responded to prior therapies

Side effects. Serious dose-limiting effects on cardiovascular and hematological systems, along with the common skin, GI, neurologic, and respiratory effects of anticancer agents.

Differentiating Agents

Tretinoin

Tretinoin is an all trans retinoic acid, which is a derivative of vitamin A.

Mechanism of action. Tretinoin induces terminal maturation of leukemic promyelocytes into polymorphonuclear monocytes in acute promyelocytic leukemia.

Uses
- Acute promyelocytic leukemia

Side effects
- Edema, arrhythmia, and blood pressure changes
- Headache, pain, fatigue, and dizziness
- Rash and dry skin
- Hypercholesterolemia and hypertriglyceridemia
- Abdominal pain, constipation, diarrhea, nausea, and vomiting
- Leukocytosis
- Upper respiratory tract disorders, dyspnea, and pneumonia

Arsenic Trioxide

Mechanism of action. Arsenic trioxide causes differentiation and apoptosis in acute promyelocytic leukemia refractory to tretinoin.

Uses
- Acute promyelocytic leukemia refractory to tretinoin

Side effects
- Chest pain, edema, and hypotension
- Headache, pain, fatigue, dizziness, and insomnia
- Rash and dry skin
- Hypo- or hyperkalemia, hyperglycemia, and hypomagnesemia
- Abdominal pain, constipation, diarrhea, nausea, vomiting, and anorexia
- Leukocytosis, anemia, and thrombocytopenia
- Upper respiratory tract disorders, cough, dyspnea, and epistaxis

Hormones and Hormone Inhibitors

Hormonal therapy is effective for some cancers (e.g., breast cancer). They may inhibit tumor growth directly or oppose the effects of endogenous hormones. Toxicities are due to hormonal effects rather than cytotoxic effects.

Corticosteroids

Corticosteroids are also discussed in Chapters 16, 26, 27, and 32.

Prednisone

Mechanism of action.   Corticosteroids are useful in cancer chemotherapy due to their lymphocytic and antimitotic actions.

Uses

— Lymphomatous cancers (in conjunction with other agents)

Antiestrogens

Testing for the presence of estrogen receptors and progesterone receptors in tumor specimens from biopsy or surgery is recommended for all patients with primary invasive breast cancer. Up to 60% of patients with metastatic breast cancer will respond to hormonal therapy if their tumors contain estrogen receptors; however, < 10% of patients with metastatic tumors that are estrogen receptor–negative respond to hormonal therapy. Up to 80% of patients with metastatic progesterone receptor–positive tumors respond to hormonal manipulation. The presence or absence of these receptors does not correlate with the response to other chemotherapies. Thus, adjuvant hormonal therapy, in combination with surgery, radiation, and/or chemotherapy, is recommended for all women whose breast cancer expresses hormone receptors.

Tamoxifen

Mechanism of action.   Tamoxifen is a partial agonist at the estrogen receptor. Its primary effect is to block the cell-proliferative effects of estrogen, but it also may inhibit replication by additional mechanisms (see Fig. 17.3, page 164). Many proteins and transcription factors interact with the estrogen receptor, so there are many downstream effects that occur because of tamoxifen's acting at the estrogen receptor, resulting in inhibition of growth-stimulatory factors, as well as activation of growth-inhibitory effects, including transforming growth factor beta (TGF-β).

Pharmacokinetics

— Given orally

Uses

— Adjuvant hormonal therapy in premenopausal women with invasive breast cancer, with or without ovarian suppression or ablation therapy
— Adjuvant hormonal therapy in postmenopausal women with invasive breast cancer

Side effects.   Nausea and vomiting, hot flashes, and hypercalcemia

Aromatase Inhibitors

Anastrozole, Letrozole, and Exemestane

Mechanism of action.   Aromatase converts the adrenal androgen androstenedione in peripheral tissue to estrone and estradiol, the main source of estrogens in postmenopausal women.
— Anastrozole and letrozole are nonsteroidal competitive inhibitors.

Fig. 34.6 ► **Aromatase inhibitors.**
Aromatase inhibitors block the conversion of androgens (testosterone and androstenedione) to estrone and estradiol in extragonadal tissue after menopause (when ovarian estrogen production ceases). In doing so, these agents inhibit the growth of estrogen-dependent breast cancers.

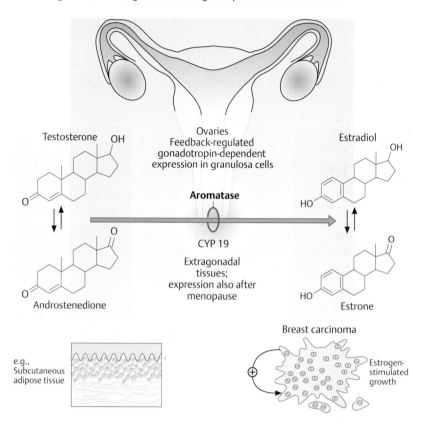

— Exemestane is a derivative of androstenedione; thus, it is a steroidal compound that acts as a false substrate for the enzyme, binding to the active site and resulting in irreversible inactivation (**Fig. 34.6**).

Uses

— For adjuvant treatment of postmenopausal women with hormone receptor–positive early breast cancer or for treatment of advanced breast cancer

Note: When an aromatase inhibitor is used in premenopausal women, a luteinizing hormone–releasing hormone (LHRH) agonist (goserelin, leuprolide, or triptorelin) is given to block ovarian estrogen production, or the ovaries are removed surgically.

Side effects.   Nausea and vomiting, hot flashes, and musculoskeletal problems

GnRH Agonist Agents

Leuprolide and Goserelin

Mechanism of action.   These agents are GnRH agonists that desensitize pituitary GnRH receptors and inhibit the release of gonadotropins (follicle-stimulating hormone [FSH] and luteinizing hormone [LH]).

Uses

— Prostate cancer treatment (in combination with an antiandrogen) to prevent the initial flare-up of the disease

Functions of the prostate gland

The prostate gland is responsible for producing a significant portion of the fluid that makes up semen. This fluid contains substances that aid sperm on their journey to the fallopian tubes during reproduction (e.g., fructose provides sperm with energy). Seminal fluid is alkaline, which neutralizes the acidity of the vagina and stops sperm death on contact. The prostate gland also plays a part in ejaculation and sealing off the urethra so that no urine is expelled at this time.

Antiandrogens

Bicalutamide, Flutamide, and Nilutamide

Mechanism of action. These agents are competitive inhibitors of dihydrotestosterone (DHT) and testosterone at receptor binding sites.

Side effects
— Hot flashes are common.
— Gynecomastia, nausea and vomiting, edema, and thrombophlebitis

34.3 Immunosuppressants

Immunosuppressants are used to prevent rejection in patients receiving organ transplants and in autoimmune diseases. Although effective in such cases, they increase the risk of infections and cancers. **Figure 34.7** illustrates the normal immune reaction and the general steps that the immunosuppressant drugs may inhibit.

Immunosuppressants have been discussed in the sections on inflammatory bowel disease, cancer chemotherapy, and rheumatoid arthritis. Those agents that have not been discussed elsewhere are included below. **Table 34.2** provides page and figure cross-references for all immunosuppressant drugs.

Table 34.2 ► **Summary of Immunosuppressants**			
Drug class	**Drugs**	**Chapter/page reference(s)**	**Figure reference(s)**
Antimetabolites	Cyclophosphamide	Chapter 34/p. 369	34.7
	Methotrexate	Chapter 27/p. 276 Chapter 33/p. 351 Chapter 34/p. 370	27.13 33.3 34.4 34.7
	Azathioprine	Chapter 27/p. 276	27.13 34.4 34.7
Calcineurin inhibitors	Cyclosporine	Chapter 27/p. 276	33.3 34.8
	Tacrolimus	Chapter 34/p. 384	34.8
Corticosteroids	Prednisone Budesonide Hydrocortisone (Cortisol) Methylprednisolone Triamcinolone Dexamethasone Betamethasone Beclomethasone Fluocinonide Ciclesonide Flunisolide Fluticasone	Chapter 16/pp. 149, 151–155 Chapter 26/p. 250 Chapter 27/p. 276 Chapter 32/p. 350 Chapter 34/p. 381	16.8–16.11 27.12 34.7
Monoclonal antibodies	Basiliximab	Chapter 34/p. 387	34.7
	Infliximab	Chapter 27/p. 274 Chapter 33/p. 358 Chapter 34/p. 387	33.4
	Muromonab-CD3	Chapter 34/p. 387	34.7
Other	Sirolimus	Chapter 34/p. 385	34.7
	Mycophenolate mofetil	Chapter 34/p. 385	34.7

▮ Humoral immunity

Humoral immunity refers to adaptive immune responses mediated by antigen-specific antibodies. Antibodies are secreted from B cells that have been activated by specific recognition of an antigen by membrane-bound antibodies expressed on the cell surface (part of the B-cell receptor [BCR]). Antibody production is supported by T helper cells (CD4+) that specifically recognize the same antigens that stimulate a given B cell, a feature termed *linked recognition*. The T cell provides cytokines that promote B-cell proliferation and differentiation. Antibodies act by binding and clearing antigens, by activating the complement pathway that promotes damage to and clearance of molecules and microorganisms, and by promoting the activities of accessory cells.

▮ Cell-mediated immunity

Cell-mediated immunity refers to adaptive immune responses mediated by T cells. Unlike B cells, T cells do not produce a secreted form of their antigen receptor, called the T-cell receptor (TCR), instead mediating their effector functions by interacting directly with other cells. Most T cells recognize peptide antigen bound by a protein complex termed the *major histocompatibility complex* (MHC). T helper cells (CD4+) interact with antigen-presenting cells displaying class II MHC. Cytotoxic T cells (CD8+) interact with cells expressing class I MHC (all nucleated cells). There are three major types of professional antigen-presenting cells: dendritic cells, macrophages, and B cells. Dendritic cells take up an antigen by receptor-mediated endocytosis or macropinocytosis and processes antigen for presentation to T cells. Macrophages take up particulate matter via phagocytosis, and B cells are involved in antigen-specific uptake via BCR-mediated endocytosis. T helper cells promote the activities of B cells and macrophages through the release of specific cytokines. Cytotoxic T cells directly kill infected cells or other abnormal cells (e.g., tumor cells) by releasing agents directly onto the target cell, which damages the integrity of the cell membrane.

Fig. 34.7 ► **Immune reaction and immunosuppressives.**
Humoral immunity (*left column*) and cell-mediated immunity (*other two columns*) are described in the call-out boxes, on this page. The far right column contains the immunosuppressant drugs with color-coded indicators of the steps in the immune reaction that they inhibit. MHC, major histocompatibility complex.

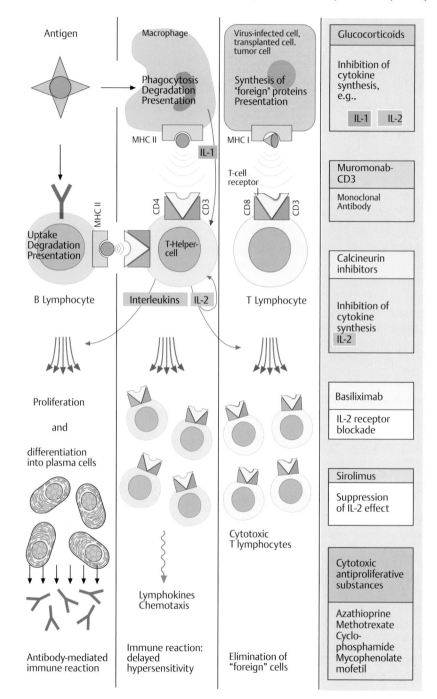

Tacrolimus

Tarcrolimus is a macrolide antibiotic produced by *Streptomyces tsukubaensis*.

Mechanism of action.   Tarcrolimus inhibits calcineurin, thus inhibiting T-cell activation (**Fig. 34.8**).

Pharmacokinetics
— Given orally or IV

Uses
— Prophylaxis of organ transplant rejection

Side effects
— *Cardiovascular:* hypertension and edema
— *Endocrine/metabolic:* hypomagnesemia, hyperglycemia, and diabetes
— *GI:* nausea, vomiting, constipation, and diarrhea
— *Hematologic:* anemia, leukopenia, and thrombocytopenia
— *Neurologic:* headache, insomnia, pain, paresthesia, and tremor

Sirolimus

Sirolimus is a macrocyclic lactone produced by *Streptomyces hygroscopicus.*

Mechanism of action.   Sirolimus inhibits T-lymphocyte activation and proliferation stimulation by interleukin cytokines (IL-2, IL-4, and IL-15) (**Fig. 34.8**).

Pharmacokinetics
— Given orally

Uses
— Prophylaxis of kidney transplant rejection

Side effects
— *Cardiovascular:* hypertension and edema
— *Dermatologic:* acne and rash
— *Endocrine/metabolic:* hyperlipidemias
— *GI:* nausea, vomiting, constipation, and diarrhea
— *Hematologic:* anemia and thrombocytopenia
— *Neurologic:* headache, insomnia, and pain

Mycophenolate Mofetil

Mycophenolate mofetil is a semisynthetic derivative of mycophenolic acid from the mold *Penicillium glaucum.*

Mechanism of action.   Mycophenolate mofetil inhibits T- and B-lymphocyte responses.

Pharmacokinetics
— Given orally or IV

Uses
— Prophylaxis of organ transplant rejection

Side effects
— *Cardiovascular:* hypertension and edema
— *Endocrine/metabolic:* hyperlipidemias
— *GI:* nausea, vomiting, constipation, and diarrhea
— *Hematologic:* anemia, severe neutropenia, and thrombocytopenia
— *Neurologic:* asthenia, headache, insomnia, pain, and tremor

Fig. 34.8 ▶ Calcineurin inhibitors and sirolimus (rapamycin).
In T-helper cells, nuclear factor of activated T cell (NFAT) promotes the expression of interleukin 2 (IL-2). NFAT is able to enter the nucleus following dephosphorylation of its phosphorylated precursor by the phosphatase calcineurin. Cyclosporine binds to the protein cyclophillin in the cell interior; this complex inhibits calcineurin, and thus the transcription and production of IL-2 are inhibited. Tarcrolimus acts like cyclosporine, but it attaches to a so-called FK-binding protein instead of cyclophillin. Sirolimus forms a complex with the FK-binding protein, changing its conformation. This complex then inhibits mTOR (mammalian target of rapamycin), which operates the signaling path leading from the IL-2 receptor to the activation of mitosis in lymphocytes, thus inhibiting lymphocyte proliferation.

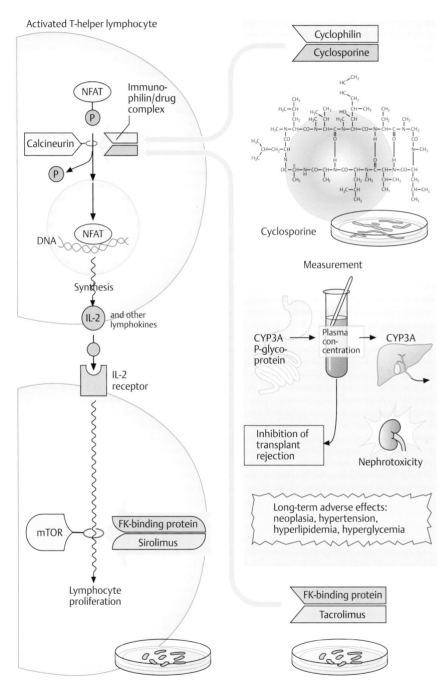

Basiliximab

Mechanism of action. Basiliximab is a recombinant anti-IL-2 receptor antibody that binds to the CD25 antigen on the IL-2 receptor and prevents IL-2 binding, thus preventing IL-2-mediated activation of lymphocytes.

Pharmacokinetics
— Given IV

Uses
— Prophylaxis of kidney transplant rejection

Side effects
— *Cardiovascular:* hypertension and edema
— *GI:* pain and vomiting
— *Hematologic:* anemia
— *Neurologic:* headache and insomnia

Infliximab

Mechanism of action. Infliximab is an antibody to tumor necrosis factor-α (TNF-α; see page 358) that blocks TNF-α from binding to TNF receptors on inflammatory cell surfaces, resulting in suppression of downstream inflammatory cytokines such as IL-1 and IL-6 and adhesion molecules involved in leukocyte activation and migration.

Muromonab-CD3

Mechanism of action. Muromonab-CD3 binds to the CD3 component of the T-cell receptor complex involved in antigen recognition, leading to rapid internalization of the T-cell receptor, thereby preventing subsequent antigen recognition.

Pharmacokinetics
— Given IV

Uses
— Acute organ transplant rejection

Side effects
— *Cytokine release reactions:* fever, chills, nausea, vomiting, diarrhea, tachycardia, and changes in blood pressure. These reactions occur in many patients following the first few doses. Anaphylactic and anaphylactoid reactions may also occur, but fatalities are rare.
— *GI:* nausea, vomiting, and diarrhea
— *Neurologic:* fever, headache, insomnia, and pain

35　Toxicology and Poisoning

Toxic reactions to drugs and other agents can occur with acute exposure to a high dose of an agent, either accidentally or intentionally administered. Chronic toxicities can be observed with long-term exposure to an agent at lower doses. These reactions may be local, following skin contact or lung inhalation, or systemic, following absorption of the toxin. In some cases, the toxicity only develops following biotransformation of the absorbed substance to toxic metabolites. The resulting toxicities may be short or long term, they may appear immediately or be delayed, and they may be reversible or irreversible.

Toxicities to specific agents have largely been dealt with along with the discussion of their pharmacological properties, but some of the more common toxic substances and poisonings are discussed in this chapter.

35.1　Nonspecific Antidotes

In cases of acute poisoning, the main goal is to minimize further exposure and enhance elimination of the toxin. Several procedures are used when specific antidotes are not available, and these are discussed below.

Gastric Lavage with Saline

Mechanism of action.　Gastric lavage (stomach pumping) involves fluid, usually saline, being sequentially administered and withdrawn via an orogastric or nasogastric tube.

Pharmacokinetics
— Given orally as a suspension in doses of up to 100 g
　Note: During this procedure, the patient's airway is protected by an endotracheal tube to prevent aspiration of the ingested substances into the lung.

Activated Charcoal

Mechanism of action.　Activated charcoal adsorbs a large number of organic and inorganic compounds and prevents their absorption from the gastrointestinal (GI) tract.

Pharmacokinetics
— Given orally or via gastric tube as a suspension in doses of up to 100 g

Syrup of Ipecac

Mechanism of action.　This is an emetic agent. Emesis used to be primary therapy but is now becoming secondary to other therapies.

Pharmacokinetics.　One ounce orally usually produces emesis within 30 minutes.

Contraindications.　Emesis is contraindicated when there is a risk of perforation of the esophagus or stomach (corrosive agents), when ingested agents may be aspirated into the lung (e.g., if the patient is comatose), or if emesis is likely to induce seizures (strychnine or CNS stimulants).

Hemodialysis

Mechanism of action.　Hemodialysis involves the use of a machine to filter waste products (e.g., creatinine and urea), salts, fluids, or drugs from the blood in kidney failure. The blood flows in the opposite direction to dialysis fluid that are separated by a semipermeable membrane. This allows substances to be cleared down their concentration gradient.

■ Emergency treatment of the poisoned patient

The procedure for the emergency treatment of the poisoned patient is as follows: (1) check respiratory function, cardiovascular function, and central nervous system (CNS) involvement; (2) stabilize the patient; (3) attempt to determine the identity and quantity of poison ingested and the time of exposure; and (4) treat with the appropriate antidote.

■ Hemoperfusion

Hemoperfusion is a technique in which large volumes of the patient's blood are passed over an adsorbent substance, e.g., resins or activated carbon, which attracts and removes toxic substances from the blood. It is used to treat overdoses of barbiturates, theophylline, digitalis, carbamazepine, methotrexate, acetaminophen, meprobamate, glutethimide, ethchlorvynol, and paraquat poisoning. Hemoperfusion may also be used to remove waste products in kidney disease and to provide supportive treatment before and after liver transplantation.

Uses. Hemodialysis is not useful for poisons with large volumes of distribution or poisons that bind tightly to plasma proteins. It is generally reserved for extreme, life-threatening poisoning with alcohol, aspirin, or CNS-active drugs.

35.2 Specific Antidotes

When the identity of the toxic substances is known or strongly suspected, it may be desirable to treat with specific antidotes.

Metal Chelating Agents

These agents are used to treat heavy metal poisoning.

Dimercaprol (British antilewisite)

Mechanism of action. Dimercaprol, or British antilewisite (BAL), protects essential enzymes by forming a stable complex with circulating metallic poison. It promotes excretion of metal in a stable complex form (**Fig. 35.1**).

Pharmacokinetics
— Given intramuscularly

Uses. Dimercaprol is an effective treatment following poisoning by mercury, arsenic, and some other less common metals, but it is not very effective for lead poisoning.

Side effects
— Increased blood pressure and heart rate, weakness, nausea, and pain at the injection site.

Calcium Disodium Edetate

Mechanism of action. Calcium disodium edetate (or ethylenediamine tetraacetic acid ($CaNa_2$ EDTA) promotes the excretion of the lead chelate.

Pharmacokinetics
— Given by intravenous (IV) infusion, as it is not effective orally

Uses
— Especially effective in lead poisoning, but may also be useful to chelate other less common metallic poisons

Side effects
— Renal damage and hypersensitivity reactions

Penicillamine

Penicillamine is a derivative of penicillin.

Mechanism of action. Penicillamine chelates copper, mercury, and lead and promotes their excretion.

Pharmacokinetics
— Administered orally

Uses
— Used to remove copper in hepatolenticular degeneration (Wilson disease)
— Used in combination, usually following EDTA, for lead poisoning
— Also useful in the treatment of rheumatoid arthritis (see **Chapter 33**)

■ Mercury poisoning

The greatest danger with mercury poisoning is damage of the GI mucosa and kidneys. Fluid loss leads to shock and death. This tends to occur with acute intoxication. Symptoms of chronic intoxication include stomatitis, excessive salivation, blue gum line, renal toxicity, and CNS symptoms (depression, weakness, headache, insomnia, irritability, and hallucinations). This is treated by giving dimercaprol.

■ Arsenic poisoning

Arsenic is considered to be a heavy metal and therefore has many toxic characteristics in common with lead and mercury. Signs and symptoms of arsenic poisoning include headache, confusion, drowsiness, abdominal pain, diarrhea, vomiting, convulsions, coma, and death. Treatment of acute arsenic poisoning is supportive and chelation therapy with dimercaprol is used to bind the arsenic and hasten excretion in all symptomatic patients.

■ Lead poisoning

Acute intoxication with lead is rare. Symptoms of chronic intoxication include spasm and hypermotility of the GI tract, which causes intense cramping and lead encephalopathy (primarily a problem in children), the early symptoms of which are nonspecific and may include decreased appetite, irritability, fatigue, abdominal pain, and vomiting, followed by drowsiness, stupor, convulsions, and coma. This may lead to mental retardation and cerebral palsies, as well as myopathy, fatigue, weakness, wrist drop, foot drop, and involvement of extraocular muscles. Other results are anemia due to impaired heme biosynthesis, porphyrinuria, basophilic stippling of erythrocytes, and gingival lead line. Blood vessel constriction causes pallor and hypertension. Initial treatment is edetate administration. Penicillamine and dimercaprol (limited effectiveness) may also be used.

Wilson disease

Wilson disease is an autosomal recessive disease that results in the accumulation of copper (that is ingested) in the liver and brain, causing cirrhosis and basal ganglia destruction. It may present in a child or young adult with neurologic signs such as tremor, seizures, mental deterioration, and weakness; or there may be signs of cirrhosis, such as jaundice, hepatomegaly (swelling of the liver), edema, and fatigue. Treatment with penicillamine is effective if given early.

Iron poisoning

Iron poisoning is the most common metallic poison, due to overdosage with oral supplements, multiple transfusions, or iron storage diseases. Acute symptoms of iron poisoning include vomiting (often bloody), gastric pain, and diarrhea. Chronic symptoms include metabolic acidosis, lethargy, which may progress to cardiovascular collapse, liver damage, and organ failure. Permanent scarring of the GI tract may occur with severe poisoning. Treatment is by desferoxamine.

Fig. 35.1 ► **Chelators.**
Dimercaprol is given by intramuscular injection to chelate various metal ions. A related compound, dimercaptopropane sulfonate (DMPS), is suitable for oral administration. Deferoxamine is highly effective at chelating iron but does not extract iron from hemoglobin or cytochromes.

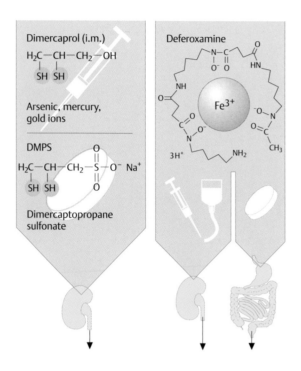

Side effects

— Hypersensitivity reactions
— Rashes
— Arthralgia
— Nephrotic syndrome

Trientine

Uses.   Trientine is an alternative copper chelating agent for patients who are hypersensitive to penicillamine.

Deferoxamine

Mechanism of action.   Deferoxamine specifically chelates iron (ferric ions and ferrous ions) and promotes its excretion. It binds free and loosely bound iron, for example, from hemosiderin and ferritin, but does not chelate iron bound to hemoglobin or cytochromes.

Pharmacokinetics.   This agent is orally effective in preventing iron absorption. It is given intramuscularly or IV for systemic toxicity.

Uses

— Acute iron toxicity and iron storage diseases (e.g., hemochromatosis)

Side effects

— Hypertension, rashes, and GI upset

Succimer

Pharmacokinetics
— Orally effective

Uses. Succimer is indicated for lead poisoning in children. It may also be effective for mercury or arsenic.

Table 35.1 summarizes other poisons and their antidotes.

Poison	Antidote	Mechanism of Action of Antidote
Belladonna (atropine)	Physostigmine (p. 47)	Anticholinesterase action
Carbon monoxide	Hyperbaric O_2	Hyperbaric O_2 increases both O_2 delivery to tissue and CO elimination.
Coumarin derivatives (e.g., warfarin)	Phytonadione (Vitamin K_1)	Vitamin K promotes hepatic synthesis of factors II, VII, IX, and X, which are needed for coagulation of the blood.
Cyanide	Sodium thiosulfate Amyl nitrite and sodium nitrite	Sodium thiosulfate increases cyanide metabolism. Amyl nitrite and sodium nitrite produce methemoglobin, which binds cyanide.
Ethylene glycol and other glycols	Ethanol (pp. 119, 120)	Ethanol is preferentially metabolized by alcohol dehydrogenase and prevents the occurrence of acidosis.
Methanol	Ethanol (pp. 121, 122)	Ethanol is preferentially metabolized by alcohol dehydrogenase and decreases the formation of both formaldehyde and formic acid from methanol.
Iodine	Starch	Starch binds iodine.
Opiates	Naloxone (p. 108)	Naloxone is a narcotic antagonist.
Nitrites	Methylene blue	Narcotic antagonist
Organophosphate	Pralidoxime	Pralidoxime is a cholinesterase reactivator.
Insecticides	Atropine (p. 49)	Atropine is an anticholinergic agent.

Table 35.1 ▶ Other Poisons and Their Antidotes

Carbon monoxide poisoning

Carbon monoxide (CO) is a colorless, odorless, tasteless, nonirritant toxic gas that is produced from the incomplete burning of fossil fuels. It binds to hemoglobin, forming carboxyhemoglobin, and in doing so, it displaces oxygen. This results in a functional anemia. Symptoms of CO poisoning include headache, dizziness, weakness, confusion, lethargy, nausea, vomiting, seizures, and, at very high concentrations, coma and death. CO poisoning is the most common cause of death from poisoning. Treatment involves removing the source of CO, 100% oxygen therapy, and hyperbaric oxygen therapy (if severe).

Electron transport chain

The electron transport chain consists of a group of complexes (CI–CV) that are located in the inner membrane of the mitochondria. It is the mechanism by which the energy needed to drive the oxidative phosphorylation of adenosine triphosphate (ATP) is generated. NADH (the reduced form of nicotinamide adenine dinucleotide) and $FADH_2$ (or 1,5-dihydro-FAD [flavin adenine dinucleotide]), derived from carbohydrate and fatty acid catabolism, are electron donors. As electrons are passed along the chain of complexes, protons (H^+ ions) are pumped into the intermembrane space at certain points (CI, CIII, and CIV). These protons cause an electrochemical gradient to form. They flow back into the mitochondrial matrix through complex V (ATP synthase), which generates ATP from adenosine diphosphate (ADP) and P_i. The electron transport chain is disrupted by toxic substances such as cyanide and CO, thus decreasing the capacity for aerobic metabolism.

Organophosphate poisoning

Organophosphates are commonly used insecticides and are one of the most common causes of poisoning worldwide. Organophosphates inhibit the action of acetylcholinesterase in nerve cells which results in excess acetylcholine. Signs and symptoms of organophosphate poisoning include salivation, lacrimation, sweating, vomiting, incontinence of urine and feces, convulsions, cyanosis, bradycardia, and hypotension. Treatment of organophosphate poisoning is with pralidoxime, a cholinesterase reactivator.

35.3   Vitamin Poisoning and Treatment

Vitamins are essential for many processes in the body, but some are highly toxic when ingested in excessive amounts. **Table 35.2** lists the toxic effects of some vitamins and the treatment that may be given.

Table 35.2 ▶ Toxic Effects of Vitamins and Treatment		
Vitamin	**Toxic Effects**	**Treatment of Toxic Effects**
Vitamin A (retinol)	Acute toxicity: dizziness, vomiting, erythema, and desquamation. Chronic toxicity: skin and hair changes, liver damage (in infants and children). Can cause pseudotumor cerebri (increased CSF fluid pressure)	Symptomatic and supportive (i.e., treatment is given to prevent, control, or relieve complications and side effects)
Vitamin D (ergocalciferol D_2, cholecalciferol D_2)	Hypercalcemia, and both mental and physical retardation	Terminate exposure to vitamin D. Initiate a low-calcium diet. Monitor urine volume, sodium, and potassium and replace lost fluids, sodium, and potassium by IV infusions.
Vitamin E (tocopherol)	Nausea, muscular weakness, fatigue, headache, blurred vision, and GI upset	None
Vitamin K	Hemolytic anemia and hyperbilirubinemia may occur in newborns and persons with glucose-6-phosphate dehydrogenase deficiency	None
Niacin (vitamin B_3, nicotinic acid, nicotinamide)	Flushing, headache, pruritus, GI irritation	Symptomatic and supportive
Pyridoxine (B_6)	Sensory neuropathy, and interference with levodopa therapy	There is no known treatment for the sensory neuropathy produced by high doses of pyridoxine. Spontaneous recovery usually occurs slowly over several months or years.
Ascorbic acid (vitamin C)	Kidney stones and rebound scurvy (seen only with huge amounts ingested)	None

Note: The vitamins that are not included here have no known toxicity.
Abbreviations: CSF, cerebrospinal fluid; GI, gastrointestinal; IV, intravenous.

Review Questions

1. Renal toxicity is associated with which of the following?
   A. Doxorubicin
   B. Fluorouracil
   C. Vincristine
   D. Cisplatin
   E. 6-mercaptopurine

2. The antineoplastic action of which drug is related to its high affinity for dihydrofolate reductase?
   A. Fluorouracil
   B. Methotrexate
   C. Mechlorethamine
   D. Dactinomycin
   E. Vincristine

3. A 62-year-old African American man undergoes a hemicolectomy to remove an invasive adenocarcinoma from his ascending colon. Pathology shows pericolic lymph node involvement but no liver metastases. Based on the stage of the tumor, a course of treatment with leucovorin calcium, fluorouracil, and irinotecan hydrochloride is undertaken. What is the purpose of including leucovorin calcium?
   A. to provide normal cells with an active form of folic acid
   B. to decrease nausea and vomiting produced by fluorouracil
   C. to activate irinotecan
   D. to increase the effectiveness of fluorouracil
   E. to increase the uptake of drug into bone to prevent metastases

4. Cardiac toxicity is associated with which of the following?
   A. Doxorubicin
   B. Fluorouracil
   C. Vincristine
   D. Cisplatin
   E. 6-mercaptopurine

5. Which one of the following drugs acts by inhibiting DNA topoisomerase?
   A. Cyclophosphamide
   B. Methotrexate
   C. Etoposide
   D. Leuprolide
   E. Fluorouracil

6. A 58-year-old woman noticed a lump in her right breast ~1 month ago. She has no pain, nipple discharge, itching, or swelling of the breast. The patient is postmenopausal and had a mammogram 2 years ago. She takes several supplements, including calcium/vitamin D and vitamin C. She also takes iron tablets for occasional mild anemia. Breast examination reveals a hard 1 cm mass in the upper right quadrant of her breast. Right axillary lymph nodes are enlarged. The mass is confirmed by mammography and needle biopsy. A test to show the level of expression of which of the following antigens would assist in determining susceptibility of the tumor to trastuzumab?
   A. CD20
   B. CD52
   C. Epidermal growth factor receptor (EGFR)
   D. HER2/neu
   E. Vascular endothelial growth factor (VEGF)

7. A 78-year-old male patient has hepatocellular carcinoma. The tumor is unresectable due to portal vein invasion. Sorafenib tosylate is a multiple tyrosine kinase inhibitor used in advanced kidney or bladder cancer that can increase survival by 6 to 9 months. What is the advantage of inhibiting multiple kinases as opposed to a single kinase?
   A. To account for genetic differences in kinases
   B. To inhibit both angiogenesis and tumor cell growth
   C. To inhibit multiple stages of blood vessel growth
   D. To inhibit multiple sites on the Raf serine/threonine kinase
   E. To ensure the drug is effective in both slow and rapid acetylators

8. A 60-year-old man reports difficulty starting his urination and poor urinary stream for the last 4 months. A digital rectal exam of the prostate reveals masses in both lobes. Serum prostate-specific antigen (PSA) is elevated. The patient is referred to a urologist, who conducts a needle biopsy and histologic grading. The decision is made to use a combination of radiotherapy and hormonal therapy. Why is flutamide administered prior to leuprolide?
   A. It prevents the breakdown of leuprolide by liver cytochrome P-450 enzymes.
   B. A positive response to flutamide may obviate the need for giving leuprolide.
   C. Ito induces receptor desensitization.
   D. Ito increases absorption from the gastrointestinal tract.
   E. Ito blocks the effect of the initial surge of hormones produced by leuprolide.

9. A 29-year-old patient has a lymph node biopsy and is diagnosed as having Hodgkin lymphoma, nodular sclerosis type. A course of therapy with doxorubicin, bleomycin, vinblastine, and dacarbazine is recommended. Before beginning chemotherapy, what steps might be taken to alleviate the most common acute toxicity of this regimen?
A. Use behavioral modification therapy.
B. Administer morphine as needed after the chemotherapy session.
C. Administer ondansetron prophylactically
D. Soak the patient's arm in Epsom salts.
E. Administer milk of magnesia.

10. A 28-year-old female patient had ingested a toxic overdose of phencyclidine, a weak base. Because of the severity of her symptoms, you rightfully conclude that almost all of the phencyclidine had been absorbed by the time she was brought to the emergency room. Which of the following actions may be effective?
A. Induce vomiting with apomorphine.
B. Alkalinize the urine with sodium bicarbonate.
C. Perform hemoperfusion.
D. Acidify the urine with ammonium chloride.
E. Perform gastric lavage with charcoal.

11. A patient who has received multiple blood transfusions may require chelation therapy with which of the following?
A. Dimercaprol
B. Succimer
C. Ethylenediaminetetraacetic acid (EDTA)
D. Trientine
E. Deferoxamine

12. A person is brought to the hospital in a coma with severely depressed respiration, no response to pain, and small pupils. A friend says the patient took some kind of drug, or drugs, but he does not know what kind. An injection of naloxone makes the pupils larger and only slightly improves respiration. Injecting more naloxone causes no further change. Of the following, what is the most probable cause of this reaction to naloxone?
A. This is probably a mixed overdose from an opioid plus another drug.
B. Naloxone was the wrong drug to use, and nalorphine should have been used.
C. The patient probably is also an amphetamine user, is tolerant to amphetamine, and would thus be cross-tolerant to the respiratory stimulation caused by naloxone.
D. This is an addict who is in a postictal state, having just suffered an opioid withdrawal convulsion.

13. A college student is brought to the emergency room. She is unconscious, with no response to painful stimuli. Deep tendon reflexes are hyperactive. Respirations are 4/min. Blood pressure is 80/50 mm Hg. The skin is cool and cyanotic. Pupils are slightly dilated with sluggish reaction to light. Her roommate reports that the patient took "about 10 or 20" capsules of chloral hydrate and "lots" of pills of codeine. An endotracheal tube is inserted. Gastric washing reveals many partially digested capsules. The resident on duty injects naloxone intravenously. After giving naloxone, respirations are still inadequate. Which one of the following measures is most appropriate to correct respiratory function?
A. Inject strychnine.
B. Inject pentylenetetrazol.
C. Inject dopamine.
D. Mechanically assist respirations.
E. Force-feed caffeine.

14. A woman is found unconscious near a bottle hand-labeled "roach poison." She is having convulsive movements and is covered with urine and feces. In the emergency room, she is cyanotic, has a pulse of 50 beats/min, blood pressure of 70/20 mm Hg, and cold, wet skin. Immediate action should include instituting artificial ventilation and which of the following?
A. Administering atropine intravenously
B. Administering edrophonium intravenously
C. Administering neostigmine intravenously
D. Ordering an assay of serum cholinesterase activity
E. Ordering a blood toxicology panel

15. Which of the following agents is useful in treating cyanide toxicity?
A. Carbon monoxide
B. Trientine
C. Sodium nitrite/sodium thiosulfate
D. Pralidoxime
E. Dimercaprol

Answers and Explanations

1. **D** Cisplatin concentrates in the kidneys and produces renal toxicity (p. 370).
A–C, E None of the other agents concentrate in the kidney and therefore do not produce renal toxicity.

2. **B** Methotrexate is a folic acid analogue that competitively inhibits dihydrofolate reductase and thus suppresses the production of purine and thymine nucleotides (p. 370).
A Fluorouracil is a pyrimidine analogue that inhibits thymidylate synthesis.
C Mechlorethamine is an alkylating agent that binds covalently to guanine nucleotides of DNA, cross-linking DNA strands, thus preventing DNA replication and transcription.
D Dactinomycin intercalates between G-C pairs in double-stranded DNA and inhibits DNA-directed RNA synthesis.
E Vincristine is an antimitotic agent that inhibits cell development.

3. **A** Leucovorin is folinic acid, the active form of folic acid that does not require dihydrofolate reductase. Leucovorin enhances the efficacy of fluorouracil, possibly by inhibiting thymidylate synthase. When given with methotrexate, leucovorin is used to provide normal cells with the active form of folic acid (p. 371).

4. **A** Doxorubicin is taken up by cardiac muscle, leading to oxidative damage of heart muscle and refractory congestive heart failure (p. 373).
B–E These agents are not cardiotoxic.

5. **C** Etoposide inhibits DNA topoisomerase II, which acts on single-stranded DNA to cause strand breakage (p. 374).
A Cyclophosphamide is a widely used alkylating agent that binds covalently to guanine nucleotides of DNA, cross-linking DNA strands, thus preventing DNA replication and transcription.
B Methotrexate is a folic acid analogue that competitively inhibits dihydrofolate reductase and thus suppresses the production of purine and thymine nucleotides.
D Leuprolide is a gonadotropin-releasing hormone (GnRH) agonist that desensitizes pituitary GnRH receptors and inhibits gonadotropin (follicle-stimulating hormone and luteinizing hormone) release.
E Fluorouracil is a pyrimidine analogue that inhibits thymidylate synthesis.

6. **D** Trastuzumab is a monoclonal antibody directed against HER2/neu. HER2/neu is a member of the epidermal growth factor family of cell membrane receptors. Trastuzumab is approved for treatment of metastatic breast cancer when HER2/neu is overexpressed (p. 377).
A Rituximab, tositumomab, ^{131}I-tositumomab, ^{111}In ibritumomab, and 90Y-ibritumomab tiuxetan bind to CD20, which is found on pre-B and mature B lymphocytes.
B Alemtuzumab binds to CD52, which is present on the surface of essentially all B and T lymphocytes, a majority of monocytes, macrophages, and NK cells, as well as a subpopulation of granulocytes.
C Cetuximab binds to EGFR, which has been detected in many human cancers, including those of the colon and rectum.
E Bevacizumab binds to VEGF and prevents the proliferation of endothelial cells and formation of new blood vessels, thus starving tumors of their blood supply.

7. **B** Sorafenib inhibits vascular endothelial growth factor receptor and (platelet-derived growth factor receptor to inhibit angiogenesis and the Raf serine/threonine kinases that mediate growth and differentiation of tumor cells (p. 379).

8. **E** The growth of prostate cells is stimulated by testosterone. Production of testosterone by Leydig cells of the testes is increased by luteinizing hormone (LH) released from the pituitary. The release of LH is regulated by gonadotropin-releasing hormone (GnRH) from the hypothalamus. Leuprolide is a GnRH-receptor agonist that initially stimulates and then desensitizes pituitary GnRH receptors. This leads to decreased gonadotropin release, decreased testosterone production, decreased prostate growth, and a beneficial effect in prostate cancer. The initial stimulation produced by leuprolide results in an initial surge in LH and testosterone release, which would have an adverse effect on prostate cancer. To block the effects of this initial surge of hormones, flutamide is given. Flutamide is a competitive antagonist of testosterone for binding to androgen receptors in the prostate gland. By doing so, it prevents them from stimulating the prostate cancer cells to grow (pp. 382 and 383).

9. **C** Nausea and vomiting are the most common side effects of this chemotherapy. Of the listed choices, the only one that could be used to address nausea and vomiting is ondansetron, which is a $5-HT_3$ receptor antagonist.

10. D Weak bases are excreted faster ("ion-trapped") if the urine is acidified with ammonium chloride.

A, E Inducing vomiting with apomorphine and performing gastric lavage with charcoal are unlikely to be effective, as the drug has already been absorbed.

B Alkalinization of the urine with sodium bicarbonate will retard elimination because phencyclidine is a weak base.

C Phencyclidine is not effectively extracted by hemoperfusion.

11. E Multiple drug transfusions can lead to iron poisoning. Deferoxamine specifically chelates iron and promotes its excretion (p. 390).

A Dimercaprol is an effective treatment following poisoning by arsenic, gold, lead, and mercury.

B Succimer is used for lead poisoning.

C Calcium disodium EDTA is used for lead poisoning.

D Trientine is a copper chelating agent.

12. A Depressed respiration, nociception, and miosis are symptoms of opiate poisoning. As a competitive antagonist of opiates, naloxone should block all of the effects of opiates, with increasing effectiveness at higher doses. The lack of further effect of naloxone suggests multiple drug use.

B–D The other possibilities are not indicated by the response to naloxone.

13. D Although naloxone will block the effects of codeine, it will not block the effects of chloral hydrate, a central nervous system depressant drug. Because there are no specific antidotes for chloral hydrate, life support measures, such as mechanical assistance of respiration, must be taken.

A Strychnine is a pesticide agent that acts by inhibiting glycine. This agent causes seizures and contractions of voluntary muscle that lead to respiratory paralysis.

B Pentylenetetrazol is an experimental drug used to induce convulsions.

C, E Neither dopamine nor caffeine would be expected to have a benefit here.

14. A These are symptoms of organophosphate poisoning. Atropine is a muscarinic receptor antagonist given to relieve the overactivation of muscarinic receptors (p. 391).

B, C Edrophonium and neostigmine are acetylcholinesterase inhibitors and would worsen the symptoms.

D, E Because this is an emergency situation, you would not have time to wait for laboratory results.

15. C Sodium nitrite produces methemoglobin, which binds cyanide. Sodium thiosulfate increases cyanide metabolism (p. 391).

A Carbon monoxide is a poisonous gas.

B Trientine is a copper chelating agent.

D Pralidoxime is a cholinesterase reactivator used in organophosphate poisoning.

E Dimercaprol is an effective treatment following poisoning by arsenic, gold, lead, and mercury.

Index

Note: Page numbers followed by "f" and "t" indicate figures and tables, respectively.
Italicized page numbers represent entries in marginal boxes.

A

Abacavir (ABC), 320
  side effects, 320t
Abciximab, 225f, 226
Abscesses, antibiotics in, *284*
Absence seizures
  features, 91t
  treatment, 97t
Absorption of drugs
  factors affecting, 1, 3
  food and, *1*
Abuse, of drugs. *See* Drugs of abuse
Acamprosate, 121
Acarbose, 175f, 176
ACE. *See* Angiotensin-converting enzyme (ACE)
      inhibitors
Acebutolol, 60, 61f
Acetaminophen, 355
Acetazolamide, 185, 186f
Acetic acids, as NSAIDs, 354, 355t
Acetylation
  in drug metabolism, 12t
  polymorphism, 27t
Acetylcholine (ACh)
  activation effects in parasympathetic system,
      44, 45t
  as central neurotransmitter, 68f, 71, 73f
  neuromuscular blockers
      depolarizing, 49, 50f, 53t
      nondepolarizing, 49, 53t
  as peripheral system neurotransmitter,
      37–38, 38f
  receptors, 40, 40f, 41t
Acetylcysteine, as mucolytic, 258
Acetylsalicylic acid. *See* Aspirin
      (acetylsalicyclic acid)
ACh. *See* Acetylcholine (ACh)
Achilles tendon reflex, 375
Acid-base balance, respiration and, *251*
Acquired immunodeficiency syndrome (AIDS).
      See HIV/AIDS
ACTH. *See* Adrenocorticotropic hormone (ACTH)
Actinomycin D (dactinomycin), 373
Action potential (AP)
  at atrial and ventricular myocardium,
      214–215, 214f
  at bundle of His, 214–215, 214f
  effects of antiarrhythmic drugs on, 217, 218f
  phases at sinoatrial (SA) node, 213–214, 214f
  at Purkinje fibers, 214–215, 214f
Activated charcoal, 388
Active transport
  in drug absorption, 3
  in proximal tubule, 12
Acyclovir, 314, 315f, 316, 319t
Aδfibers, in pain pathways, *103*, 103f
Adalimumab
  for inflammatory bowel disease, 274, 276
  for rheumatoid arthritis, 358–359, 359f
Addisonian crisis, *154*
Adefovir dipivoxil, 319
Adenosine, as antiarrhythmic, 221

Adenosine triphosphate (ATP) hydrolysis, drug
      absorption and, 3
Adenylate cyclase system, in signal
      transduction, 23, 23f
ADH. *See* Antidiuretic hormone (ADH)
ADHD (attention deficit/hyperactivity disorder),
      123
Administration of drugs
  calculating amount from V_d, 8
  in children, 27
  continuous IV infusion, kinetics of, 15–16,
      16f
  distribution in body following, 4, 5f
  in elderly, 28
  enteral, 1, 2f, 2t
  in hepatic disease, 19
  inhalation, 2t
  for local anesthetics, 79t
  parenteral, 1, 2f, 2t
  in pregnancy, 29–30
  in renal disease, 19
  repeated dosing, kinetics of, 16–18, 16t, 17f,
      18t, 19f
  routes, 1, 2t
      as antimicrobial selection factor, 284t
      in dosing regimen selection, 18t
      ferrous sulfate, 233f
      time course of plasma concentration in, 2f
  topical, 2t
  transdermal, 2t
  via endotracheal tube, *249*
Adrenal crisis, acute, *154*
Adrenal gland
  embryology, *35*
  hormonal secretions, 151f. *See
      also* Adrenocortical
      hormones; Glucocorticoids;
      Mineralocorticoids
Adrenal insufficiency, primary and secondary,
      139
Adrenergic agents
  depleting catecholamines, 62, 62f
  sympatholytics, 60–61, 61f
  sympathomimetics
      catecholamine, 54–58
      non-catecholamine, 58–59
Adrenergic neuron blockers
  clonidine, 58–59, 58f
  guanethidine, 62, 62f
  in hypertension therapy, 198–199
  methyldopa, 58f
  reserpine, 62, 62f
Adrenergic receptor agonists (β_2), 251
Adrenergic receptors, 41, 41t
  β_2-, interaction with epinephrine, 63t
  drug interactions with, 63t
Adrenocortical hormones, 150–156
  glucocorticoids, 151–156
  mineralocorticoids, 156
Adrenocorticotropic hormone (ACTH), 139
  cosyntropin and, 139
  disorders, 139

Adsorbents, as antidiarrheals, 271, 272f
Aerosols, as drugs of abuse, 126
Affinity, of agonists, 24
Afterload, cardiac, *204*
Age of patient, as antimicrobial selection factor,
      284t
Agonists
  adrenergic receptor activation by, 63t
  cannabinoid, as antiemetics, 265, 266t
  and competitive antagonists, 24, 25f
  described, 24
  inverse, 24
  opiate, 102, 104–107. *See also* Morphine
      mixed agonist-antagonists, 107
  prolactin-inhibiting hormone, 166
Agranulocytosis, typical *vs.* atypical
      antipsychotics and, 101t
AIDS. *See* HIV/AIDS
Albumin, drug distribution and, *4*, 4t
Albuterol
  adrenergic receptor interaction with, 63t
  for asthma and COPD, 251
  as directly acting sympathomimetic, 59
Alcohol
  as anxiolytic/sedative-hypnotic, 84–85
  as drug of abuse, 119–122
Alcoholism
  drug management, 121
  vitamin deficiencies in, *121*
Aldosterone, in renin-angiotensin-
      aldosterone system, 183, 183f
Alemtuzumab, 376–377, 378t
Alendronate, 149
Aliskiren, 194
Alkaline phosphatase, *149*
Alkylating agents, as cancer chemotherapy, 367,
      368f, 369–370
Allergens
  in asthma immunopathogenesis, 250f
  as asthma trigger factors, 249f
Allergic rhinitis, 254f
  decongestants for symptomatic relief,
      255–256
  H_1 antihistamines for, 256, 256f
  intranasal steroids for, 257
  mast cell stabilizers for, 255f, 257
Allergy
  atopy and antiallergy therapy, *252*f
  histamine and, *344*. *See also* Histamine
Allopurinol, for acute gout, 360f, 361
Almotriptan, 340–341
α_1 acid glycoprotein, *4*, 4t
α_1/α_2 receptors, 41, 41t
α_2-adrenergic receptor agonists, 199–200
α_1-adrenergic receptor-blocking agents. *See*
      α-blockers
α_1-antitrypsin deficiency, *249*
α-blockers
  in hypertension therapy, 198
  inhibiting sympathetic function, 60
α-glucosidase inhibitors, as oral hypoglycemic
      agents, 175f, 176

α$_1$-proteinase inhibitors, for COPD, 254
Alprazolam, 82–83
    as drug of abuse, 122
    mechanism of action, 82, 84f
    uses for, 82t
Alprostadil, 349
Alteplase, 230–231
Aluminum hydroxide, 260f, 261
Alzheimer disease, 115
    drug therapy for, 115
Amantadine, 317, 319t
    as antiparkinsonian drug, 113, 114f
Amebicidal drugs, 327–328, 328t
Amides, as local anesthetic
    mechanisms of action, 79, 80f
    pharmacokinetics, 80, 80t
    side effects, 81
Amikacin, 300–301
Amiloride, 188–189, 188f
Amino acids, in drug metabolism, 12t
Aminocaproic acid, 231
Aminoglutethimide, 156
Aminoglycosides, 300–301
    therapeutic use, 302f
Aminosalicylates, for ulcerative colitis, 273, 274f
Amiodarone, as antiarrhythmic, 220–221
Amitriptyline, 86–87, 87f, 267
Amlodipine, 196, 197f
    electrophysiological and hemodynamic
        effects, 198t
Amobarbital
    as anxiolytic/sedative-hypnotic, 83–84, 84t
        mechanism of action, 84f
    as drug of abuse, 122
Amoxapine, 88
Amoxicillin, 290, 291f, 292
    uses for, 291
Amphetamine(s)
    as CNS-acting appetite suppressant, 277
    as drugs of abuse, 123–124
    as mixed acting sympathomimetic, 59
Amphotericin B, 324, 325f
Ampicillin, 290, 292
    uses for, 291
Amprenavir, 322
    side effects, 323t
Amyl nitrate, in angina therapy, 209, 210f
Amylin analogue, as oral hypoglycemic agents,
        176
Anabolic effects, of testosterone, 166t
Anabolic steroids, 167
Anaerobic bacteria, 306
Anaerobic infections, 306
Anakinra, 359
Analgesics
    acetaminophen, 355–356
    NSAIDs. See Nonsteroidal antiinflammatory
        drugs (NSAIDs)
    opioid. See Opioids
Anastrozole, as cancer chemotherapy agent, 381
Androgenic effects
    anabolic steroids, 167
    testosterone, 166t
Androgens, synthetic, 167
Anemia
    blood smear in, 232
    hemolytic, 27t
    iron deficiency, 232
    megaloblastic, 232
        drug therapy for, 234
    signs and symptoms, 232

Anesthesia
    agents for. See Anesthetics
    defined, 75
    goals, 75, 75f
    malignant hyperthermia and, 76
Anesthetics
    adjuncts to, 75t
    dissociative, 77–78
    dosing standard for, 75
    inhalation agents, 75–77, 76t
    intravenous agents, 77–79. See also
            Barbiturates; Benzodiazepines
    local, 79–81, 80t
Angina
    classic, pathogenesis in coronary sclerosis,
            208, 209f
    drug management, 208
    myocardial oxygen demand and, 208, 208f
    types, 208
Angiotensin antagonists
    in heart failure therapy, 205
    for hypertension, 191, 193f, 194, 202t
Angiotensin I/Angiotensin II, 191, 193f, 194
    in renin-angiotensin system, 181, 183f
Angiotensin II receptor antagonists, 194
Angiotensin-converting enzyme (ACE)
            inhibitors, 191, 193f, 194
    in heart failure therapy, 204
Anidulafungin, 327
Anistreplase, 230
ANS. See Autonomic nervous system (ANS)
Antabuse (disulfiram), for alcoholism
            management, 121
Antagonists
    adrenergic receptor activation by, 63t
    angiotensin. See Angiotensin antagonists
    as antiemetics
        dopamine, 266, 266t
        5-HT$_3$, 266–267, 266t
        NK$_1$, 264–265, 266t
    competitive, 24, 25f
    described, 24
    estrogens, 163–164, 164f
    glycoprotein IIb/IIIa, 226
    H$_2$ receptor, effects on GI system, 259f, 261
    mixed. See Labetalol
    opiate, 108
        mixed agonist-antagonists, 107
    progesterone, 165, 165f
    testosterone, 168f
    vasopressin, 190
    of vitamin K, 228, 229f, 230f
Anthraquinones, 268
Antiallergy therapy, atopy and, 252f
Antiandrogens, 167
    as cancer chemotherapy, 383
Antianemia drugs (hemantics), 232, 233f, 234
Antianginal drugs
    beta-blockers, 211, 212t
    calcium channel blockers, 211, 212t
    vasodilators (nitrates), 209, 210f, 211,
            212t
Antiarrhythmic agents
    adenosine, 221
    class I, 217, 217t, 218f
    class IA, 217, 217t
    class IB, 217t, 219, 219f
    class IC, 217t, 219–220
    class II, 217t, 220
    class III, 217t, 220
    class IV, 217t, 220–221

Antibacterial drugs, 287–312
    antileprotic, 311
    antimycobacterial, 308–309, 309t, 310f
    antiseptics, 311–312, 312t
    disinfectants, 311–312, 312t
    inhibitors of bacterial cell wall synthesis,
            287–296
    inhibitors of folate metabolism, 304, 305f,
            306
    inhibitors of nucleic acid metabolism, 302,
            303f, 304
    inhibitors of protein synthesis, 296–302
    microorganisms targeted by, 307t
    miscellaneous, 306
    modes of action, protein synthesis and,
            298f
    site of action, 287f
Antibiotic-associated pseudomembranous
            colitis, 295
Antibiotics. See also specific classes of antibiotics
    in abscesses, 284
    as cancer chemotherapy, 368f, 372–374
    contraceptive pill efficacy and, 309
    penetration into cerebrospinal fluid, 292
Antibody, anti-IgE, 253, 346
Anticancer agents, 365. See also Cancer
            chemotherapy
    cell cycle and, 365, 365f
    in combination therapy, attributes of,
            366–367
    resistance to, 367, 367f
    toxicity, 366, 366f
Anticholinergic drugs
    as antiemetics, 265, 266t
    for asthma and COPD, 251
Anticholinesterases, 44f, 47–48
Anticoagulants, 226–231
Anticonvulsants, 91–97
Antidepressants
    first-generation, 86–88
    second-generation, 88
    third-generation, 89
Antidiarrheals, 270–271
    site of action, 272f
Antidiuretic hormone (ADH), 142
    syndrome of inappropriate secretion, 190
    synthesis and secretion, stimuli for, 142
Antidotes
    metal chelating agents, 389–391
    nonspecific, 388–389
    specific, 391t
Antiemetic effects, of antipsychotic agents, 98
Antiemetics, 264–267, 266t
Antiepileptic drugs, 91–97, 97t
    sites of action
        in GABAergic synapse, 95f
        neuronal, 92f
Antiestrogens
    as cancer chemotherapy, 381
    in reproductive endocrinology, 164
Antifungal drugs, 324–327, 325f
    echinocandins, 327
    imidazole, 324, 325f, 326
    polyene, 324, 325f
    tetrazole, 326
    other, 326–327
Antihistamines
    as antiemetics, 265–266, 266t
    for cough, 257
    H$_1$, 256, 256f, 344–345
    H$_2$, 346

Antihyperlipidemic therapy, 237
    bile acid sequestrants, 239–240, 239f
    fibrates, 240–241
    nicotinic acid (niacin), 240
    statins, 237, 238f
Antihypertensives, 191, 202t
    angiotensin antagonists, 191, 193f, 194, 202t
    direct vasodilators, 200–201, 200f, 202t
    diuretics, 191, 202t
    sympatholytics, 194–200, 202t
    therapeutic indications, 191
Antihypoglycemics, 177
Anti-IgE antibody, 253, 346
Antiinfective activity, in combination therapy, 285
Antiinflammatory drugs. *See* Nonsteroidal antiinflammatory drugs (NSAIDs)
Antileprotic drugs, 310f, 311
Antimalarial drugs, 329, 330f, 331–332
Antimanic drug, 89–90
Antimetabolites
    as antibacterial agents, 304, 305f, 306
    as cancer chemotherapy, 368f, 370–372
    as immunosuppressants, 383t
    for inflammatory bowel disease, 276–277, 276f
    virustatic, chemical structure of, 315f
Antimicrobial drugs
    for bacterial infections. *See* Antibacterial drugs
    bacteriostatic *vs.* bactericidal, 281–282, 281f
    combination therapy with, 285
    empiric therapy with, 285
    for fungal infections. *See* Antifungal drugs
    mechanism of action, 281, 281t
    for parasitic infections. *See* Antiparasitic drugs
    selection factors
        drugs, 284, 284t
        microorganisms, 282–284, 283t
        patients, 284, 284t
    spectra, 282
    susceptibility to, 282
    therapeutic principles, 281–286
    for viral infections. *See* Antiviral drugs
Antimitotics, as cancer chemotherapy, 374–375
Antimycobacterial agents, 308–309, 309t, 310f
Antiparasitic drugs
    for metazoan infections, 332–333
    for protozoan infections, 327–331, 328t, 330f
Antiparkinsonian drugs, 111–113, 112t, 114f, 115
Antiplatelet drugs, 224–226, 225f
Antipsychotic agents
    atypical, 100–101
        comparison with typical agents, 101t
        drug interactions with, 99
        effects, 98, 99t
        mechanism of action, 98
        pharmacokinetics, 98
        side effects, 99
        tolerance, dependence, and withdrawal, 99
    typical, 100
        comparison with atypical agents, 101t
        drug interactions with, 99
        effects, 98, 99t
        mechanism of action, 98
        pharmacokinetics, 98
        side effects, 99
        tolerance, dependence, and withdrawal, 99

Antipyretics
    acetaminophen, 355–356
    fever and, *352*
    NSAIDs. *See* Nonsteroidal antiinflammatory drugs (NSAIDs)
Antiseptics
    external, 312, 312t
    urinary, 311–312
Antituberculosis drugs, 308–309
    treatment protocol, 309t
Antitussives, 257
Antiviral drugs, 313–323
    in HIV/AIDS management. *See under* HIV/AIDS
    inhibitors of nucleic acid synthesis, 314–317, 315f
    mechanism of action, 313f
    neuraminidase inhibitors, 318
    viral M2 protein blockers, 317, 318f
Anxiolytics, 82–85
AP. *See* Action potential (AP)
Apnea, succinylcholine, 27t
Appetite enhancers, 278
Appetite suppressants, 277
Aprepitant, 264–265
Aralast™, for COPD, 254
Argatroban, 228
Aripiprazole, 100–101
Aromatase inhibitors, as cancer chemotherapy, 381–382, 382f
Aromatic L-amino decarboxylase inhibitors, for Parkinson disease, 112–113, 114f
Arsenic poisoning, *389*
Arsenic trioxide, 380
Articaine, as local anesthetic, 79–81, 80f, 80t
Ascorbic acid
    redox reactions, *39*
    toxic effects and treatment, 392t
Aspartate, as central neurotransmitter, 68f, 71, 73t
Aspirin (acetylsalicylic acid), 353
    as antiplatelet drug, 224–225, 225f
    contraindicated for gout, 361
    mechanism of action, 351
    as prostaglandin antagonist, 350
Asthma, 249
    atopy and, *249*
    genetic predisposition and trigger factors, 249f
    immunopathogenesis, 250f
    treatment, 250–254
Atazanavir, 322
    side effects, 323t
Atenolol
    adrenergic receptor interaction with, 63t
    as β-blocker, 60, 61f
    for hypertension, 194–196, 195f
    for hypothyroidism, 145
Atonic seizure
    features, 91t
    treatment, 97t
Atopy
    and antiallergy therapy, 252f
    asthma and, *249*
Atorvastatin, 237
Atovaquone, 330f, 331
Atrial fibrillation, 216t
Atrial flutter, 216t
Atrial myocardium, action potential phases at, 214–215, 214f
Atrioventricular (AV) node, action potential phases at, 214, 214f
Atropine, 49, 52, 53t
    poisoning, antidote for, 391t

Attention deficit/hyperactivity disorder (ADHD), *123*
Autocoids, 340–350
    bradykinin and related drugs, 342–343
    eiscosanoids and related drugs, 347, 348f, 349–350
    histamine and related drugs, 343–346, 347t
    leukotrienes and related drugs, 350
    serotonin and related drugs, 340–342, 342t
Autonomic nervous system (ANS)
    adrenergic receptors, 41, 41t
    cholinergic receptors, 40, 40f, 41t
    disorders, *42*
    divisions, 35, 35t
    innervation of target organs by, 35, 36t
    neurotransmitters, 37–39
    physiologic responses, 41, 42t–43t
Azathioprine, 276–277, 276f
Azidothymidine (zidovudine), 320
    in HIV/AIDS management, 320t
Azithromycin, 297
AZT (zidovudine), 320, 320t
Aztreonam, 295

B

Baclofen, 116
Bacteria
    anaerobic, *306*
    gram negative, 286t
    gram positive, 286t
    resistance to antimicrobial agents, 282–284, 283f, 283t
    specific agents targeting, 307t
Bacterial cell wall
    gram-negative, *287*
    structure, *287*
    synthesis, inhibitors of, 287–296
Bacterial enzymes, *283*
Bacterial growth, oxygen levels and, *282*
Bacterial toxins, *283*
    exotoxins, *284*
Bactericidal agents, 281f, 282
Bacteriostatic agents, 281f, 282
Ballismus, *98*
Balsalazide, 273
Barbiturates
    as antiepileptics, sites of action of
        in GABAergic synapse, 95f
        neuronal, 92f
    as anxiolytics/sedative-hypnotics, 83–84, 84f, 84t
    as intravenous anesthetic agents, 78–79
    therapeutic index for, 82
Baroreceptor reflex, *54, 191*
Basal ganglia, in Parkinson disease, *111*, 111f
Basiliximab, 387
Beclomethasone, 250–251
Belladonna. *See* Atropine
Benserazide, 112–113
Benzocaine, as local anesthetic, 79–81, 80f, 80t
Benzodiazepine receptor agonists, nonbenzodiazepine, 83
Benzodiazepines
    as antiepileptics, 94–95
        neuronal sites of action, 92f
        sites of action in GABAergic synapse, 94, 95f
    as anxiolytics/sedative-hypnotics, 82–83, 82t, 84f
    cross-tolerance with alcohol, 120

Benzodiazepines (*cont.*)
    as drugs of abuse, 122
    as intravenous anesthetic agents, 78–79,
       82–83, 82t
    therapeutic index for, 82
Benztropine, 51f, 52, 53t
    as antiparkinsonian drug, 114f, 115
Beractant, 254
β$_2$ agonists, 251
β-adrenergic receptor agonists, 206
β-adrenergic receptor antagonists, 220
β-blockers
    in angina therapy, 211, 211t, 212t
    in heart failure therapy, 205
    for hypertension, 194–196, 195f
    inhibiting sympathetic function, 60–61, 61f
β-lactam antibiotics, 287–295, 287t. *See also*
       Cephalosporins; Penicillin(s)
    cell-wall synthesis inhibition and, 287,
       287f–288f
    chemical structure, 288f
    mechanism of action, 287, 288f
β-lactamase inhibitors, 295
β-receptors, 41, 41t
Betamethasone, 152, 154
Bethanecol, 46
Bevacizumab, 377, 378t
Bicalutamide, 383
Biguanides, as oral hypoglycemic agents, 174, 175f
Bile acid sequestrants, for lowering plasma
       cholesterol levels, 239–240, 239f
Bimatoprost, 349
Bioavailability (*F*), 3
    in dosing regimen selection, 18t
Bisacodyl, 268
Bismuth subsalicylate
    as antidiarrheal, 271
    effect in GI system, 262–263
Bisphosphonates, 149
    and osteonecrosis of jaw, *149*
Bivalirudin, 228
Bleeding, drug therapy for, 231
Bleomycin, 373–374
Blood, drugs affecting, 223–235
    antianemia drugs (hemantics), 232, 233f, 234
    anticoagulants, 226–231
    antiplatelet drugs, 224–226, 225f
    hematopoietic growth factors, 235
Blood dyscrasia, *357*
Blood flow, drug distribution and, 4
Blood smear, in anemia, *232*
Blood-tissue barriers, 6f
"Blue bloaters," *250*
Bone marrow function, *369*
    components, *147*
Bone metabolism
    calcitonin effects on, 148
    estrogen effects on, 157t
    magnesium and, *147*
    pituitary hormone effects on, 146, 146f,
       147t, 148
    vitamin D effects on, 148
Bone remodeling regulation, 150f
Bortezomib, 380
Botulinum toxin, *53*
Bradykinin
    antagonists, 343
    effects, 343, 347t
Brain
    effect of progesterone on, 159t
    effects of estrogen in, 157t

Bran, as laxative, 270
Breast milk, drug secretion into, 30, 30f
Breasts, progesterone effects on, 159t
British antilewisite (BAL), as chelating agent,
       389, 390f
Bromocriptine, 166
    as antiparkinsonian drug, 113, 114f
Bronchial tone, β-blockers effect on, 61f
Bronchospasm, NSAID-induced, *249*
Broth dilution tests, *283*
Buccal drug administration, 2t
    distribution in body following, 5f
Budesonide
    for asthma, 250–251
    for inflammatory bowel disease, 276
Bulk-forming laxatives, 270, 270f
Bumetanide, 185, 187
Bundle of His, action potential phases at,
       214–215, 214f
Bupivacaine, as local anesthetic, 79–81, 80f, 80t
Buprenorphine, 107, 109t
Bupropion, 88
    for smoking cessation, 125
Buserelin, 141
Buspirone, 85
Busulfan, 370
Butyrophenone antipsychotics, 100

C

C fibers, in pain pathways, *103, 103f*
Cabergoline, 166
CABG (coronary artery bypass graft), *208*
Caffeine, as drug of abuse, 123
Calcineurin inhibitors, 383t, 386f
Calcitonin, bone metabolism and, 147f, 148–149
Calcium (Ca^{2+})
    homeostasis, hormonal regulation, 146f
    physiological roles, *147*
Calcium carbonate, 260, 260f
Calcium channel blockers
    in angina therapy, 211, 212t
    electrophysiological and hemodynamic
       effects, 198t
    in hypertension therapy, 196, 197f
Calcium disodium edetate, as chelating agent,
       389
Cancer, genes critical for, *365*
Cancer chemotherapy, 365–383
    alkylating agents, 367, 368f, 369–370
    antiandrogens, 383
    antibiotics, 368f, 372–374
    antiestrogens, 381
    antimetabolites, 368f, 370–372
    antimitotics, 374–375
    aromatase inhibitors, 381–382, 382f
    corticosteroids, 381
    differentiating agents, 380
    general principles, 365–367, 366f
    GnRH agonist agents, 382
    hormones and hormone inhibitors, 381
    monoclonal antibodies, 375–378, 378t
    taxanes, 375
    topoisomerase inhibitors, 368f, 374
    tyrosine kinase inhibitors, 378–380, 379f
Candesartan, 194
Cannabinoid agonists, as antiemetic, 265, 266t
Cannabis
    as drug of abuse, 125
    medical uses, 278
Capecitabine, 372
Capillaries, glomerular *vs.* systemic, *181*

Capillary endothelial cells, drug
       distribution and, 4, 6f
Captopril, 191, 193f, 194
Carbachol, 46
Carbamazepine, 92–93
    drug interactions with, 93
    neuronal sites of action, 92f
Carbidopa, 112–113, 114f
Carbidopa, for Parkinson disease, 112–113,
       114f
Carbon monoxide poisoning, *391*
    antidote for, 391t
Carbonic anhydrase inhibitor diuretics, 185,
       186f
Carboplatin, 370
Carboprost tromethamine, 349–350
Carcinogenesis, chemical, *365*
Carcinoid tumors, and serotonin
       syndrome, *340*
Cardiac action potential phases, 213–215, 214f
Cardiac arrhythmias, 216
    classification, 216t
    as digoxin side effect, 206
    drug therapy for, 217–221, 217t
    nondrug therapies for, *221*
Cardiac axis, *215*
Cardiac enzymes, *209*
Cardiac muscle metabolism, *208*
Cardiovascular system
    acetylcholine effects in, 45t
    autocoid effects on, 347t
    catecholamine effects on, 54f, 55f
    drugs acting upon
       antianginals, 208–212
       antiarrhythmics, 213–221
       antihyperlipedemics, 236–241
       antihypertensives, 191–202. *See also*
       Diuretics
       blood agents, 223–235
       in heart failure, 203–207
    morphine effects on, 105t
Cardioversion, *216*
Carmustine, 369
Carpal tunnel syndrome, *138*
Caspofungin, 327
Castor oil, 268
Catabolism, alcohol, 120f
Catecholamines
    cardiac effects, 55f
    drugs that deplete, 62, 62f
    endogenous, 54–57
    metabolic effects, 55f
    synthetic, 57–58
    vascular smooth muscle effects, 54f
Cathartics
    contact (stimulant-irritant), 268
    saline (osmotic), 269
    uses and contraindications, 268t
CD4 cells, *320*
CD8 cells, *320*
Cefaclor, 293
Cefadroxil, 292–293
Cefamandole, 293
Cefapime, 294
Cefazolin, 292–293
Cefixime, 293–294
Cefmetazole, 293
Cefonicid, 293
Cefoperazone, 293–294
Cefotaxime, 293–294
Cefotetan, 293

Cefoxitin, 293
Cefpodoxime proxetil, 293
Cefproxil, 293
Ceftazidime, 293–294
Ceftizoxime, 293–294
Ceftriaxone, 293–294
Cefuroxime/Cefuroxime axetil, 293
Celecoxib, 355
Cell cycle, anticancer agents and, 365, 365f
Cell lysis, 287
Cell wall synthesis inhibitors
    bacitracin, 296
    β-lactam antibiotics, 287, 287f–288f.
        See also β-lactam antibiotics;
        Cephalosporins; Penicillin(s)
Cell-mediated immunity, 382
Central autonomic control, disorders of, 38
Central nervous system (CNS)
    appetite suppressants and, 277
    autocoid effects on, 347t, 349t
    drugs acting on. See also individually named
        drugs; specific drug classes
        abuse of, 118–126
        anesthetics, 75–81
        anticonvulsants, 91–97
        antidepressants/antimanics, 86–90
        antipsychotics, 98–101
        anxiolytics/sedative-hypnotics, 82–85
        in neurodegenerative diseases,
            110–117
        neuropharmacological principles,
            67–74. See also Central
            neurotransmitters; individually
            named neurotransmitters
        opiate receptor agonists/
            antagonists, 102–109
    ethanol intoxication effects, acute and
        chronic, 119t
    local anesthetic effects on, 81
    morphine effects on, 105t
Central neurotransmitters, 67–74, 68f, 73t.
        See also individually named
        neurotransmitters
Cephalexin, 292–293
Cephalosporins, 292–294
    first-generation, 292–293
    fourth-generation, 294
    second-generation, 293
    side effects, 292
    third-generation, 293–294
Cephalothin, 292–293
Cephapirin, 292–293
Cephradine, 292–293
Cerebrospinal fluid, antibiotic penetration into,
        292
Certain safety factor, in dose-response
        relationship, 26
Certolizumab pegol, 274, 276
Cestode infections, treatment of, 333
Cetirizine, 344–345
Cetrorelix, 141
Cetuximab, 377, 378t
Chagas disease, treatment of, 328t
Charcoal, activated, 388
Chelators, 389–391, 390f
Chemical carcinogenesis, 365
Chemokine coreceptor antagonist, 323
Chemotherapy. See also Cancer chemotherapy
    wafer implants for, 369
CHF (congestive heart failure), 203f
Children. See Pediatric patients

Chloramphenicol, 300f, 301
    therapeutic use, 300f
Chloroguanide, 331–332
7-Chlorolincomycin, 297–299
Chloroquine, 329, 330f
Chlorothiazide, 187
Chlorpheniramine
    for cough, 257
    as H₁ antihistamine, 344–345
Chlorpromazine, 100
Chlorpropamide, 174
Chlorthalidone, 187
Cholecalciferol D₃, 147
    toxic effects and treatment, 392t
Cholera, 299
Cholesterol
    in dyslipidemia, 236, 236
        drugs for lowering levels. See
            Antihyperlipidemic therapy
        metabolism in liver, 239, 239f
        steroid synthesis and, 156
Cholesterol levels
    drugs for lowering. See Antihyperlipidemic
        therapy
    estrogen effects on, 157t
Cholestyramine, 239, 239f
Choline magnesium salicylate, 354
Cholinergic agonists, 44–48. See also
        Parasympathomimetics
Cholinergic antagonists, 48–53, 53t
    muscarinic receptor antagonists, 49, 51f,
        52–53, 53t
    nicotinic receptor antagonists, 48–49, 50f,
        53t
Cholinergic receptors, 40, 40f, 41t
Cholinomimetics. See
        Parasympathomimetics
Chronic obstructive pulmonary disease (COPD),
        249
    clinical signs, 250
    treatment, 250–254
Ciclesonide, 250–251
Cidofovir, 317
Cimetidine, 346
    gastrointestinal system effects, 259f, 261
Cinacalcet, 147
Ciprofloxacin, 302, 303f, 304
Circulatory systems, portal, 3
Cirrhosis of liver, 120f
Cirtirizine, 256, 256f
Cisplatin, 370
cis-retinoic acid, heterodimeric receptors with,
        22f
Citalopram, 89
Citric acid cycle. See Krebs cycle
Cladribine, 372
Clarithromycin, 297
Clavulanic acid, 295
Clearance (CL), in dosing regimen selection, 18t
Clindamycin (7-chlorolincomycin), 297
Clofazimine, 311
Clofibrate, 240–241
Clomiphene, 164
Clomipramine, 90
Clonazepam, 82–83
    as drug of abuse, 122
    mechanism of action, 82, 84f
    uses for, 82t
Clonic seizure
    features, 91t
    treatment, 97t

Clonidine
    adrenergic receptor interaction with, 63t
    as directly acting sympathomimetic, 58–59,
        58f
    in hypertension therapy, 199–200
Clopidogrel, 225–226, 225f
Clotrimazole, 324, 326
Clotting cascade inhibition, 226, 228f
Clotting tests, 229
Cloxacillin, 289
Clozapine, 100–101
Cluster headaches, 341
CMV (cytomegalovirus), 316
CNS. See Central nervous system (CNS)
CoA (coenzyme A), 38
Coagulation
    anticoagulants and, 226–231
    disseminated intravascular, 343
Cocaine, as drug of abuse, 123–124
Codeine
    as antidiarrheal, 271
    for cough, 257
    as drug of abuse, 118
    withdrawal symptoms, 119t
Coenzyme A (CoA), 38
Colchicine, 359, 360f, 361
Colestipol, 239
Colfosceril, 254
Colistin, 306
Colitis, pseudomembranous,
        antibiotic-associated, 295
Combination therapy
    anticancer agents in, attributes of, 366–367
    antimicrobial agents, 285
Competitive antagonism, 24, 25f
Compulsive drug abuse/use, defined, 118t
Conduction system, of heart, 213, 213f
Congestive heart failure (CHF), 203f
Conjugation reactions, in drug
        metabolism, 9f, 11, 12t
Continuous IV infusion, steady-state
        concentration in, 15–16, 16f
Contraception, hormonal. See Hormonal contra-
        ception
Contraceptive pill, antibiotics and, 309
Contractility, cardiac, 204
COPD. See Chronic obstructive pulmonary
        disease (COPD)
Copper poisoning (Wilson disease), 391
Coronary artery bypass graft (CABG), 208
Coronary blood flow, 208
Coronary intervention, percutaneous, 227
Coronary sclerosis, classic angina
        pathogenesis in, 208, 209f
Corticorelin, 139
Corticosteroids
    for asthma, 250–251
    as cancer chemotherapy, 381
    effect on respiratory burst, 152
    effects and side effects, 275f
    as immunosuppressants, 383t
    for inflammatory bowel disease, 276
    as prostaglandin antagonists, 350
Cortisol (hydrocortisone), 152, 154
    bone metabolism and, 149
    modification by glucocorticoids, 155f
Cosyntropin, ACTH and, 139
Co-trimoxazole, tetrahydrofolate synthesis
        inhibition and, 305f
Cough, treatment of, 257
Coumarin derivatives, antidote for, 391t

COX-2 selective inhibitors, as NSAIDs, 355
COX-1/COX-2 (cyclooxygenase enzymes) inhibition. See Nonsteroidal antiinflammatory drugs (NSAIDs)
Creatinine, drug elimination and, 12
Crohn's disease, 273, 273f
    drug therapy for, 274f
Cromolyn sodium, 346
    for allergic rhinitis, 255f, 257
    for asthma, 253
Cryptosporidiosis, treatment of, 328t
Curare, 49, 53t
Cushing syndrome, 139
Cyanide poisoning, antidote for, 391t
Cyclooxygenase enzymes (COX-1/COX-2) inhibition. See Nonsteroidal antiinflammatory drugs (NSAIDs)
Cyclopentolate, 52, 53t
Cyclophosphamide, 369
Cystic fibrosis, 258
Cytarabine, 368f, 372
Cytochrome P-450 enzyme(s), 8
    abnormalities in, 27t
    drug interactions involving, 8, 10f, 13f
    inducers and inhibitors, 10f
    oxidations, 11t
    synthesis in liver, 10f
Cytomegalovirus (CMV), 316
Cytostatic resistance mechanisms, 367, 367f
Cytotoxicity, cancer chemotherapy drugs, 368f

D

Dactinomycin (actinomycin D), 373
DAG system, in signal transduction, 23, 23f
Danazol, 167
Dantrolene, 117, 117f
Dapsone (diaminophenylsulfone [DDS]), 311
Darunavir, 322
    side effects, 323t
Darvon (propoxyphene), 107
Dastinib, 378–379
Daunorubicin, 373
Debrisoquine-4-hydroxylase deficiency, 27t
Decongestants
    for cough, 257
    for rhinitis symptomatic relief, 255–256
Deep vein thrombosis (DVT), 227
Deferoxamine, as chelating agent, 232, 390, 390f
Delavirdine, 321–322
Delayed gastric emptying, drug therapy for, 267
Deliriant hallucinogens, as drugs of abuse, 124
Delirium tremens, 120
    management, 120
δ receptors, actions mediated by, 102, 102t
Demeclocycline, 190, 299–300
Dental injections, facial palsy with, 79
Dependence
    amphetamines, 124
    antipsychotics, 99
    barbiturates, 122
    benzodiazepines, 122
    caffeine, 123
    cannabis, 125
    cocaine, 124
    defined, 118t
    deliriant hallucinogens, 124
    ethanol, 120
    nicotine, 125
    psychedelic hallucinogens, 124

Depot contraceptive injections, 163
Depression
    symptoms, 86t
    treatment. See Antidepressants
Desflurane, 76, 76t
Desipramine, 86–87, 87f
Desmopressin (antidiuretic hormone), 189f, 190.
        See also
        Antidiuretic hormone (ADH)
    for treatment of bleeding, 231
Detoxification, 118
Dexamethasone, 152, 154
Dexfenfluramine, 277
Dextromethorphan, 108, 109t
    for cough, 257
Diabetes mellitus, 170, 171f
    antihypoglycemic drugs for, 177
    gestational, 172
    insulin/insulin preparations for, 170–174
    nephrogenic, treatment of, 189
    oral hypoglycemic drugs, 174–177, 175f
    osmotic diuresis with, 184
    signs, symptoms, and complications, 170t
    type I, 170, 170
    type II, 170
        oral hypoglycemic drugs for, 174, 175f, 176–177
    types of, 170
    typical vs. atypical antipsychotics and, 101t
Diabetic ketoacidosis (DKA), 170
Diabetic nephropathy, 184
Diamorphine
    as drug of abuse, 118
    withdrawal symptoms, 119t
Diarrhea, drug treatment for. See Antidiarrheals
Diazepam
    as anxiolytic/sedative-hypnotic, 82–83
        mechanism of action, 82, 84f
        uses for, 82t
    as drug of abuse, 122
    as intravenous anesthetic agents, 79
    for spasticity and muscle spasms, 116, 117
Diazoxide, 201
Diclofenac, 355t
Dicloxacillin, 289
Didanosine (ddl), 320
    side effects, 320t
Dietary fiber, 270
    as laxative, 270
Diethylstilbestrol, 157
    bone metabolism and, 149
Differentiating agents, as cancer chemotherapy, 380
Diffusion hypoxia, with nitrous oxide, 77
Diflunisal, 354
Digoxin (digitalis), in heart failure therapy, 205–206
    effects, 205
    mechanism of action, 205
    side effects, 206
    toxicity and drug interactions, 206
Dihydroergotamine mesylate, 341
Dihydrofolate reductase inhibitors, 331–332
Dihydrotestosterone (DHT), 166, 168f
Diiodohydroxyquinolone (iodoquinol), 328
DIL (drug-induced lupus erythematosus), 27, 27t
Diltiazem, 196, 197f
    electrophysiological and hemodynamic effects, 198t

Dimercaprol, as chelating agent, 389, 390f
Dimercaptopropane sulfonate, 390f
Dinoprostone, 349–350
Dipeptidyl peptidase 4 (DPP-4) inhibitors, 176–177
Diphenhydramine
    as antiparkinsonian drug, 115
    as anxiolytic/sedative-hypnotic, 85
    for cough, 257
    as H_1 antihistamine, 344–345
Diphenoxylate, 271, 272f
Diphenylmethanes, 268
Direct thrombin inhibitors, 228–230, 229f, 230f
Direct-acting parasympathomimetics
    bethanecol, 46
    carbachol, 46
    characteristics, 44f, 45
    contraindications, 45
    methacholine, 45–46
    pilocarpine, 46
Directly acting sympathomimetics, 58–59
Disease-modifying antirheumatic drugs (DMARDs), 356–358
Disinfectants, external, 312, 312t
Disk diffusion test, 283
Disopyramide, as antiarrhythmic, 217
Disseminated intravascular coagulation, 342
Dissociative anesthetic, ketamine as, 77–78
Distal tubule, drug reabsorption in, 12
Distribution of drugs
    factors affecting, 4
    fluid compartments for, 7, 7f
    volume, 4, 7–8, 7f, 7t
Disulfiram (Antabuse), for alcoholism management, 121
Diuretics
    carbonic anhydrase inhibitors, 185, 186f
    in heart failure therapy, 204, 204f
    in hypertension management, 191
    loop (high-ceiling), 185, 186f, 187
    osmotic, 184, 185f
    over-the-counter drugs as, 189
    potassium-sparing, 188–189, 188f
    renal action, 183, 184f
    thiazides, 186f, 187
DKA (diabetic ketoacidosis), 170
DNA
    antibacterial dug action on, 303f
    spontaneous mutations in, bacterial resistance and, 283
Dobutamine
    as adrenergic agent, 58
    in heart failure therapy, 206
Docetaxel, 375
Docusate, 269
Dolasetron, 266–267
Donepezil, 115
Dopamine
    as adrenergic agent, 57
    adrenergic receptor interaction with, 63t
    as central neurotransmitter, 67, 68f, 73t
    release, inactivation, and pharmacological uses, 69f
    as therapeutic agent, 57f
Dopamine antagonists, as antiemetics, 266, 266t
Dopaminergic tracts, 67
Dose-response relationship
    certain safety factor, 26
    potency, 25, 25f
    therapeutic index, 26

Dosing regimens
    fixed-dose/fixed-time-interval, 16–17, 16t, 17f
    irregular, 18, 19f
    loading dose in, 17–18
    selection factors, 18t
Doxazosin
    as α-blocker, 60
    in hypertension therapy, 198
Doxorubicin, 373
Doxycycline, 299–300
Doxylamine, 85
Dronabinol
    as antiemetic, 265
    as appetite enhancer, 278
Drug(s)
    abnormal pupillary reactions to, *105*
    absorption, 1, *1*, 3
    as adjuncts to anesthetics, 75t
    administration. *See* Administration of drugs
    delivery. *See* Administration of drugs
    nonmedical use. *See* Drugs of abuse
    teratogenicity, 30
Drug abuse, defined, 118t. *See also* Drugs of abuse
Drug addiction, defined, 118t
Drug classification, by interaction with receptors, 24, 25f
Drug delivery. *See* Administration of drugs
Drug interactions
    with antipsychotic agents, 99
    cytochrome P-450 enzymes and, 8, 10f
    digitalis, 206
    in dosing regimen selection, 18t
    felbamate and, 96
    gabapentin and, 96
    with grapefruit, *8*
    involving cytochrome P-450 enzyme, 13f
    with levodopa, 112
    with MAOIs, 88
    with meperidine, 106
    with opioids, 106
    with phenobarbital/primidone, 93
    with phenytoin, 92
    with receptors. *See* Drug-receptor interactions
    stage and mechanism, 13, 13t
    with tricyclic antidepressants, 87
    with triptans, 341
    with valproic acid, 94
Drug misuse, defined, 118t
Drug-induced lupus erythematosus (DIL), *27*, 27t
Drug-metabolizing enzymes, induction of, 27t
Drug-receptor interactions, 20–24, 20f–23f, 24t, 25f
    drug classification based on, 24, 25f
Drug-resistant genes, transfer of, *283*, 283t
Drug-response relationship, 25–26, 25f
Drugs of abuse
    alcohol, 119–122, 119t, 120f
    barbiturates, 122
    benzodiazepines, 122
    opioids, 118–119, 119t
    quaaludes, 123
    stimulants, 123–124
    terms related to, definitions, 118t
d4T. *See* Stavudine (d4T)
Ductus arteriosus, *350*
Duloxetine, 88
DVT (deep vein thrombosis), *227*
Dynorphins, *106*

Dyscrasia, blood, *357*
Dyslipidemia, 236. *See also* Hyperlipidemic diseases
    therapy for, 237
    typical *vs.* atypical antipsychotics in, 101t

E
ECG. *See* Electrocardiogram (ECG)
Echinocandins, 327
Edema
    mobilization of fluid by diuretics, 204f
    pulmonary, *187*
Efferent neurons, in autonomic and somatic nervous systems, 37f
Eicosanoids
    prostaglandin agonists, 349–350
    prostaglandin antagonists, 350
    synthesis, 347, 348f
Elderly patients, prescribing drugs for, 28
Electrical activity, of heart
    action potential phases, 213–215, 214f
    cardiac axis, *216*
    excitation-contraction coupling, *196*, *215*
    measuring, 215–216, 215f
Electrocardiogram (ECG)
    interpretation, 215–216
    recording, 215, 215f
Electrochemical coupling, inhibition of, 117f
Electrolytes, *268*
Electron transport chain, *391*
Eletriptan, 340–341
Elimination of drugs
    after cessation of continuous IV infusion, 15, 16f
    first-order kinetics, 14, 14f
    hepatic, 13
    renal, 12–13
    zero-order kinetics, 14–15, 15f
Embolism, 224, 224f
    pulmonary, *230*
Embryology, adrenal gland, *37*
Emergency hormonal contraception, 162
Emesis, drug therapy for causes of, 264–267, 266t
Empiric therapy, antimicrobial agents, 285
Emtricitabine (FTC), 320
    side effects, 320t
Enalapril, 191, 193f, 194
Endocarditis, *289*
Endocrine disorders, drugs used in treatment of. *See also individually named drugs; individual drug classes*
    hypothalamic, pituitary, thyroid, and adrenal disorders, 136–156
    insulin, hypoglycemic, and antihypoglycemic drugs, 170–177
Endogenous catecholamines, 54–57
Endogenous opioids, for pain modulation, 104, *104*, 104f
Endometriosis, *141*
End-organ damage, in hypertension, *191*
Endorphins, *106*
Endothelial cells
    capillary, drug distribution and, 4, 6f
    role in preventing thrombus formation, *223*
Endotoxins, *284*
Endotracheal tube, drug delivery via, *249*
Enflurane, 76, 76t
Enfuvirtide, 323
Enkephalins, *106*
Enoxaparin, 227–228

Entacapone, 113, 114f
Entamoeba histolytica infection, drug therapy for, 327–328, 328t
Entecavir, 319
Enteral drug administration, 1, 2t
    time course of plasma concentration in, 2f
Enteric nervous system, 37
Entry (fusion) inhibitor, in HIV/AIDS management, 321f, 323
Enzyme-linked membrane receptor, 21, 21f
Enzymes
    bacterial, *283*
    cardiac, *209*
    drug-metabolizing, induction of, 27t
    pancreatic, replacement of, 264
    phosphorylation, 23, 23f
    5α-reductase, testosterone and, 166, 168f
Ephedrine
    as CNS-acting appetite suppressant, 277
    as mixed acting sympathomimetic, 59
EPI. *See* Epinephrine (EPI)
Epidural anesthesia, administration method for, 79t
Epilepsy, 91
    drug therapy for, 91–97, 97t. *See also* Antiepileptic drugs
Epinephrine (EPI), 39, 55–56
    adrenergic receptor interaction with, 63t
    interaction with β₂-adrenergic receptor, 56f
    structure-activity relationship, 56f
Epiphyseal plates, growth at, *138*
Epoetin alfa, 235
EPS. *See* Extrapyramidal system (EPS)
Eptifibatide, 225f, 226
Ergocalciferol D₂, 147, 148
    toxic effects and treatment, 392t
Ergonovine, 169
Ergot alkaloids
    for migraine, 341
    uterine effects, 169
Ergotamine, 341
Erlotinib, 379
Erythrocyte sedimentation rate (ESR), *234*
Erythromycin, 296–297
    for increased GI motility, 267
Erythropoietin, *235*
Esmolol
    as antiarrhythmic, 220
    as β-blocker, 60, 61f
    for hypothyroidism, 145
Esomeprazole, 259–260, 259f
ESR (erythrocyte sedimentation rate), *234*
Esters, as local anesthetic
    mechanisms of action, 79, 80f
    pharmacokinetics, 80, 80t
    side effects, 81
Estradiol, 157, 158f
    bone metabolism and, 149
Estrogens, 157–159
    antagonists, 163–164, 164f
    bone metabolism and, 149
    effects, 157t
    side effects, 159
    uses for, 158–159
Eszopiclone, 83
Etanercept, 358–359, 359f
Ethacrynic acid, 185, 187
Ethambutol, 308, 309t
Ethanol, as sedative-hypnotic, 85
Ethanol toxicology, 119–120
    acute and chronic intoxication effects, 119t

Ethinyl estradiol, 157
    bone metabolism and, 149
    intravaginal ring, 162–163
    in transdermal patch contraceptives, 162
Ethosuximide, 95
    neuronal sites of action, 92f
Ethyl glycol toxicity, antidote for, 391t
Ethylene glycol toxicology, 122
Etidronate, 149
Etodolac, 355t
Etonogestrel, as contraceptive
    intravaginal ring, 162–163
    subdermal implant, 162
Etoposide, 374
Etravirine, 322
Excess mucus production, treatment of, 258
Excitation-contraction coupling, in cardiac
        muscle, 196, 215
Exemestane, 381–382
Exenatide, 176–177
Exotoxins, 284
Expectorants, 258
Extended-spectrum penicillins, 290–292
External antiseptics/disinfectants, 312,
        312t
Extrapyramidal system (EPS), 98
    effects of antipsychotic agents on, 98
    in Parkinson disease, 111
    side effects with antipsychotic agents, 99,
        99t, 101t
Exudates, 262
Eye, acetylcholine effects in, 45t
Ezetimide, 239f, 240

F
Facial palsy, from dental injections, 79
Famciclovir, 314, 316
Famotidine, 346
    effect on gastrointestinal system, 259f, 261
Fast-acting insulin, 173f, 174
    pharmacokinetic properties, 173t
Fasting blood sugar test, 170
Febrile convulsions/seizures
    NSAIDs for, 93
    recurrent, antiepileptics for, 97t
Feedback, negative, 137
Feflunomide, 358
Felbamate, 96
    drug interactions and, 96
    neuronal sites of action, 92f
Fenfluramine, 277
Fenoprofen, 355t
Ferrous sulfate, for iron deficiency anemia, 232
    administration routes, 233f
Fetal alcohol syndrome, 119
Fetal lung maturity, test for, 254
Fetus
    chronic ethanol intoxication effects on, 119t
    drug exposure and damage in, 29–30, 29f
Fever, antipyretic drugs and, 352
Fexofenadine
    for allergic rhinitis, 256, 256f
    as H$_1$ antihistamine, 344–345
Fiber. See Dietary fiber
Fibrates, as cholesterol-lowering agents,
        240–241
Fibrillation, atrial and ventricular, 216, 216t
Fibrinogen, 225f
Fibrinolysis, 231f
    myocardial infarction and, 230
Filgrastim, 235

Finasteride, 167
Finger clubbing, 250
First-generation cephalosporins, 292–293
First-order kinetics, of elimination, 14, 14f
First-pass metabolism, bioavailability and, 3
5-HT. See Serotonin (5-HT)
Fixed-dose/fixed-time-interval regimens, 16–17,
        16t, 17f
Flatworm infections, treatment of, 333
Flecainide, 219–220
Fluconazole, 327
Flucytosine, 325f, 326
Fludarabine, 372
Fludrocortisone, 156
Fluid compartments, for drug distribution, 7, 7f
    drug features and, 7t
Flumazenil, 83
Flunisolide, 250–251
Fluocinonide, 152, 154
Fluoride, bone metabolism and, 150
Fluoroquinolones, 302, 303f, 304
Fluorouracil, 371–372
Fluoxetine
    as antidepressant, 87f, 89
    for obsessive-compulsive disorder, 90
Fluoxymesterone, 167
Fluphenazine, 100
Flurazepam, 82–83
    as drug of abuse, 122
    mechanism of action, 82, 84f
    uses for, 82t
Flurbiprofen, 355t
Fluticasone, 250–251
Fluvastatin, 237, 238f
Fluvoxamine
    as antidepressant, 89
    for obsessive-compulsive disorder, 90
Folate metabolism
    inhibitors. See Antimetabolites
    vitamin B$_{12}$ and, 234f
Folic acid, for neural tube defects prevention, 234
Folinic acid (leucovorin), 234
Follicle-stimulating hormone, 139, 140f, 141
Follitropin, 165–166
Fomivirsen, 317
Food(s)
    and drug absorption in stomach, 1
    tyramine-containing, MAOI interaction
        with, 88
Formoterol, 251
Foscarnet, 316, 319t
Fourth-generation cephalosporins, 294
Frank-Starling mechanism, 203
Frovatriptan, 340–341
FTC. See Emtricitabine (FTC)
Fungal infections, 324
    drug therapy for. See Antifungal drugs
Fungi
    pathogenic, 324
    reproduction, 324
Furosemide, 185, 186f, 187

G
G proteins
    interaction with ion channels, 23f, 24
    phosphorylation, 23, 23f
    in signal transduction, 21–24, 22f, 23f
GABA. See Gamma-aminobutyric acid (GABA)
GABAergic synapse, antiepileptic site of action
        in, 95f

Gabapentin, 96
    drug interactions and, 96
    sites of action
        in GABAergic synapse, 95f
        neuronal, 92f
Galantamine, 115
Gallstones, 159, 264
Gallstones, drugs to dissolve, 263–264
Gamma-aminobutyric acid (GABA)
    characteristics, 68f, 73t
    GABAergic synapse, antiepileptic site of
            action in, 95f
    pathways and functions, 73
    receptors, 72
    synthesis, 72, 72, 72f
Ganciclovir, 316, 319t
Ganglionic blocking agents, 48, 53t
    in hypertension therapy, 199
Ganirelix, 141
Gasoline, as inhalant, 126
Gastric acid
    drugs neutralizing, 260–261, 260f
    histamine and, 346
    secretion, autocoid effects on, 349t
Gastric acid production, 260
    drugs lowering, 259–260, 259f
Gastric antacids, 260–261, 260f
    nonsystemic, 260–261
    systemic, 260, 261
Gastric emptying, delayed, drug therapy for,
        267
Gastric lavage with saline, 388
Gastric pH, and mucosal protection, 260
Gastric ulcer formation, with NSAIDs, 262
Gastroesophageal reflux disease (GERD), 260
Gastrointestinal system, drugs/agents
            affecting, 259–278
    acetylcholine, 45t
    antidiarrheals, 270–271, 272f
    antiemetics, 264–267
    in appetite suppression and enhancement,
        277–278
    autocoid, 347t
    ethanol intoxication, acute and chronic,
        119t
    in gallstone dissolution, 263–264
    gastric antacids, 260–261, 260f
    in H. pylori eradication, 263
    histamine (H$_2$) receptor antagonists, 261
    in inflammatory bowel disease, 273–277
    laxatives and cathartics, 267–270
    morphine, 105t
    mucosal protective agents, 262–263,
        262f–263f
    pancreatic enzyme replacements, 264
    parathyroid hormone, 147t
    prokinetics, 267
    proton pump inhibitors, 259–260
    vitamin D, 148
Gastroparesis, drug therapy for, 267
Gefitinib, 379
Gemcitabine, 372
Gemfibrozil, 240–241
Gemifloxacin, 302, 303f, 304
Gemtuzumab ozogamicin, 378, 378t
Generalized seizures
    features, 91t
    treatment, 97t
Genes
    critical for cancer, 365
    drug-resistant, transfer of, 283, 283t

Genetics
  asthma predisposition and, 249f
  role in hyperlipidemic diseases, 237
Gentamicin, 300–301, 302f
GERD (gastroesophageal reflux disease), 260
Gestational diabetes, 172
GH. See Growth hormone (GH)
Giardiasis, treatment of, 328t
Glaucoma, primary open-angle, 46
Glial cells, drug-sensitivity and, 74t
Glial degradative enzymes, drug-sensitivity and, 74t
Glibenclamide, 174, 175f
Glimepiride, 174
Glipizide, 174
Glomerular capillaries, 181
Glomerular filtration, drug elimination and, 12
Glucagon, as antihypoglycemic drug, 177
Glucagon-like peptide 1 (GLP-1) agonists, 176–177
Glucocorticoids, 151–156
  bone metabolism and, 149
  duration of action, 154t
  effects, 152t
  immune system effects, 153f
  mechanism of action, 151–152
  principal and adverse effects, 153f
  receptors and second messengers, 152f
  side effects, 154, 156
  uses for, 154t
Glucose tolerance test, 170
Glucose-6-phosphate dehydrogenase, 27
  deficiency in, 27t
Glutamate, as central neurotransmitter, 68f, 71, 73t
Glutamine, hydrolysis of, 72f
Glutathione, in drug metabolism, 12t
Glyburide, 174
Glycated hemoglobin (AC1) test, 170
Glycine, as central neurotransmitter, 73, 73t
Glycol poisoning, antidote for, 391t
Glycopeptide antibiotic, 295–296
Glycoprotein IIb/IIIa
  antagonists, 226
  in platelet aggregation, 224f
Glycopyrrolate, 52–53, 53t
GnRH agonist agents, as cancer chemotherapy, 382
Gold salts, 358
Goldie–Coldman hypothesis, 367
Gonadotropins, 139, 140f, 141
  as ovulatory agents, 165–166
Goserelin, 141, 382–383
Gout
  aspirin contraindicated for, 361
  drug therapy for, 359, 360f, 361
GPCR. See G-protein coupled receptors (GPCR)
G-protein coupled receptors (GPCR), 21, 41
  drug-sensitivity and, 74t
  opiate receptors, 102
Grading, of tumors, 371
Gram staining, 282
Gram-negative cell wall, 287
Granisetron, 266–267
Grapefruit, and drug interactions, 8
Griseofulvin, 325f, 326–327
Growth hormone (GH)
  disorders, 138
  effects of, 138t
  hypothalamic regulation, 137

and nitrogen balance, 138
  receptors, 137
  secretion of, factors affecting, 138
Guaifenesin, 258
Guanethidine, 62, 62f
  in hypertension therapy, 198–199
Gyrase inhibitors, 302, 303f, 304
  action on DNA, 303f

H
H_1 antihistamines, 344–345
  for allergic rhinitis, 256, 256f
H_2 antihistamines, 346
H_1 receptors, 343, 344f
H_2 receptors, 343, 344f
  antagonists, effects on GI system, 259f, 261
H_3 receptors, 343, 344f
H_4 receptors, 343
HAART (highly active antiretroviral therapy), 320, 323
Half-life of drug
  in dosing regimen selection, 18t
  effect of V_d on, 8
  elderly patients and, 28
  elimination, 14
  methadone and levo-α-acetylmethadol, 106–107
  steady-state concentration and, 15
Hallucinogens, as drugs of abuse, 124
Haloperidol, 100
Halothane, effects of, 76, 76t
Hashish. See Cannabis
hCG. See Human chorionic gonadotropin (hCG)
Head injury management, mannitol in, 184
Heart
  action potential phases in, 213–215, 214f
  beta-blockers effect on, 61f
  cardiac axis, 216
  catecholamine effects on, 55f
  conduction system, 213, 213f
  electrophysiology, 213–216
  excitation-contraction coupling in, 215
  lithium salts side effects on, 90
  local anesthetic side effects on, 81
  measuring electrical activity, 215–216, 215f
  rate/rhythm abnormality. See Cardiac arrhythmias
Heart failure, 203f
  drug management, 203
  etiology, 203
  stages, 207
Helicobacter pylori
  diagnosis, 263
  eradication of, drug therapy for, 263
Hemantics (antianemia drugs), 232, 233f, 234
Hematocrit, 232
Hematopoietic growth factors, 235
Hemochromatosis, 233
Hemodialysis, 388–389
Hemolytic anemia, 27t
Hemolytic jaundice, 296
Hemoperfusion, in vitamin poisoning, 388
Hemophilia A and B, 231
Hemostasis, platelet-mediated, 223, 223f
Henderson-Hasselbalch equation, 3
Heparin, 226–227, 227f
  thrombocytopenia induced by, 227f
  use in pregnancy, 226
Heparin-associated conditions
  hyperkalemia, 226
  osteoporosis, 226

Hepatic disease
  antimicrobial selection factors in, 284t
  drug dosage in, 19
Hepatic jaundice, 296
Hepatitis A, 319
Hepatitis B, 319
  drug therapy for, 318–319
Hepatitis C, drug therapy for, 318–319, 319
Hepatocellular jaundice, 296
Heroin. See Diamorphine
Herpes simplex virus (HSV), 315
Herpes zoster (shingles), 315
Heterodimeric receptors, 21, 22f
Hexamethonium, 48, 53t
High-density lipoproteins (HDLs), 236, 236f
Highly active antiretroviral therapy (HAART), 320, 323
His, bundle of, action potential phases at, 214–215, 214f
Histamine, 343–344, 344f
  allergy and, 344
  anti-IgE antibody, 346
  effects, 343, 347t
  gastric acid and, 346
  H_1 antihistamines, 344–345
  H_2 antihistamines, 346
  inhibitors, 346
  receptors for, 343
Histamine (H_2) receptor antagonists, gastrointestinal system effects, 261
HIV/AIDS
  drug therapy for, 320–323, 321f
    chemokine coreceptor antagonist, 323
    entry (fusion) inhibitor, 321f, 323
    HAART, 320, 323
    integrase inhibitor, 323
    nonnucleoside reverse transcriptase inhibitors, 320–322, 321f
    nucleoside reverse transcriptase inhibitors, 320, 320t, 321f
    protease inhibitors, 321f, 322, 323t
  replication of HIV virus, 321
H^+-K^+ ATPase, 260
  inhibitors. See Proton pump inhibitors
hMG. See Human menopausal gonadotropin (hMG)
HMG-CoA reductase inhibitors, hepatic effects, 238f
Hodgkin disease, 369
Homatropine, 51f, 52, 53t
Homeostasis
  Ca^{2+}, hormonal regulation of, 146f
  negative feedback in, 137
Homodimeric receptors, 21, 22f
Hormonal contraception, 160–163
  emergency, 162
  by injection, 163
  intrauterine, 163
  intravaginal ring, 162–163
  oral, 160, 161f
  subdermal implant, 162
  transdermal patch, 162
Hormone receptors, 136
Hormone replacement therapy, 159
Hormones/hormone inhibitors, as cancer chemotherapy, 381
Horner syndrome, 36
HSV (herpes simplex virus), 315
5-HT. See Serotonin (5-HT)

Human chorionic gonadotropin (hCG), 141
  as ovulatory agents, 165–166
Human immunodeficiency virus (HIV).
        See HIV/AIDS
Human menopausal gonadotropin (hMG), 141
  as ovulatory agents, 165–166
Humoral immunity, 382
Huntington disease, 71
Hydralazine
  in heart failure therapy, 207
  in hypertension therapy, 200–201
Hydrochlorothiazide, 186f, 187
Hydrocortisone, 152, 154
  modification by glucocorticoids, 155f
Hydrolysis
  in drug metabolism, 8, 11
  glutamine, 72f
Hydroxychloroquine, 356–357
3-Hydroxy-3-methylglutaryl-CoA
        reductase inhibitors, hepatic
        effects, 238f
5-Hydroxytryptamine type 3 (5-HT$_3$) antagonists,
        as antiemetics, 266–267, 266t
Hyperkalemia, 188
  heparin-associated, 226
Hyperlipidemic diseases
  drug therapy for
    bile acid sequestrants, 239–240, 240f
    fibrates, 240–241
    nicotinic acid (niacin), 240
    statins, 237, 238f
  role of genetics in, 237
Hypersensitivity
  delayed-type, 288
  immediate, 288
  to local anesthetics, 81
  type I (allergy), 344
Hyperstimulation syndrome, ovarian, 141
Hypertension
  causes and mechanisms, 191, 192f
  drug management in, 191, 202t
    angiotensin antagonists, 191, 193f, 194,
        202t
    direct vasodilators, 200–201, 200f, 202t
    diuretics, 191, 202t
    indications, 191
    sympatholytics, 194–200, 202t
  end-organ damage in, 191
Hypertensive crisis
  clonidine withdrawal precipitating,
        200
  with MAOIs, 88
  triptans and, 341
Hyperthermia, malignant, 76
Hyperthyroidism, 145
Hypoalbuminemia, 4
Hypoglycemic drugs, oral, 174, 175f, 176–177
Hypotension, counterregulatory responses in,
        200, 200f
Hypothalamic hormones, 137f
  drugs affecting, 143t
  second messengers used by, 136t
  target organs, 136t
Hypothyroidism, 144
  treatment, 144–145
Hypoxia, diffusion, with nitrous oxide, 77

I
I^{131}, 145
Ibendronate, 149
IBS (irritable bowel syndrome), 271

Ibuprofen, 355t
Idarubicin, 373
Ifosfamide, 369
Imatinib, 378, 379f
Imidazole antifungals, 324, 325f, 326
Imipenem with cilastin, 294–295
Imipramine, 86–87, 87f
Immune reaction, immunosuppressives and,
        384f
Immune system
  glucocorticoid effects on, 153f
  status of, as antimicrobial selection factor,
        284t
Immunity
  cell-mediated, 382
  humoral, 382
Immunopathogenesis, asthma, 250f
Immunosuppressants, 383–387, 383t, 384f, 386f
  for inflammatory bowel disease, 276
Inamrinone, 206
Indinavir, 322
  side effects, 323t
Indirect-acting parasympathomimetics
  ambenonium, 47
  characteristics, 44f, 47
  edrophonium, 47–48
  isoflurophate, 48
  neostigmine, 47
  parathion, 48
  physostigmine, 47
  pyridostigmine, 47
Indium 111 ibritumomab, 376, 378t
Indomethacin, 354
  for acute gout, 361
Infection(s). See also Superinfections
  anaerobic, 306
  Entamoeba histolytica, drug therapy for,
        327–328, 328t
  fungal, 324. See also Antifungal drugs
  metazoan, drug therapy for, 332–333
  Plasmodium spp. See Malaria
  prophylaxis
    bacterial infection, 285
    for viral flu, 317, 318f
  protozoan, drug therapy for, 327–331, 328t,
        330f
  site of, as antimicrobial selection factor, 284t
  viral, 313, 314t. See also Antiviral drugs
Infiltration administration method, for local
        anesthetic, 79t
Inflammation
  autocoid effects on, 347t, 349t
  drugs reducing. See Nonsteroidal
        antiinflammatory drugs (NSAIDs)
Inflammatory bowel disease
  drug treatment for, 273–277
  types, 273, 273f
Inflammatory mediators, 351
Infliximab
  as immunosuppressant, 387
  for inflammatory bowel disease, 274, 276
  for rheumatoid arthritis, 358–359, 359f
Influenza, 318
Influenza A viruses
  neuraminidase inhibitors for, 318, 319t
  prophylaxis for, 317, 318f
Influenza B viruses, neuraminidase
        inhibitors for, 318, 319t
Inhalants, as drugs of abuse, 126
Inhalation anesthetic agents, 75
  effects, 76, 76t, 77

induction rate, factors influencing, 76, 76t
Inhalation drug administration, 2t
  distribution in body following, 5f
Injectable hormonal contraception, 163
Inotropic agents, positive, 205–206
Inotropic glutamate receptors, 68f, 71, 73t
Insecticide ingestion, antidote for, 391t
Insulin
  deficiency effects, 171f
  effects, 172t
  K$^+$ balance and, 172
  mechanism of action, 170, 172f
  modified preparations, 173, 173t
  side effects, 172
  synthesis, 170
  therapeutic methods, 173f
Insulin aspart, 174
Insulin detemir, 174
Insulin glargine, 174
Insulin glulisine, 174
Insulin lispro, 174
Integrase inhibitor, in HIV/AIDS
        management, 323
Interferon alfa, 318–319, 319f
Interleukin-1 (IL-1) antagonist, 359
Interleukin II (opreleukin), 235
Intermediate-acting insulin, 173f, 174
  pharmacokinetic properties, 173t
International Normalized Ratio (INR), warfarin,
        228
Interstitial fluid, in drug distribution, 7, 7f
  drugs favoring, 7t
Intervals, on ECG recording, 215f, 216
Intoxication
  acute effects
    ethanol, 119t
    stimulants, 123
  benzodiazepines, 122
  chronic effects
    ethanol, 119t
    stimulants, 123
  hallucinogens, psychedelic and deliriant, 124
  inhalants, 126
  nicotine, 124
Intracellular fluid, in drug distribution, 7, 7f
  drugs favoring, 7t
Intracellular receptors, 21, 22f
Intramuscular drug administration, 2t
  distribution in body following, 5f
  time course of plasma concentration in, 2f
Intranasal steroids, for allergic rhinitis, 257
Intrauterine contraceptive devices, 163
Intravaginal ring contraceptives, 162–163
Intravascular fluid, in drug distribution, 7, 7f
  drugs favoring, 7t
Intravenous anesthetic agents, 77–79
  redistribution effects, 78f
Intravenous drug administration, 2t
  distribution in body following, 5f
  time course of plasma concentration in, 2f
Inverse agonists, 24
Iodine, 145
  antidote for, 391t
Iodine 131 tositumomab, 376, 378t
Iodoquinol (diiodohydroxyquinolone), 328
Ion channels
  drug-sensitivity and, 74t
  G proteins interaction with, 23f, 24
  ligand-gated, 21, 21f
  voltage-dependent, 21
Ionization, effect on drug absorption, 3

IP$_3$ system, in signal transduction, 23, 23f
Ipecac, syrup of, 388
Ipratropium, 52, 53t
    for asthma and COPD, 251
Irinotecan, 374
Iron deficiency anemia, 232
    drug therapy for, 232
Iron dextram, 232
Iron poisoning/overload, 391
    antidote for, 232
Irregular dosing regimens, 18, 19f
Irritable bowel syndrome (IBS), 271
Isoflurane, 76, 76t
Isoniazid (isonicotine hydrazine [INH]), 308, 309t
Isoproterenol
    as adrenergic agent, 57
    adrenergic receptor interaction with, 63t
    for hypertension, 195f
Isosorbide dinitrate
    in angina therapy, 209, 210f
    in heart failure therapy, 207
Isosorbide mononitrate, in angina therapy, 209, 210f
Itraconazole, 327
Ivermectin, 333

J
JAK–STAT pathway, 137
Jaundice, 296
Jaw osteonecrosis, bisphosphonates and, 149
Jugular venous pressure, 203

K
K$^+$ balance, insulin and, 172
Kallikrein inhibitors, 343
Kanamycin, 300–301
Kaolin, 271
κ receptors, actions mediated by, 102, 102t
Ketamine, 77–78
    as drug of abuse, 124
Ketoconazole, 326
Ketone formation, 171
Ketoprofen, 355t
Ketorolac, 355t
Kidney. See also Renal entries
    autocoid effects on, 349t
    calcitonin effects on, 148
    diuretic actions in, 183, 184f
    drug elimination and, 12–13
    functions, 182f
    parathyroid hormone effects on, 147t
    urine formation in, 182f
    vasa recta in, 181
    vitamin D effects on, 148
Kidney stones, 185
Krebs cycle, 72
    GABA "shunt" in, 72

L
LAAM (levo-α-acetylmethadol), 106–107, 109t
Labetalol
    as β-blocker, 61
    for hypertension, 195f
Lactation, as antimicrobial selection factor, 284t
Lactulose, 269
Lamivudine (3TC), 319
    in AIDS/HIV management, 320, 320t
Lamotrignine, 96
    neuronal sites of action, 92f

Lanreotide, 138
Lansoprazole, 259–260, 259f
Latanoprost, 349
Laxatives
    bulk-forming, 270, 270f
    lubricant, 269
    uses and contraindications, 268t
L-dopa. See Levodopa
Lead poisoning, 389
Leishmaniasis, treatment of, 328t
Lennox-Gastaut syndrome, 96
Lepirudin, 228
Leprosy, drug therapy for, 310f, 311
Letrozole, 381–382
Leucovorin (folinic acid), 234
Leukotriene(s), 350
    as antagonists, 251, 252f
    as modifiers, for asthma, 251, 252f, 253
    release from mast cells, 346
    synthesis inhibitors, 251, 252f
Leuprolide, 141, 382–383
Levalbuterol, 251
Levetiracetam, 97
Levo-α-acetylmethadol (LAAM), 106–107, 109t
Levodopa, for Parkinson disease, 111–112, 114f
    side effects, 112t
    systemic effects, 112t
Levofloxacin, 302, 303f, 304
Levonorgestrel, intrauterine contraceptive device, 163
Levothyroxine, 144
Lewy body dementia, 110
Lidocaine
    as antiarrhythmic, 219, 219f
    as local anesthetic, 79–81, 80f, 80t
Ligand-gated ion channels, 21, 21f
    drug-sensitivity and, 74t
Lincomycin, 297
Lipids, 236
    abnormalities in. See Dyslipidemia
Lipoproteins, 236
    metabolism, 236f
    optimal levels for, 236
Lisinopril, 191, 193f, 194
Lithium carbonate, 190
Lithium salts, as antimanic drug, 89–90
Liver
    cholesterol metabolism in, 239, 239f
    chronic ethanol intoxication effects on, 119t, 120f
    cirrhosis, 120f
    cytochrome P-450 enzyme synthesis in, 8, 10f
    drug elimination and, 13
    effects of HMG-CoA reductase inhibitors in, 238f
Loading dose, 17–18
Local anesthetic agents
    administration methods, 79t
    antiarrhythmic (class I) agents as, 217, 218f
    dental injections, 79
    mechanism of action, 79, 80f
    pharmacokinetics, 80, 80t
    side effects, 81
    vasoconstrictors in, 79
Lomustine, 369
Long-acting insulin, 173f, 174, 174f
    pharmacokinetic properties, 173t
Loop (high-ceiling) diuretics, 185, 186f, 187
Loperamide, 271, 272f
Lopinavir, 323t
Loracarbef, 293

Loratadine
    for allergic rhinitis, 256, 256f
    as H$_1$ antihistamine, 344–345
Lorazepam
    as anxiolytic/sedative-hypnotic, 82–83
        mechanism of action, 82, 84f
        uses for, 82t
    as drug of abuse, 122
    as intravenous anesthetic agents, 79
Losartan, 194
Lovastatin, 237, 238f
Low-density lipoproteins (LDLs), 236, 236f
Loxapine, 100
LSD (d-lysergic acid diethylamide), as drug of abuse, 124
Lubricant laxatives, 269
Lugol solution, 145
Lung maturity, in fetus, test for, 254
Lupus erythematosus, drug-induced, 27, 27t
Luteinizing hormone, 139, 140f, 141
d-Lysergic acid diethylamide (LSD), as drug of abuse, 124

M
Macrolide antibiotics, 296–299, 298f
Magnesium, bone metabolism and, 147
Magnesium hydroxide
    as cathartic, 269
    as gastric antacid, 260f, 261
Malaria, 329
    plasmodial life cycle in, 330f
    treatment, 329, 330f, 331
Malignant hyperthermia, 76
Mania
    symptoms, 86t
    treatment, 89–90
Mannitol
    in head injury management, 184
    as osmotic diuretic, 184, 185f
Maprotiline, 88
Maraviroc, 323
Marijuana. See Cannabis
Mast cell stabilizers
    for allergic rhinitis, 255f, 257
    for asthma, 253
Mast cells, leukotriene release from, 346
Matabotropic glutamate receptors, 68f, 71, 73t
MDR (multidrug resistance), 284
Mebendazole, 332
Mechlorethamine, 369
Medroxyprogesterone/Medroxyprogesterone acetate, 159
    as contraceptive injection, 163
Mefloquine, 330f, 331
Megaloblastic anemia, 232
    treatment, 234
Megestrol, 278
Meglitinides, as oral hypoglycemic agents, 176
Meloxicam, 355t
Memantine, 115
Membrane receptor, enzyme-linked, 21, 21f
Meningitis, 294
Menstrual cycle, 140
    hormonal control, 140f
Meperidine, 106, 109t
    drug interactions with, 106
    as drug of abuse, 118
    withdrawal symptoms, 119t
Mercaptopurine, 368f, 371
    for inflammatory bowel disease, 276–277, 276f

Mercury poisoning, *389*
Mesalamine, 353–354
  tetrahydrofolate synthesis inhibition and, 305f
  for ulcerative colitis, 273
Mescaline, as drug of abuse, 124
Mesolimbic-mesocortical dopaminergic tract, 67
Mestranol, 157
  bone metabolism and, 149
Metabolic acidosis, *185*
Metabolic disturbances, typical *vs.* atypical antipsychotics and, 101t
Metabolic syndrome, *237*
Metabolism of drugs
  hydrolysis reactions, 11
  morphine, 104, 105f
  oxidation reactions, 8, 10f, 11t
  phase 1 (transformation) reaction, 8, 9f–10f, 11, 11t
  phase 2 (conjugation) reactions, 9f, 11, 12t
  reduction reactions, 11
Metal chelating agents, 389–391, *390*
Metaproterenol
  for asthma and COPD, 251
  as directly acting sympathomimetic, 58
Metaraminol, as directly acting sympathomimetic, 58
Metazoan infections, drug therapy for, 332–333
Metformin, 174, 175f
Methacholine, 45–46
Methacycline, 299–300
Methadone, 106–107, 109t
  as drug of abuse, 118
  withdrawal symptoms, 119t
Methamphetamine, as mixed acting sympathomimetic, 59
Methanol toxicology, 121–122
  antidote for, 391t
Methaqualone, as drug of abuse, 123
Methemoglobinemia, *329*
Methicillin, 289
Methicillin-resistant *Staphylococcus aureus* (MRSA), *289*
  alternative drug therapy for, 292
Methimazole, 144–145
Methohexital
  as anxiolytic/sedative-hypnotic, 83–84
    mechanism of action, 84f
    use, 84t
  as drug of abuse, 122
  as intravenous anesthetic agents, 78–79
Methotrexate
  as cancer chemotherapy agent, 368f, 370–371
  as DMARD, 356
  for inflammatory bowel disease, 276–277, 276f
Methoxamine, as directly acting sympathomimetic, 58
Methylation, in drug metabolism, 12t
Methylcellulose, as laxative, 270
Methyldopa, 58f
  in hypertension therapy, 198
Methylergonovine, 169
Methylphenidate, 277
Methylprednisolone, 152, 154
Methyltestosterone, 167
Methylxanthines, 253
Metoclopramide, 267

Metoprolol
  adrenergic receptor interaction with, 63t
  as β-blocker, 60, 61f
  for hypertension, 194–196
  for hypothyroidism, 145
Metronidazole
  action on DNA, 303f
  as amebicidal, 327–328
  as antibacterial, 306
Mexiletine, 219, 219f
Micafungin, 327
Miconazole, 324, 326
Microorganisms
  antibacterial agents targeting, 307t
  as factor in antimicrobial selection
    resistance, 282–284, 283f, 283t
    species susceptibility, 282
Midazolam
  as anxiolytic/sedative-hypnotic, 82–83
    mechanism of action, 82, 84f
    uses for, 82t
  as drug of abuse, 122
  as intravenous anesthetic agents, 79
Mifepristone, 165, 165f
Miglitol, 176
Migraine, *341*
Milk of magnesia. *See* Magnesium hydroxide
Milrinone, 206
Mineral oil, as laxative, 269
Mineralocorticoids, 156
Minimum alveolar concentration (MAC),
    as anesthetic dosing standard, 75
"Minipills," progestin-only, 160, 161f
Minocycline, 299–300
Minoxidil, 200–201
Mirtazapine, 88
Misoprostol, 350
  effect in GI system, 262, 263f
Mixed antagonists. *See* Labetalol
Mometasone, 250–251
Monoamine oxidase inhibitors (MAOIs), 87–88
  drug interactions with, 88
  hypertensive crisis with, *88*
Monoclonal antibodies
  as cancer chemotherapy, 375–378, 378t
  as immunosuppressants, 383t, 387
Montelukast, 251, 252f, 253
Moricizine, 219–220
Morphine, 102
  as antidiarrheal, 271
  compounds related to, 102
  as drug of abuse, 118
  effects on organ systems, 105t
  indications for, 109t
  mechanism of action, 102, 104
  metabolism, 104, 105f
  pharmacokinetics, 104, 105f
  withdrawal symptoms, 119t
Motor systems, in Parkinson disease, *111*
Movement, in Parkinson disease, *111*
Moxifloxacin, 302, 303f, 304
MRSA. *See* Methicillin-resistant *Staphylococcus aureus* (MRSA)
Mucolytic drugs, 258
Mucosal irritation, peristalsis stimulated by, 268, 268f
Mucosal protective agents, effects in GI system, 262–263, 262f–263f
Mucus, excess production, treatment of, 258
Multidrug resistance (MDR), 284
Multiple endocrine neoplasia type 1 (MEN1), *148*

μ receptors, actions mediated by, 102, 102t
Muromonab-CD3, 387
Muscarinic receptor antagonists, 49, 51f, 52–53, 53t
Muscarinic receptors, 40, 40f, 41t
Muscle
  chronic ethanol intoxication effects on, 119t
  smooth. *See* Smooth muscle
Muscle fibers, cardiac, membrane potential changes at, 213–215, 214f
Muscle spasms
  inhibition of neuromuscular transmission/ electrochemical coupling and, 117f
  treatment, 116–117, 116f
Muscular dystrophy, *117*
Myasthenia gravis, *48*
Mycophenolate mofetil, 383t, 385
Myocardial infarction, *209*
  fibrinolysis and, 230
Myocardium, atrial and ventricular, action potential phases at, 214–215, 214f
Myoclonic seizure
  features, 91t
  treatment, 97t
Myxedema (hypothyroidism), *144*

N
Na⁺-iodide pump, *145*
Nabumetone, 355t
Na⁺-channel blocking drugs, in arrhythmia therapy, 218f, 219f
Nadolol
  adrenergic receptor interaction with, 63t
  as β-blocker, 60, 61f
Nafcillin, 289
Nalmefene, 108, 109t
Naloxone, 108, 109t
Naltrexone, 108
  for alcoholism management, 121
Naphazolinem, 255–256
Naproxen, 355t
Naratriptan, 340–341
Narcolepsy, *123*
Nateglinide, 176
National Notifiable Diseases Surveillance System (NNDSS), *302*
Natural penicillins, 289, 290f, 291f
Nausea, drug therapy for causes of, 264–267, 266t
NE. *See* Norepinephrine (NE)
Necrotizing fasciitis, *296*
Nedocromil sodium, 346
  for allergic rhinitis, 255f, 257
Negative feedback, *137*
Nematode infections, treatment of, 332–333
Neomycin, 300–301, 302f
Neonates
  breastfeeding and, 30, 30f
  drug withdrawal effects in, 30
  physiology, *30*
  respiratory distress syndrome in, 254
Nephroblastoma (Wilms tumor), *374*
Nephrogenic diabetes mellitus, treatment of, *189*
Nephropathy, diabetic, 184
Nephrotic syndrome, *187*
Nephrotoxic drugs, *19*
Nerve blockers
  administration methods, 79t
  nerve fiber sensitivity to, *80*

Nerve fiber, sensitivity to nerve blockers, *80*
Neuraminidase inhibitors, for influenza A and B, 318, 319t
Neuritis, retrobulbar, *308*
Neurodegenerative diseases, treatment of, 110–117
    Alzheimer's disease, 115
    Parkinson disease, 110–115
    spasticity and muscle spasms, 116–117
Neuroleptic effects, of antipsychotic agents, 98
Neuroleptic malignancy syndrome (NMS), *99*
Neurologic effects, lithium salts, 90
Neuromuscular blockers of acetylcholine
    depolarizing, 49, 50f, 53t
    nondepolarizing, 49, 53t
Neuromuscular transmission, inhibition of, 117f
Neuronal communication, *37*
Neurons, drug-sensitivity and, 74t
Neuropeptide neurotransmitters, 74
    pain caused by, *106*
Neurotransmitters. *See also individually named neurotransmitters*
    adrenergic receptors, 41, 41t
    of autonomic and somatic nervous system, 37–39
    in central nervous system, 67–74, 68f, 73t. *See also* Central neurotransmitters; *individually named neurotransmitters*
    cholinergic receptors, 40, 40f, 41t
Neutral Protamine Hagedorn (NPH) insulin, 174
Nevirapine, 322
Niacin (nicotinic acid)
    as cholesterol-lowering agent, 240
    toxic effects and treatment, 392t
Nicardipine, 196, 197f
    electrophysiological and hemodynamic effects, 198t
Nicotinamide, 392t
Nicotine
    as drug of abuse, 125
    replacement therapy, 125
Nicotinic acid (niacin)
    as cholesterol-lowering agent, 240
    toxic effects and treatment, 392t
Nicotinic receptor antagonists
    depolarizing neuromuscular blockers of acetylcholine, 49, 50f, 53t
    ganglionic blocking agents, 48, 53t
    nondepolarizing neuromuscular blockers of acetylcholine, 49, 53t
Nicotinic receptors, 40, 40f, 41t
Nifedipine, 196, 197f
    electrophysiological and hemodynamic effects, 198t
Nigrostriatal tract/Nigrostriatal dopaminergic tract, 67
    Parkinson disease and, 111, 111f
Nilutamide, 383
Nitrates, in angina therapy, 209, 210f, 211, 212t
Nitric oxide, *344*
Nitrite poisoning, antidote for, 391t
Nitrofurantoin, as urinary antiseptic, 311–312
Nitrogen balance, growth hormone and, *138*
Nitroglycerin
    in angina therapy, 209, 210f
    in heart failure therapy, 207
Nitroprusside, 207
Nitrous oxide
    diffusion hypoxia with, *77*
    as drug of abuse, 126

effects, 76, 76t
    uses and side effects, 77
Nizatidine, 346
    effect on gastrointestinal system, 259f, 261
NK$_1$ antagonists, as antiemetics, 264–265, 266t
NMS (neuroleptic malignancy syndrome), *99*
NNDSS (National Notifiable Diseases Surveillance System), *302*
Nonbenzodiazepine benzodiazepine receptor agonists, 83
Non-catecholamine sympathomimetics, 58–59
Nonnucleoside reverse transcriptase inhibitors, in HIV/AIDS management, 320–322, 321f
Nonsteroidal antiinflammatory drugs (NSAIDs)
    acetic acids, 354, 355t
    for acute gout, 360f, 361
    as analgesic, 351
    as antipyretic, 351
    bronchospasm induced by, *249*
    contraindications, 351, 353
    COX-2 selective inhibitors, 355
    for febrile convulsions/seizures, *93*
    gastric ulcer formation with, *262*
    mechanism of action, 351, 352f
    as prostaglandin antagonists, 350
    for rheumatoid arthritis, *46,* 356, 356f
    salicylates/salicylic acid salts and derivatives, 353–354
    side effects, 351, 352f
    uses, 351
Nonsystemic antacids, 260–261, 260f
Norelgestromin, in transdermal patch contraceptives, 162
Norepinephrine (NE)
    as adrenergic agent, 54
    as central neurotransmitter, 67, 68f, 73t
    as peripheral system neurotransmitter, 38–39, 39f
Norethindrone, 159
Norfloxacin, 302, 303f, 304
Norgestrel, 159
Nortriptyline, 86–87, 267
Notifiable diseases, *302*
NRDS (neonatal respiratory distress syndrome), 254
NSAIDs. *See* Nonsteroidal antiinflammatory drugs (NSAIDs)
Nucleic acid
    metabolism inhibitors, 302, 303f, 304
    synthesis inhibitors, as antivirals, 314–317, 315f
Nucleoside reverse transcriptase inhibitors
    in HIV/AIDS management, 320, 321f
    side effects, 320, 320t
Nystatin, 324, 325f

O

Obsessive compulsive order, medication for, 90
Obstructive jaundice, *296*
Octreotide, 138
Ofloxacin, 302, 303f, 304
Olanzapine, 100–101
Olsalazine, 353–354
    for ulcerative colitis, 273
Omalizumab, for IgE-mediated allergic asthma, 253, 346
    atopy and, *252f*
Omeprazole, gastric acid production and, 259–260, 259f
Oncogenes, *365*

Ondansetron, 266–267
Open-angle glaucoma, primary, *46*
Opiate agonists
    endogenous, 104, 104f
    exogenous, 102, 104, 104f
    mixed opiate agonist-antagonists, 107
Opiate antagonists, 108
    mixed opiate agonist-antagonists, 107
Opiate poisoning, antidote for, 391t
Opiate receptors
    actions mediated by, 102, 102t
    actions of endogenous and exogenous opioids at, 104, 104f
    signal transduction, *102*
Opiates, for cough, 257
Opioid poisoning, *108*
Opioids
    as antidiarrheals, 271, 272f
    as drugs of abuse, 118
    for pain modulation, 102, 103f. *See also* Morphine
    contraindications, 106
    drug interactions with, 106
    effects on organ systems, 105t
    endogenous, 104, *104,* 104f
    exogenous, 102, 104, 104f
    indications for, 109t
    side effects, 106
    uses for, 106
    withdrawal symptoms, 119t
Opreleukin (interleukin II), 235
Oral contraceptives
    combination type, 160, 161f
    progestin-only, 160, 161f
Oral drug administration, 1, 2t
    distribution in body following, 5f
    time course of plasma concentration in, 2f
Oral glucose tolerance test, *170*
Oral hypoglycemic drugs, 174, 175f, 176–177
Organ rejection, immunosuppressants for prevention of, 383–387, 383t, 384f, 386f
Organic nitrates, in angina therapy, 209, 210f, 211, 212t
Organophosphate poisoning, *391*
    antidote for, 391t
Orlistat, 277
Oseltamivir, 318
Osmotic diuretics, 184, 185f
Osteonecrosis of jaw, bisphosphonates and, *149*
Osteoporosis, heparin-associated, *226*
Otitis media, *292*
Ovarian hyperstimulation syndrome, *141*
Over-the-counter (OTC) drugs, as diuretics, 189
Ovulation
    agents promoting, 165–166
    effects of estrogen on, 157t
Oxacillin, 289, 291f
Oxaliplatin, 370
Oxandrolone, 167
Oxaprozin, 355t
Oxazepam, 82–83
    as drug of abuse, 122
    mechanism of action, 82, 84f
    uses for, 82t
Oxidation reactions, in drug metabolism, 8, 9f–10f, 11, 11t
Oxitropium, 251
Oxymetazoline, 255–256

Oxymetholone, 167
Oxytetracycline, 299–300
Oxytocin, 142, 169

P

P35 gene, *365*
Paclitaxel, 375
Paget disease, *149*
Pain
   neuropeptide neurotransmitters causing, *106*
   opioids modulating. *See under* Opioids
Pain pathways, *103,* 103f
Paliperidone, 100–101
Palonosetron, 266–267
Pamidronate, 149
Pancreatic enzymes, replacement of, 264
Pancreatitis, chronic, *264*
Pancrelipase, 264
Pantoprazole, 259–260, 259f
Pantothenic acid, as coenzyme A precursor, *38*
Parasympathetic division, autonomic nervous
     system, 35, 35t
   efferent neurons, 37f
   innervation of target organs by, 35, 36f
   physiologic responses, 41, 42t
Parasympathomimetics
   direct-acting, 44f, 45–46
   indirect-acting, 44f, 47–48
Parathyroid hormone, 146f, 147t
Paregoric (tincture of opium), 271, 272f
Parenteral drug administration, 1, 2t
   time course of plasma concentration in, 2f
Parkinson disease, *67,* 110, 110f
   drug therapy for, 111–113, 112t, 114f, 115
   nigrostriatal tract and, 111, 111f
Paromomycin, 328
Paroxetine, 89
Partial seizures
   features, 91t
   treatment, 97t
Passive diffusion, in drug absorption, 1
Pathogenic fungi, *324*
Patient, factors in antimicrobial selection, 284,
     284t
Pectin, 271
Pediatric patients, prescribing drugs for, 27
Pegvisomant, 139
Pelvic inflammatory disease (PID), *163*
Penciclovir, 314, 316
Penicillamine, 389
Penicillin(s), 289–292
   extended-spectrum, 290–292
   natural, 289, 290f, 291f
   penicillinase-resistant, 289
   resistance to, 290f
   side effects, 289
Penicillin G, 289
   derivatives, 291f
   disadvantages, 290f
Penicillin V, 289, 291f
Penicillinase-resistant penicillin, 289, 291f
Penicillin-binding proteins (PBPs), *287*
   cell-wall synthesis inhibition and, 287
Pentazocine, 107, 109t
Pentobarbital
   as anxiolytic/sedative-hypnotic, 83–84
     mechanism of action, 84f
     use, 84t
   as drug of abuse, 122
Pentoxyfylline, for treatment of bleeding, 231
Pepsin, *1*

Peptic ulcers, *261*
Percutaneous coronary intervention, *227*
Peripheral nervous system (PNS)
   autocoid effects on, 347t, 349t
   divisions, 35–37. *See also* Autonomic
     nervous system (ANS); Somatic
     nervous system
   drugs acting on. *See* Adrenergic agents;
     Cholinergic agonists; Cholinergic
     antagonists
Peristalis stimulation
   by bulk-forming laxatives, 270, 270f
   in diarrhea, 272f
   by intraluminal bolus, 270f
   by mucosal irritation, 268, 268f
Peristaltic reflex, *268*
Permeability, capillary wall, drug distribution
     and, 4, 6f
Perphenazine, 100
Pharmacodynamics. *See* Dose-response
     relationship; Drug-receptor
     interactions
Pharmacogenetics
   defined, 27
   disorders, 27t
   elderly patients and, 28
   pediatric patients and, 27
Pharmacokinetics, 1–19
   absorption, 1, 3
   administration. *See* Administration of drugs
   defined, 1
   distribution. *See* Distribution of drugs
   elimination, 12–13
   genetic variants in, 28f
   interactions. *See* Drug interactions
   of local anesthetics, 80, 80t
   metabolism. *See* Metabolism of drugs
   plasma concentration and dosing, 14–15,
     14f–15f
   short-acting insulin, 173t
Phencyclidine, as drug of abuse, 124
Phenobarbital, 93
   as anxiolytic/sedative-hypnotic, 83–84
     mechanism of action, 84f
     use, 84t
   drug interactions with, 93
   as drug of abuse, 122
   neuronal sites of action, 92f
Phenothiazine antipsychotics, 100
Phenoxybenzamine
   adrenergic receptor interaction with, 63t
   as α-blocker, 60
Phentermine, 277
Phentolamine
   adrenergic receptor interaction with, 63t
   as α-blocker, 60
Phenylephrine
   adrenergic receptor interaction with, 63t
   for cough, 257
   as directly acting sympathomimetic, 58
   for rhinitis symptomatic relief, 255–256
Phenylpropanolamine, 277
Phenytoin, 91–92
   drug interactions with, 92
   neuronal sites of action, 92f
Pheochromocytoma, *60*
Phosphodiesterase inhibitors, in heart failure
     therapy, 206
Phosphorylation
   of enzymes, 23, 23f
   of G proteins, 23, 23f

Phytonadione (vitamin K$_1$), as warfarin
     antagonist, 229
PID (pelvic inflammatory disease), *163*
Pilocarpine, 46
Pimozide, 100
Pindolol, 194–196, 195f
"Pink puffers," *250*
Pioglitazone, 176
Piperacillin, 292
Piperazine, 333
Piroxicam, 355t
Pituitary hormones, 136–142, 137f
   drugs affecting, 143t
   target organs, 136t
Placenta, drug passage through, 29, 29f
Plasma drug concentration
   determinants, 14–15, 14f–15f
   in irregular dosing, 18, 19f
   loading dose and, 17–18
   steady-state
     achieving rapidly, loading dose and, 17–18
     in continuous IV infusion, 15–16, 16f
     in dosing regimen selection, 18t
     in oral administration, 16–17, 16t, 17t
   time course of, enteral *vs.* parenteral
     administration, 2f
Plasma protein binding, drug distribution and,
     4, 4t
Plasmodium spp. infection. *See* Malaria
Plasticity, synaptic, *67*
Platelet aggregation, 224f
   autocoid effects on, 347t, 349t
   inhibitors, 224–226, 225f
Platelet-mediated hemostasis, 223, 223f
Pneumocystosis, treatment of, 328t
PNS. *See* Peripheral nervous system (PNS)
Poisoning. *See also* Toxicology
   acute, with tricyclic antidepressants, *86*
   antidotes for, 391t
   arsenic, *389*
   carbon monoxide, *391*
   copper (Wilson disease), *391*
   emergency treatment for, *388*
   iron, *391*
   lead, *389*
   mercury, *389*
   opioid. *See* Opioid poisoning
   vitamin, treatment for, 392, 392t
Polydipsia, lithium salts and, 90
Polyene antifungals, 324, 325f
Polyethylene glycol, 269
Polymorphism, acetylation, 27t
Polymyxin B, 306
Polypharmacy, elderly patients and, 28
Polyuria, lithium salts and, 90
Porphyrias, *27*
   barbiturate use and, 83
Portal circulation, *3*
Positive inotropic agents, 205–206
Post-hepatic jaundice, *296*
Potassium iodide, 145
Potassium-sparing diuretics, 188–189, 188f
Potency, in dose-response relationship, 25, 25f
Pramipexole, 113
Pramlintide, 176
Pravastatin, 237
Praziquantel, 333
Prazosin
   adrenergic receptor interaction with, 63t
   as α-blocker, 60
   in hypertension therapy, 198

Prednisone, 152, 154
    as cancer chemotherapy agent, 381
    for inflammatory bowel disease, 276
    as prostaglandin antagonist, 350
Pregnancy
    antihypertensives contraindicated in, 194
    antimicrobial selection factors in, 284t
    drug administration in, 29–30
    heparin therapy in, 226
    physiological changes in, 30
Pre-hepatic jaundice, 296
Preload, cardiac, 203
Premarin™, 157
    bone metabolism and, 149
Presynaptic synthetic pathways, drug-sensitivity
            and, 74t
Primaquine, 329, 330f
Primary open-angle glaucoma, 46
Primidone, 94
    drug interactions with, 93, 94
Probenecid, 361
Procainamide, as antiarrhythmic, 217
Procaine
    as antiarrhythmic, 219f
    as local anesthetic, 79–81, 80f, 80t
Procarbazine, 370
Prochlorperazine, 266
Procyclidine, 115
Progabide, sites of action in GABAergic synapse,
            95f
Progesterone, 157, 158f, 159
    antagonists, 165, 165f
    effects, 159t
Progestins, 159
    "minipills," 160, 161f
    in oral contraceptive, 160, 161f
    in transdermal patch contraceptives, 162
Proguanil, 330f, 331
Prolactin, 142
    disorders, 142
Prolactin-inhibiting hormone agonists, 166
Prolastin™, 254
Promethazine, 344–345
Propafenone, 219–220
Prophylaxis
    with antimicrobial agents, 285
    for viral flu, 317, 318f
Propofol, 77
Propoxyphene (Darvon), 107
Propranolol
    adrenergic receptor interaction with, 63t
    as antiarrhythmic, 220
    as β-blocker, 60, 61f
    for hypertension, 194–196, 195f
    for hypothyroidism, 145
Propylthiouracil, 144–145
Prostacycline, 349t
Prostaglandins (PGs)
    actions, 349t
    agonists, 349–350
    antagonists, 350
    in sperm, 349
Prostate gland, 382
Protamine sulfate, as heparin antidote, 227
Protease inhibitors, in HIV/AIDS
            management, 321f, 322, 323t
Protein synthesis, 296
    inhibitors, 296–302
Proteins, penicillin-binding. See Penicillin-
            binding proteins (PBPs)
Protirelin, 142

Proton pump inhibitors, gastrointestinal system
            effects, 259–260, 259f
Proto-oncogenes, 365
Protozoan infections, drug therapy for, 327–331,
            328t, 330f
Proximal tubule, active transport in, 12
Pseudoephedrine
    for cough, 257
    for rhinitis symptomatic relief, 255–256
Pseudomembranous colitis, antibiotic-associated,
            295
Psilocybin, as drug of abuse, 124
Psychedelic hallucinogens, as drugs of abuse,
            124
Psyllium preparations, as laxative, 270
Puberty, estrogen effects at, 157t
Pulmonary edema, 187
Pulmonary embolism, 230
Pulmonary surfactant, 254
Purines, 356
Purkinje fibers, action potential phases at,
            214–215, 214f
Pyramidal motor systems, in Parkinson disease,
            111
Pyrantel, 332
Pyrazinamide, 309, 309t
Pyridoxine, 392t
Pyrimethamine, 330f, 331–332

Q
Quaaludes, 123
Quadriplegia, 35
Quetiapine, 100–101
Quinidine, 217
Quinine, 329, 330f, 331
Quinolones, 302, 303f, 304

R
Rabeprazole, 259–260, 259f
Radioiodine, 145
Radiotherapy
    local effects, 366
    systemic effects, 366
Raloxifene
    bone metabolism and, 149
    in reproductive endocrinology, 163, 164f
Raltegravir, 321f, 323
Ramelteon, 85
Random blood sugar level, 170
Ranitidine, 346
    gastrointestinal system effects, 259f, 261
    for lowering gastric acid production, 259f
Rapamycin. See Sirolimus
Rasagiline, 115
Receptors
    drug interactions with. See Drug-receptor
            interactions
    G protein signal transduction and, 21–24,
            22f, 23f
    growth hormone, 137
    for histamine, 343
    types, 21, 21f–22f, 24t
    typical vs. atypical antipsychotics and, 101t
Rectal drug administration, 2t
    distribution in body following, 5f
Recurrent febrile seizures, treatment of, 97t
Redistribution effects, intravenous
            anesthetic agents, 78f
Redox reactions, ascorbic acid, 39
5α-Reductase enzyme, testosterone and, 166,
            168f

Reduction reactions, in drug metabolism, 8, 11
Reflection coefficient, 4
Reflex(es)
    Achilles tendon, 375
    baroreceptor, 54
    peristaltic, 268
    vomiting, 265
Renal disease
    antimicrobial selection factors in, 284t
    drug dosage in, 19
Renal failure
    acute, 187
    chronic, 150
Renal osteodystrophy, 150
Renal pharmacology
    antidiuretic drugs, 189–190
    diuretics, 183–189. See also Diuretics
    renal physiology and, 181, 182f–183f, 183
    vasopressin antagonists and, 190
Renal transport system, 181, 182f
Renin
    direct inhibitors, 194
    in renin-angiotensin-aldosterone system,
            181, 182f
Renin-angiotensin-aldosterone system, 156
    ACE inhibitors and, 191, 193f, 194
    aldosterone relationship in, 183, 183f
    renin relationship in, 181, 182f
Repaglinide, 176
Reproduction, effects of estrogen on, 157t
Reproductive disorders, drug used in treatment
            of, 136–156. See also individually
            named drugs; Reproductive
            endocrinology, drugs used in;
            individual drug classes
Reproductive endocrinology, drugs used in,
            157–169
    anabolic steroids, 167
    androgens, 166–167
    antiandrogens, 167, 168f
    estrogen antagonists, 163–164
    estrogens, 157–159
    hormonal contraception, 160–163
    ovulatory agents, 165–166
    progesterone antagonists, 165
    progestins, 159
    uterine actions, 169
Reserpine, 62, 62f
    in hypertension therapy, 198–199
Resistance
    to anticancer agents, 367, 367f
    to antimicrobial agents, 282–284, 283f,
            283t. See also Methicillin-
            resistant Staphylococcus aureus
            (MRSA)
    combination therapy and, 285
    cytostatic, 367, 367f
    multidrug, 284
Respiration, and acid-base balance, 251
Respiratory burst, effect of corticosteroids on,
            152
Respiratory depression, drugs causing, 249
Respiratory distress syndrome, neonatal, 254
Respiratory syncytial virus (RSV), 316
Respiratory system
    acetylcholine effects in, 45t
    drugs affecting, 249–258
Responses, to drugs, 25–26, 25f
Reteplase, 230–231
Reticular activating system, 124
Retinol, toxic effects and treatment, 392t

Retrobulbar neuritis, *308*
Reuptake mechanisms, drug-sensitivity and, 74t
Reverse transcriptase inhibitors, in HIV/AIDS management
    nonnucleoside, 320–322, 321f
    nucleoside, 320, 321f
Rhabdomyolysis, *237*
Rheumatoid arthritis, 355–356
    drug therapy for, 356, 357f
        DMARDs, 356–358
        IL-1 antagonist, 359
        NSAIDs, *46*, 356, 356f
        TNF-α inhibitors, 358–359, 359f
    pathogenesis, *356*
Rhinitis, 254. *See also* Allergic rhinitis
    decongestants for symptomatic relief, 255–256
Rhythm disturbance, in heart. *See* Cardiac arrhythmias
Riatriptan, 340–341
Ribavirin, 316, 319t
    for hepatitis C, 319
Rifampin
    action on DNA, 303f
    as antituberculosis drug, 309, 309t
Rimantadine, 317, 319t
Risedronate, 149
Risperidone, 100–101
Ritinavir, 322
    side effects, 323t
Rituximab, 376, 378t
Rivastigmine, 115
Rofecoxib, 355
Ropinirole, 113
Rosiglitazone, 175f, 176
Rosuvastatin, 237
Roundworm infections, treatment of, 332–333
RSV (respiratory syncytial virus), *316*

S
Salicylates, 353–354
Salicylic acid salts and derivatives, 353–354
Saline, gastric lavage with, 388
Salmeterol, 251
Salsalate, 354
Saquinavir, 322
Sargramostim, 235
Schizophrenia
    signs and symptoms, *100*
    typical *vs.* atypical antipsychotics for, 101t
Scopolamine, 51f, 52, 53t
Secobarbital
    as anxiolytic/sedative-hypnotic, 83–84
        mechanism of action, 84f
        use, 84t
    as drug of abuse, 122
Second messengers
    used by glucocorticoids, 152f
    used by hypothalamic hormones, 136t
Second-generation cephalosporins, 293
Secretions, acetylcholine effects on, 45t
Sedative-hypnotic drugs, 82–85
Segments, on ECG recording, 215f, 216
Seizures
    antiepileptic drugs for, 91–97, 97f
    types, 91, 91t
Selective estrogen receptor modulators (SERMs)
    bone metabolism and, 149
    in reproductive endocrinology, 163, 164f
Selective serotonin reuptake inhibitors (SSRIs), 87f, 89

Selegiline, 114f, 115
Sepsis, *342*
Serotonin (5-HT), 340
    agonist drugs, 340–341, 342t
    antagonist drugs, 342t
    effects, 340, 347t
    mixed drugs, 341
Serotonin (5-HT), as central neurotransmitter, 68f, 69, 73t
    drug influence on, 70f
Serotonin syndrome
    carcinoid tumors and, *343*
    triptans and, 341
Sertraline, 89
Set point temperature, *351*
Sevoflurane, 76, 76t
Shingles (herpes zoster), *315*
Short-acting insulin, pharmacokinetic properties, 173t
SIADH (syndrome of inappropriate secretion of antidiuretic hormone), *190*
Signal transduction
    adenylate cyclase system, 23, 23f
    DAG system, 23, 23f
    G proteins, 21–24, 22f, 23f
    Insulin, 172f
    IP_3 system, 23, 23f
    opiate receptor, *102*
    receptors, 21, 21f–22f
Simvastatin, 237
Sinoatrial (SA) node, action potential phases at, 213–214, 214f
Sirolimus, 383t, 385, 386f
Sitagliptin, 177
Sjögren's syndrome, *46*
Smooth muscle, autocoid effects on, 347t, 349t
Sodium bicarbonate, as gastric antacid, 260f, 261
Sodium carboxymethylcellulose, as laxative, 270
Sodium iodide, 145
    pump, *145*
Sodium nitroprusside, in hypertension therapy, 201
Sodium phosphate, as cathartic, 269
Solvents, as drugs of abuse, 126
Somatic nervous system, 36
    efferent neurons, 37f
    neurotransmitters, 37–39
Somatomedins, 138
Somatotropin, 138
Sorafenib, 379
Sotalol, 220–221
South American trypanosomiasis, treatment of, 328t
Spasticity
    inhibition of neuromuscular transmission/electrochemical coupling and, 117f
    treatment for, 116–117
        mechanisms influencing, 116f
Spectinomycin, 301–302
Sperm, prostaglandins in, *349*
Spinal anesthesia, administration method for, 79t
Spironolactone, 188, 188f
Staging, of tumors, *371*
Staphylococcus aureus, methicillin-resistant, *289*
Starling forces, *181*
Statins, for lowering plasma cholesterol levels, 237, 238f

Status asthmaticus, *251*
Status epilepticus, *91*
    treatment for, *91*, 97t
Stavudine (d4T), 320
    side effects, 320t
Steady-state plasma concentration
    in continuous IV infusion, 15–16, 16f
    in dosing regimen selection, 18t
    and IV anesthetic agent redistribution effects, 78f
    in oral administration, 16–17, 16t
Steatorrhea, *264*
Steroid(s)
    anabolic, 167
    intranasal, for allergic rhinitis, 257
    perioperative coverage, *154*
    synthesis, cholesterol and, *156*
Stimulants, as drugs of abuse, 123–124
Stool softeners, 269
Streptokinase, 230
Streptomycin, 300–301
Stroke, *225*
Subcutaneous drug administration, 2t
    time course of plasma concentration in, 2f
Subdermal implant contraceptives, 162
Subitramine, 277
Sublingual drug administration, 2t
    distribution in body following, 5f
Succimer, 391
Succinylcholine, 49, 50f, 53t
    apnea and, 27t
Sucralfate, effect in GI system, 262, 262f
Sulbactam, 295
Sulfacytine, 304, 305f, 306
Sulfadiazine, 304, 305f, 306
Sulfamethizole, 304, 305f, 306
Sulfamethoxazole, 304, 305f, 306
    tetrahydrofolate synthesis inhibition and, 305f
Sulfasalazine, 353–354
    as DMARD, 357
    tetrahydrofolate synthesis inhibition and, 305f
    for ulcerative colitis, 273, 274f
Sulfation, in drug metabolism, 12t
Sulfinpyrazone, 361
Sulfisoxazole, 304, 305f, 306
Sulfonamides (sulfas), 304, 305f, 306
Sulfonylurea derivatives, 174, 175f
Sulindac, 355t
Sumatriptan, 340–341
Sunitinib, 379–380
Superantigens, *284*
Superinfections, *282*
    combination therapy in, 285
Surfactant, pulmonary, *254*
Susceptibility, to antimicrobial agents, 282
Sympathetic division, autonomic nervous system, 35, 35t
    efferent neurons, 37f
    innervation of target organs by, 35, 36f
    physiologic responses, 41, 43t
Sympathetic function, drugs inhibiting, 60–61, 61f
Sympathetic tone, inhibitors of
    clonidine, 58–59, 58f
    guanethidine, 62, 62f
    in hypertension therapy, 198–199
    methyldopa, 58f
    reserpine, 62, 62f

Sympatholytics, 60–61, 61f
    for hypertension, 194–200, 202t
Sympathomimetics
    catecholamine, 54–58
    directly-acting, 58–59
    mixed acting, 59
    non-catecholamine, 58–59
Synaptic plasticity, 67
Synaptic transmission, drug-sensitive sites in, 74t
Syndrome of inappropriate secretion of anti-diuretic hormone (SIADH), 190
Synovial membranes, in rheumatoid arthritis, 356, 356, 357f
Synthetic catecholamines, 57–58
Syrup of ipecac, 388
Systemic antacids, 260, 260f, 261
Systemic capillaries, 181

T
Tacrine, 115
Tacrolimus, 385
Tamoxifen
    as cancer chemotherapy agent, 381
    in reproductive endocrinology, 163, 164f
Tardive dyskinesia, 99
Taxanes, as cancer chemotherapy, 375
Tazobactam, 295
TB. See Tuberculosis (TB)
Teeth, tetracycline staining of, 300
Telbivudine, 319
Temazepam
    as drug of abuse, 122
    effects, 82
    mechanism of action, 82, 84f
    uses for, 82t
Temperature, set point, 351
Temperature regulation, 351
Tenecteplase, 230–231
Teniposide, 374
Tenofovir, 319
    in HIV/AIDS management, 320, 320t
Teratogenicity, drug, 30
Terazosin
    as α-blocker, 60
    in hypertension therapy, 198
Terbinafine, 327
Terbutaline
    adrenergic receptor interaction with, 63t
    for asthma and COPD, 251
    as directly acting sympathomimetic, 58
Teriparatide, 147
Testosterone
    anabolic effects, 166t
    androgenic effects, 166t
    metabolism, 166, 168f
    production, 166
    synthetic esters, 166–167
Testosterone cypionate, 166–167
Testosterone enanthate, 166–167
Tetracaine, as local anesthetic, 79–81, 80f, 80t
Tetracyclines, 299–300, 300f
    staining of teeth by, 299
Tetrahydrofolate synthesis, inhibitors of, 305f
Tetrazole antifungals, 326
Theophylline, 253
Therapeutic index (TI)
    barbiturates vs. barbiturates, 82
    in dose-response relationship, 26
    in dosing regimen selection, 18t
Thiabendazole, 332

Thiamylal, 78–79
Thiazide diuretics, 186f, 187
Thiazolidinediones, 175f, 176
Thiethylperazine, 266
Thioguanine, 368f, 371
Thiomylal
    as anxiolytic/sedative-hypnotic, 83–84, 84f, 84t
    as drug of abuse, 122
Thiopental
    as anxiolytic/sedative-hypnotic, 83–84, 84f, 84t
    as drug of abuse, 122
    as intravenous anesthetic agent, 78–79
Thioridazine, 100
Thiothixene, 100
Thioxanthenes, 100
Third-generation cephalosporins, 293–294
3TC. See Lamivudine (3TC)
Thrombocytopenia, 227, 354
    heparin-induced, 227f
Thrombolytic drugs, 230–231
Thrombosis, 224, 224f
    deep vein, 227
Thromboxanes, 349t
Thrombus formation, role of endothelial cells in preventing, 223
Thyroid gland, origins, 141
Thyroid hormones, 143–144
    effects, 143f, 144t
    release and degradation, 143f
    synthesis, 143
    TSH stimulating release, 141t
Thyroid-stimulating hormone (TSH), 141–142
    disorders, 142
    release of thyroid hormones and, 141t
Thyrotoxicosis (hyperthyroidism), 145
Thyrotropin, 142
TI. See Therapeutic index (TI)
Tiagabine, 97
    sites of action
        in GABAergic synapse, 95f
        neuronal, 92f
Ticarcillin, 290, 292
    uses for, 291
Ticlopidine, 225–226, 225f
Tiludronate, 149
Timolol
    adrenergic receptor interaction with, 63t
    as β-blocker, 60, 61f
    for hypertension, 194–196, 195f
Tiotropium, 251
Tipranavir, 322
    side effects, 323t
Tirofiban, 225f, 226
Tissue binding, in drug distribution, 7, 7f
    drugs favoring, 7t
Tissue plasminogen activators (t-PA), 230–231
Tobacco, as drug of abuse, 125
Tocainide, 219
Tocopherol, 392t
Tolazamide, 174
Tolbutamide, 174
Tolcapone, 113
Tolerance
    amphetamines, 124
    antipsychotics, 99
    barbiturates, 122
    benzodiazepines, 122
    caffeine, 123
    cannabis, 125

    cocaine, 124
    defined, 118t
    deliriant hallucinogens, 124
    ethanol, 120
    nicotine, 125
    organic nitrates, 211
    psychedelic hallucinogens, 124
Tolmetin, 355t
Tonic seizure
    features, 91t
    treatment, 97t
Tonic-clonic seizure
    features, 91t
    treatment, 97t
Topical drug administration, 2t
    local anesthetic, 79t
Topiramate, 96–97
Topoisomerase, 374
    inhibitors, as cancer chemotherapy, 368f, 374
Topotecan, 374
Toremifene, 163
Torsade de points, 217
Tositumomab, 376, 378t
Toxic reactions to drugs. See Toxicology
Toxicity
    acetaminophen, 356
    aminoglycosides, 302f
    of anticancer agents, 366, 366f
    aspirin, 353
    chloramphenicol, 301f
    digitalis, 206
    of ergotamine, 341
    as H₁ antihistamines, 345
    levothyroxine, 144
Toxicology
    acute vs. chronic toxicities, 388
    antidotes
        nonspecific, 388–389
        specific, 389–391
    ethanol, 119–120
    ethylene glycol, 122
    methanol, 121–122
Toxins, bacterial, 283
    exotoxins, 284
Toxoplasmosis, treatment of, 328t
t-PA (tissue plasminogen activators), 230–231
Tramadol, 108, 109t
Tranexamic acid, 231
Transdermal drug administration, 2t
    distribution in body following, 5f
Transdermal patch contraceptives, 162
Transformation reactions, in drug metabolism, 8, 9f–10f, 11, 11t
Transplant rejection, immunosuppressants for prevention of, 383–387, 383t, 384f, 386f
Transudates, 262
Trastuzumab, 377, 378t
Travoprost, 349
Trazadone, 88
Tretinoin, 380
Triamcinolone, 152, 154
    for asthma, 250–251
Triamterine, 188–189, 188f
Triazolam, 82–83
    as drug of abuse, 122
    mechanism of action, 82, 84f
    uses for, 82t
Tricarboxylic cycle. See Krebs cycle
Trichomoniasis, treatment of, 328t

Tricyclic antidepressants, 86–87, 87f
acute poisoning with, *86*
as antiemetics, 266t, 267
drug interactions with, 87
Trientine, 390
Trifluridine, 317
Trigger factors, for asthma, 249f
Trihexyphenidyl, 115
Trimethaphan, 48, 53t
in hypertension therapy, 199
Trimethoprim
as antimalarial, 331–332
tetrahydrofolate synthesis inhibition and, 305f
as urinary antiseptic, 311
Triptans, 340–341
Trypanosomiasis, treatment of, 328t
TSH. *See* Thyroid-stimulating hormone (TSH)
Tuberculosis (TB), 308
drug therapy for, 308–309
protocol, 309t
Tuberoinfundibular dopaminergic tract, 67
Tumor development, *365*
Tumor markers, *366*
Tumor necrosis factor (TNF)-α inhibitors
for inflammatory bowel disease, 274, 276
for rheumatoid arthritis, 358–359, 359f
Tumor suppressor genes, *365*
Tumors
benign *vs.* malignant, *367*
grading, *371*
staging, *371*
Tyramine, 59
Tyrosine kinase inhibitors, as cancer chemotherapy, 378–380, 379f

U
Ulcerative colitis, 273, 273f
drug therapy for, 274f
Ultrafiltration, *181*
Uricosurics, for gout, 360f, 361
Urinary antiseptics, 311–312
Urinary tract, acetylcholine effects in, 45t
Urine formation, 182f
Urofollitropin, 165–166
Urokinase, 230
Ursodiol, 263–264
Uterus
anatomy and innervation, *169*
drugs acting on, 169
Uterus, effect of progesterone on, 159t

V
Valacyclovir, 314, 316
Valdecoxib, 355
Valganciclovir, 316, 319t
Valproic acid, 94
drug interactions with, 94
neuronal sites of action, 92f
Valsalva maneuver, *216*
Valsartan, 194
Vancomycin, 295–296
Varenicline, for smoking cessation, 125
Vasa recta, *181*
Vascular smooth muscle, catecholamines effects on, 54f

Vascular tone, beta-blockers effect on, 61f
Vasoactive intestinal peptide (VIP), *138*
Vasoconstrictors, in local anesthetic agents, 79
Vasodilators
in angina therapy, 209, 210f, 211, 212t
in heart failure therapy, 207, 207f
in hypertension therapy, 200–201, 200f, 202t
arterial and venous vasodilators, 201
arterial vasodilators, 200–201
Vasopressin (antidiuretic hormone), 189, 189f.
See also Antidiuretic hormone (ADH)
antagonists, 190
Vecuronium, 49, 53t
Venlafaxine, 89
Ventricular fibrillation, 216t
Ventricular myocardium, action potential phases at, 214–215, 214f
Ventricular premature beats, 216t
Ventricular tachycardia, 216t
Verapamil, 196, 197f
electrophysiological and hemodynamic effects, 198t
Vertigo, *266*
Very-low-density lipoproteins (VLDLs), 236, 236f
Vigabatrin, sites of action
in GABAergic synapse, 95f
neuronal, 92f
Vinblastine, 375
Vincristine, 374–375
Vinorelbine, 375
VIP (vasoactive intestinal peptide), *138*
Viral flu, *318*
prophylaxis for, 317, 318f
Viruses, 313
infections caused by, 313, 314t
drug therapy for. *See* Antiviral drugs
replication, 313, 313f
Virustatic antimetabolites, chemical structure of, 315f
Vitamin(s)
deficiencies in alcoholism, *121*
toxicology and treatment, 392, 392t
Vitamin A, 392t
Vitamin B$_3$, 392t
Vitamin B$_5$, *38*
Vitamin B$_6$, 392t
Vitamin B$_{12}$
absorption, *234*
folate metabolism and, 234f
for megaloblastic anemia, 234
Vitamin C
redox reactions, *39*
toxic effects and treatment, 392t
Vitamin D
bone metabolism and, 147–148
metabolism, 148f
toxic effects and treatment, 392t
Vitamin E, 392t
Vitamin K
antagonists, 228, 229f, 230f
toxic effects and treatment, 392t
Volatile solvents, abuse of, 126

Voltage-dependent ion channels, 21
drug-sensitivity and, 74t
Volume of distribution (V_d), 4, 7–8
calculating amount of drug needed from, 8
in dosing regimen selection, 18t
effect on drug half-life, 8
fluid compartments and, 7f, 7t
Vomiting, drug therapy for causes of, 264–267, 266t
Vomiting reflex, *265*
von Willebrand disease, *231*
von Willebrand factor (vWF), 223, 223f

W
Wafer implants, chemotherapy, *369*
Warfarin, 228–229, 229f, 230f
coumarin derivatives, antidote for, 391t
heritable insensitivity to, 27t
and International Normalized Ratio, 228
Waves, on ECG recording, 215, 215f
Weight gain, typical *vs.* atypical antipsychotics and, 101t
Weight loss medication, peripherally acting, 277
WHI (Women's Health Initiative), *159*
Wilms tumor, 374
Wilson disease, *391*
Withdrawal, defined, 118t
Withdrawal effects/symptoms
amphetamines, 124
antipsychotics, 99
barbiturates, 122
benzodiazepines, 122
caffeine, 123
cannabis, 125
cocaine, 124
deliriant hallucinogens, 124
ethanol, 120
in neonates, 30
nicotine, 125
opioids, 119t
psychedelic hallucinogens, 124
Wolff-Chaikoff effect, *145*
Women's Health Initiative (WHI), *159*

Y
Yohimbine, adrenergic receptor interaction with, 63t
Yttrium 90 ibritumomab tiuxetan, 376, 378t

Z
Zafirlukast, 251, 253
Zaleplon, 83
Zanamivir, 318
Zemaira™, 254
Zero-order kinetics, of elimination, 14–15, 15f
Ziconotide, 108–109, 109t
Zidovudine (azidothymidine; AZT), 320
in HIV/AIDS management, 320t
Zileuton, 251, 252f, 253
Ziprasidone, 100–101
Zoledronate, 149
Zollinger–Ellison syndrome, *261*
Zolmitriptan, 340–341
Zolpidem, 83
Zonisamide, 97